Visual evoked potentials in man
New developments

Visual evoked potentials in man: new developments

Methodology of patterned visual stimulation
Neurophysiology of visual functions in man
Clinical applications

EDITED BY

JOHN E. DESMEDT

Professor of Neurophysiology and of Pathophysiology of the Nervous System
Director of the Brain Research Unit, University of Brussels

CLARENDON PRESS · OXFORD

1977

Oxford University Press, Walton Street, Oxford OX2 6DP

OXFORD LONDON GLASGOW NEW YORK
TORONTO MELBOURNE WELLINGTON CAPE TOWN
IBADAN NAIROBI DAR ES SALAAM LUSAKA ADDIS ABABA
KUALA LUMPUR SINGAPORE JAKARTA HONG KONG TOKYO
DELHI BOMBAY CALCUTTA MADRAS KARACHI

ISBN 0 19 857393 6

Text set in 10/12 pt. IBM Press Roman, printed by photolithography, and bound in Great Britain at The Pitman Press, Bath

Preface

The object of this book is to provide a comprehensive presentation of the most recent data on visual functions studied electrophysiologically in normal man and in patients. Its 35 chapters deal with the visual evoked potential (abbreviated VEP) method in which the electrical potentials generated in the occipital cerebral cortex as a result of appropriate photic stimulation of the eyes are recorded from the intact scalp and averaged by a digital computer. The text emphasizes the critical evaluation of the state of the art in this fast-growing area of human neurophysiology, as well as the clinical uses of VEPs both for assisting clinical diagnosis and for pathophysiological investigations of patients with disordered visual functions. Without attempting to present the earlier literature in detail, the various chapters concentrate on the new results and on current issues which have to be resolved if the VEP method is to become a widely used and essential procedure for all those concerned with visual functions in man (for example, in neurology, ophthalmology, the neurosciences, optometry, clinical pharmacology, and psychology).

The project embodied in this book received considerable momentum from the Brussels Symposium on Cerebral Evoked Potentials (April 1974), which assembled for the first time most of the active VEP investigators and also provided them with enough time for discussion. The idea, in fact, was not to publish the proceedings emanating from a symposium (such volumes frequently lack perspective and consistency), but on the contrary to emphasize the publication project and to design a discussion workshop as one of the mechanisms for enlarging the scope of the proposed book.

The various methodologies for patterned visual stimulation were assessed carefully on the basis of a report drawn up (and subsequently up-dated: see Chapter 1) by a working party chaired by Dr. Martin Halliday. This part of the project should no doubt considerably help progress in the development of versatile and consistent procedures for the pattern VEP which is now superseding the simple flash VEP techniques. Dr. Henk Spekereijse agreed to elaborate an overview (Chapter 2 of this book) which draws freely on the extensive data assembled by his group in Amsterdam over the years, but also incorporates many of the ideas emerging from the workshop discussions. Indeed, several chapters of this book present fresh experimental results which were stimulated by, and actually obtained after, the Brussels conference.

I am grateful to Dr. Martin Halliday (London), Dr. Henk Spekreijse (Amsterdam), and Professor Geoffrey Arden (London) for friendly advice, and indeed to all the contributors whose enthusiastic participation resulted in a book that will, I believe, be unique and should set new standards for the study of visual functions in man.

Brussels
September 1976

J.E.D.

Contents

NOTE ON UNITS

In the experimental work described in this book, the units used for luminance are foot-Lamberts (ft-L) and log foot-Lamberts.

One apostilb (asb) is the luminance of a uniformly diffusing surface that emits 1 lumen per square metre.

Abbreviation for trolands: td

List of contributors

G. B. ARDEN	Department of Visual Sciences, Institute of Ophthalmology, Judd Street, London WC1H 9QS, U.K.
J. C. ARMINGTON	Department of Psychology, Northeastern University, Boston, Massachusetts 02115, U.S.A.
A. ATKIN	Department of Ophthalmology, Mount Sinai School of Medicine, Fifth Avenue and 100th Street, New York 10029, U.S.A.
G. BARRETT	Institute of Neurology, National Hospital, Queen Square, London WC1N 3BG, U.K.
E. C. BECK	Neuropsychology Research, Veterans Administration Hospital, 500 Foothill Drive, Salt Lake City, Utah 84113, U.S.A.
I. BODIS-WOLLNER	Department of Neurology, Mount Sinai School of Medicine, Fifth Avenue and 100th Street, New York 10029, U.S.A.
R. P. BORDA	Department of Neurophysiology, The Methodist Hospital, 6516 Bertner Boulevard, Houston, Texas 77030, U.S.A.
B. A. BROOKS	Department of Physiology, University of Texas, Health Science Center, 7703 Floyd Curl Drive, San Antonio, Texas 78284, U.S.A.
J. H. COOK	Department of Visual Sciences, Institute of Ophthalmology, Judd Street, London WC1H 9QS, U.K.
D. H. CROWELL	Newborn Psychological Research Laboratory, University of Hawaii Manoa, 2538 The Mall, Honolulu, Hawaii 96822, U.S.A.
J. E. DESMEDT	Brain Research Unit of the University of Brussels, 115 Boulevard de Waterloo, B 1000 Brussels, Belgium.
M. DIMITRAKOUDI	Neuropsychology Unit, University of Aston, Gosta Green, Birmingham B4 7ET, U.K.
R. E. DUSTMAN	Neuropsychology Research, Veterans Administration Hospital, 500 Foothill Drive, Salt Lake City, Utah 84113, U.S.A.
O. ESTEVEZ	The Netherlands Ophthalmic Research Institute Laboratory of Medical Physics, University of Amsterdam, 196 Herengracht, Amsterdam, The Netherlands.
M. FEINSOD	Department of Neurosurgery, Hadassah University, Jerusalem, Israel.
A. M. HALLIDAY	Institute of Neurology, National Hospital, Queen Square, London WC1N 3BG, U.K.
E. HALLIDAY	Institute of Neurology, National Hospital, Queen Square, London WC1N 3BG, U.K.
A. HARDEN	Department of Neurophysiology, Hospital for Sick Children, Great Ormond Street, London WC1N 3JH, U.K.

G. F. A. HARDING — Neuropsychology Unit, University of Aston, Gosta Green, Birmingham B4 7ET, U.K.

M. R. HARTER — Department of Psychology, University of North Carolina, Greensboro, North Carolina 27412, U.S.A.

C. D. HENDLEY — Department of Physiology, Mount Sinai School of Medicine, Fifth Avenue and 100th Street, New York 10029, U.S.A.

J. R. HERON — Department of Communication, University of Keele, Newcastle-under-Lyme, Staffordshire ST5 5BG, U.K.

W. T. HOYT — Neuro-ophthalmology Unit, Department of Neurosurgery, University of California, Medical Centre, San Francisco, California 94142, U.S.A.

D. A. JEFFREYS — Department of Communication, University of Keele, Newcastle-under-Lyme, Staffordshire ST5 5BG, U.K.

R. W. KATAOKA — Human Factors Technology Division, Naval Electronics Laboratory Center, San Diego, California 92152, U.S.A.

J. KULIKOWSKI — Department of Ophthalmic Optics, University of Manchester, Institute of Science and Technology, P.O. Box 88, Sackville Street, Manchester M60 1QD, U.K.

D. KURTZBERG — Departments of Pediatrics and Neuroscience, Albert Einstein College of Medicine, 1300 Morris Park Avenue, Bronx, New York, 10461, U.S.A.

E. G. LEWIS — Neuropsychology Research, Veterans Administration Hospital, 500 Foothill Drive, Salt Lake City, Utah 84113, U.S.A.

W. I. MCDONALD — The National Hospital, Queen Square, London WC1N 3BG, U.K.

L. MAFFEI — Laboratory of Neurophysiology, CNR, Via S. Zeno 51, 56100-Pisa, Italy.

M. M. MARCUS — Brain Behavior Research Center, Sonoma State Hospital, Eldridge, California 95431, U.S.A.

J. I. MARTIN — Human Factors Technology Division, Naval Electronics, Laboratory Center, San Diego, California 92152, U.S.A.

J. G. MAY — Department of Psychology, University of New Orleans, Lake Front, New Orleans, Louisiana 70122, U.S.A.

W. F. MICHAEL — Institute of Neurology, National Hospital, Queen Square, London WC1N 3BG, U.K.

M. MILLODOT — Department of Optometry, UWIST, Cardiff CF1 3NU, U.K.

B. A. MILNER — Department of Communication, University of Keele, Newcastle-under-Lyme, Staffordshire, ST5 5BG, U.K.

J. MUSHIN — Medical Research Council, Institute of Neurology, The National Hospital, Queen Square, London WC1N 3BG, U.K.

G. PAMPIGLIONE — Department of Neurophysiology, Hospital for Sick Children, Great Ormond Street, London WC1N 3JH, U.K.

D. REGAN — Department of Psychology, Dalhousie University, Halifax, N.S. B3H 4J1, Canada.

D. REITS — The Netherlands Ophthalmic Research Institute, Wilhelmina Gasthuis, 104 Eerste Helmerstraat, Amsterdam, The Netherlands.

T. SCHENKENBERG — Neuropsychology Research, Veterans Administration Hospital, 500 Foothill Drive, Salt Lake City, Utah 84113, U.S.A.

V. B. SHEOREY — Department of Visual Sciences, Institute of Ophthalmology, Judd Street, London WC1H 9QS, U.K.

S. SOKOL — Department of Ophthalmology, Tufts–New England Medical Center Hospital, 171 Harrison Avenue, Boston, Massachusetts 02111, U.S.A.

H. SPEKREIJSE — Laboratory of Medical Physics, University of Amsterdam, 196 Herengracht, Amsterdam, The Netherlands.

J. P. SPIRE — Neuro-ophthalmology Unit, Department of Neurosurgery, University of California, Medical Center, San Francisco, California 94142, U.S.A.

H. G. VAUGHAN Jr — Departments of Neuroscience and Neurology, Albert Einstein College of Medicine, 1300 Morris Park Avenue, Bronx, New York 10461, U.S.A.

C. T. WHITE — Speech, Hearing and Neurosensory Center, 8001 Frost Street, San Diego, California, 92123, U.S.A.

B. W. WILSON — Neuro-ophthalmology Unit, Department of Neurosurgery, University of California, Medical Center, San Francisco, California 94142, U.S.A.

Part 1 New methodologies and the physiological analysis of visual processes in man

1. Methodology of patterned visual stimulation

(Report of the Brussels Symposium ad-hoc committee)

G. B. ARDEN, I. BODIS-WOLLNER, A. M. HALLIDAY (Chairman), A. JEFFREYS, J. J. KULIKOWSKI, H. SPEKREIJSE AND D. REGAN

Introduction

Patterned visual stimulation has been assuming increasing importance in recent work on visual evoked potentials and at the Brussels Symposium a Working Party was set up to review and report on the currently available methods. This chapter aims to compare these methods and to make clear the relative merits and demerits of each technique. No one technique is equally good for all applications, and the choice of method to be used must depend to a large extent on the type of investigation being undertaken. For instance, speed and simplicity are important features for a routine screening test to be used in a busy eye clinic, whereas fine accurate quantitative control of stimulus parameters (such as brightness, contrast, pattern element size, colour, etc.) may be much more important in the context of a fundamental research project in this field.

In this chapter each member of the Working Party has contributed an account of the particular method of pattern stimulation which is familiar to him, attempting to assess objectively its relative advantages and disadvantages (including cost and ease of setting up) as compared with other methods. Among the methods dealt with are oscilloscope displays (Kulikowski, Bodis-Wollner), slide projectors with either shutters or rotating mirrors (Halliday), rotating polaroid discs (Arden), fluorescent tubes either with patterned mirrors (Spekreijse) or a tachistoscopic display (Jeffreys).

The experimenter has to decide whether to record responses to low-frequency stimulation (e.g. 2 per s) or to higher frequency stimulation (e.g. 10 per s or more). The latter type of response, because of its somewhat simpler quasi-sinusoidal waveform, has the advantage that measurement of overall amplitude or phase is relatively easy and does not involve any decisions about the identification of components or the way in which they are to be measured (e.g. peak to baseline, or peak to peak). On the other hand, the resolution of latency changes may be much

Visual evoked potentials in man: new developments (ed. J. E. Desmedt), pp. 3–15. Clarendon Press, Oxford 1977.

less accurate than with the well-defined peaks of the components of the response to infrequent stimuli, and harmonic distortion of the sinusoidal waveform may prove troublesome. An alternative approach when recording the steady-state response is to employ Fourier analysis rather than averaging (see Chapters 2 and 4).

Terminology

There are so many varieties of pattern stimulation in use that it is particularly important in working in this field to give an accurate description of the stimulus. Clichés which obscure the precise meaning should be avoided. In the current literature several different terms are used for the same thing and this makes the terminology unnecessarily confusing. There would clearly be advantages in a single set of generally accepted terms for the responses obtained to various forms of spatially patterned visual stimulation. The Working Party considered a number of the labels currently used and recommends some from among these for general adoption by workers in this field. VEP stands for visual evoked potential throughout this book.

'Pattern VEP' is to be preferred to 'spatial contrast VEP' because it is simpler and more immediately intelligible. 'Pattern onset–offset' is preferable to 'pattern appearance–disappearance' because it is more precise and does not confuse the objective stimulus parameters with questions of subjective perception, which may be an independent variable (e.g. in threshold experiments). The term 'contrast increase–decrease' should preferably be used only for responses to modulation of the contrast depth of a steadily presented pattern and not as an alternative to 'pattern onset–offset'. 'Pattern reversal' is preferable to 'alternating pattern' as it is less ambiguous.

Some authors have subdivided responses into 'pattern-related' and 'non-pattern-related' components. Among the former they have attempted to distinguish those which are 'contour (outline) specific' from those which are 'contrast specific'; the latter are almost by definition 'luminance related', but may nonetheless be distinct from other components related to the *overall* luminance (Jeffreys, Chapter 6 of this book). In practice, these theoretically valid distinctions are not always firmly established by the experimental findings and they should be used only with caution. The size of the pattern element (spatial frequency) is a key variable in this context. For instance, responses to sinusoidal gratings of less than 1 cycle per degree are largely luminance responses (Kulikowski 1974). For checkerboard patterns, check sizes of greater than 25′ subtense can give VEPs contaminated by luminance-related responses (Spekreijse 1966). For example, blurring a pattern of large checks can *increase* rather than decrease VEP amplitude, probably as a result of luminance contamination (Regan and Richards 1973).

Kulikowski suggests that luminance-transient responses may be identified experimentally by the observation that (1) they are identical for pattern onset and pattern offset, provided the space average luminance is held constant. This is because the luminance detectors, which do not respond to low temporal frequencies, are insensitive to baseline level of luminance and hence cannot distinguish between a bright bar or check being turned on and a dark one being turned off; (2) they give equivalent responses for pattern reversal at *half* the contrast for pattern onset–offset because these stimuli produce the same transient change in local luminance; (3) they are unaffected by pre-adaptation to a steady pattern of similar spatial frequency and orientation, which attenuates the pattern response (Kulikowski 1974).

It should be pointed out that the usual method of identifying and labelling components in the VEP waveform by means of their polarity and latency may run into difficulties in the case of pattern-related components, as the polarity of these components may change according to the location of both the recording electrode and the retinal stimulus (Halliday and Michael 1970; Jeffreys 1971*b*; Lesevre and Rémond 1972).

Saturation level

The amplitude of most VEPs show a ceiling effect when saturation level is reached, and those working with these responses should know and state whether the responses they are recording are below or above saturation level. This is particularly important when comparing amplitudes for different experimental conditions.

Stimulus parameters

Pattern VEPs depend critically on an unusually large number of stimulus para meters. Among those that should be controlled and specified are the following.

1. *Stimulus intensity.* Both the latency and amplitude of pattern responses varies with brightness.

2. *Choice of pattern* (e.g. checkerboard or grating, etc.). Where appropriate the orientation of the pattern should also be stated.

3. *The size of the pattern elements.* This can mean the dimensions of individual checks or the spatial frequency of gratings. This parameter is most usefully specified in terms of visual angle (e.g. 50′ squares or a 10 cycles per degree grating).

4. *Total field size and shape and its relation to the fixation point.* Again this is best specified in terms of visual angle and retinal eccentricity. The waveform of the pattern response depends critically on the area of visual field stimulated.

5. *Method of presentation of the pattern.* This could be, for example, pattern reversal or brief pattern onset–offset in a blank field of the same mean luminance, etc. The presentation rate and the duration of the different phases should be specified. Different methods of presentation of the same pattern produce large changes in the VEP (Jeffreys, Chapter 6 of this book).)

Recording conditions

Fixation should be controlled and monitored by direct visual inspection or via closed-circuit television. It should be clearly stated whether stimulation is binocular or monocular, and, if the latter, what precautions have been taken to occlude vision in the other eye. This is particularly important in flash stimulation. The nature of the surround to the stimulus area should be indicated where appropriate. Recording conditions, e.g. ambient light level, state of dark adaptation, use of mydriatic drops, etc. should be fully described.

Electrode montage

The electrode montage and polarity convention (e.g. negative upward) should be clearly stated. The word 'indifferent' should not be used in describing the reference electrode, as it begs the question. The ear electrode, commonly designated a 'reference', is frequently anything but a passive reference in relation to the occipital response. Considerable care may be needed to identify the contribution of each electrode to the recorded response. The use of more than one reference in different recordings may give valuable information in this regard (Michael and Halliday 1971).

Flashed-pattern stimulation

A number of studies have been published in which the stimulus was a patterned field illuminated intermittently by a stroboscopic flash tube (e.g. Spehlmann 1965; Rietveld, Tordoir, Hagenouw, Lubbers, and Spoor 1967; Harter and White 1968). This has the disadvantage that the response is a mixed one, partly to the abrupt luminance changes introduced by the flash and partly to the pattern stimulation itself. All the other methods considered in this chapter allow the presentation of a pattern stimulus under conditions of constant mean luminance. Patterned flash stimulation has been reported to be particularly effective in some clinical applications (Jeavons, Harding, Panayiotopoulos, and Drasdo 1972).

There are a number of minor drawbacks to the use of flash tube stimulators. Some flash tubes produce a click when they are fired, and hence are a potential source of auditory responses. When used in low ambient light conditions, particularly if they have been in use for some time, they may not trigger reliably. This can often be overcome by arranging for a local source of ions, which can be conveniently supplied, for instance, by a dimly lit neon tube placed next to the flash tube itself. Where different rates of stimulation are used, the light output may vary with the flicker rate. Ideally the output of the flash tube should be constantly monitored to ensure that it is performing properly.

Oscilloscope displays

The main advantage of oscilloscope displays is their versatility. Brightness, contrast, field size, and pattern size can be easily altered or can even be computer-controlled. Grating or checkerboard patterns can be readily generated with either a sinusoidal or a square-wave luminance profile. The total flux can be held constant while contrast is modulated, either by turning the pattern on and off (pattern onset–offset) or by reversing the bright and dark elements (pattern reversal). The grating has a special advantage over the checkerboard in activating neurones which are orientation specific.

One version of the oscilloscope technique (Kulikowski and Leisman 1973) employs an oscilloscope with a time base, one generator for a triangular vertical raster and one to generate grating patterns whose contrast is adjusted using an attenuator. An ordinary cheap oscilloscope – e.g. the Telequipment D61 – can be used without modification. The cost rises if a more sophisticated display, e.g. Tektronix 604/4, is employed. This display has a green phosphor (P31) and a screen size of about 10 x 8 cm or slightly less. This is adequate for testing the visual capacity in clinical conditions. If this colour is not acceptable, the Tektronix 604 can be ordered with a 'silver' phosphor P4 (blue–yellow) without extra charge, but if a wider screen is required another display scope is needed. There is the rather expensive Hewlett Packard display 1300 series, which may be provided with the silver phosphor P4 and whose screen is 50·8 cm (20 in) wide. Viewed at a distance of 57 cm, this subtends 30° of visual angle, and 1 cm on the screen corresponds to 1°. The model 1300 must be provided with a separate time-base.

One of the main limitations of the oscilloscope technique is the maximum field size imposed by the dimension of the cathode-ray tube face, and the maximum brightness, allowing for the rapid scan of the tube face required to produce a steady pattern display.

As well as generating 'pattern onset–offset' or 'pattern-reversal' responses, the oscilloscope method can be used to record the responses to varying the depth of contrast of a steadily presented pattern. Such contrast modulation consists of the successive presentation of the same grating pattern at higher and lower contrast, without altering either the mean spatial or temporal luminance of the pattern. Both the modulation depth and the mean contrast can be independently varied. In the version of this technique used by Bodis-Wollner, vertical gratings with a sinusoidal luminance profile are generated on the cathode-ray tube of a Tektronix 561 oscilloscope with a P4 phosphor (Chapter 35 of this book). The cathode-ray tube is surrounded by a screen which is back-illuminated at about the same brightness and hue as the cathode-ray tube. The mean contrast of the grating can be modulated in steps of 0·05 log units from full modulation downwards. The spatial frequency of the steady grating is determined by the frequency of a carrier sine wave, derived from, for example, a Wavetek 136 generator, and the amplitude of this signal determines the mean contrast of the grating. This carrier wave is further amplitude-modulated by a square-wave signal, the amplitude of which determines the depth of contrast modulation ($\Delta C/C$, where C is the mean contrast and ΔC the contrast increment). The modulating square wave can attenuate the carrier frequency from 100 per cent down to 0 per cent for pattern onset–offset responses. Separate potentiometers allow the modulation depth ΔC and carrier amplitude C to be independently varied.

In order to achieve perfect synchronization between the sweep rate, carrier frequency, and modulating frequency the following method is used. A constant-frequency master clock (e.g. sweep generator Wavetek 134) is suitably divided down to control the horizontal sweep rate of the display cathode-ray tube and to produce the required frequencies for both amplitude modulation of the carrier and frequency modulation of the carrier. The carrier signal is phase locked to the master signal by feed-back from a phase comparator circuit. The amplitude of the carrier is multiplied by the voltage of the amplitude-modulating signal through the analog circuit of the Wavetek 136 generator. This amplitude signal is used after suitable amplification for z-axis modulation of the d.c.-coupled Tektronix 561 oscilloscope.

There is increasing evidence that in the human visual system two types of detector mechanisms exist which are analogous to 'sustained' and 'transient' detectors in the cat's visual system. It has been suggested that contrast-modulated gratings are particularly suited to study responses which might arise in these two types of detectors, since temporal flicker and spatial contrast can be independently varied in the same pattern (Bodis-Wollner *et al.*, Chapter 35 of this book).

Pattern displays using commercial television sets

Electromagnetic tubes produce larger, brighter displays than those obtainable from electrostatic display tubes. The limitations are in the design of the field coils, and if significant departures from standard commercial television specifications are required the apparatus will be costly. However, Arden reports that it is possible to obtain patterned displays with a reversal rate up to 16 Hz with commercial sets. Spatial frequencies obtainable are so high that they are not a limiting factor. Thus it is possible to obtain all the patterns which have been used in published work from a cheap commercial television (excluding tilted gratings for which one can use a Dove prism to view the screen). A simple version of the equipment is in clinical use and gives results which are better than the rotating polaroid technique (Arden *et al.*, Chapter 3 of this book). Additional advantages of using the television set are that the checkerboard pattern can be mixed with an 'off-air' signal, e.g. to attract the attention of children. Providing the contrast of the stimulus and the off-air signal are approximately equal and about 50 per cent contrast ratio, no interference results. It is not necessary to lock the pattern-reversal rate to the television frame rate for clinical work. The apparatus compares favourably in price with any other equipment, and is more versatile: the stimulator can be readily adapted for producing 'split fields' or four stimuli in independent quadrants: square and sinusoidal gratings can be generated, and contrast, temporal, and spatial frequencies easily changed. Some of the techniques for altering the display parameters are suitable for computer control. Colour television sets can be used, but careful blanking of the stimulus is required. Chrominance changes can be separated from luminance changes if the appropriate signals are injected after decoding.

Slide-projector technique

Halliday has used an ordinary 5 x 5 cm slide projector (Kodak Carousel) as a pattern stimulator in two different ways. In the first method (Halliday and Michael 1970) two similar projectors are used, to each of which a fast shutter has been fitted. For pattern reversal the slide of a grating or checkerboard is placed in one projector and a slide of the complementary pattern (negative) in the other. The two projectors are focused in register on the back of a translucent screen, viewed by the subject, and the two slides are then alternately projected, the shutters being controlled by square waves derived from suitable timing circuits, e.g. a Digitimer. To attain fast shutter speeds (less than 8 ms from fully open to fully closed) the shutter itself is also constructed of two checkerboard slides, working on the Venetian-blind principle, one slide being moved across the other by a small electro-mechanical transducer to occlude or open the light path. Speed is attained at the cost of cutting down the maximum luminance of the projector by a little more than 50 per cent. Pattern onset responses can be recorded with the same equipment by replacing the slide in the second projector with a slide of a uniform grey field of equal mean luminance.

In an alternative projector method (Halliday, McDonald and Mushin 1972) the image is directed to the screen via a rotatable mirror, placed near the projector, and controlled by a small electro-mechanical transducer. By turning the mirror through a small angle, the pattern can be moved from side to side across the screen. The rapid displacement of a vertical grating or checkerboard through one half-cycle produces a reversal of the pattern. Provided this is sufficiently fast (less than 10 ms) the response is to all appearances identical to a reversal response produced by the alternating shutter method. If the mirror movement takes longer than 10 ms, however, the response shows an increased latency.

Among the advantages of the projector method are its relatively low cost and the ease and convenience with which slides can be made and changed to vary the pattern (e.g. providing grating or checkerboard stimuli of different spatial frequency and check size). The moveable screen allows great flexibility of viewing distance and field size. Different parts of the field can be stimulated using different cardboard screens with suitably located translucent segments. These screens slide quickly and easily out of a screen holder constructed out of dural. A small fixation light is provided in the centre of the screen by an independent projector.

One version of the pattern-reversal mirror stimulator which is available commercially from Digitimer Ltd. consists of a standard 5 x 5 cm slide projector mounted next to a high-speed mirror galvanometer. This apparatus is available in two forms. In one the projector and mirror galvanometer are mounted available in two forms. In one the projector and mirror galvanometer are mounted on a base which can be used with the experimenter's own screen, either for back or front projection as required. In the other the basic unit can be obtained mounted in the cabinet incorporating a screen 17·5 x 17·5 cm on which the image is back-projected. The galvanometer used to move the pattern on the screen carries a mirror of 3·5 x 3·5 cm and with a suitable driving amplifier is able to cause a checkerboard reversal in 5 ms or less. A suitable drive amplifier is available which will accept either an input waveform from an external source or is capable of free running and generating square waves, triangular waves, or ramp waveforms to cause varying rates of pattern displacement. In the free running mode a trigger signal is available to synchronize averager or other apparatus to the pattern movement. The trigger signal may be switched to coincide with the start of movement of the pattern to either the left or right.

Among the disadvantages of this method are the difficulty of controlling contrast, and the limited maximum luminance available, which is determined by the projector lamp. Although it is convenient that the pattern slides can be made by photography, the non-linearity of the photographic emulsion poses problems in achieving the required luminance levels, and these problems become more acute with colour slides. In the shutter method difficulties may be encountered in matching the light sources of the two projectors for both brightness and colour, and the projector lamps tend to change colour with age. It is also difficult to get complementary images of the two checkerboards in register over a large field. For whole-field stimulation the mirror method has practical advantages.

Rotating polaroid method

Arden has used screens made of polaroid squares (Behrman, Nissim, and Arden 1972). These may be bought (as Vectorgraphs to special order) or can be constructed out of strips of polaroid. The thicker material is preferred. Strips 5 mm thick are cut, and from these 5 mm squares can be made; alternatively, the squares may be punched from a sheet with a special punch. The squares are assembled on a plate of glass with a brush (it helps to wear polaroid spectacles). The assembly can be sprayed with an acrylic aerosol, so that the squares stick together; they are then mounted between two glass plates bound with tape. A 30 x 30 array can be made in two days; a grating can be made in a couple of hours. The pattern reversal occurs when the array is viewed through a second polaroid disc spun before the eye. It is simple to change the contrast of the squares with wave plates, or to change from pattern reversal to pattern onset–offset with additional stationary polaroids.

A disadvantage of the technique is that only sinusoidal changes in contrast can be produced. The advantages are that (1) the system is robust and portable, (2) pattern reversal occurs automatically and precisely, and (3) at high contrast imperfections in the display can be ignored.

Responses obtained are large and the waveform is simple, approximating to a sinusoid with a fundamental 4 times the speed of rotation of the disc. It is thus rather easy to use the system in conjunction with a phase-sensitive detector. The responses obtained come from the fovea and the parafovea if the square size is 10 min or less. However, if the square size is greater (and this is easily achieved by bringing the screen nearer to the patient), responses are derived from more peripheral areas of the retina.

By comparison, other methods of obtaining pattern-reversal responses (e.g. with pen motors and projectors or by the use of vibrators) are not self-adjusting; and the patterned mirrors used by Spekreijse and Van der Tweel (see below) are more complex to set up, more fragile, and less easily modified. Since the presence of imperfections on the display does not abolish the polaroid responses, while this does occur with the responses to the patterned mirror stimulus used by the Dutch group, these two methods evidently do not measure the same phenomenon.

In addition to the advantages listed above, a pleasing feature of this system is that fixation is not necessary and that interpretation of the response depends upon amplitude and phase information only. In testing patients, there is a definite time limit and this simple technique provides worthwhile and reliable clinical results on a routine basis, without fatiguing the patient.

Pattern mirror method

The pattern stimulus used by Spekreijse is formed by the reflecting and transparent elements of a patterned mirror (Spekreijse 1966; Van der Tweel and Spekreijse 1969). The luminance of the two sets of elements are provided by separate light sources, two fluorescent tubes, the brightness of which can be modulated independently. Fundamental to this technique is the separation of luminance and spatial parameters (the latter being determined by the pattern of reflecting surfaces on the mirror). The advantages and disadvantages of this technique as compared with other methods of pattern stimulation can be related to the luminance and the pattern elements respectively.

With regard to the luminance elements the method has the advantage that (1) a large range of luminance levels can be produced with a high photopic upper limit (10 000 asb); (2) the waveform of temporal modulation is easily controlled, with depths up to 100 per cent and rise times below 2 ms; (3) luminance modulation and spectral composition are easily and independently controlled for each of the sets of spatial elements; and (4) the homogeneity of the stimulus field is better than 0·05 neutral density over an area with a diameter of 16 cm.

However, to reach these specifications, bulky light sources (integrating spheres) are needed and considerable technical skill is required both for the production of the lamps and maintenance of specifications.

As regards the pattern element, the choice of spatial configuration is restricted only by the graphical techniques employed in the fabrication of the mirrors. In practice 24 edges per minute are feasible. This sets the limit for spatial gradients, so that sine-wave patterns are rather difficult to fabricate.

Among advantages of this technique are: (1) switching from pure luminance to pattern stimulation (pattern onset) is done electronically, rather than mechanically, as in the projector and rotating polaroid method; (2) contrast thresholds as low as 0·05 per cent can be determined accurately; (3) it is easy to produce dichoptic stimuli in which the two separate images are automatically aligned. Among disadvantages of the method are: (1) the pattern is set at an angle of 45° which limits the useful visual angle; (2) the spatial parameters cannot be changed during stimulation without additional optical equipment; (3) there are slight colour differences between the transmitted and reflected lights.

Choice of pattern

In Spekreijse's experiments a checkerboard pattern is the preferred stimulus because an analysis of, for example, the influence of the size of the pattern elements is best performed if the shape of the elements fits the generally assumed circular shape of the integrative or receptive fields. Polygons of higher order are of course more disc-like, but such polygons will have more than four neighbours so that they are not feasible for counterphase experiments.

Bar patterns provide a simpler situation if concepts of spatial Fourier analysis are employed, but they behave as a contrast stimulus in only one direction.

Versatility of stimulus

If both sets of checks are modulated equally (generally square wave) and in counterphase, the total amount of light falling on the eye remains constant. However, the spatial-contrast stimulus differs depending on the mean intensities of the two sets of checks.

1. *Pattern reversal* is obtained when both sets of checks have the same mean intensity. The 'bright' and 'dark' checks interchange rhythmically at twice the temporal modulation frequency. Hence only response components which are even multiples of the stimulus frequency can be obtained, regardless of their luminance or contrast origin.
2. *Pattern onset–offset* is achieved by adjusting the intensities of the two sets of checks in such a way that they are equal during half the stimulus period. The checkerboard pattern first appears, then disappears to leave a blank field, once during each stimulus cycle.

Sometimes it is useful to modulate only one light source, in which situation the net luminance of the stimulus changes rhythmically. In the pattern onset–offset situation two conditions can be distinguished.

3. *Onset of pattern at luminance increase.*
4. *Onset of pattern at luminance decrease.*

Condition 1 is useful in clinical studies where experimental duration is of importance, but it should be realized that the separate components can no longer be identified.

Condition 2 is most appropriate if one wants to study the characteristics of the onset and offset response with the least contamination by luminance components.

Conditions 3 and 4 are especially useful to establish a contrast origin of the response (ERG (electroretinogram) and VEP). If different responses are elicited by the onset and offset of the pattern, but these responses remain the same regardless of the direction of the luminance change, a contrast origin seems established.

Chromatic contrast (chromatic pattern) stimulation

Spekreijse's patterned-mirror technique can be adapted to give either pattern reversal or contrast increase–decrease accompanied by no changes of either luminance or luminance contrast. For example, equiluminant red–green checks either exchange places or appear and disappear. This stimulus is pure chromatic contrast and gives VEPs distinct from luminance-contrast VEPs (Regan 1973). Chromatic-contrast stimuli seem to be more useful than monochromatic patterns in studying colour blindness (Regan and Spekreijse 1974).

Tachistoscopic display method

The system employed by Jeffreys (1968, 1971*a*) consists of four oval perspex fields, each one back-illuminated by three (15·3 cm; 6 in) blue fluorescent tubes and optically superimposed by half-silvered mirrors. Each field is independently switched by externally controlled bistable units. The basic stimulus is the alternation of a test field (pattern) and a reference field (blank or pattern). Small crosses in the centre of each field are aligned to produce a steady fixation mark in the centre of the uniformly illuminated 12-cm diameter field. Viewing distance is 75 cm. Typical luminance 1·8 log ft-L (with mirrors). Fine 'brightness controls' are used to match the luminance of each field.

Among advantages of the method are that:

1. different types of pattern stimulus are possible at constant luminance, e.g. pattern onset–offset, pattern reversal, or pattern displacement;
2. different forms of pattern can be presented in any prescribed region of the field;
3. different patterns can be presented in the same run, e.g. for 'adaptation' studies;
4. there is accurate control of duration with switching times of less than 1 ms;
5. high contrast levels are achieved;
6. it can be adapted for dichoptic stimulation;
7. it is easy to use and little maintenance is required.

Among disadvantages of the method are that:

1. although the timing and order of presentation are easily varied, the spatial configuration of the pattern cannot be externally controlled, e.g. by computer;
2. pattern alignment presents some difficulty;
3. background illumination changes on switching; this can be reduced by the use of a steady surround field;

4. each individual pattern has to be drawn or prepared photographically;
5. although contrast variation is possible with polaroids (at reduced luminance) it is difficult to control contrast precisely by this method;
6. the use of fast-switching (blue) tubes makes it unsuitable for colour experiments.

Commercial tachistoscopes are available but are often less flexible than 'custom-built' models. Such models are fairly straightforward to build and are inexpensive.

Maxwellian-view stimulator

Armington has employed a pattern stimulator using Maxwellian-view optics. The subject views the stimulus through an eye lens that forms an image of the light source within the pupil. The subject sees a bright field of light which fills this lens. Maxwellian-view stimulators, then, are to be distinguished from those in which the stimulus is projected onto a screen or in which the subject directly views the light source.

There are several advantages claimed for Maxwellian-view stimulators. They are more efficient than other stimulators in getting light from the source to the retina and, in particular applications, the amount of light falling on the retina is independent of the size of the subject's pupil. They also permit ready control of stimulus parameters such as luminance, field size, focus, duration, etc. Among disadvantages of Maxwellian-view stimulators are the fact that they are relatively complicated to construct and require that the subject's eye be accurately aligned with their optics. A description of a Maxwellian-view stimulator for producing pattern-reversal stimuli may be found elsewhere in this book (Chapters 14 and 11). An excellent review of the principles involved and the methods for calibrating these stimulators has been prepared by Westheimer (1966).

The optical efficiency of a Maxwellian-view stimulator can be high enough to use monochromatic stimulus patterns at daylight (photopic) illumination levels even in the far red and blue. However, the large effect of the eye's chromatic aberration upon pattern VEPs may then be troublesome (Regan 1973*a*). For small (foveal) stimulus fields, one of the ocular achromatizing lenses will counter chromatic aberration, but for field sizes exceeding 1°–2° other methods are necessary (Regan, Chapter 11 of this book).

Matrix of light-emitting diodes

Another method for producing a patterned visual stimulus has been to employ a matrix of light-emitting diodes of the type described by Evans, Binnie, and Lloyd (1974). The advantage of this particular technique is in the ability to switch sets of linked elements in the diode matrix electronically. In this way either an alternating pattern or a pattern onset–offset stimulus can readily be produced. Among disadvantages of the method are the limited maximum brightness available from the diode elements and their fixed dimensions and colour characteristics.

Fibre optic display

Any desired pattern display (e.g. a checkerboard) can also be built up from an array of fibre optics, illuminated from two or more suitably modulated light sources. The technique is convenient to use, but the absolute size and arrangement of the pattern elements is fixed, and the apparent size of the elements can only be altered by changing the viewing distance, with a consequent change in the overall size of the display.

Stereoscopic pattern stimulation

Pattern stimulators have been built that produce small, controllable changes in the *relation* between stimulus patterns viewed by the left and right eyes. Consequently the subject has the illusion that a single stimulus pattern moves backwards and forwards in depth, and VEPs may be recorded that reflect the activities of neurones concerned with stereoscopic depth perception. Three Julesz patterns may be used with three projectors that are switched on and off in sequence (Regan and Spekreijse 1970); alternatively, two identical stimulus patterns may be mounted on vibrators or viewed through rotatable mirrors (Regan and Beverley 1973*a*). In order to eliminate artifacts due to monocular pattern stimulation, the stimulus patterns must be aligned very carefully (1 minute of arc or better) and relative rotation avoided. Alignment can be a problem. One counter is to use optical path lengths of several metres.

When two gratings are viewed, one with each eye, and when their relative spatial frequencies are changed, the subject sees a single grating that tilts in depth. Fiorentini and Maffei (1970*b*) used this technique to explore the effect upon grating-reversal VEPs of tilting the grating in depth.

2. Visual evoked potentials and the physiological analysis of visual processes in man

H. SPEKREIJSE, O. ESTEVEZ, and D. REITS

The Netherlands Ophthalmic Research Institute and *The Laboratory of Medical Physics, Amsterdam*

Introduction

The perception of light and spatial contrast are the primary functions of the visual system. In man information may be obtained on both and also on higher-order functions such as depth and colour perception by not only psychophysical techniques, but also by means of the occipital evoked potentials (VEPs) to various forms of light, colour, and contrast stimulation.

It is the purpose of this chapter to illustrate how, by application of some advanced tools of system analysis, the human visual system can be divided into various elements which can, in turn, be arranged into a logical functional sequence. We will also discuss how, by comparing normal visual functioning with some forms of visual defects, one can gain further insight on the organization of this part of the nervous system.

The chapter is divided in four sections covering luminance VEPs, spatial nonlinear analysis, pattern VEPs, and isolated colour mechanisms, and there is a final mathematical section devoted to the analysis of visual evoked responses.

The first section gives the current state of luminance VEP research. It will be shown how the VEPs to homogeneous field stimulation can be distinguished on the basis of different temporal frequency responsiveness, distribution on the skull, binocular interactions, etc. Three subsystems can be identified in the frequency domain: a high-frequency subsystem, which underlies the primary response originating in the striate cortex; a medium-frequency subsystem associated with the secondary response originating in area 18 and possibly in 19; and a low-frequency subsystem, which generates the late response that cannot be attributed to a specific cortical region. In this analysis the human visual system is purposely oversimplified into a N-channel model with identical, independent pathways.

In the second section it will be demonstrated that sequential analysis may also offer a powerful tool for the study of the location and the characteristics of spatial interactions. It will be concluded that the potentials evoked in man by

Visual evoked potentials in man: new developments (ed. J. E. Desmedt), pp. 16–89. Clarendon Press, Oxford 1977.

presentation of a pattern stimulus cannot be described on the basis of receptor summation pools. These pools, however, probably 'shape' the input to the contrast generating mechanism. Two extreme situations can account, then, for a reduction in visual acuity: either larger-than-normal receptive fields feeding into a fully developed contrast mechanism (distal defect), or normal receptive fields acting as input to a malfunctioning contrast mechanism (central defect). Psychophysical as well as VEP measurements suggest that the first situation dominates in rod-monochromacy and the second one in amblyopia.

In the third section we attempt to highlight those points concerning pattern VEPs which seem to us the better established and which may be used as keystones in the description of the mechanisms responsible for the pattern VEP generation. It is concluded that in the appearance response to a checkerboard pattern, three components with different latencies can be distinguished. The finding that the dipole representations of CI, the earliest component, and of the high-frequency luminance subsystem (cf. next section) overlap, suggests that the response to a contrast stimulus may contain an appreciable luminance contribution, thus controls for establishing a luminance or contrast origin are discussed. On the other hand component CII (latency 100–120 ms) can be clearly associated to changes in spatial contrast, especially around sharp contours. Component CIII might also be related to the same parameter. It is not certain whether CIII should be considered as an independent component or as an after-effect of CII.

Regan and Spekreijse (1974) found that a checkerboard pattern consisting of red and green fields of equal luminance does not elicit a pattern VEP in colour-normal subjects. They suggested that the contrast-generating mechanism must be fed by independent 'colour-coded channels'. On the basis of the experiments described in the fourth section the hypothesis is advanced that the CII component is generated by a *single* cortical *contour* mechanism which can be independently reached by either of the long wavelength cone channels and that once one of these inputs attains a certain value, the contrast mechanism blocks the input of the other cone system. This scheme can explain a number of electrophysiological findings and seems also to be consistent with some psychophysical facts pertaining to both colour and contrast vision.

In the mathematical section a survey will be given of some system analysis techniques that are commonly used to study both the spontaneous EEG data and VEPs. This section was included in the hope that it might make physiologists currently engaged in VEP research aware of the tremendous analytical potential lying in these mathematical tools and which, thanks to widespread use of modern general purpose digital computers, have become easily available at most laboratories.

Luminance VEPs

The study of the human visual system by means of scalp-recorded potentials evoked by luminance stimulation is favoured by the availability of an extensive body of knowledge on system analysis. Before the late 1950s the choice of stimulus was frequently determined, not by analytical reasons, but by technical feasibility, which accounts for the use of flash stimulation in the early studies.

VEPs to flash stimulation

Flash VEPs present several components with different latencies. These components have been associated with different functions of the visual system and/or with different locations within the brain. For example, Ciganek (1961), relying on the superposition technique of Dawson (1947) and averaging VEPs by hand, studied 75 subjects and proposed a scheme (Fig. 2.1) in which three components are

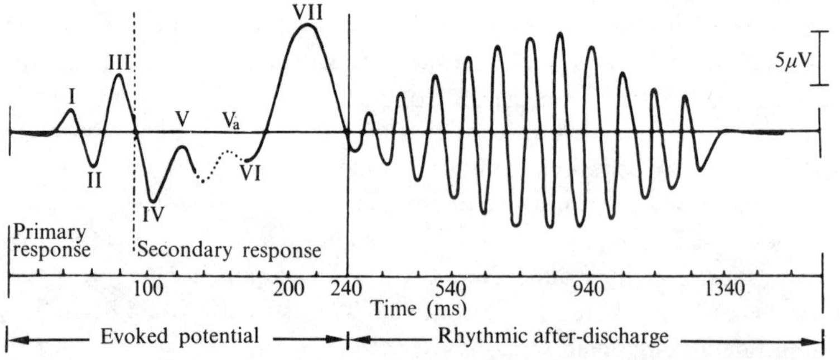

Fig. 2.1. Schematic representation of the human flash VEP. Three components can be recognized: a primary response, a secondary response, and a rhythmic after-discharge. Note the different time-scales. Symbols I–VII indicate the successive components of the VEP.

distinguished: a 'primary' component (latency 29 ± 2 ms) with a minimum of inter-individual variability, a secondary component (latency about 90 ms) which is more variable, and a rhythmic after-discharge with enormous variability within and among subjects (latency 135–350 ms, with an average of 250 ms). Owing to the overlap of the various components and the lack of knowledge about their waveforms, latencies could be estimated with accuracy only for the primary component. Since the primary component does not change when the subject is alert or in the various states of sleep and remains present at high flash frequencies (up to 35 Hz) where the secondary component and after-discharge have become negligible, it was considered to originate in the primary visual cortex (Brodmann's area 17). In man, most of the optic nerve fibres are thinner than 1 μm (Chacko 1948). For a myelinated fibre with a diameter of 1 μm, the propagation velocity of nerve impulses is about 6 m s^{-1}. If the total length of the direct pathway from the eye to the visual cortex is about 20 cm then the time between the onset of the photoreceptor response and the arrival of the volley in area 17 will be about 35 ms (adding a few milliseconds to include synaptic delays). This value corresponds to the latency observed for the primary VEP component.

Topological studies of flash VEP with simultaneous recording from various regions of the scalp in order to relate the components with particular areas of the cerebral cortex should be performed, since surprisingly few data are available (see Vaughan 1969). With midline electrodes Rémond (1969) found that the initial positive waves in the flash VEP are largest just anterior to the inion. Components with latencies between 50 ms and 100 ms are largest a little farther forward and the after-discharge is maximal about 8 cm anterior to the inion.

VEPs to sine-wave-modulated light

In the studies of the scalp potentials evoked by variation of the intensity of wide unstructured stimulus fields, the VEP system is analysed in a 'single-channel' manner which neglects the fact that the normal retina includes four different photoreceptor populations, each with a different retinal distribution and numerosity. The flash VEPs may not fit into a 'single-channel' simplification, since this form of stimulation initiates some interaction mechanisms along the visual pathway. To further complicate matters, different rates of flash presentation will make the visual system pass through different states of light adaptation. For these reasons the flash VEP cannot be a simple function of the intensity of the stimulus.

Some of these disadvantages can be overcome by the application of small modulations of the signal, such as sine-wave modulation superposed on a continuous steady field. With such stimuli the effects of luminance change and mean luminance level can be studied separately. Similarly to the 'component' analysis of the flash VEP, one might expect, by classifying the VEPs to sine-wave stimulation as a function of temporal frequency, to be able to associate different frequency regions with different cortical locations and/or brain functions.

(a) *The high- and low-frequency region.* When the human visual system is stimulated with sine-wave modulated light of constant mean luminance and modulation depth, and the amplitude of the fundamental VEP component in the VEP (i.e. with the same frequency as the stimulus) is plotted as a function of stimulus frequency, an amplitude versus frequency function with a characteristic shape generally emerges (Fig. 2.2 (a)). Starting at frequencies as low as 3 Hz, the response first grows with increasing frequency to reach a maximum amplitude around 10 Hz, then decays to a minimum (which can be close to zero) in the range of 25–40 Hz, increases again to reach a generally less pronounced maximum in the range of 45–60 Hz and finally decreases monotonically for still higher stimulus frequencies. Two different regions can also be distinguished in the phase characteristic, where the phase difference between stimulus and fundamental VEP component is plotted versus stimulus frequency (Fig. 2.2 (b)). For frequencies up to about 20 Hz the phase lag increases more rapidly with frequency than for frequencies above 20 Hz. From the slope of the phase plot an estimate of latency can be obtained as follows. If the phase of the VEP were determined solely by a pure delay time (latency) of τ seconds then τ could be calculated from the formula $\tau = -\Delta\phi/2\pi\Delta f$ in which $\Delta\phi$ is the phase difference in radians associated with Δf in hertz. However, since amplitude variations due to integrative or differentiative processes cannot exist

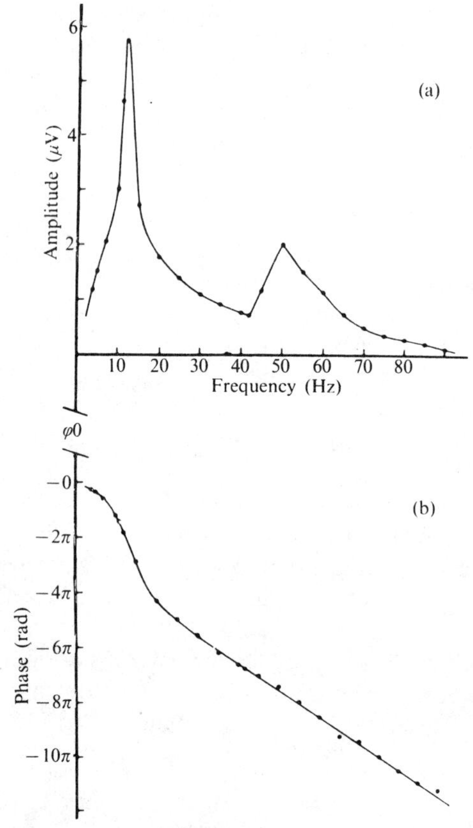

Fig. 2.2 (a). Amplitude and (b) phase characteristics of the fundamental component in the VEP (inion–vertex derivation) to a binocularly presented sine-wave modulated stimulus field of 20°. Note the linear frequency-scale. The luminance of the stimulus field seen in Maxwellian view was 10 000 asb.

without variations in phase, some part of the phase plot must be associated to the amplitude plot. If the assumption is made that the amplitude and phase characteristics of the human VEP system can be described by a linear minimum-phase-shift system plus the fixed delay described above, then the real delay time can be estimated from the phase plot once corrected for the phase shift associated to the amplitude plot. Without such correction the latency would be overestimated. For the low-frequency branch of the phase plot, the latency estimates range from 120 ms to 220 ms when retinal illumination is reduced from 150 000 td to 4 td. The latencies deduced from the high-frequency part of the phase plot vary from 48 ms to 62 ms for retinal illuminations of 150 000 td down to about 120 td (Van der Tweel and Verduyn Lunel 1965; Spekreijse 1966).

The fact that the high-frequency VEP always has a much shorter delay than the low-frequency VEP can be interpreted as a reflection of different transfer processes along the visual pathway. These two processes may also project to different cortical areas, as is directly evident from the midline recordings presented in Fig. 2.3. These recordings, obtained in the same subject, show that the VEP to

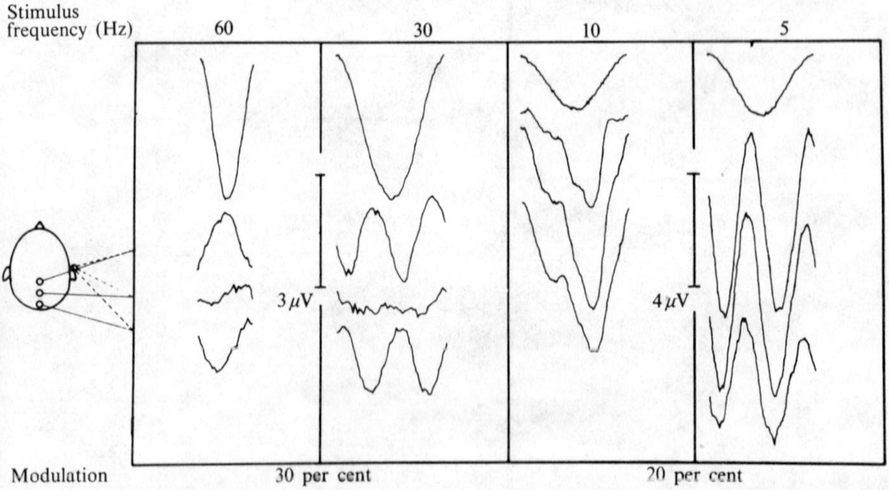

Fig. 2.3 'Monopolar' midline recordings of the VEPs to a sine-wave modulated stimulus field of 20° seen in Maxwellian view. Mean luminance of the binocularly presented stimulus is 10 000 asb. The fundamental and second harmonic components in the response to low-frequency stimulation (10 Hz and 5 Hz respectively) have the same phase irrespective of electrode position. The responses to high stimulus frequencies (60 Hz and 30 Hz) can have an opposite phase at different electrode positions.

high-stimulus frequencies can have an opposite phase at different electrode positions, whereas those to low-frequency stimulation have the same phase and approximately the same amplitude. Since these topological differences hold irrespective of stimulus frequency, they point to a different cortical localization for the short-latency, high-frequency responses and for the long-latency, low-frequency responses. The data in Fig. 2.4 suggest in addition that both types of responses are differentially treated even at an early stage in the retina–cortex system. These data were obtained in a patient whose right visual pathway was affected with retrobulbar neuritis. During a follow-up study of 4 weeks the VEP measurements showed no differences between the low-frequency VEPs of the strongly and the less affected eye. This is in contrast to the high-frequency VEPs, which could not be obtained from the affected eye at the first session. However, as the visual acuity improved, the high-frequency responsiveness of the affected eye also increased, as is shown, for example, in the recordings of the fourth and last session.

(b) *The medium-frequency region.* In addition to the low-frequency and high-

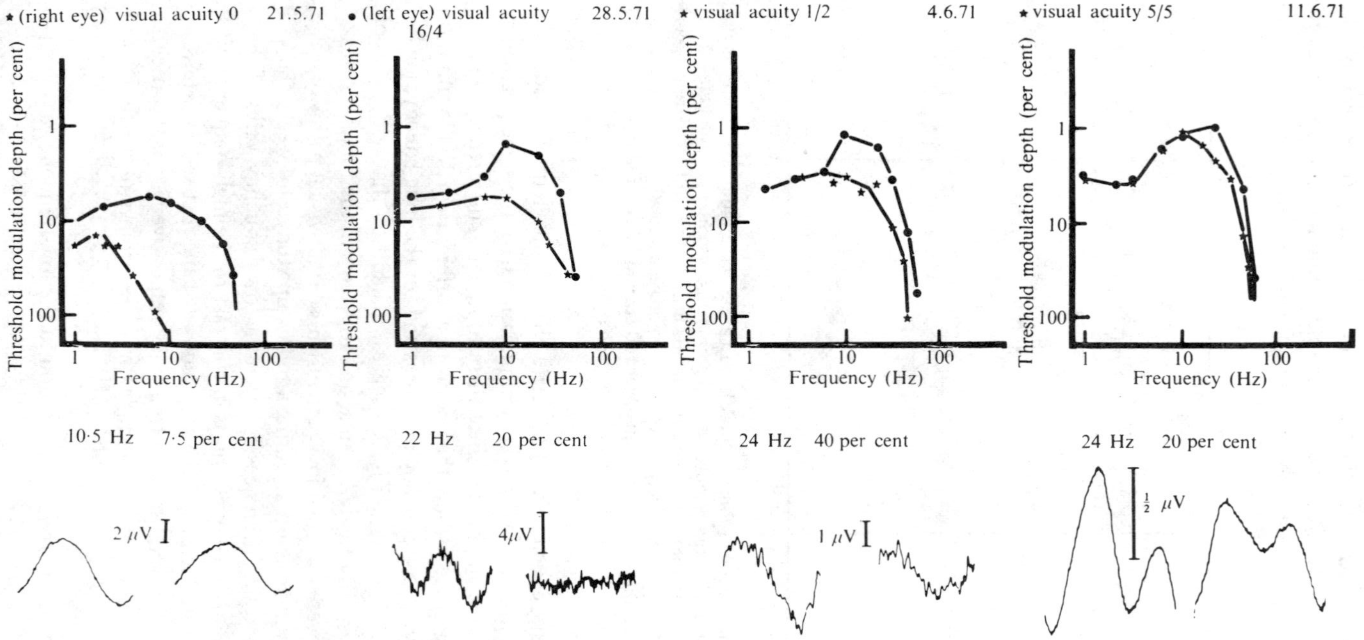

Fig. 2.4 Psychophysics (top row) and electrophysiology (bottom row) of a patient with a right eye (circles) affected with retrobulbar neuritis. With the recovery of visual acuity the high-frequency tails of the flicker fusion curves of the right eye become progressively (weekly sessions) more similar to those of the left eye (stars). The first picture in the bottom row shows the low-frequency (10·5 Hz) occipital response of each eye to sine-wave modulated light. From the first session on, these responses were similar for both eyes. The other pictures show the high-frequency (22–24 Hz) responses. Whereas at the first session to such response could be obtained with the affected eye, at the fourth and last session the two eyes do not differ much. The mean luminance is 5 000 asb.

frequency responses that can be discriminated both by cortical representation and stimulus processing, Regan (1968*c*) reported a VEP peaking in the 12–25 Hz range that seems not to be related to the other two components since: (a) these medium-frequency VEP components are more colour-dependent than either the low- or high-frequency components; (b) their topological distribution differs from that of the low-frequency responses; and (c) in patients with multiple sclerosis, medium-frequency responses may be delayed in the affected eye (without changing VEP amplitude) whereas the high-frequency responses are not delayed (Milner, Regan, and Heron 1974; Regan, Milner, and Heron, Chapter 29). From the slope of the phase plots Regan estimates that the apparent latency of the medium-frequency response lies between 100 ms and 140 ms.

VEPs to Gaussian-noise-modulated light

The advantages of sinusoidally modulated light (small signal, steady adaptation level) are somewhat counteracted by the need of presenting a number of frequencies to obtain insight in the behaviour of the low-, medium- and high-frequency VEPs. Since these frequencies must be applied in sequence and the system allowed to reach a stationary state, the interpretation may give problems if the VEP system is non-stationary. This difficulty can be overcome by the use of the Gaussian-noise-modulated light technique introduced in VEP research by Lopes da Silva (1970). A white Gaussian-noise-modulated stimulus has the advantage that all frequencies are presented simultaneously (which is also the case with flash stimulation, since theoretically a brief pulse contains all frequencies to the same extent). However, with noise stimulation all frequencies are continuously present while the state of adaptation remains constant during the entire recording period. Thus, even if the overall gain of the VEP system was changing during a recording session the VEPs to all frequencies would be influenced in the same way, leaving the shape of the amplitude and phase characteristics invariant. Therefore the VEP amplitudes at different frequencies can be compared better with each other than in the case of sinusoidal stimulation presented serially.

The luminance variation $L(t)$ of a white Gaussian noise stimulus can be expressed as: $L(t) = L_0\{1 + mx(t)\}$, where L_0 is the mean luminance level and $x(t)$ is a stochastic signal that is characterized by a flat power spectral density (white noise) with the amplitude probability density function (Gaussian)

$$p(x) = \frac{1}{\sigma\sqrt{2\pi}} \exp\,(-x^2/2\sigma^2),$$

where σ^2 is the power of the Gaussian noise signal. The modulation depth m of a Gaussian-noise-modulated light can be defined as $m = \sigma/L_0$. The highest modulation depth that can be applied before the stimulus becomes asymmetrical (since absence of light is an absolute minimum) depends on the amplitude limitation of the noise generator used. For a commercial noise generator like the Hewlett Packard 3722 A, the nearly Gaussian amplitude distribution is limited between $+2{\cdot}5\sigma$ and $-2{\cdot}5\sigma$. Hence with such a generator the highest modulation depth that can be chosen without clipping is $\sigma/2{\cdot}5\sigma = 40$ per cent.

A disadvantage of noise stimulation is the fact that more sophisticated equipment is needed to analyse the VEPs, since the cross-spectra or cross-correlation functions between the noise stimulus and the EEG signals have to be calculated. For such an analysis, correlators or general-purpose computers are needed, whereas VEPs to sine-wave-modulated light and flashes can be obtained with averagers that are readily available in most VEP research laboratories and clinics. However, averagers may be useful to compute cross-correlation functions when they are used in a special way (triggered correlation; de Boer and Kuyper (1968); Reits (1975); and the last section of this chapter).

The interpretation of the cross-correlation function between the noise signal and the EEG relies on the fact that for a linear system or a system that contains a static nonlinearity such as saturation or a threshold, the cross-correlation function $R_{xy}(\tau)$ between a white Gaussian-noise stimulus $x(t)$, and the response $y(t)$ is directly proportional to the impulse function of the (linear elements of the) system (Bussgang 1952). As an example, in Fig. 2.5 the correlation 'responses' are shown for a number of midline derivations. In these cross-correlation functions three components can be distinguished: an early component with peaks between 30 ms and 80 ms, a secondary component with peaks in the range of 60 ms to 150 ms and an after-discharge-like wave which becomes evident after 90 ms. The values of the correlation responses at negative times (left side of Fig. 2.5) give a measure for the 'variance' of the response due to the finite time-lengths (4 min) of the EEG recordings that were used. To demonstrate the improvement of the signal-to-noise ratio with recording length, in Fig. 2.5 the correlation response of a 13 min EEG record (curve B) is also shown. Comparison of the 13 min and 4 min records indicates that – in agreement with observations for the flash response – the first two components show less variability than the after-discharge since the prominent after-discharge in the response is no longer significant when the signal length is increased to 13 min. By plotting the peak-to-peak values of the components versus electrode position, Reits (1975) reached the conclusion that the amplitude distributions of the three components differ, suggesting that they originate in different cortical areas.

While on the one hand the cross-correlation responses may be compared under certain conditions to the flash VEPs, by taking their Fourier transform, they can also be compared to the amplitude and phase characteristics obtained with sine-wave-modulated light. An example is shown in Fig. 2.6. The correlation responses for two occipital derivations appear in Fig. 2.6(a). In these 'responses' the early and the secondary component can be distinguished easily, but no after-discharge is evident. It is interesting to note that in the spontaneous EEG of this subject almost no alpha activity was present. Fourier transformation of these responses resulted in the cross-power and phase spectra depicted in Fig. 2.6(b) and (c). The two

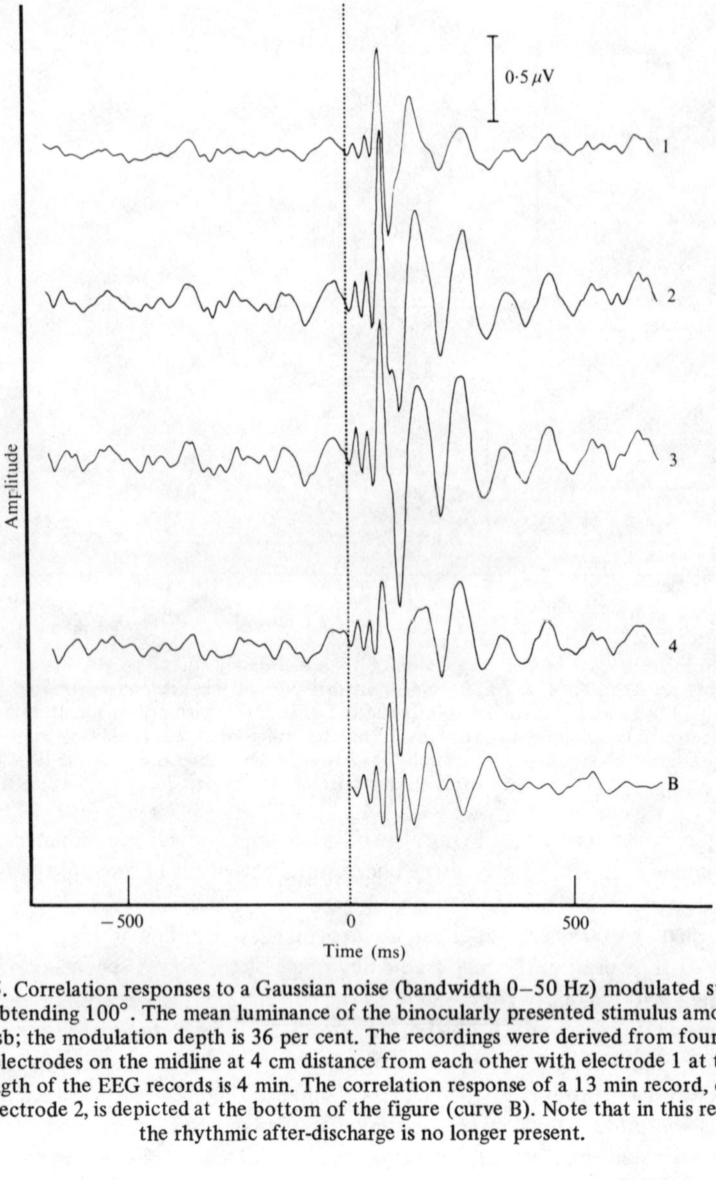

Fig. 2.5. Correlation responses to a Gaussian noise (bandwidth 0–50 Hz) modulated stimulus field subtending 100°. The mean luminance of the binocularly presented stimulus amounts to 2700 asb; the modulation depth is 36 per cent. The recordings were derived from four 'monopolar' electrodes on the midline at 4 cm distance from each other with electrode 1 at the inion. The length of the EEG records is 4 min. The correlation response of a 13 min record, derived from electrode 2, is depicted at the bottom of the figure (curve B). Note that in this response the rhythmic after-discharge is no longer present.

components in the correlation function express themselves as two peaks in the power spectra: one in the range of 14–20 Hz and the other in the range of 30–45 Hz. These peaks become particularly evident in the coherence spectra (Fig. 2.6(d)) where the cross-spectra are compensated for background activity. This compensation affects mainly the low-frequency part of the spectrum (whose

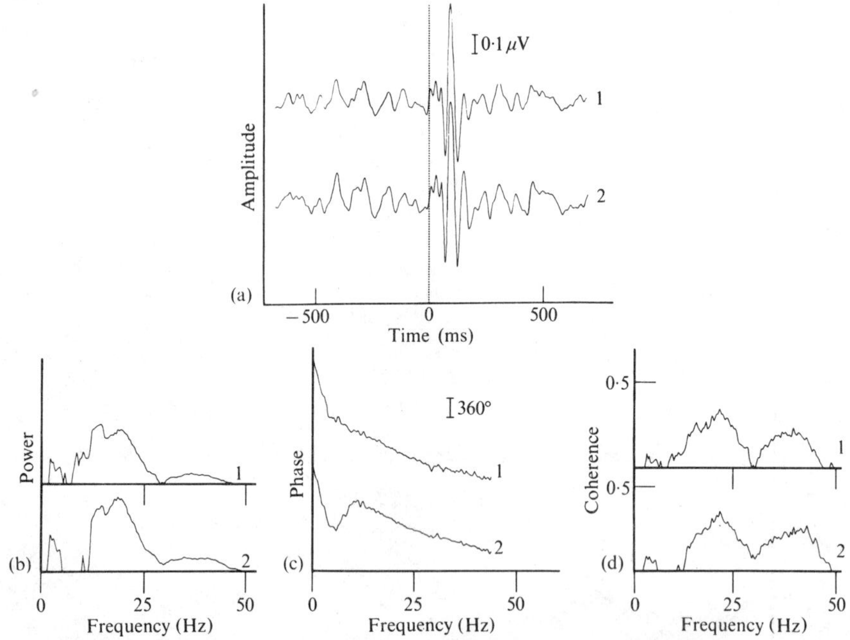

Fig. 2.6. Correlation responses (a) to a Gaussian noise modulated stimulus field. For stimulus specifications see legend of Fig. 2.5. Fourier transformation of these responses resulted in the cross-power and phase spectra depicted in (b) and (c). From the cross-power spectra the coherence spectra depicted in (d) were obtained. In these coherence spectra the two components of the correlation response express themselves as two maxima, one in the range of 14–20 Hz and the other in the range of 30–45 Hz.

variability becomes also evident from the phase characteristics) and enhances the high-frequency part, since most of the background activity is in the low-frequency range.

In the phase spectra two slopes can be recognized, one below 30 Hz and another above 30 Hz. The peak in the high-frequency range of the power spectra corresponds mainly to the 'early component' in the correlation 'response' since this component consists of waves with shorter periods – i.e. of higher mean frequency – than the other component. Furthermore if the latency of this component is estimated from the high-frequency slope of the phase plot, delays of 40–60 ms are found. These values are similar to the latencies determined with sinusoidal stimulation. When the phase plots are corrected for the minimum phase shift of the VEP system, pure latencies of the order of 30 ms are found, which corresponds with the onset of the primary flash VEP. The peak in the amplitude characteristic near 16 Hz corresponds to the secondary component in the correlation 'response'. The latency of this component can be estimated from the low-frequency tail of the phase spectrum at 90–110 ms, a value of the same order as found for the secondary component in the flash VEP.

Conclusions On the basis of the VEPs to homogeneous field stimulation with flashes, sinewave and Gaussian-noise-modulated light, the picture emerges that through scalp electrodes at least three signals with different cortical origin can be derived from the human visual system:

(a) The first signal expresses itself in the time domain as an early component with a latency of about 30 ms. In the frequency domain this signal dominates in the frequency range of 40–60 Hz.

(b) The second signal has a latency of 100–120 ms and dominates the medium frequency range (14–20 Hz) of the frequency domain.

(c) The peak frequency of the third signal coincides with the alpha frequency (9–12 Hz). In the time domain this signal has a latency of 120–200 ms.

In the next section the probable cortical origin of each of these signals and their dependence on stimulus parameters will be discussed. On the basis of this analysis a sequential model for the human evoked response system to luminance stimulation will be developed, consisting of a number of linear and nonlinear processes. By comparing the properties of these processes with those of retinal ganglion cells in goldfish and of single cells in the lateral geniculate of macaque monkey, the sequential model can be projected along the visual pathway.

The primary response; the high-frequency subsystem

Topology. Both the studies of Cigánek (1961) and Reits (1975) suggest that the short-latency response is generated in the primary receiving area of the visual radiation from the lateral geniculate nucleus. In this visual area (Brodmann's area 17), the meridional projection of the retina lies along a longitudinal infolding on the medial and cerebellar surfaces of the occipital lobe (the calcarine fissure) in such a way that the macula is represented posteriorly in the occipital lobe. In man only the first 2° of the macular area (the forea) is arranged in concentric bands on the free surface of the occipital cortex (Teuber 1961). At larger eccentricities the retino-cortical projection is as indicated in Fig. 2.7(a) with a decreasing surface area devoted to each degree of visual field when moving from the fovea to the periphery (Daniel and Whitteridge 1961). The vertical halves of the visual fields are projected in the contra-lateral hemispheres, with the upper and lower half visual fields represented below and above the calcarine fissure respectively. If the assumption is made that the surface potential field produced by cortical activity has properties similar to those of a corresponding dipole sheet (for a discussion see MacKay (1969)), then the symmetrical arrangement of the striate cortex will result in potentials of opposite polarity for upper and lower or right and left half-field stimulation, since the equivalent dipole direction is perpendicular to the cortical surface. Prediction by this model is in accordance with the polarity that is observed for the primary component in the cross-correlation response to Gaussian-noise-modulated light (see Table 2.1 and Fig. 2.8). Note the asymmetrical representation of left and right half-field stimulation in the contralateral

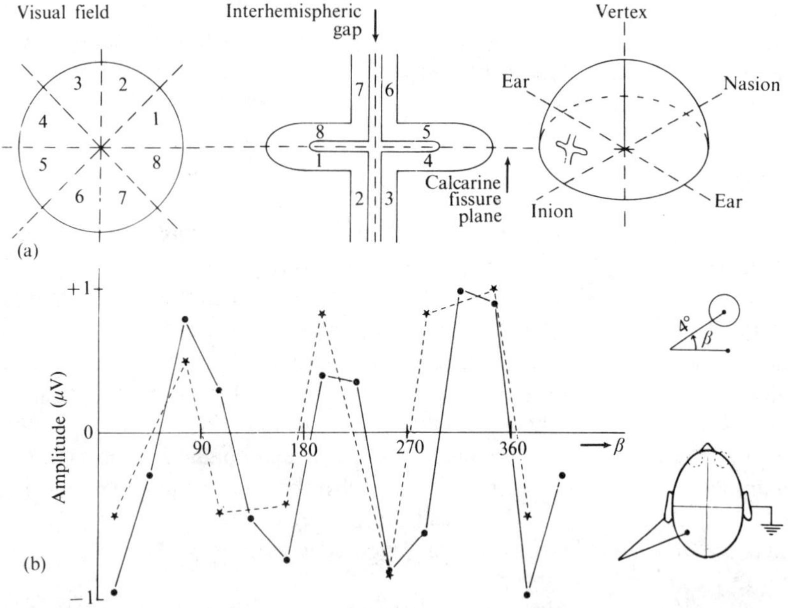

Fig. 2.7. A schematic and idealized layout of the visual field on the striate cortex around the interhemispheric gap and the calcarine fissures (a). The centre figure in (a) gives the backview of the transverse cross-section of this arrangement. In the right-hand figure of (a) this cortical layout is further simplified into a dipole sheet positioned in a spheric, homogeneous medium. For the electrode position indicated, this dipole model resulted in the potential depicted by a dashed line in (b), where the actual VEP data are represented by a solid line. These data were obtained with a high-frequency sine-wave modulated 2° stimulus positioned at an eccentricity of 5° in the visual field.

hemispheres and the larger responses to lower than to upper half-field stimulation. The example depicted in Fig. 2.8 shows that in accordance with the retino-cortical projection, simultaneous stimulation of the left and right visual half-fields in counterphase results in counterphase primary responses at the left and right hemispheres.

TABLE 2.1

Stimulus situation	Peak amplitude primary response† (μV)
Lower half-field	+ 0·20
Upper half-field	− 0·16
Both fields in phase	+ 0·08
Both fields in counterphase	+ 0·37

†Midline electrode positioned 6 cm above inion

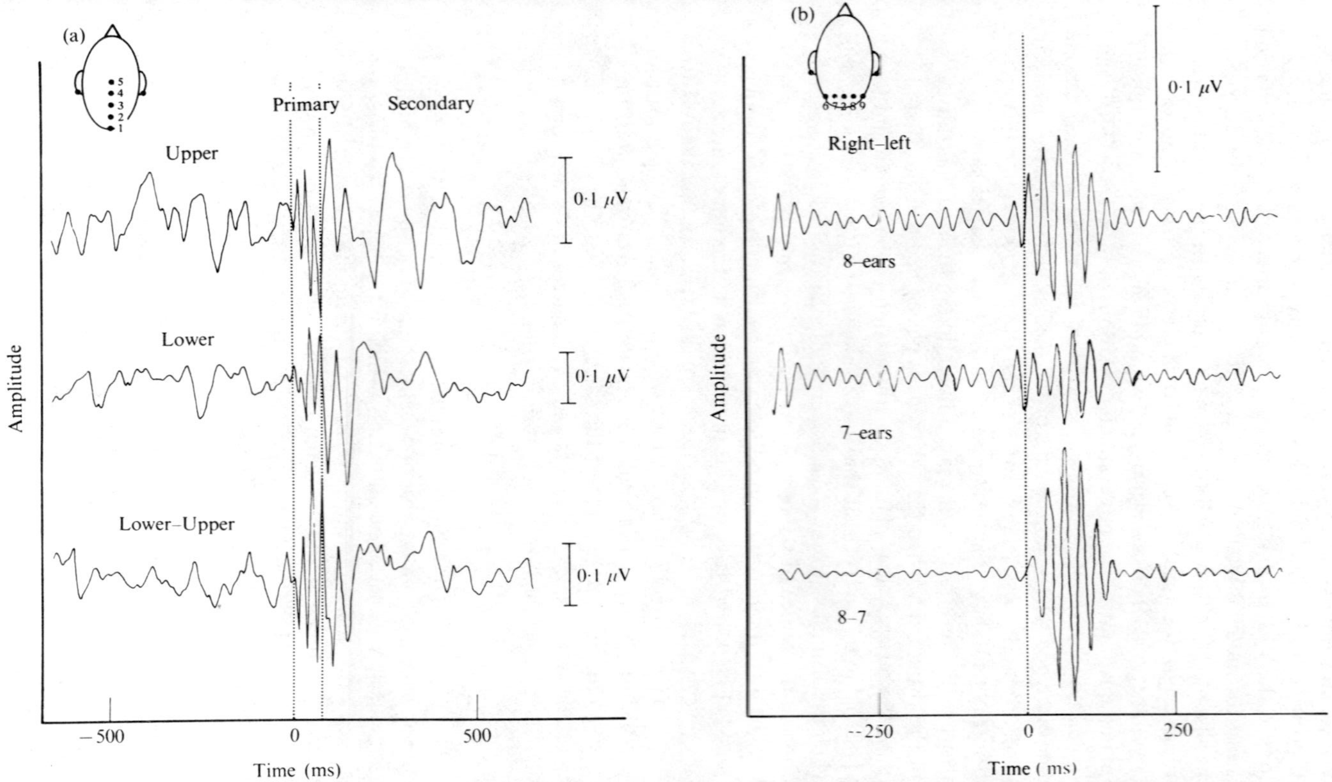

Fig. 2.8. Cross-correlation responses from monopolar electrode derivation 3 to upper half-field, lower half-field and to simulation of both fields in counterphase (a). Note that, in contrast to the secondary response, the primary responses to the two half-field stimulations are in counterphase. This is emphasized in the bottom figure of (a) where the primary response is enhanced whereas the secondary response is reduced.

In (b) the responses for counterphase stimulation of left and right half-fields are shown. By filtering the EEG records (bandwidth 30–50 Hz) mainly the primary component is left in these figures. Since the 'monopolar' responses are in counterphase a larger response is obtained for the bipolar derivation (bottom figure). For stimulus specifications see legend of Fig. 2.5.

A more crucial test for the model is the potential distribution of the response to a relatively small stimulus field located at a fixed eccentricity as a function of the angular position in the visual field. The eccentricity is chosen so as to avoid contributions to the VEP from regions on the exterior surface of the occipital lobe. On the basis of the model it would be expected that for almost every electrode position the sign of the response will flip over six times when the stimulus field rotates through a full 360° in the visual field. If the retino-cortical projection were completely symmetrical, then reversal of sign would take place whenever the stimulus moves from one quadrant to the next (angular positions of 90°, 180°, 270°, and 360°). Two additional reversals of sign will take place depending on the location of the recording electrode relative to the axes of the medial surfaces of the hemispheres in and around the calcarine fissures. When the electrode is in either the second or fourth quadrant of the transverse cross-sectional plan (back view) of the striate cortex, the reversals occur upon stimulation in the first and third quadrant of the visual field. When the electrode is placed in either the first or third quadrant the reversal takes place upon stimulation in the second and fourth quadrant. This is due to the fact that the dipole associated with the response will flip over when the stimulus crosses the axis perpendicular to the line connecting the electrode and the centre of the retinal representation. In Fig. 2.7(b) the amplitude of the high-frequency response to a sine-wave modulated 3° stimulus field positioned at an eccentricity of 4° is presented as a function of angular location for two subjects. Both the number of polarity reversals and the relative amplitudes of the responses are in accordance with the model. Taking into account the considerable inter-individual variability in the detailed arrangement of the striate cortex and in the configuration of the calcarine fissures, the good correspondence between the experimental and expected results is such that it can be taken that the primary high-frequency response indeed originates in the area striata.

Saturation. The VEPs to high-frequency luminance modulation show that the amplitude of the response follows proportionally the modulation depth of the sine-wave stimulus up to a certain modulation, which is the higher the lower the mean luminance level, and then starts to flatten ('saturate') (Spekreijse 1966).

Since in case of monocular and binocular stimulation, saturation becomes evident at the same modulation depth (Fig. 2.9(a)) and since the saturation point does not depend on stimulus field size (Fig. 2.9(b)), the saturating element must be assumed to occur early in the visual pathway and certainly at a site preceding the binocular interaction.

Since the assumption seems to hold that the saturation is frequency independent (static) (Spekreijse 1966) the dependence of saturation on stimulus frequency can provide information about distal dynamic processing. If, for example, high-frequency attenuation occurs before the saturating element, then the saturation point will be reached at higher modulation depth for increasing

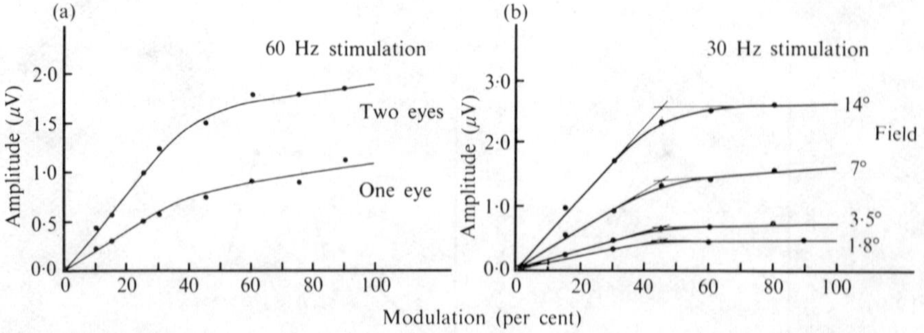

Fig. 2.9. Amplitude of the primary response as a function of modulation depth in case of one- and two-eye stimulation (a) and for various sizes of the stimulus field (b). (a) gives the amplitude of the fundamental component and (b) that of the second harmonic. The mean luminance of the stimulus field was 10 000 asb; The pupils were dilated.

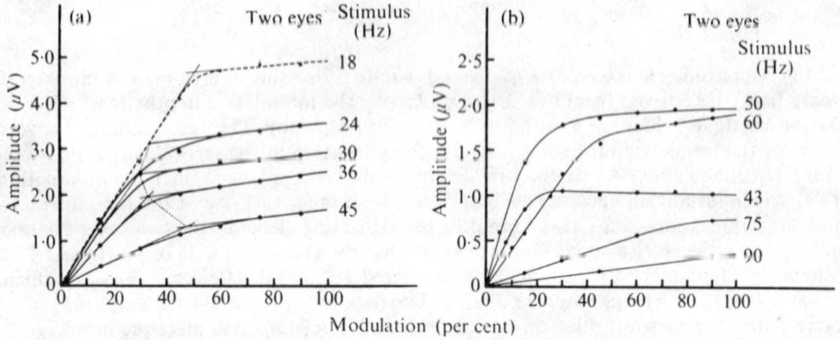

Fig. 2.10. Saturation of the primary response as a function of the frequency of a sine-wave modulated 20° Maxwellian field. The mean luminance was 10 000 asb: the pupils were dilated. (a) gives the amplitude of the second harmonic and (b) that of the fundamental component in the response. For clarity the saturation curve to the 18 Hz stimulus is doubled in amplitude. (dotted line).

stimulus frequency. The data of Fig. 2.10 show that the high-frequency VEP saturates at increasingly higher modulation depths for stimulus frequencies below and above 30 Hz, indicating that low- and high-frequency attenuation occurs before the saturation. It should be noted that this conclusion can be drawn only from the dependence of the saturation point on stimulus frequency and not from the actual size of the response. In the latter, dynamic processing is also reflected, which occurs after the saturation and which accounts for the fact that the response to 60 Hz stimulation is larger than that to, for example, 43 Hz.

If the modulation depths at which saturation occurs are plotted as a function of stimulus frequency, one gets the amplitude characteristic depicted in Fig. 2.11(a) (full line). This amplitude characteristic resembles the characteristics that can be calculated under comparable conditions on the basis of linearizing experiments (Van der Tweel and Spekreijse 1969) or from the correlation responses to Gaussian-

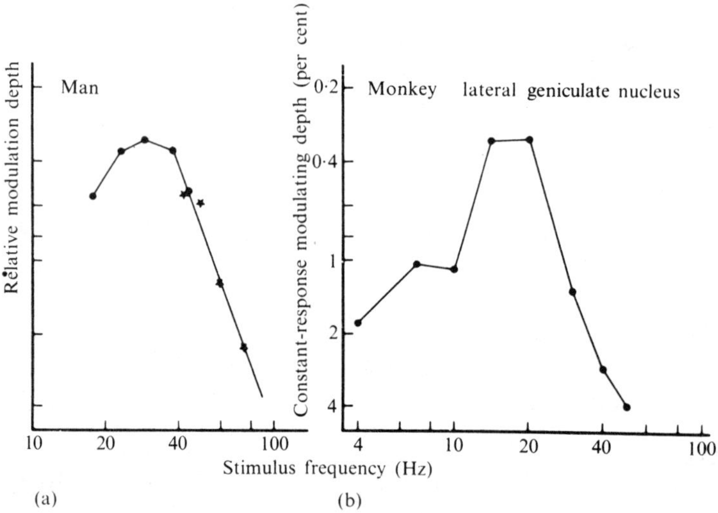

Fig. 2.11. Amplitude characteristics of distal dynamic processing in man (a) and monkey (b). The data in (a) are derived from Fig. 2.10 by plotting the modulation depths at which saturation becomes evident as a function of stimulus frequency. The curve comprises two sets of data: for the frequency range of 18–45 Hz the saturation of the second harmonic is used, and for frequencies above 43 Hz the fundamental data are employed. Since the modulation depth at which saturation becomes evident depends on the actual size of the fundamental and second harmonic components at the input of the saturating element, the two sets of data may be shifted along the vertical axis. This is done so that the saturation data of 43 Hz and 45 Hz coincide. The luminance of the binocularly presented 20° stimulus field seen in Maxwellian view was 10 000 asb. The pupils were dilated. The data in (b) represent the amplitude characteristics of yellow-off, blue-on lateral geniculate nucleus cell in macaque monkey determined with blue sinusoidally modulated light at a retinal illumination of 480 td. This amplitude characteristic is obtained by plotting the modulation depth required for each stimulus frequency to reach a constant response criterion. The Maxwellian field subtended 15°.

noise-modulated light (Reits 1975). It might be of interest to compare these curves with the amplitude characteristics of lateral geniculate cells. By plotting as a function of stimulus frequency the modulation depths that are required to reach in single lateral geniculate nucleus cells of macaque monkey an arbitrary spike-discharge pattern evoked by sinusoidal luminance modulation, Fig. 2.11(b) was obtained (Spekreijse, Van Norren, and Van den Berg 1971). The overall similarity to the human electrophysiological curves is clear.

Rectification. The spike responses at various stages along the visual pathway show an essential form of distortion. What this means becomes clear by observing Fig. 2.12, where the spike responses derived from retinal ganglion cells in goldfish and from lateral geniculate cells in the monkey are depicted as a function of the modulation depth of a sine-wave stimulus. In both situations sine-wave stimulation produces, for modulation depths exceeding a small but definite value, a burst of action potentials only *once* during each stimulus cycle. The average responses in

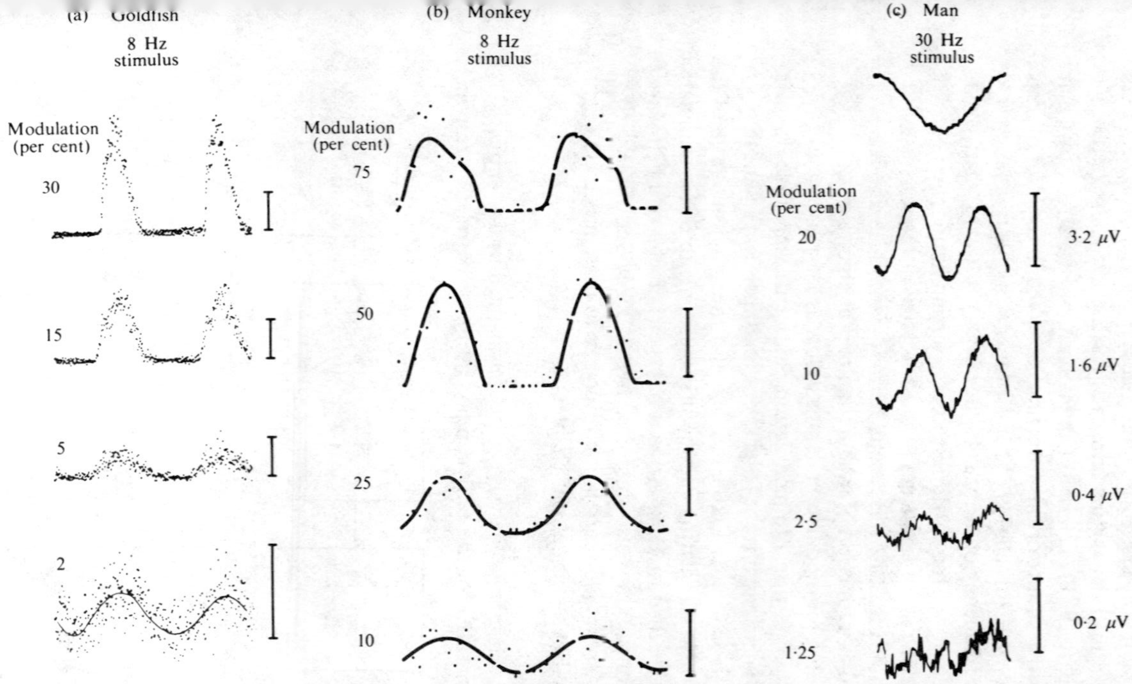

Fig. 2.12. Spike responses from retinal ganglion cells in goldfish and from lateral geniculate cells in monkey are depicted as a function of the modulation depth of a sine-wave stimulus. In the first two columns the responses to two complete stimulus periods are presented. In the third column the primary response (inion–vertex derivation) is shown as a function of the modulation depth of a 30 Hz sine-wave modulated field. This response consists mainly of a second harmonic component, whose amplitude grows proportionally to modulation depth.

(a) Average spike response of a red-off centre process to a 650 nm stimulus with a mean intensity of about 1 $\mu W\ cm^{-2}$. The number of summations with the CAT (computer of average transients) computer is 300. Calibration bars are 20 spikes per bin. Bin duration for averaging is 625 μs.

(b) Average spike responses of the excitatory component of a green-on, red-off lateral geniculate nucleus cell of macaque monkey. The number of summations is 100; the mean retinal illumination amounts to 480 td. Calibration bars are 20 spikes per s.

(c) VEPs to a white 20° sine-wave modulated field seen in Maxwellian view. The number of summations is inversely proportional to modulation depth. The luminance is 10 000 asb.

Fig. 2.12 show that during half the stimulus period the density distribution of the nerve impulses has roughly the same shape as the sinusoidal stimulus and that during the other half of the stimulus cycle no spike discharge can be observed at all. Note that at high modulation depths all responses saturate. These data suggest that a half-wave rectifier can model the distortions observed in the discharge pattern of retinal ganglion cells in goldfish and of lateral geniculate nucleus cells in macaque monkey to small signal stimulation (Spekreijse 1969; Spekreijse, Van Norren, and Van den Berg 1971). The right-hand column of Fig. 2.12 shows that a similar model can also account for the distortions observed in the VEP of man to high-frequency sine-wave stimulation. When a proper stimulus frequency is chosen (about half the frequency of the peak of the primary response) then, owing to the frequency selectivity of the cortical process, a second harmonic (i.e. a component with twice the input frequency) can be isolated in the response. In the right-hand column of Fig. 2.12 this second harmonic to 30 Hz sine-wave stimulation is depicted as a function of modulation depth. Since a second harmonic can be detected for modulation depths as low as 2·5 per cent and since the amplitude is proportional to modulation depth (the amplitude doubles when the modulation is increased from 10 per cent to 20 per cent) a linear rectifier can describe these results. Taking into account the amplitude ratio of the second harmonic to 30 Hz stimulation and the first harmonic to 60 Hz stimulation, the conclusion can be reached that this element has the character of a half-wave linear rectifier. This conclusion is also supported by the behaviour of the early component in the (bi- and mono-)correlation responses to noise-modulated light (Reits (1975), and the last section of this chapter).

Conclusions: a model. The above analysis can be summarized in the sequential model presented in Fig. 2.13 for the early component in the correlation response

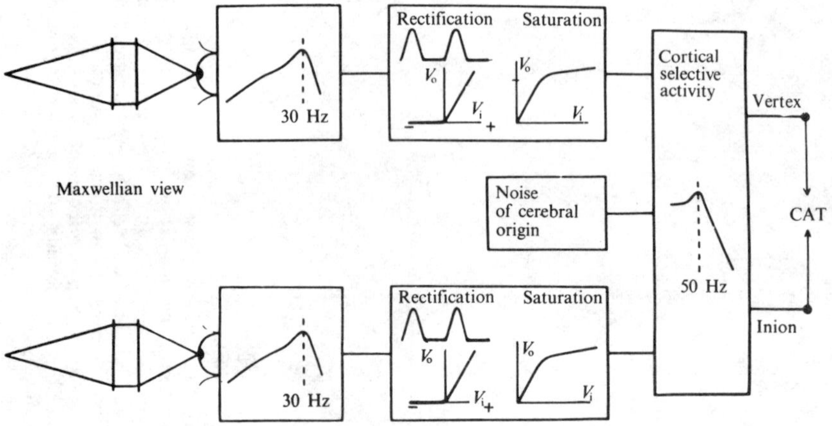

Fig. 2.13. A simplified model of the main processes in the human primary response system to luminance stimulation.

to noise stimulation or the high-frequency part of the amplitude characteristic to sine-wave stimulation. It should be realized that in this model the visual system is oversimplified into a N-channel model, with identical independent pathways feeding into the area striata in correspondence with the retino-cortical projection. Interactions among channels or between channels of different systems have been left out of this scheme on purpose.

The secondary response; the medium-frequency subsystem

Topology. The studies of Spekreijse (1966), Regan (1968), and Reits (1975) indicate that the VEP components in the range of roughly 12–25 Hz have a more restricted occipital representation than the low- and high-frequency responses. The largest medium-frequency responses are found with electrode positions at the occipital regions at about 5 cm above the inion and 4 cm to the left and the right of the midline. Since the equivalent dipole for the secondary response lies above area 17, Reits (1975) suggested that this component originates in the secondary cortex (areas 18 and 19).

Zeki (1969) has shown that the prestriate cortex of the monkey seems to be largely occupied by a representation of the central 4–5° of the visual field in such a way that there is a mirror-like retinotopic arrangement across the striate-prestriate boundary (Cowey 1964). Furthermore there is evidence that there may be some asymmetry about the projection into the calcarine fissure. It seems that in man the upper visual field extends further forward on the lower wall than the lower visual field on the upper wall of the calcarine fissure (Whitteridge 1973). These anatomical findings point to a second representation of the macular area lateral and anterior to area 17.

If this secondary projection were the source of generation of the secondary response or medium-frequency response, then it could be expected that stimulation of the lower half of the visual field would result in a more anteriorly positioned and larger medium-frequency response than that to upper half-field stimulation. The data in Fig. 2.8 and Table 2.2 show that this is indeed the case. Moreover, the correlation responses to upper and lower half-field stimulation are in phase, so that the response to full-field stimulation is about the sum of the responses to half-field stimulation. This additivity of the half-field responses, which contrasts greatly with the behaviour of the high-frequency responses, is also in accordance with the retinotopic arrangement in the prestriate cortex, if the assumption is made that the equivalent dipole direction is perpendicular to the cortical surface.

The results of stimulation of the left and right visual half-fields are more difficult to interpret. The data in the bottom half of Table 2.2 indicate that the medium-frequency responses dominate at the electrode placed over ipsilateral hemisphere. On first view this observation suggests an ipsilateral representation of the macular region in area 18. Although connections from area 17 in one hemisphere through the corpus callosum to area 18 in the other hemisphere are mentioned, this pathway seems rather controversial (Doty and Negrao 1973). Furthermore, if the medium-frequency responses would follow such a pathway then there should be a sequential relationship between the high- and medium-

TABLE 2.2

Stimulus situation	Peak amplitude secondary response† (μV)	
Lower half-field	+ 0·50	
Upper half-field	+ 0·15	
Both fields in phase	+ 0·85	
Both fields in counterphase	+ 0·35	
	Electrode on† right hemisphere (μV)	Electrode on‡ left hemisphere (μV)
Left half-field	+ 0·08	+ 0·21
Right half-field	+ 0·33	+ 0·15
Both fields in counterphase	0·25	0·17

†Midline electrode positioned 6 cm above inion.
‡Electrodes were positioned 4·5 cm lateral from the midline and 4·5 cm above the inion.

frequency responses, unless the cells in area 17 that link the medium-frequency system to area 18 do not themselves contribute to an area-17 response. The latter we consider rather unlikely. A sequential link between the high- and medium-frequency systems is, however, in conflict with clinical observations since in patients with optic-nerve atrophy, the medium-frequency response may be delayed whereas the high-frequency response remains unaffected (Regan, Milner, and Heron, Chapter 29 of this book). It therefore seems likely that the medium- and high-frequency responses are mediated by channels that are separated as early as the retinal ganglion cell level. There is histological evidence in favour of such a parallel pathway both at optic nerve and optic radiation level: e.g. areas 18 and 19 in the cat receive retinal afferents that come particularly from the pulvinar of the dorsal thalamus (Poggio 1968); such collaterals of the retino-geniculate fibres are well known (Ramón y Cajal 1955; Meikle and Sprague 1964). Moreover there is electrophysiological evidence in dogs for a pathway to areas 18 and 19 that parallels the direct specific visual pathway. Lopes da Silva, Van Rotterdam, Storm van Leeuwen, and Tielen (1970) found in awake dogs with implanted electrodes that distorted responses to sine-wave-modulated light can be recorded simultaneously in the lateral geniculate nucleus and the calcarine regions, but not in area 18. Furthermore they found that the latter responses are generated by a 'beta' frequency-selective system that has a clear-cut topological distribution that is restricted primarily to area 18 and possibly to 19.

This parallel pathway has, however, a predominantly contra-lateral representation. Therefore, if the medium-frequency response in man reflects activity of this pathway, then the observed ipsilaterality of the response should not be taken as implying a response generator in the ipsilateral hemisphere. With the secondary macular representation anterior and lateral of the occipital lobe, partly on the exterior and partly on the medial surface of the occipital cortex, the resultant dipole may point to the other hemisphere, in such a way that the VEP will show a seemingly ipsilateral representation. This conclusion, although in accordance with anatomy, needs further experimental verification.

Nonlinear behaviour. The characteristics of the medium-frequency or secondary response have not been studied as extensively as those of the low- and high-frequency responses. Using sine-wave stimulation, it has been observed by both Spekreijse (1966) and Regan (1968), in man, and by Lopes da Silva *et al.* (1970), in the dog, that this response is rather undistorted. The ratio between the fundamental and second harmonic component can be as large as 8:1 (Regan 1968), so that the fundamental component gives a good description of the medium-frequency VEP. This finding contrasts with the study of Reits (1975), who found a medium-frequency response in the bicorrelation function between a Gaussian-noise-modulated stimulus and the VEP, even at modulation depths as low as 4 per cent. This would indicate that a nonlinearity with a rectifying nature is situated in the pathway that results in the medium-frequency response. The reason for the discrepancy between the sine-wave and noise data is not clear, but caution is needed in the interpretation of the bicorrelation functions, since, due to overlap in time and frequency content, the low- and medium-frequency components cannot easily be distinguished from each other.

With regard to saturation from both the sine-wave and noise data the same picture emerges. Most of the saturation takes place before the signals of the two eyes merge together. In this respect, and also in the amplitude dependence of the response on mean luminance level, the medium-frequency response resembles the high-frequency one. On the other hand the medium- and high-frequency components differ in that the medium-frequency component depends on the spectral composition of the stimulus light. Regan (1968) reported that the frequency selectivity near 16 Hz may be enhanced by superposing the stimulus, preferably blue, on a steady red or yellow background. This suggests that a receptor with a blue sensitivity may be involved, although it is not clear whether this response is initiated by blue cones or by the rod system. The latter seems less likely since the medium frequency responses can also be obtained at high photopic intensities.

The distal linear process. In the last section of this chapter it will be shown how a system consisting of two linear processes with transfer functions $H_1(j\omega)$ and $H_2(j\omega)$ respectively that are linked by a static nonlinearity such as a rectifier, can be analysed by means of the correlation technique. In this section such an analysis will be applied to estimate the amplitude characteristic of the linear process preceding the static nonlinearity.

For the above system the cross-bicorrelation spectrum will be proportional to

$$H_2\{j(\omega_1+\omega_2)\}H_1(j\omega_1)H_1(j\omega_2) \tag{2.1}$$

(see the section on analysis of evoked responses). In Fig. 2.14 an example of such a spectrum is given in the form of equipotential lines expressed in relative values of

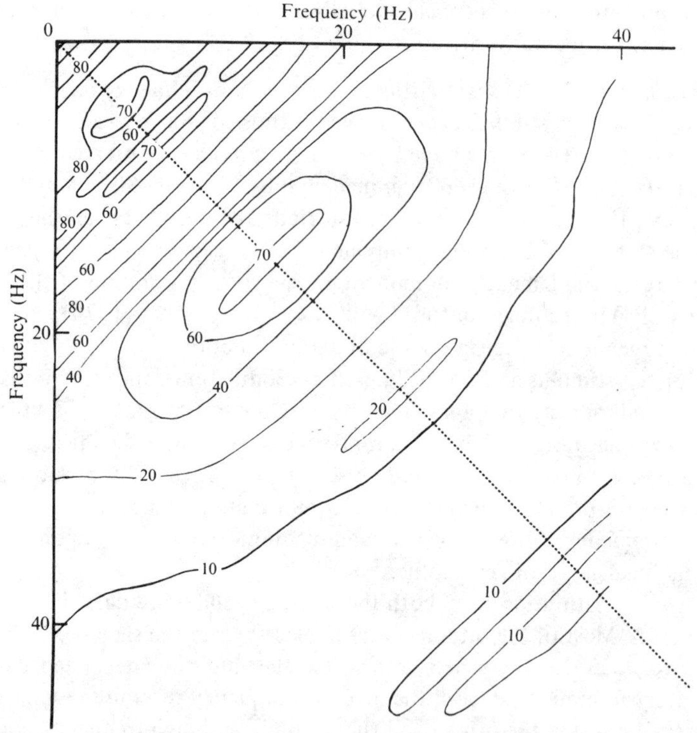

Fig. 2.14. Cross-bipower spectrum calculated for a 13 min EEG record derived from a 'mono-polar' midline electrode positioned 3 cm above the inion. The modulation depth of the Gaussian noise (bandwidth 0–50 Hz) modulated stimulus field is 36 per cent. The mean luminance is 2700 asb. The spectrum is drawn in the form of equipotential lines in the plane $(\omega_1/2\pi, \omega_2/2\pi)$. The values along the equipotential lines are the relative amplitudes in per cent of peak amplitude of the cross-bipower spectrum.

the maximum value (= 100) of the spectrum. Along the line $\omega_1+\omega_2$ = constant (dotted) the values of the cross-bispectrum do not depend on $H_2(j\omega)$ but only on $H_1(j\omega)$. Furthermore along this line $H_1(j\omega_1)H_1(j\omega_2)$ has a derivative which is zero for $\omega_1=\omega_2$. This can be easily understood by substituting in (2.1): $\omega_1=\omega+h$ and $\omega_2=\omega-h$ and taking the derivative d/dh. Since a maximum is nearly always found for $\omega_1 = \omega_2$, it can be concluded that $H_1(j\omega)$ has at most one clear maximum. This maximum can be read off by determining the line $\omega_1 + \omega_2 =$ constant, along which the curvature of the bispectrum is the steepest. This can be understood if one realizes that for $h \to 0$ the product $H_1(j(\omega - h))\, H_1(j(\omega + h))$ grows the quickest for values of $(\omega - h)$ and $(\omega + h)$ below and above the peak frequency of $H_1(j\omega)$. This is the region of the amplitude characteristic where the curvature is the strongest. If on the other hand the frequencies $(\omega - h)$ and $(\omega + h)$ were on those regions of the slopes of the amplitude characteristic where the attenuation per octave is constant, then the product would have been constant. For the bispectrum depicted in Fig. 2.14 this analysis results in an estimate for the maximum of $H_1(j\omega)$ between 15 Hz and 20 Hz. An estimate of the shape of the amplitude characteristic of $H_1(j\omega)$ can be obtained as follows. If one chooses $H_1(2\pi) = 1$ and $H_1(4 \times 2\pi) = A$ then the value of $H_1(6 \times 2\pi)$ can be estimated by determining along for instance the line $\omega_1 + \omega_2 = 2\pi \times 8$ the values at $H_2(8 \times 2\pi)$ $H_1(2\pi \times 6) H_1(2 \times 2\pi)$ and $H_2(2\pi \times 8) H_1^2(2\pi \times 4)$. By continuing this procedure one can estimate that the low-frequency attenuation of $H_1(j\omega)$ is about 6 dB per octave and that the high-frequency attenuation lies in the range of 12–18 dB per octave.

Conclusions: a model. The clinical data of Milner, Regan, and Heron (1974), in particular, seem to point to a separation of the channels by which the early and high-frequency responses are mediated at a stage as distal as the retinal ganglion cells. If the assumption is valid that the nonlinearity reflects the on and off nature of ganglion cell activity then it cannot be excluded that the first linear element in the sequential model is shared by both subsystems. On first view the amplitude characteristics of these distal elements seem not to support this hypothesis. It should, however, be realized that the high-frequency data were obtained at an approximately 1000 times higher luminance level than the medium-frequency data. This could account for the higher peak frequency of the high-frequency subsystem in accordance to the shift in peak frequency of the MTF (modulation transfer function) plots with mean luminance level (Kelly 1961). Furthermore, when the medium- and high-frequency responses are analysed at the same luminance level, then similar distal amplitude characteristics are found (Reits 1975). However, in the cross-correlation functions the medium- and low-frequency subsystems can be confused easily.

With regard to the nonlinearity, there is no consensus about its shape. It may behave like a half-wave linear rectifier, as is the case for the high-frequency subsystem, or it may even be of a weaker nonlinear nature. All in all many gaps remain to be filled in our knowledge about the medium-frequency subsystem.

On the other hand, the medium-frequency region is rather suitable for studying general aspects, such as latency and amplitude fluctuations in the VEP, since the measurements are not influenced by the frequency selectivity of the low-frequency system and larger responses can be obtained than at high frequencies.

In EP studies it is frequently assumed that the average evoked potential is an exact replica of the response to a single stimulus. The validity of this assumption cannot easily be verified since the time course of possible fluctuations in the response is unlikely to be lower or of the same order as the recording length needed in the averaging process. In searching for such fluctuations a different approach must be chosen. A suitable technique could be the analysis of power spectra, since amplitude and/or phase fluctuations in periodic signals result in sidebands (provided the rate of variation exceeds the spectral resolution). The power spectrum of an EP recording in Fig. 2.15 shows that such sidebands are in fact present. By analysing the

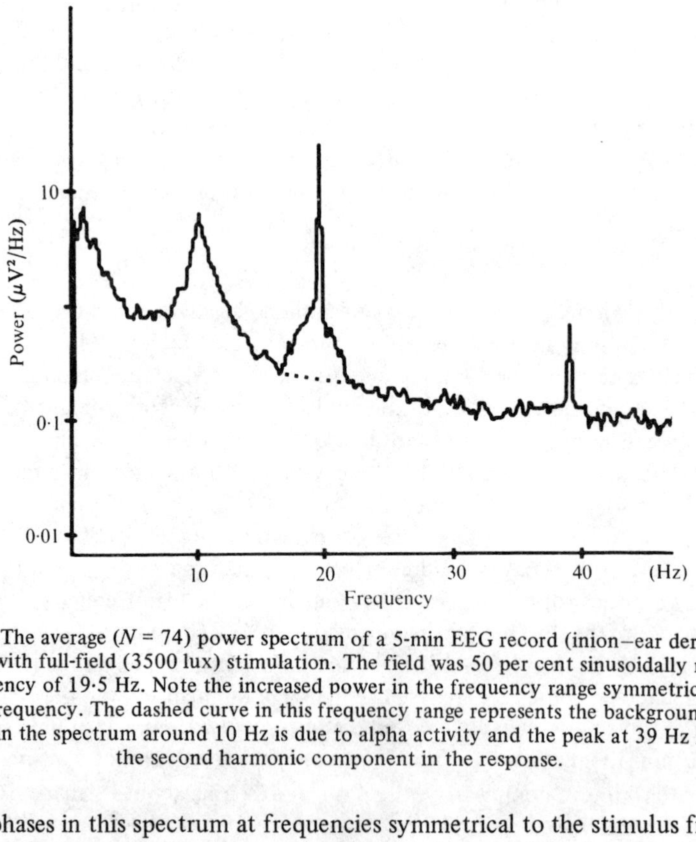

Fig. 2.15. The average ($N = 74$) power spectrum of a 5-min EEG record (inion–ear derivation), obtained with full-field (3500 lux) stimulation. The field was 50 per cent sinusoidally modulated at a frequency of 19·5 Hz. Note the increased power in the frequency range symmetrical to the stimulus frequency. The dashed curve in this frequency range represents the background power. The peak in the spectrum around 10 Hz is due to alpha activity and the peak at 39 Hz reflects the second harmonic component in the response.

relative phases in this spectrum at frequencies symmetrical to the stimulus frequency it could be concluded that in this particular example the sidebands have to be attributed to amplitude fluctuations of the order of 70 per cent with frequencies up to 2·5 Hz. For high and low stimulus frequencies it is more difficult to reach a similar conclusion, owing to the smaller response amplitude and larger noise (alpha-rhythm) respectively. It seems, however, not unlikely that here also fluctuations may occur which could account in part for the variability in the waveform of flash-evoked responses.

The late response; the low-frequency subsystem

Contrary to the primary and secondary responses, the late response seems not to originate in the visual cortex. This conclusion is already indicated by the observation that the potential distribution of the late response coincides with that of the alpha rhythm, which is known from depth recordings also to be present outside the visual cortex. More direct evidence offers the position of the equivalent dipole which gives the potential distribution of the late response over the scalp. This dipole lies near the centre of the head, far from the cortex. This suggests that in reality the sources of the late response cover a substantial part of the cortex and that this response cannot be attributed to a specific region.

Signal processing preceding the rectifier. In the section on 'the analysis of evoked responses' (p. 76) it is shown that the masking or linearizing property of noise or an auxiliary signal can be used to determine the functional sequence of linear and nonlinear transformations in a system that contains a nonlinearity. Furthermore the linearizing phenomenon can be used to determine the characteristics of the individual elements (Spekreijse and Oosting 1970). This possibility will be applied to determine the amplitude characteristic of the distal linear process in the low-frequency subsystem.

For this purpose a sinusoidal auxiliary signal is preferred since it passes undisturbed through a linear system. The advantage of this feature is that, if the nonlinearity is preceded by a linear process, then an auxiliary sine wave $B \sin \beta t$ added to the sinusoidal stimulus $A \sin \omega t$, results in an incoming signal to the nonlinearity which still consists of two sine waves but with amplitudes A^* and B^*. As long as B^* sufficiently exceeds A^* the auxiliary signal will mask the nonlinearity and an almost undistorted response will be obtained. It should be realized that period-averaging is required to reduce the amount of auxiliary signal in the final recording, and that the sinusoidal stimulus $A \sin \omega t$ must retain the same frequency in the successive experiments in order to keep the influence of proximal frequency-dependent processes constant.

Suppose that the linear process has a high-frequency cut-off, then for increasing frequencies β the amplitude B^* will be progressively reduced. Therefore, if the sinusoidal stimulus $A \sin \omega t$ retains the amplitude, a progressively more distorted response will be obtained for increasing frequencies β. With this method it is possible to determine the attenuation of a linear process which precedes the nonlinearity. One way of determining this initial linear attenuation is to choose for each frequency β such an amplitude B that the response contains a constant amount of distortion. This means that B^* is constant at the input of the nonlinearity. By plotting B against β on logarithmic scales (just as in the case of the flicker fusion curves), the amplitude characteristic of the first linear process can be obtained. This method is illustrated in Fig. 2.16, where the linearizing effect of high-frequency auxiliary signals upon the low-frequency VEP is shown.

From this type of experiment one may conclude that a high-frequency attenuation of 18 dB per octave exists prior to the nonlinear stage. The cut-off frequency lies between 20 Hz and 30 Hz, and a low-frequency attenuation of 6 dB per octave is found.

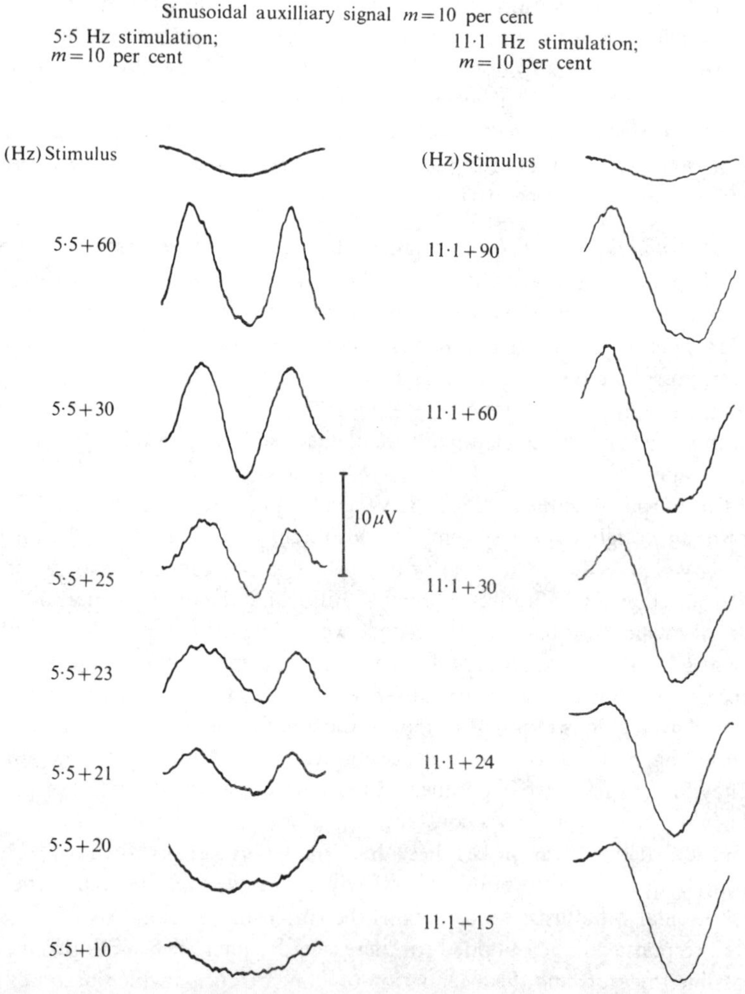

Fig. 2.16. The late responses to sinusoidally modulated light with frequencies of 5·5 Hz (left-hand column) and 11·1 Hz (right-hand column). Added to this stimulus is a sinusoidal auxiliary signal with the same modulation depth ($A/B = 1$). The left-hand column shows that the effect of decreasing the frequency of this auxiliary signal is to enhance the linearizing effectiveness of the auxiliary signal. This indicates at once that high-frequency attenuation precedes the distorting stage. Since the auxiliary signal has scarcely any influence on the amplitude of the fundamental component in the response (right-hand column), the distortions in the human low-frequency subsystems can be ascribed to linear rectification. The VEPs were derived with midline electrodes (inion–vertex). The diffuse stimulus field was binocularly presented; the luminance was 200 asb.

Proximal selective process. The relationship between the late response and the stimulus is also determined by a proximal process which shows frequency-selective behaviour. In a number of subjects a good correspondence can be found between the amplitude characteristics of the low-frequency subsystem and the amplitude spectrum of the alpha rhythm. In case the selectivity is high, other frequency-dependent processes along the visual pathway can even be neglected near the resonance frequency.

Rhythmic phenomena have been basic to EEG work, and especially the relationship of the alpha rhythm to VEPs has been discussed many times. For instance, much attention has been given to the after-discharges of a rhythmic character, the so-called ringing phenomena, that can be found after light-flash stimulation (Barlow 1962; Walter 1962; Cohn 1964). A number of theories has been advanced to explain the origin of the rhythmic phenomena. Some of them explicitly mention relaxation oscillations (Dewan 1964); others suggest this by the use of terminology such as photic driving, synchronization, entrainment, etc.

Experiments with relaxation oscillators indicate that certain pseudo-linear and pseudo-resonance effects can be mimicked when a weaker stimulus is used than that needed for full synchronization. An interesting and important difference between the relaxation oscillator and a passive resonance filter can be found when the relaxation oscillator is influenced near twice its natural frequency. In this case a kind of frequency selectivity is also found, but at the influencing frequency (Van der Tweel and Boon 1970). In the synchronized state the locking occurs at each of two periods, resulting in a response at half of the influencing frequency. A selectivity at twice the frequency of the peak of the resonance curve was not demonstrated in our subjects. On the other hand Fig. 2.17 shows that subharmonic responses are found in contrast to the expectations in a passive model. Such a result cannot easily be obtained in a regular viewing situation, since eye blinks might disturb the phase locking between subharmonic components in subsequent sections of the record. This figure does not show an average response of the total EEG record but the amplitude spectrum of averaged sections, each containing 40 stimulus periods. This representation is chosen because it allows a better discrimination between response and background activity than can be obtained with the classical averaging technique. This becomes clear if one realizes that the response components to periodic stimulation can be present only at discrete points (e.g. 1/3, 1/2, 1, 2 times the stimulus frequency) along the frequency axis. Hence, if at these points the amplitude of the spectrum exceeds that in neighbouring points, then the existence of a particular (sub)harmonic component is demonstrated. These results indicate that for the description of the frequency selectivity of the VEPs a more elaborate model is needed, to account for the subharmonic generation. Such a model should include, for example, a nonlinear feedback loop as was proposed by Lopes da Silva (1970).

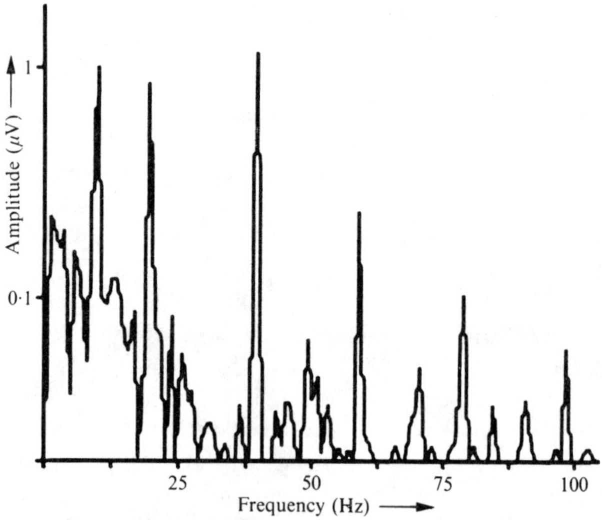

Fig. 2.17. The spectrum of 90 subsequent EEG records (vertex–ear derivation) each record containing 40 stimulus periods. The subject was stimulated through the eyelids with a sinusoidally modulated light (modulation depth is 50 per cent and stimulus frequency is 19.5 Hz). Note the peaks in the spectrum at 1/2, 1, 2, 3, 4, and 5 times the sumulus frequency. With normal observation the subharmonic is easily lost since owing to eye blinks the phase of this particular subharmonic component can jump 180°.

Conclusions: a model. Fig. 2.18 gives a simplified version of the model that accounts for the luminance VEPs of the low-frequency subsystem. This model can be distinguished in two essential points – saturation and rectification – from the models for the medium- and high-frequency subsystems. From the ratio of fundamental to second harmonic component in the response to sine-wave modulated light or from the ratio of mono- to bi-cross-correlation functions to

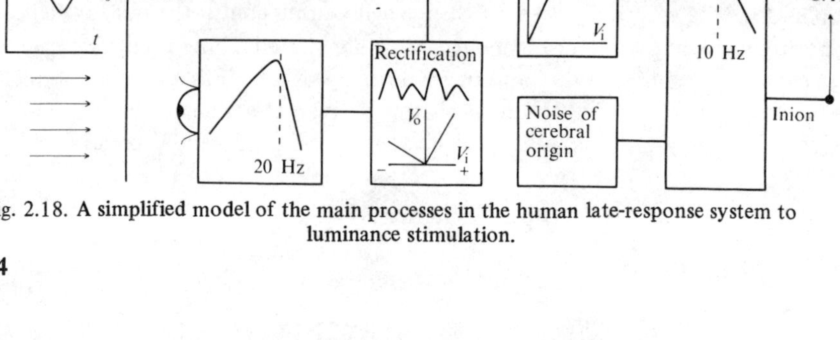

Fig. 2.18. A simplified model of the main processes in the human late-response system to luminance stimulation.

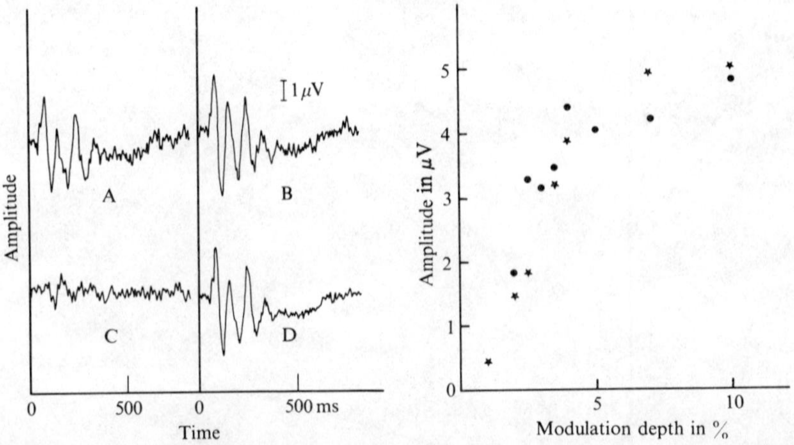

Fig. 2.19. Responses of bright and dark pulses with a time course (sin 100 πt)/100 πt and 5 per cent modulation depth. Inion–ear derivation; full-field stimulation with a mean luminance of 2700 asb. Left: A, average response to 400 bright pulses; B, the same to 400 dark pulses; C, the difference between the top two responses (divided by 2 to facilitate comparison of the records); D, half the sum of A and B. Right: peak-to-peak value of the responses to bright (*) and dark (•) pulses measured 100 ms after the stimulus onset. The responses can be seen to saturate at about 5 per cent modulation depth.

Gaussian-noise-modulated light, it can be deduced that the nonlinear element has the nature of a slightly asymmetric full-wave linear rectifier. Hence the distortion is most outspoken for the low-frequency subsystem.

The enigma of the saturation has not been solved. The data in Fig. 2.20 indicate on the one hand that the saturation of the low-frequency responses occurs at increasingly higher modulation depths as the size of the stimulus field is decreased and on the other hand that the signals from both eyes feed the saturating element jointly. The simplest explanation would be that saturation is a property of the alpha-frequency selective process. This, however, can be ruled out since (a) the modulation depth at which the low-frequency response starts to saturate is not related to the alpha frequency and (b) an increase in the power of the background activity does not shift the saturation point to lower modulation depths. It had therefore to be concluded that saturation occurs preceding the proximal frequency selective process.

Final remarks

In the foregoing sections three models are presented for the human evoked response system to account for the responses obtained with sinusoidal and Gaussian noise modulated homogeneous fields. The question can be raised whether these models can also give a complete description of the human evoked response system to any other type of light modulation. As stated in the introduction, these models would not apply to the case when strong stimuli, as for example flashes, are applied since

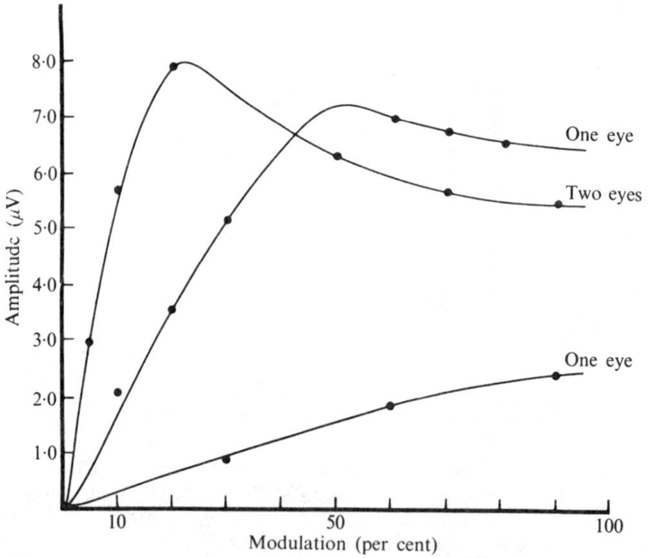

Fig. 2.20. Amplitude of the late component in the VEP as a function of modulation depth in case of one- and two-eye stimulation (diffuse field) and to a monocularly presented 2° stimulus field, surrounded by a steady field of the same luminance. In the latter situation a steady field of similar luminance (200 asb) was presented to the fellow eye. The stimulus frequency was 5 Hz.

the models are based on a small signal approach. With strong stimuli other non-linearities, not necessarily those already specified, may also play a role (the models are, however, good enough to account for the gross features of flash responses). These observations apply also to the case of responses to pulse-modulated light (Reits 1975). To enable comparison of the pulse response and the responses to noise-modulated light, bright and dark pulses were presented alternately, once per second, and with pulse-shapes that were identical to the time course of the autocorrelation function of the Gaussian-noise-modulated light:

$$h(t) = \frac{\sin 2\pi\nu t}{2\pi\nu t}, \text{ with } \nu = 50 \text{ Hz.}$$

The data depicted in Fig. 2.19 show that the responses to such bright and dark pulses have the same polarity, as has been observed before by Clynes, Kohn, and Lifshitz (1964), and also the same size. Furthermore, they saturate in a similar way at low modulation depths. The most striking feature of these responses is their relatively large amplitude: the amplitude of the sum of the responses to bright and dark pulses is always much larger than the amplitude of the cross-bicorrelation function. For the example given in Fig. 2.19 they exceed the amplitude of the noise 'response' by a factor of more than 10. The models in the sections above cannot account for these properties of the pulse-modulated light responses. To achieve this they would have to be extended with a low-pass filter – with a time constant smaller than 1 second – followed by a saturating full-wave rectifier. This extension does not influence the input–output relation for continuous small signals like sinusoids and noise-modulated light.

The models presented in this chapter thus do not offer a unique description of the human evoked response system. The final form of a model is largely determined by the way the question about the sequential organization of the system was originally phrased. The basic assumption that underlies the parameter estimation is that a single essential nonlinearity is sufficient to describe the nonlinear behaviour of each of the three subsystems. All other questions concerning the characteristics of the dynamic processing preceding and following this nonlinearity are a logical consequence of this assumption.

Spatial nonlinear analysis

In the sequential analysis of the luminance VEPs in the previous section the human visual system was purposely oversimplified into an *N*-channel model with identical, independent pathways.

For the study of, for example, the flicker sensitivity to large homogeneous fields this simplification may be justified, but as soon as small fields are considered, the spatial integrative properties of the visual system have to be taken into account. Spatial integration relates to one of the most important features of the visual system. Even at the retinal level there are special elements, such as horizontal and amacrine cells, whose major task seems the spreading of nervous influences in the plane of the retina. In this section it will be demonstrated that sequential analysis may also offer a powerful tool for the study of the location and the characteristics of spatial interactions.

In this analysis colour coding will be neglected. Since spatial and spectral coding are interrelated, it should be realized that the picture that will be unfolded in the next paragraphs cannot be complete. In the section on isolated colour mechanisms the interrelation between spectral and spatial coding will be treated more fully.

Receptive field concepts based on animal experiments

Moving along the visual pathway, spatial coding becomes more elaborate at subsequent stages. Starting as distally as the horizontal cells which the outputs of the receptors feed into, there seems to be pure summation over rather extensive retinal areas. For example, in carp retina, stimulus area and intensity can be interchanged for stimulus fields with diameters extending up to 50° (Norton, Spekreijse, Wolbarsht, and Wagner 1968). As shown in Fig. 2.21 the so-called Ricco's law, i.e. that a constant luminous flux (intensity times stimulus area) gives a constant response, holds for the horizontal cell responses in carp retina for stimulus diameters up to 5 mm. To maintain a constant response in this area, a reduction of stimulus intensity by a factor of 4 can be compensated by an increase of stimulus diameter with a factor of 2.

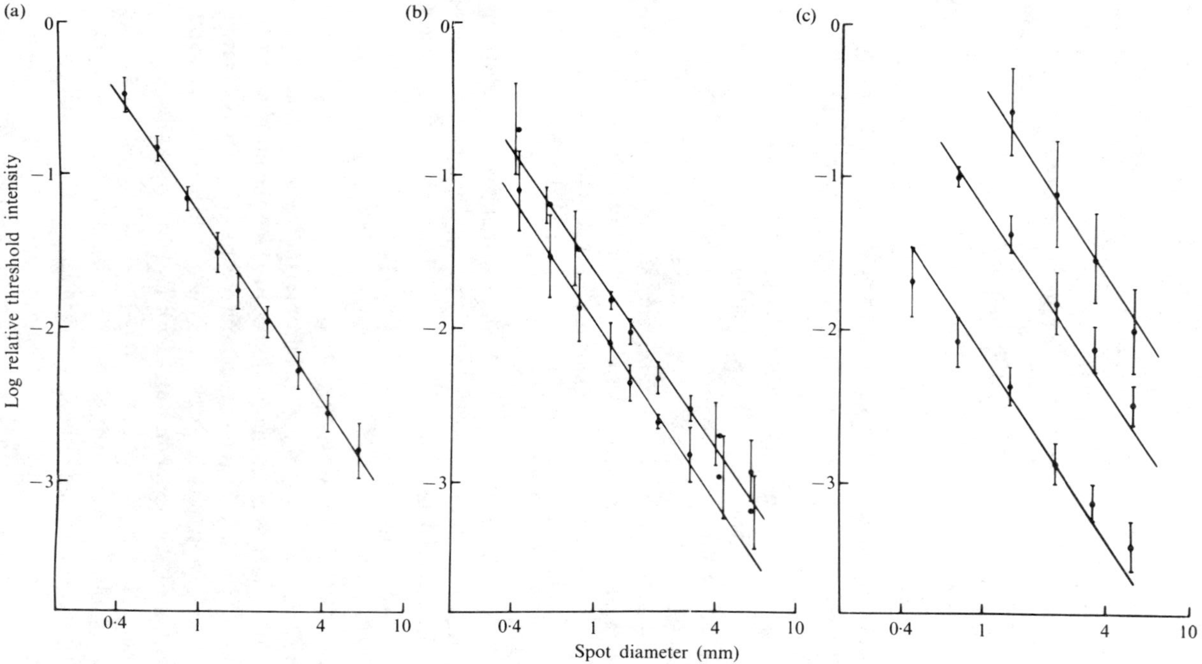

Fig. 2.21. Area–intensity relationship for constant threshold responses of horizontal cells in carp retina. The stimuli were circular and concentric with the micropipette tip. Zero log intensity is approximately 55 μW cm^{-2}. Repetitive flashes, each with a duration of 0·5 s, were followed by dark intervals of 1·5 s. The horizontal axis gives the diameter of the spot focused on the retina. The straight lines of the three graphs represent the relation: intensity × area = constant (Ricco's law). The vertical bars are the standard deviation for each data point. (a) The results for 11 monophasic units; (b) results for 8 biphasic units; (c) results for 8 triphasic units. The data in (a) are obtained by stimulating with 625 nm; in (b) with 700 nm (upper data points) and 500 nm (lower data points); in (c), from top to bottom, with 680 nm, 580 nm, and 480 nm, respectively.

The spot diameters in (c) are the outer diameter of an annulus minus the 0·75 mm diameter of a central stop.

At ganglion cell level, the last stage of retinal processing, not only is the size of the Ricco or full summation fields strongly reduced, but moreover these can be surrounded by a summation field which opposes the action of the central field. An illustration is given in Fig. 2.22 which gives the stimulus intensity versus

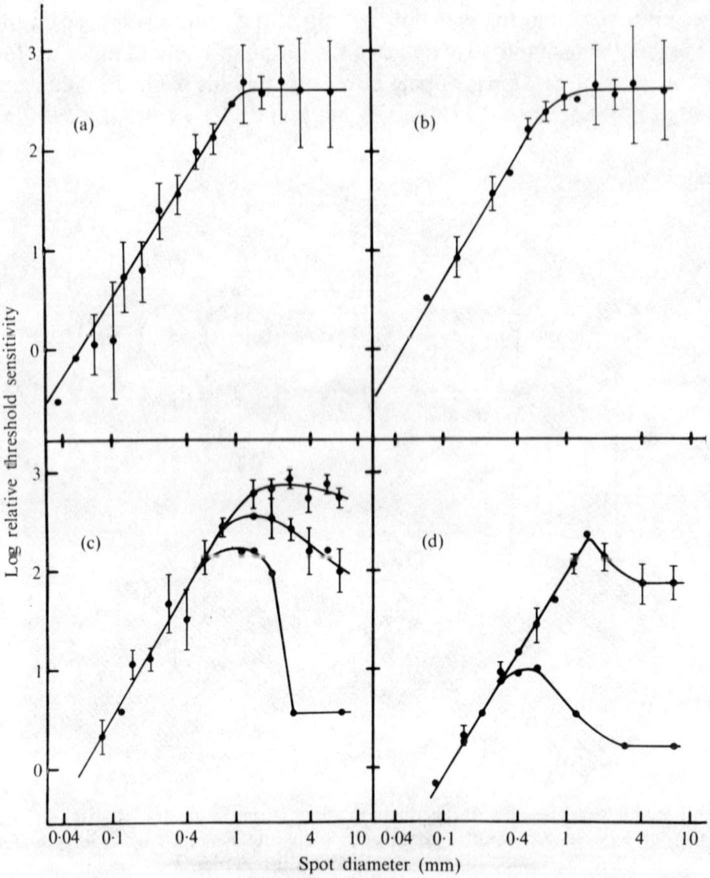

Fig. 2.22. (a) and (c) The averaged area–intensity relationship for the monochromatic types and the red components of the bichromatic ganglion cells in goldfish retina. (b) and (d) The same relationship for the green components of the bichromatic ganglion cell response types. (a) and (b) are the averaged full-summation plot for units without an antagonistic peripheral information channel; (c) and (d) are similar plots for units with such a peripheral field. The averaged curve in (a) is based on 14 units, in (b) on 6 units, in (c) on 9 units (top) and 5 units, and in (d) on 6 units. Zero log threshold sensitivity is approximately 10^{13} quanta cm^{-2} s^{-1}; the vertical bars represent the standard deviations (2σ).

stimulus diameter relationship for ganglion cell responses in goldfish retina. Irrespective of the colour coding of a particular unit, Ricco's law holds for diameters up to 1 mm in the plane of the retina, equivalent to a visual field of 7°

(Spekreijse, Wagner, and Wolbarsht 1972). For larger stimuli, either the increase in spot diameter does not affect the response at all (Fig. 2.22(a) and (b)), or an increase of stimulus intensity is required to reach the response criterion ((c) and (d)). The latter indicates the existence of an antagonistic receptive field organization with a surrounding process of lower sensitivity than the central process since, for spot sizes up to 5 mm in the plane of the retina, the central response dominates. At a subsequent stage (and now we leave the retina of fish and move on to the lateral geniculate of cat) a regrouping of receptive fields seems to take place as is illustrated in the scheme developed by Maffei (1972). In this model (Fig. 2.23)

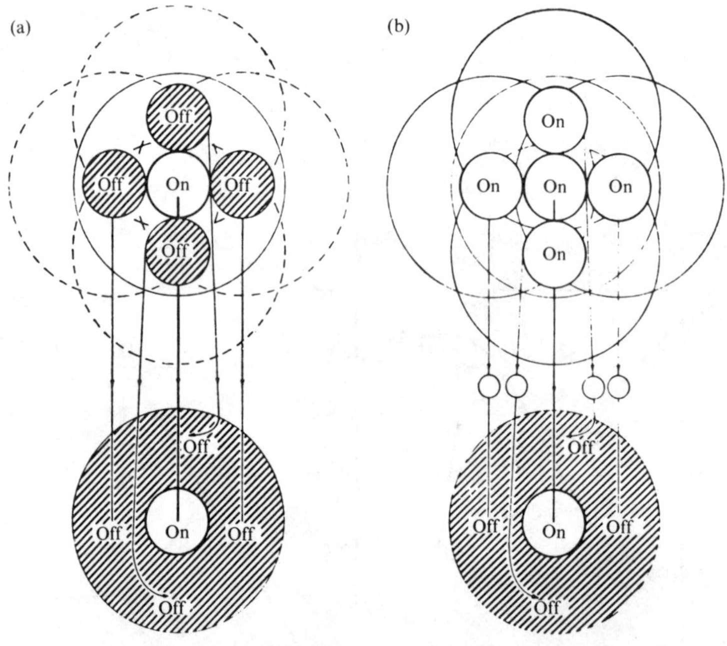

Fig. 2.23. Possible schemes of retino-geniculate connections as given by Maffei and Fiorentini (1972). In each scheme an on-centre lateral geniculate nucleus receptive field is depicted with some retinal receptive fields projecting on it.

it is assumed that a pool of central retinal processes forms the surround. This implies that at the lateral geniculate the spatial tuning will be greatly enhanced. In addition there will be a third, although weak, surround with the same sign as the central process, as has indeed been found (Maffei 1972).

Whereas at lateral geniculate nucleus level there still is a circular receptive field organization this is no longer so in the primary visual cortex. There elongated receptive fields seem to dominate, which in addition frequently exhibit directional sensitivity. Similar receptive fields can also be found in the tectum opticum of goldfish; an example is depicted in Fig. 2.24.

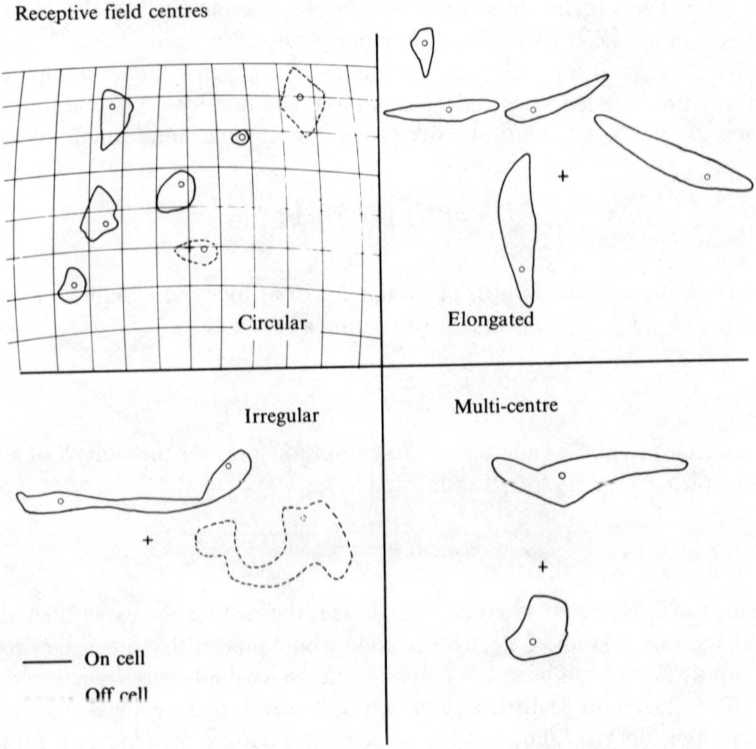

Fig. 2.24. Examples of receptive field organizations of neurones in the tectum opticum of goldfish. The fields are depicted in the form of equisensitivity lines (70 per cent of peak sensitivity). A graticule unit represents 5° in the visual field.

The finding that at various stages along the visual pathway the spatial integration can be described by Ricco's law has been frequently interpreted as implying that receptive fields have a constant sensitivity profile. If this is the case, stimulus intensity and stimulus area can be interchanged while maintaining the strength of the response at a fixed level. The constant sensitivity profile, however, is in discrepancy with direct estimates of receptive field sensitivity made by spot displacement measurements. If the local sensitivity within a receptive field is determined as a function of the position of a small stimulus spot, always a monotonically decaying (e.g. Gaussian shaped) profile is found with a maximum of sensitivity in the centre of the receptive field. Ricco's law can, however, also be obtained with any type of sensitivity profile if one realizes that the excitation strength E that results from Ricco-type experiments with a centered stimulus spot of radius R can be characterized by

$$E = 2\pi \int_0^R f(I, r)\, w(I, r)\, r dr,$$

a formula which contains the spatial weighting function $w(I,r)$, but also introduces the effects of a local intensity transformation $f(I,r)$.

If, for the sake of simplicity, the assumption is made that the local intensity transformation is independent of the position r, and that the weighting function does not depend on stimulus intensity I, then the formula above simplifies to

$$E = 2\pi f(I) \int_0^R w(r)\, r\mathrm{d}r,$$

One can usually approximate $f(I)$ by a simple power function I^n and $w(r)$ by a power function r^{-k} $(k < 2)$, so that this formula becomes

$$E = \frac{2\pi}{2-k} I^n \,.\, R^{2-k}.$$

For a constant response experiment this expression gives for the slope S of a Ricco plot in which log $1/I$ is plotted against log R:

$$S = \frac{2-k}{n}.$$

So a slope of 2 will result when $2n = 2 - k$, as is the case for the experimental results depicted in Figs 2.21 and 2.22. This relation would predict that a constant response field profile ($k = 0$) can be inferred only when the local intensity transformation is linear ($n = 1$). A more realistic assumption is, however, that the local response $f(I)$ is not proportional to I, but that the shape of $f(I)$ flattens with increasing intensity. In the latter case the receptive field should have a monotonically decreasing sensitivity profile in order to maintain the validity of Ricco's law. As can be seen from Fig. 2.25, a local intensity transformation $f(I) = \sqrt{I}$ and a weighting function $w(r) = r^{-1}$ can describe quite well both the Ricco plots and the spot displacement data of the ganglion cell responses in isolated goldfish retina.

Spatial dynamic interactions

The brief outline above points to progressively more elaborate spatial processing along the visual pathway in all animal work. In this section it will be shown that lateral interactions also play a role in human visual perception.

1. It is well established that the shape of the flicker fusion curves in man depends on retinal illumination. On the other hand, both Kelly (1959) and Van der Tweel (1961) have shown that these curves are also a function of the spot size used.

In Fig. 2.26(a) two flicker fusion curves are presented. At first glance one would guess that these curves were determined at different luminance levels. This is not, however, the case; luminance was kept constant, but stimulus field size increased from 2·2′ to 22′. The increase in flicker sensitivity with field size suggests that not luminance by itself, but luminance integrated over a certain area sets the

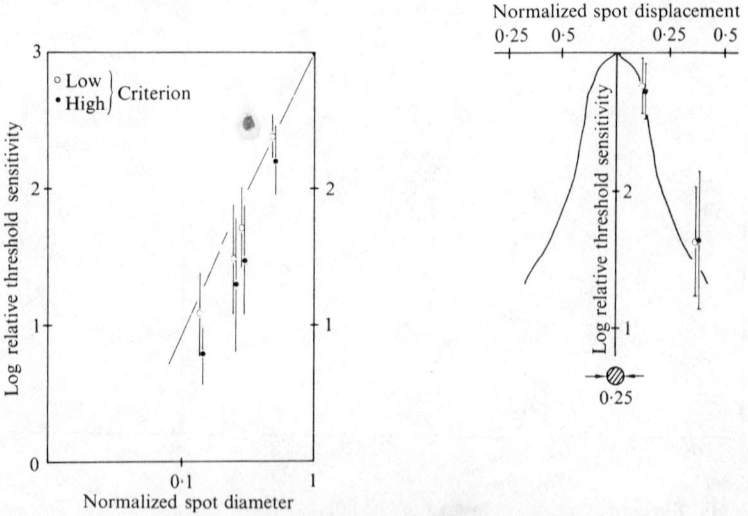

Fig. 2.25. Averaged Ricco plot (left) and averaged spot displacement measurement (right) based on extracellular recordings of 15 ganglion cells in isolated goldfish retina. The data plotted as filled circles were obtained with a 3 times higher spike response criterion than the data plotted as open circles. The difference between these two sets of data seems to indicate that the power n of $f(I) = I^n$ is not constant over the intensity range used but is approximated by $n = \frac{1}{2}$ in this figure. The spatial weighting function $w(r) = r^{-1}$ is truncated for values of $r \leqslant 0{\cdot}01$. This results in a slight flattening at the top of the sensitivity profile and in a slightly steeper slope of the Ricco plot for small spot diameters. For larger diameters this slope is 2. The bars give one standard deviation on each side of the mean.

shape of the flicker fusion curves. To test this hypothesis the dynamic characteristics of retinal ganglion cells in goldfish were determined as a function of stimulus intensity and spot size (Fig. 2.26(b)). This figure shows that the shape of the amplitude characteristics depends on the luminous flux falling within a receptive field rather than on the intensity of the stimulus spot since the same amplitude characteristic can be obtained by increasing the stimulated retinal area by a factor of 32 and diminishing the intensity by the same factor or vice versa (curves 2 and 3). This means that first the output signals of the early retinal processes are summed, and next the system is 'tuned' – the term Ratliff, Knight, and Graham (1969) use for the Limulus eye – according to the absorbed light power.

2. The psychophysical finding that a small flickering field is best perceived when it is surrounded by a homogeneous field of the same luminance can be understood if the assumption is made that also in man antagonistic spatial processing takes place. The apparent reduction of the luminance level of the test field by the presence of a surround fits into this concept. Furthermore, a gap between stimulus and surrounding field should shift the point of highest sensitivity to higher intensities of the surround, as has been found indeed (Fig. 2.27).

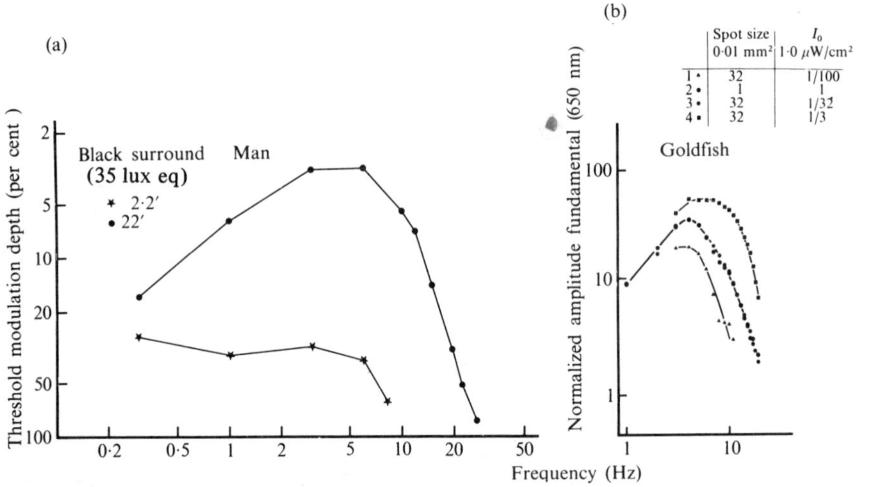

Fig. 2.26. (a) Flicker fusion curves in man for stimulus fields of 2·2′ and 22′. (b) The amplitude characteristics of the central red-off, green-on process of a spontaneous ganglion cell in goldfish retina depicted as a function of the luminous flux (power) of a Gaussian noise modulated (σ = 40 per cent) stimulus spot. A constant flux $E = AI_0$, where A is the stimulus area and I_0 the mean stimulus intensity, gives identical curves (2 and 3).

3. In view of the linearizing effect of external or internal noise upon the response of a nonlinear system, the luminance VEPs presented in the first section of this chapter indicate that in the human visual system spatial summation takes place. Because of the quantal character of light, quantal noise will exceed the induced

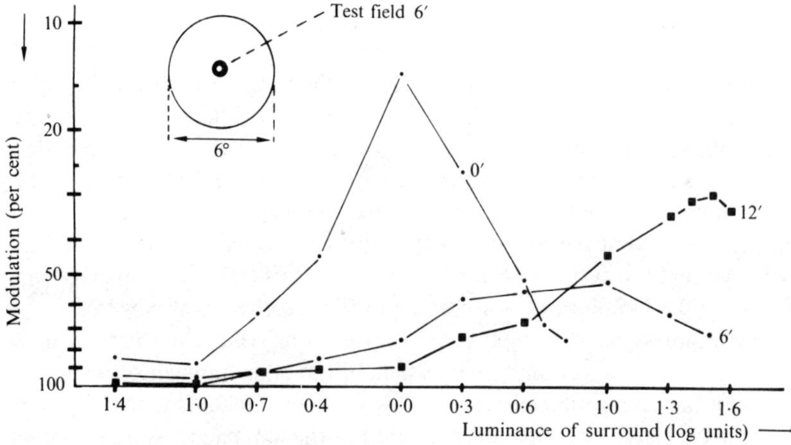

Fig. 2.27. Threshold modulation depth of a 16 Hz sine-wave modulated test field of 6′ as a function of the luminance of a surround subtending 6°. At zero log luminance the luminances of both fields are identical and amount to 1800 asb. When test field and surround are separated by a black annulus of 6′ and 12′ respectively, the point of highest sensitivity is reached at increasingly higher luminances of the surround.

light variations for sufficiently small modulation depths. Estimation, with acceptable visual parameters, of the magnitude of this noise per receptor, indicates that it overpowers the modulation at depths where there is still considerable distortion in the VEP. Therefore to account for the appearance of second harmonics in the occipital response for modulation depths as low as 2 per cent, it was necessary to postulate that the receptors would interact in order to improve the signal-to-noise ratio at the input of the rectifying process, so that the linearizing effect of the quantal noise would become negligible. On theoretical grounds it was deduced that these electrophysiological summation fields had to be of the order 20′ (Spekreijse 1966).

Search for receptive fields in man

To obtain an objective estimate of receptive field size in man, we used a spatial contrast stimulus formed by the reflecting and transparent elements of a checkerboard-patterned mirror. Polygons of higher order would of course approximate more closely to the generally assumed circular shape of the integrative fields, but such polygons would have more than four neighbours so that they are not feasible for counterphase experiments. (For further details on experimental design and choice of stimulus configuration see Chapter 1 of this book).

If the checks are considerably smaller than the hypothesized peripheral summation fields, no response at all should be found when the two sets of checks are modulated in counterphase. In this case the flicker signals from adjacent checks would cancel before reaching the rectifying stage (first column of Fig. 2.28). On the other hand, for comparatively large checks, the second harmonic should resemble that elicited by an unpatterned stimulus field. Note that with this kind of counterphase stimulation the average illumination of the eye remains constant.

As can be seen in the second column of Fig. 2.28 this approach proved fruitful in the analysis of spatial interaction in the goldfish retina (Spekreijse and Van den Berg 1971). Counterphase checkerboard stimulation within the receptive field of a ganglion cell in this retina did not result in a spike discharge at all. This means that the goldfish retina treats each patch of light in the same way irrespective of whether neighbouring patches are modulated in phase (homogeneous field stimulation) or in counterphase (pattern reversal). The algebraically summed reactions to all patches falling within a receptive field determines the strength of the ganglion cell discharge. In its most simple form this luminance model predicts that the response to counterphase stimulation can never exceed the response to homogeneous field stimulation. For the VEP in man this simple model does not apply since counterphase stimulation resulted in a much larger evoked response than homogeneous field stimulation (third column of Fig. 2.28).

This observation can have two implications: either the receptive-field model is too simple, and centre–surround interactions, for example, should be taken into account, or the VEP exhibits a new component that cannot be extrapolated from the luminance model. In the first situation the response (consisting of only even

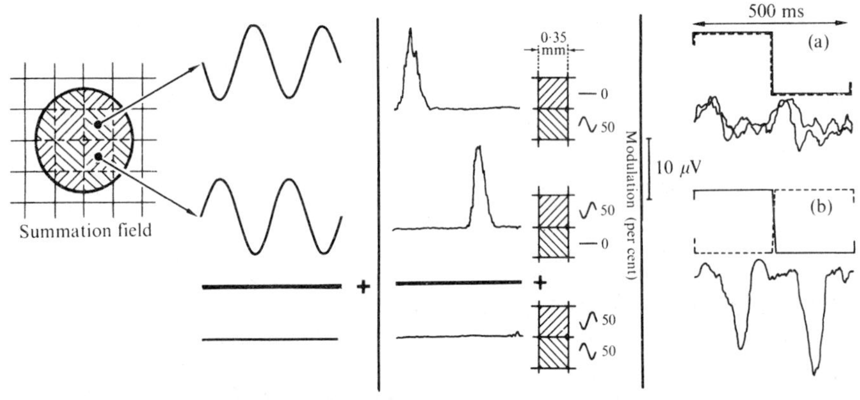

Fig. 2.28. *Left*: schematic representation of spatial summation between counterphase signals generated by the two sets of counterphase-modulated squares of a checkerboard pattern. No response will be obtained for the depicted case with spatial summation preceding the rectifying element.
Middle: period-averaged spike data for a green-off, red-on centre process of a ganglion cell in goldfish retina. The top figure gives the average spike response to sine-wave modulation (50 per cent) of one set of squares (0·35 mm width in the plane of the retina). The other set of squares is not modulated at all, but has a steady intensity identical to the mean intensity of the modulated set. Reversing the condition and modulating the other set of squares with the same depth, but in counterphase, results, of course, in the same rectified sinusoid but shifted 180° in phase (middle figure). Simultaneous counterphase modulation of both sets of squares does not result in a spike discharge at all (bottom figure). The mean intensity of the stimulus light passing through an Ealing FTP interference filter (530 nm) is approximately 4 μW cm^{-2}. The number of summations is 100; the modulation frequency is 5 Hz. The patterned spot focused on the retina has a diameter of 2 mm.
Right: period-averaged occipital responses in man to in-phase (homogeneous field) and counterphase (switching of spatial contrast) modulation of the two sets of squares. If both responses had the same origin, then the size of response (b) should be equal or smaller than that of response (a). The reverse is the case, which indicates that the two responses originate from different systems. The stimulus field with a mean luminance of 5000 asb extends 6°; the check size is 15′: inion–vertex derivation.

harmonics) may be larger than the contribution of the even harmonics of the response elicited by a patterned stimulus field if the checks equal the extension of the receptive field centre, because for this spatial frequency the antagonistic influence of the surround will be minimized by counterphase stimulation. The data in Fig. 2.29 leaves no doubt that a centre–surround model cannot account for the VEP to contrast stimulation. In the situation depicted the luminance of one set of checks remained constant, whereas the other set was square-wave modulated so that during half the stimulus period no pattern was visible. In the first instance, if luminance processing were the origin of the VEP then a similar response would have been expected at, for example, the increase of mean luminance irrespective of

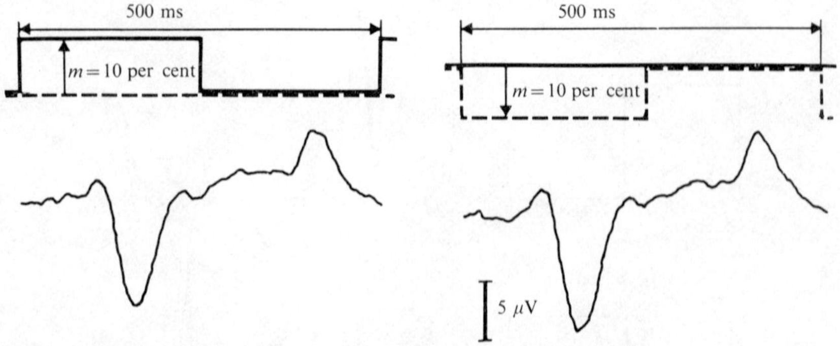

Fig. 2.29. The second row shows contrast VEPs (inion–vertex derivation) to an appearing–disappearing checkerboard with 20′ checks of 10 per cent modulation. The continuous line in the first row indicates the luminance modulation of one set of checks, the dashed line that of the other set.

the luminance level of the steady set of checks. The data show, however, that a similar response is obtained at the appearance of the pattern irrespective whether this condition is reached by an increase or by a decrease of mean luminance level. A pure pattern origin for the VEPs in man to checkerboard stimulation seems established.

It is interesting to note that in the human ERG no contrast component can be demonstrated, but that the ERG to pattern reversal is mainly caused by luminance distortion (Figs. 2.30 and 2.31). Fig. 2.30(a) shows the ERG of an 8° field, square-wave modulated with a modulation depth of 90 per cent. Fig. 2.30(b) gives the same response but the trigger of the averager has been shifted half the period; i.e. the response is shifted 180° in phase.

Summation of both responses results, of course, in a symmetrical response (Fig. 2.30(c)). In Fig. 2.31 this response is compared with that to a checkerboard-reversal stimulus. To make comparison easier and to decrease the duration of the experiment the averager was triggered twice per period; hence only even harmonics remain in the average. As can be seen, the shape and latency of both responses are similar. This holds irrespective of stimulus frequency. Therefore most if not all of the ERG to high-contrast pattern reversal can be considered as the net result of the addition of responses to luminance increase and decrease. The lack of a spatial contrast component in the ERG indicates that the contrast pathway separates from the luminance pathway after the structures that generate the ERG.

Two reasons for a reduced visual acuity

The finding that in the human ERG no appreciable contrast component is present is not so surprising if one realizes that contrast processing must be preceded at least partly by luminance processing.

In this respect the electrophysiology of two subjects that we studied, both with

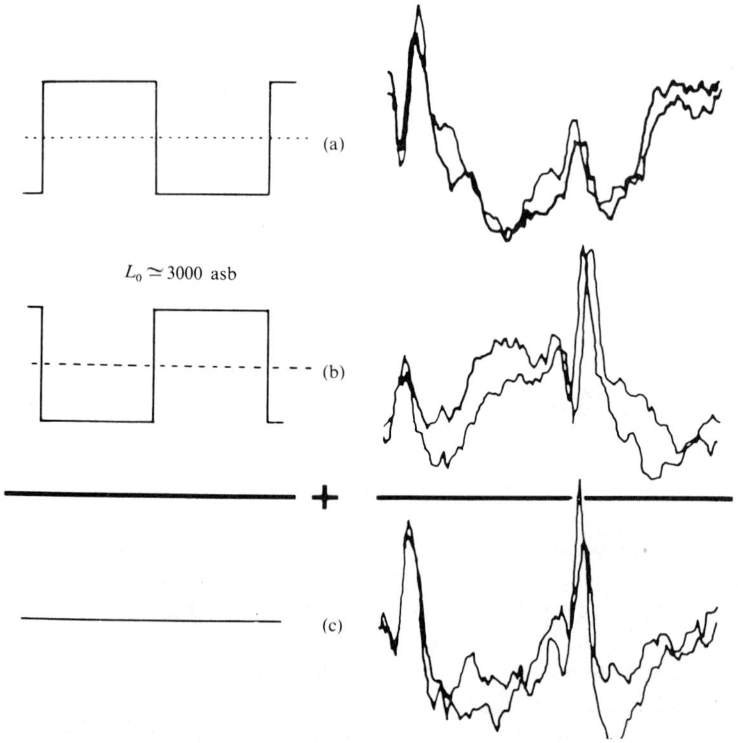

Fig. 2.30. ERGs to a 8° field, square-wave modulated with a modulation depth of 90 per cent. (a) and (b) ERGs to the same stimulus but with the trigger of the averager at either the increase (a) or at the decrease (b) of the luminance stimulus. (c) gives the summed response of (a) and (b).

a reduced visual acuity of about $\frac{1}{6}$, might be interesting. The VEPs of both subjects were rather normal to homogeneous field stimulation but to contrast stimulation they could be clearly distinguished (Fig. 2.32). One of them, a rod achromat, showed a normal contrast VEP, although with a longer latency. The other one, an amblyope (ex anisometria) gave a distorted contrast VEP for the amblyopic eye. It seems that only one component of the response of the normal eye of this subject is present in the amblyopic eye response. According to the topological studies of Jeffreys and Axford (1974) this component has a parafoveal origin. Therefore the reduced visual acuity in these two subjects has a different basis: in the amblyopic subject it is probably due to malfunctioning of the foveal contrast mechanism; in the achromat it seems due to a deviation in receptive field size. These conclusions are substantiated by the psychophysics of these two subjects to luminance and contrast stimulation (Fig. 2.33).

In Fig. 2.33(a) and (b) the psychophysics, obtained under similar conditions, of the rod achromat (a) and a normal subject (b) are compared. The shape of both

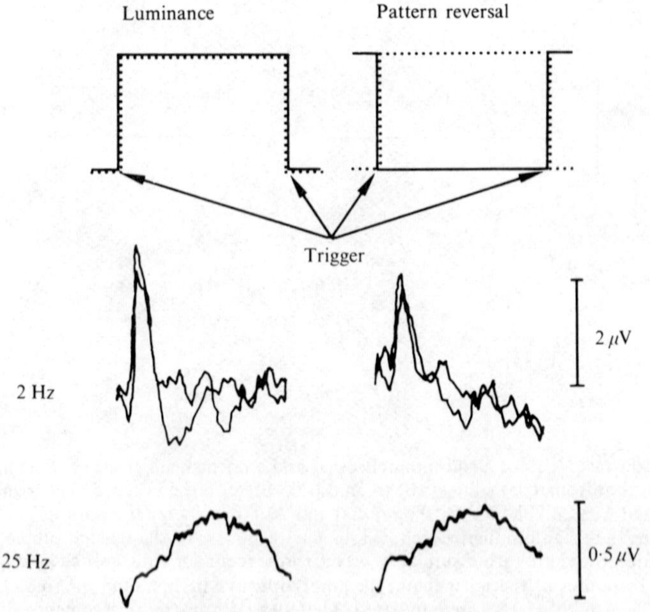

Fig. 2.31. ERGs to luminance modulation and pattern reversal. The averager is triggered twice per period. Identical responses are obtained irrespective of stimulus frequency. Mean luminance is 3000 asb; modulation depth is 90 per cent, check size 60′. The stimulus field extends 8° and is surrounded by a steady field of equal luminance to minimize stray light.

sets of curves is similar. However, the thresholds to checkerboard stimulation are much higher for the achromat. This reduction in contrast sensitivity is greater for decreasing check sizes. These findings can be described by the assumption of larger summation pools in the achromat than in the normal. Such excessive fields will diminish the effective input to the contrast mechanism.

In Fig. 2.33(c) and (d) the psychophysics of the amblyopic (c) and normal (d) eye of the amblyopic subject are shown. Both eyes give the same flicker fusion curves for homogeneous field stimulation. The curves to checkerboard stimulation deviate at the low-frequency side: the amblyopic eye curve keeps the shape of the homogeneous field curve whereas the normal eye shows the increase in sensitivity due to contrast perception. The similarity of the two curves in Fig. 2.33(c) is the psychophysical expression of the absence of a spatial-contrast processing mechanism in the amblyope. At the same time the presence of contrast processing in the normal eye indicates that the contrast mechanism as such is not affected.

Conclusion

It seems beyond doubt that a pattern stimulus can evoke an occipital potential that cannot be described on the basis of receptive field concepts. On the other

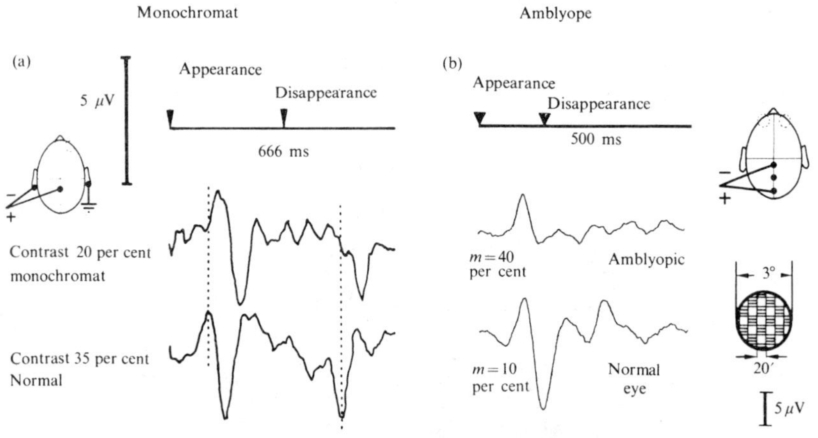

Fig. 2.32. Contrast VEPs of a rod monochromat and a normal subject (a) and an amblyopic (amblyopia ex anisometria) subject (b) to an onset–offset checkerboard. The responses in (a) were obtained with 50′ checks for the normal and 200′ checks for the monochromatic subject. In both cases the mean luminance was 12 asb. The responses of the normal subject and the monochromat are rather similar in waveform, except for a difference in latency.
(b) The responses of the normal and the amblyopic eye of an amblyope to a checkerboard pattern of 3° with 20′ checks are compared. These waveforms (mean luminance 5000 asb) differ.

hand, the response to a contrast stimulus with even a constant luminance flux may contain an appreciable luminance contribution. Controls for the latter are indicated whenever the response tends to become symmetrical and also when coarse, high-contrast patterns are needed, as is often the case in studies of deteriorated vision. The usefulness of these controls has already been demonstrated in the judgement of the cortical potentials in monkey to patterned stimuli (Padmos, Haaijman, and Spekreijse 1973).

The second purpose of this section was to clarify that there can be two extreme causes for a reduction in visual acuity: either large receptive fields which reduce the input to the spatial-contrast mechanism or normal receptive fields feeding into a malfunctioning contrast mechanism.

The latter conclusion – if correct – has direct implications for the interpretation of the amplitude of the contrast VEP as a function of check size. In many publications it is suggested that the maximum amplitude of the occipital VEP in man to checks of 15–20′ is related to average (retinal) receptive field size. Such a correlation is not self-evident if one realizes that a given stimulus field contains 9 times as many checks of 10′ than of 30′. It has therefore been argued (Spekreijse, Van der Tweel, and Regan 1973) that no attention should be paid to the peak in the response curve as a function of check size. In this discussion it was, however, overlooked that the spatial-contrast mechanism is not activated directly but through spatial summation pools. Hence given a fixed number of contrast-

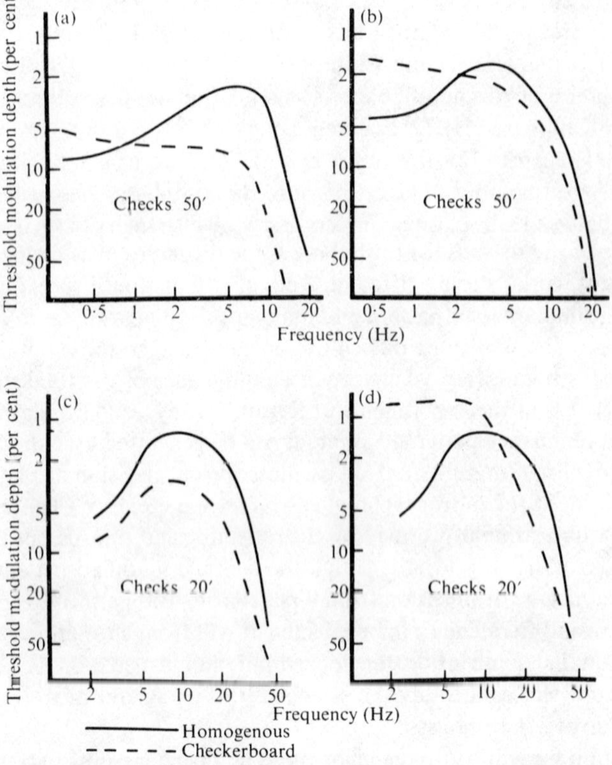

Fig. 2.33. Luminance and pattern modulation versus frequency curves for a corrected subject with amblyopia ex anisometria, a rod achromat, and a normal at the luminance used for the achromat. (A) Rod achromat; natural pupil (approx. 3 mm); luminance 1·5 asb. (B) Same condition for a normal subject, artificial pupil (3 mm). (C) Amblyopic eye, 5000 asb, natural pupil. (D) Normal eye, 5000 asb, natural pupil.

sensitive elements that contribute to the contrast VEP, the amplitude of this VEP will reflect the strength of the input signal feeding into the contrast mechanism. The latter will depend on the ratio of check size to receptive field diameter. Therefore the maximal response amplitude as a function of check size, although not being evoked by a luminance channel but by a spatial-contrast mechanism, may still bear the characteristics of the summation pools which form the first stage in spatial processing along the visual pathway.

Pattern VEPs

Ever since Marshall and Harden (1952) first recorded in man cortical potentials evoked by means of a spatially structured stimulus, a number of workers have been studying the properties of pattern VEPs.

Among the many parameters studied which, in one way or another, determine these responses are: pattern configuration (Rietveld *et al.* 1967; Jeffreys 1971*a*), retinal-site stimulated (Harter and White, 1968, 1970; Harter, 1970, 1971*b*; Jeffreys, Chapter 6 of this book), contrast-modulation depth (Spekreijse 1966; Campbell and Kulikowsky 1972; Spekreijse *et al.* 1973), and temporal frequency and waveform (Regan 1972*a*; Spekreijse *et al.* 1973; Estévez and Spekreijse 1974*a*). In spite of the great amount of effort put into these studies, a clear-cut picture of the relations between stimulus parameters and VEP characteristics has not yet emerged. One of the reasons for this failure is the difficulty in assessing and comparing results of workers using different types of stimulation. Especially the results obtained with simultaneous 'pattern and luminance' stimulation, as in the extensive studies of Harter and White, are difficult to be compared to those obtained with a purer 'contrast' stimulus (e.g. where the mean luminance of the total stimulus field is kept constant) as in the experiments of Regan, Jeffreys, and our group.

A constant-luminance patterned stimulus can be generated by either using a tachistoscopic substitution method, an oscilloscope or television display, a rotating polaroid, or the mirror technique, which we prefer (see Chapter 1 of this book). The pattern stimulus, formed by the reflecting and transparent elements of a patterned mirror, has the advantage that the contrast-modulation depth can be set with a great degree of precision from 0 per cent to 100 per cent. Furthermore both waveform and frequency can be selected at will from a function generator and, in addition, independent or time-locked pure luminance modulation can be introduced if one wishes to study the effects of this parameter or to compare luminance and pattern responses.

In this section we will try to highlight those points concerning pattern VEPs which seem to us the better established and which may be used as keystones in the description of the mechanisms responsible for the pattern VEP generation. Most of the results discussed were obtained with a checkerboard pattern configuration presented centrally with the rows of checks oriented along the vertical and horizontal axes relative to the observer's eyes. Similar results can, however, also be demonstrated with other orientations and/or stimulus configurations, as well as with eccentric fixations.

Contrast dependency of the pattern VEPs

The occipital VEP to an onset–offset pattern contains two main wave-complexes, one following the onset and another following the offset of a pattern (Fig. 2.29). Both appearance responses in Fig. 2.29 are similar, in spite of the fact that the pattern arises in the first case by an increase and in the second by a decrease of the luminance of one set of checks. In both cases the luminance of the other set of elements remains constant in time. This finding indicates immediately that these VEPs are due to a mechanism that reacts to changes in spatial contrast, i.e. differences in luminance over the visual field, independently of the direction in which these luminance changes take place.

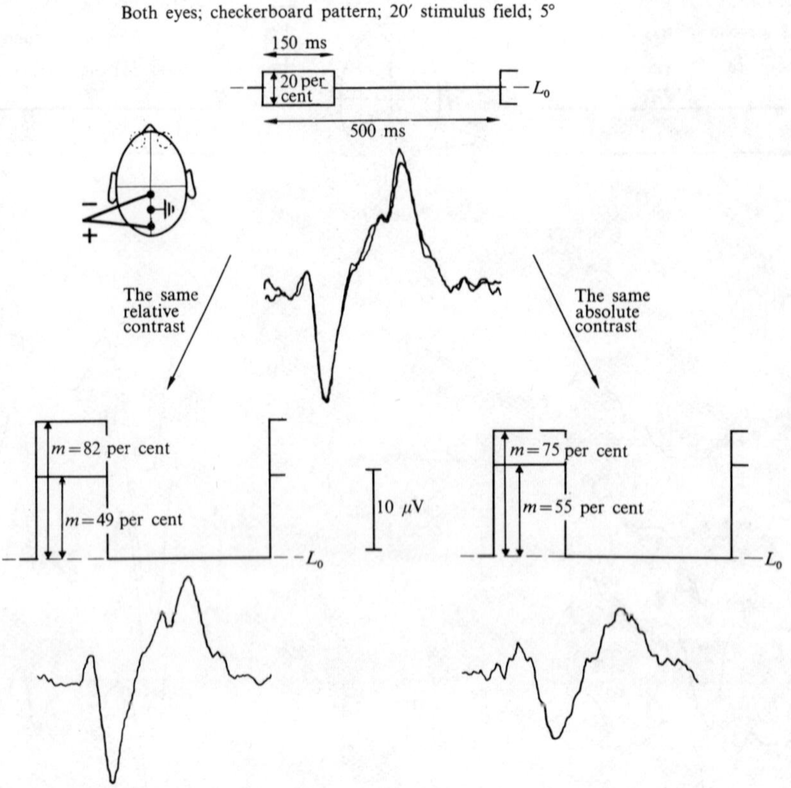

Fig. 2.34. Contrast VEPs to an onset–offset checkerboard (*top*). A simultaneous jump in luminance does not affect this response as long as the relative contrast remains constant (*bottom left*). To a similar luminance jump, but with a constant absolute difference, the response becomes smaller and broader (*bottom right*).

Furthermore if an increase (or decrease) in the average luminance takes place simultaneously with the appearance of a pattern (bottom row of Fig. 2.34) then the VEP will diminish (or increase) unless the luminance step is so re-adjusted that the instantaneous contrast ($\Delta L/L$) remains constant. In other words, the VEP to pattern presentation seems to be generated by a system computing the relative contrast of a pattern, i.e. the luminance differences between the two sets of elements. This behaviour, comparable to a 'logarithmic differential amplifier', can be clearly established without need to introduce a measure of the response; a 'constant waveshape' criterion is sufficient.

For quantitative studies, choices have to be made as to what and how to measure them. The first problem encountered is that both wave complexes change not only in overall size but also in form as a result of a change in stimulus parameter, such as contrast depth and check size (Fig. 2.35). This can be under-

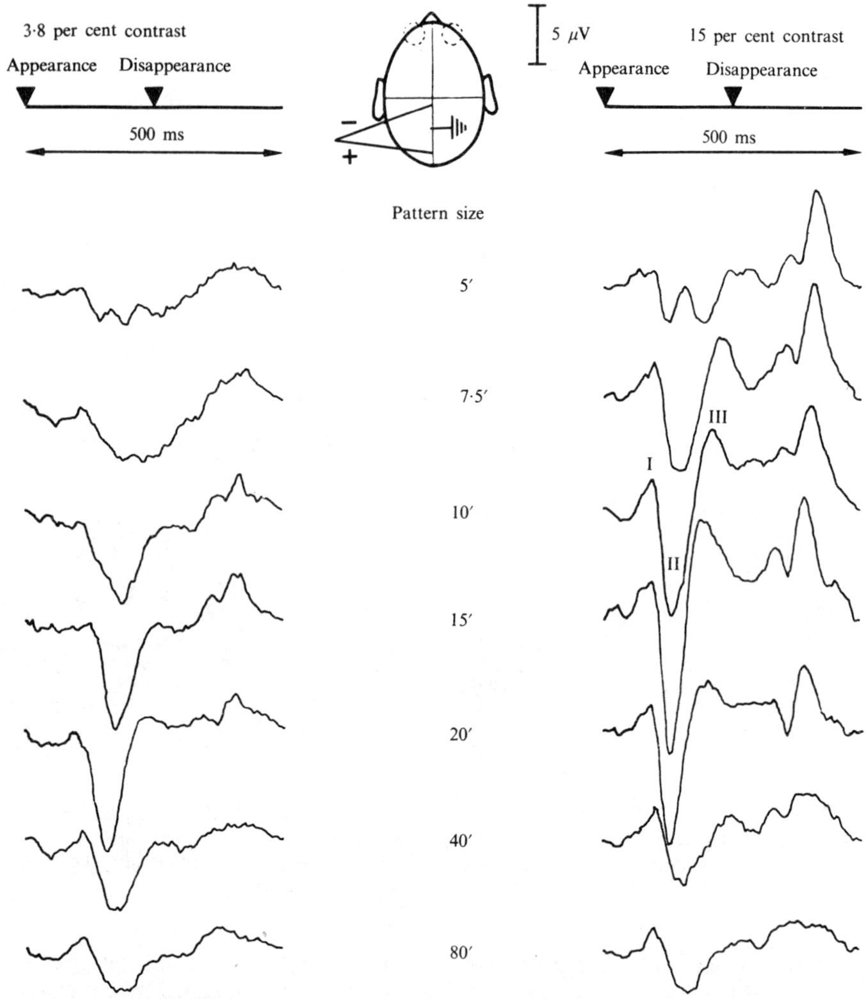

Fig. 2.35. Occipital responses to the appearance and disappearance of a checkerboard of 3·8 per cent (left) and 15 per cent (right) contrast as a function of check size. Central fixation.

stood only if the assumption is made that different cortical mechanisms contribute to the onset and offset VEPs and react to the various aspects of the pattern in different ways.

The onset VEP contains components similar to those obtained by short presentations of a pattern and identified by Jeffreys (Chapter 6 of this book) as CI (65–80 ms) and CII (90–120 ms). The disappearance or 'off' VEP can contribute to and interact actively with the appearance VEP in the pattern-reversal situation if these reversals take place abruptly (within 50 ms) (Spekreijse *et al.*

1973; Estévez and Spekreijse 1973). However, the link between the different mechanisms may not be a sequential one, since it is possible to select the stimulus so that either one of the VEPs will be selectively enhanced or diminished (Fig. 2.35).

An analysis of the work of Jeffreys, Michael and Halliday (1971), and Estévez and Spekreijse (1973) leads to the following (admittedly simplified) picture:

(a) The appearance response to long presentations can contain the CI and CII components of the short presentation responses. The 100–120 ms negative peak recorded near inion can be identified with CII, a mainly foveal component of extrastriate origin. CI, not always present when small field sizes (2° or less) and central fixation are used, has a more extended representation over the cortex including areas of the medial face and depth of the calcarine fissure. (For further details see Jeffreys, Chapter 6 of this book.)

(b) The component measured by Halliday and Michael (1971) is probably identical with the positive peak of the 'off' response (Estévez and Spekreijse 1973) and is definitely not arising in the striate areas. An extrastriate origin overlapping with that of CII, or surrounding it, seems likely (see also Halliday, McDonald, and Mushin, Chapter 5 of this book).

The distinction in topological representation over the skull and in dependence on stimulus parameters supports the idea that the three 'components' (CI, CII, and 'off') may represent activity of different populations of cortical cells involved in processing different aspects of a patterned stimulus. Since, on the one hand, CI is not usually present for central small field (less than 2° field) stimulation, and, on the other hand, the 'off' components seems a rather unspecific response signalling solely abrupt reduction in contrast (Spekreijse *et al.* 1973) we will concentrate in the remaining part of this section on component CII, the foveal response evoked near and around the occipital pole which seems to correlate the strongest with the spatial 'contrast' parameter. Jeffreys calls this component the contour-specific component.

Contrast VEPs

When a centrally viewed 2–3° checkerboard field with 15–20′ checks is modulated sinusoidally (or by triangular waveshape), only the VEP component that can be identified as CII, remains (Estévez and Spekreijse 1973). In this situation the measurements can be carried out in a simple and straightforward manner: amplitude, phase, and, eventually, harmonic distortion are sufficient to completely characterize the response (Fig. 2.36).

In Fig. 2.37 the amplitude of the VEP is plotted as a function of the logarithm of the contrast-modulation depth. For contrasts below 20–30 per cent the data can be fitted by a straight line. For higher contrasts the VEP 'saturates', i.e. it no longer grows with increasing contrast. The intersection of the straight line has been shown to correlate rather well with the psychophysical threshold for

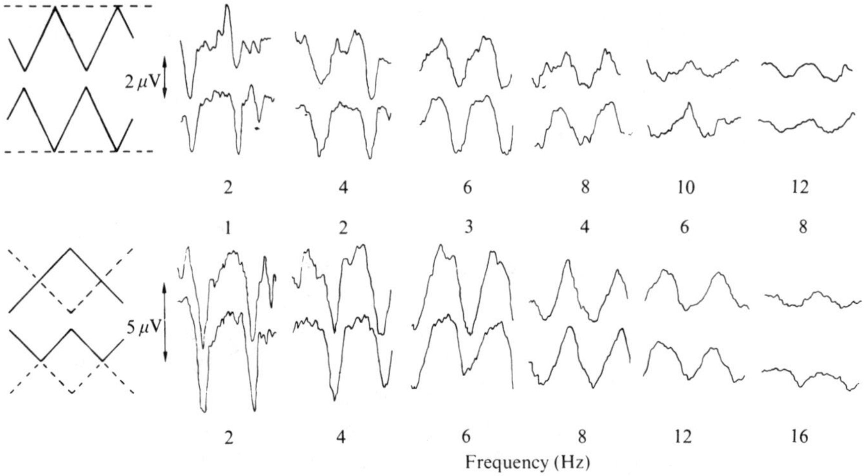

Fig. 2.36. VEPs (inion–vertex derivation) to a centrally fixated 3° checkerboard with 15′ checks that are triangularly modulated. At a given stimulus frequency the various stimulus situations, which are comparable from a contrast point of view but differ in luminance sense, result in rather similar responses. This establishes at once a contrast origin of these responses over the frequency range depicted.

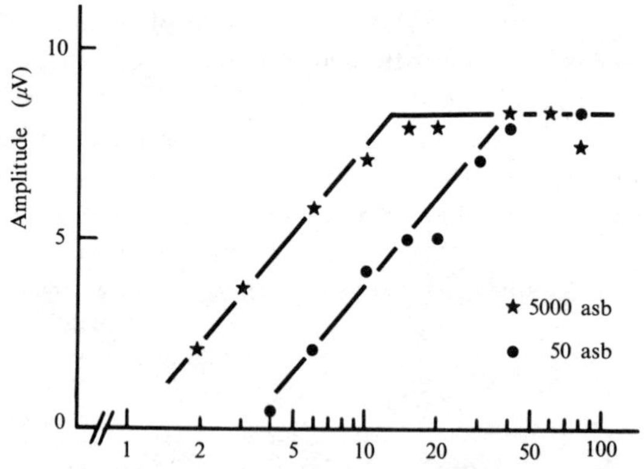

Fig. 2.37. Amplitude of the appearance response as a function of contrast for two levels of retinal illumination. For low contrasts the response to the appearance of a 3° checkerboard with 20′ checks seems to increase logarithmically with contrast; saturation becomes evident at lower contrasts the higher the mean luminance.

perception of the pattern (Campbell and Maffei 1970). Since this correlation is valid over a wide range of temporal frequencies (Cavonius 1972), the data suggest that this VEP is generated by a cortical 'contrast' mechanism. Also, the VEP data on the effects of defocusing (Spekreijse 1966; Regan and Richards 1971), monoptic standing contrast (Spekreijse *et al.* 1973; Jeffreys 1971*a*), and dichoptically presented standing contrast (Spekreijse, Khoe, and Van der Tweel 1972) point in the same direction.

The data in Fig. 2.38 indicate that the modulation of sharp gradients of luminance acts as stimulus for these VEPs. In this Figure the amplitude and phase characteristics of the VEP to checkerboard reversal are compared to those obtained

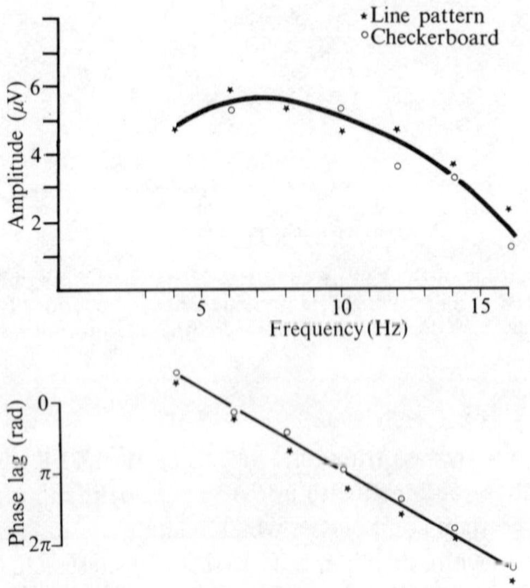

Fig. 2.38. Amplitude and phase of the VEPs to sine-wave reversal of a checkerboard with 15′ checks and of a grid consisting of 1′ lines at distances of 15′. Since both stimulus situations result in rather similar characteristics it seems established that the contours act as stimulus. The slope of the phase characteristic gives a latency of 115 ms, which is in accordance with the proposed CII dominance in these responses.

by sole modulation of a grating of lines (1′ width). These lines had the same separation as the check width (15′) and the enclosed fields were not modulated. Since the two characteristics are identical, these data suggest that the same mechanism is responsible for the generation of both VEPs. Other experiments indicated that gradients up to 5′ activate this mechanism. Since furthermore a 'suppressing' pattern produces the same effect whether it is presented to the same or to the fellow eye (Fig. 2.39) it can be concluded that the generator of CII must be located at least after the signals of the two eyes have come together: the cortical cells generating the response must be of the 'binocular' type. In view of the rather small retinal distances over which these cells seem to operate it is rather surprising to find an optimum for 15′ checks as a function of check size. This seeming discrepancy seems to be related to the 'luminance' receptive field size of the channels feeding into the spatial-contrast mechanism (see the section on spatial nonlinear analysis (p. 83).

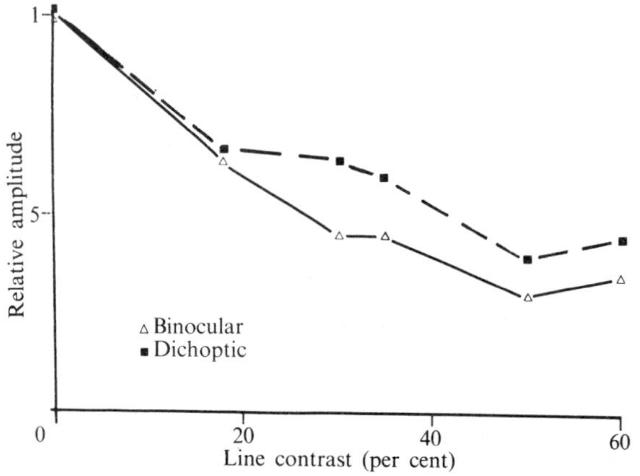

Fig. 2.39. Relative amplitude of the VEP to an onset–offset checkerboard (with 20′ checks) as a function of the contrast of an outlining grid presented either dichoptically or physically superimposed. The 20 per cent contrasting checks were presented for 60 ms at a rate of 2 Hz.

Conclusion

The presentation of a patterned stimulus evokes a cortical VEP which differs in many aspects from those obtained with homogeneous light stimulation. The pattern VEP, however, may contain components which relate more to the luminance changes occurring in the stimulus than to spatial contrast as such. The component CII (120 ms) is the clearest component which one can associate to the changes in spatial contrast, especially around sharp contours. Component CIII, which sometimes follows CII, might also be related to the same parameter, and could be in part an after-effect of CII, or its continuation.

It seems to us that although CI and the 'off' complex do relate to contrast, they nevertheless show the most dependence on pure luminance changes.

Whether CI represents a pre-processing leading to the generators of CII is not certain. It is, in any case, clear that the dipole representations of CI and those of the high-frequency luminance responses overlap to a great extent and probably coincide. This does not mean necessarily that the same neural process generates both responses, but it does suggest a strong relationship between the corresponding mechanisms.

Our work on isolated colour mechanisms suggests to us a possible construction: CI could be generated independently by each colour system and then feed into a higher-order contour mechanism which would receive binocular contributions and could be entered by any of the 6 systems (8 systems if we include the scotopic system).

The CII contour response would then signal that within any of the inputs a sharp image has been formed. More evidence for this idea may be found in the section on isolated colour systems; we want here to point out that such a CI → CII relationship could help to explain a number of electrophysiological findings and would also be consistent with many psychophysical facts pertaining to both colour and contrast vision. An example of this could be the McCree effect (see Regan 1972*a*): when the chromatic aberration of the eye is corrected by means of a special lens, both the psychophysical thresholds rise and the contrast VEP to a checkerboard decrease.

With our scheme this could be explained if there was a single contour mechanism and competitive access to it from every colour system. When a sharp image formed within one colour system, this would preferably input the contour box and block the others actively. Then, if accommodation is controlled by the output of the contour box, whenever this sharp image is found, accommodation would stop and all other inputs would no longer contribute to sharpness. Attempts, by artificial means, to sharpen simultaneously two or more images would favour only an active competition for the 'contour' box between the two colour systems, leading to deterioration of vision rather than to improvement, as it is found in practice.

Isolated colour mechanisms

As has been shown in the preceding sections, both the luminance and the contrast VEPs represent a photopic mechanism which may, at least in principle, involve the three types of cones normally present in the retina. For further analysis of the photopic system it is necessary to understand the ways in which the different cone populations contribute to the response, which sort of interactions must be accounted for in the processing schemes and, eventually, how the colour of the stimulus is encoded in the VEP. The latter cannot be neglected since the receptors which give rise to the luminance and contrast VEPs are also responsible for colour perception. One expects, rather naturally, the correspondent to this percepted attribute to be encoded in some way in the VEPs. Studies relating 'hue' or 'colour' to some characteristic of the VEPs have so far delivered contradictory results (Shipley, Jones, and Fry 1965, 1968; Cigánek and Ingvar 1969; Cigánek and Shipley 1970; see also White *et al.*, Chapter 12 of this book).

To approach the above problems we have developed a technique to modulate selectively the three photopic systems independently of each other. By combining the inputs in different ways, an analysis as outlined in the preceding sections for white light can also be performed for the colour channels.

The 'spectral compensation' method

When confronted with the problem of selective stimulation of a single-cone system, it has been customary to apply the two-colour adaptation technique developed by Stiles (1939, 1959), De Vries (1948), and Wald (1964). This technique is based on the fact that each cone mechanism can be independently 'adapted' by an intense stimulus: i.e. the response of a single cone population to a test light may become weaker as the mean background level is increased. By selecting the spectral composition of the background light to adapt two of the three cone systems it is possible to modulate the remaining, less adapted, mechanism. Although this technique was primarily intended to reveal the spectral sensitivities of the cone mechanisms over the whole of the visible spectrum, it has also been used in psychophysics to determine the dynamic properties (spatial and temporal transfer functions) of the isolated cone systems (Green 1968, 1969; Kelly 1974). For the study of the interactions between the various colour channels, however, the two-colour method is not the most appropriate tool, since the selective modulation of one system is achieved by driving the others into saturation. Furthermore, owing to the extensive overlap of the cone spectral sensitivities, the studied system will also be partly adapted to some unknown degree. The behaviour of the system under zero adapting light condition can then be inferred only by repeating the measurements with different amounts of adapting light and then extrapolating the data to the zero condition. This procedure may not always be warranted and can, under certain circumstances, lead to serious mistakes in the extrapolated results (Cavonius and Estévez 1975).

A technique better suited for the selective modulation task is the 'spectral-compensation' method (Estévez and Spekreijse 1974). In this method the ratio of modulation of two coloured lights is so adjusted that for one type of cone the effective input remains constant (Fig. 2.40). For a cone system with a different

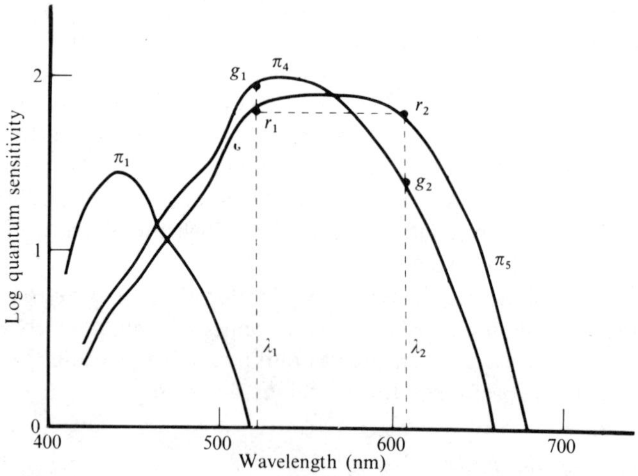

Fig. 2.40. Stiles' π_μ spectral sensitivity functions are shown to illustrate the spectral compensation idea. Wavelengths λ_1 and λ_2 are chosen to stimulate equally π_5 (see intercepts at r_1 and r_2); alternation of lights λ_1 and λ_2 with the same intensity will cause constant quantum catch in π_5. Since π_4 is unequally sensitive to these lights (see intercepts g_1 and g_2), the same stimulus will result in a modulated quantum catch. In practice the lights used are wide-band and the *intensities* adjusted for equal quantum catch in either the π_4 or π_5 mechanism.

spectral sensitivity the alternation of the two lights cannot result in complete cancellation and it will therefore be modulated to some extent. The amount of effective modulation can be easily calculated from the sensitivity function of the non-compensated system. It should be realized that in this manoeuvre the levels of adaptation of both the compensated and the modulated system do not play a role. By properly choosing the colour and the relative intensities of the lights it is in fact possible to adjust the levels independently of each other within wide limits. Furthermore, since the selectiveness of stimulation is achieved by compensation at the input where linearity still holds, the solutions to the compensation equations are all linear and can be additively combined to form other solutions. In practical terms this means that one can *simultaneously* modulate two types of photoreceptors with two completely different stimuli such as two different waveforms, same waveform but different modulation, in-phase and out-of-phase, etc. An application of this will be discussed below in connection with the contrast VEPs.

Since the success of the compensation technique depends strongly on the validity of the spectral sensitivity curves used for calculation of the modulation ratios, a control experiment has been carried out to measure whether the sensitivity functions of the mechanisms stimulated correspond to the expected forms of the isolated cone sensitivities (Estévez, Spekreijse, Van den Berg, and Cavonius 1975). For these experiments a checkerboard pattern-reversal stimulus was prepared by means of the compensation technique to be seen either by one of the long-wavelength or the short-wavelength cones. Both the electrophysiological and psychophysical results suggest that the mechanisms being stimulated are those identified by Stiles as π_1 (or π_3), π_4, and π_5 (Fig. 2.41). Furthermore, by com-

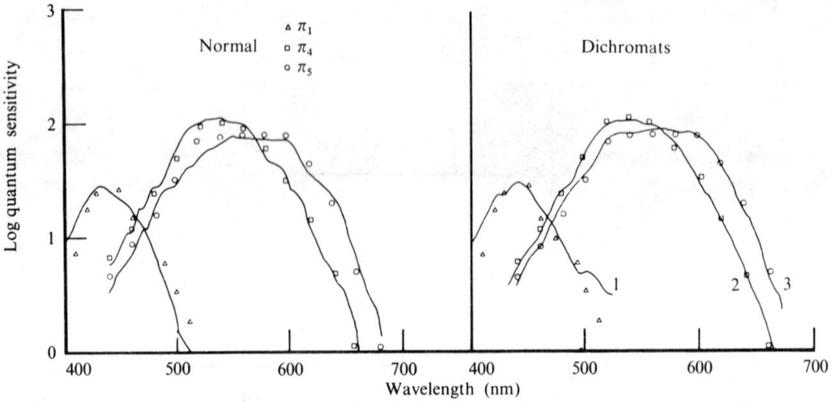

Fig. 2.41. Contrast VEP determined spectral sensitivity functions (continuous lines) in a normal (*left*) and two dichromats (*right*): one aprotanope (sensitivity function 2) and one deuteranope (sensitivity function 3). The short-wavelength function (1) was obtained in the deuteranope; the protanope short-wavelength function was similar to the one shown here. The symbols in both sides are Stiles' functions.

paring data obtained in dichromats and normal trichromats it could be concluded that the separation ratio achieved with this technique was better than 6 to 1 when the stimulus was adjusted using Wald's data (Wald 1964) and better than 10 to 1 when the corresponding Stiles' data were used.

Contrast VEPs from the isolated-cone systems

The results from the above-described control experiment confirmed that, when properly stimulated, all cone systems can independently evoke a contrast response similar to that obtained with white-light stimulation. Furthermore, while the 'blue' cones required a larger check size, both long-wavelength systems responded better to the 15–20′ check sizes which are also the white-light optimum.

The fact that all three cone types are capable of evoking a contrast response means that either the contrast VEP stage can be entered by all three systems, or that each cone system remains separated up to and including an individual contrast processing mechanism at cortical level. To further analyse this question we concentrated on the two long-wavelength systems that seem to produce most, if not all, of the normal white-light photopic response.

The first question one may ask is to what extent do the responses from the

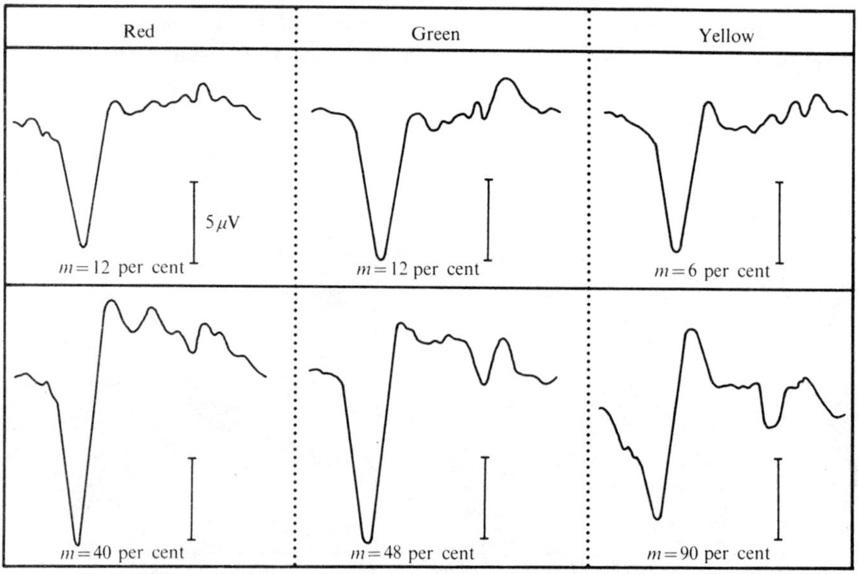

Fig. 2.42. Responses to contrast modulation of the isolated red and green cone systems and the two simultaneously in phase: 'yellow' condition. At low modulations the responses seem to indicate full summation, 6 per cent for the 'yellow' condition gives the same response as 12 per cent for either the red or the green cone systems. At higher modulation depths the isolated conditions give larger responses than the largest that can be obtained in the 'yellow' condition (second row).

isolated mechanisms differ from each other and from those to white light. In Fig. 2.42 the responses to three situations are depicted: isolated red, isolated green, and yellow stimulation. This last situation can be effectively compared to the usual white-light activation. It can be seen that neither the responses from the isolated systems differ among them nor from the 'yellow' condition. An important feature of these responses is their 'completeness' in terms of components: all components characterized in the white-light responses are present in the responses of the isolated cone systems. An interesting finding forms the fact that, while the yellow appearance responses saturate at about 8 per cent modulation depth, the responses of both the isolated red and green systems show no sign of saturation: even for modulations as large as 50 per cent the isolated red response keeps increasing (Fig. 2.43). On the other hand, for small modulation depths there seems

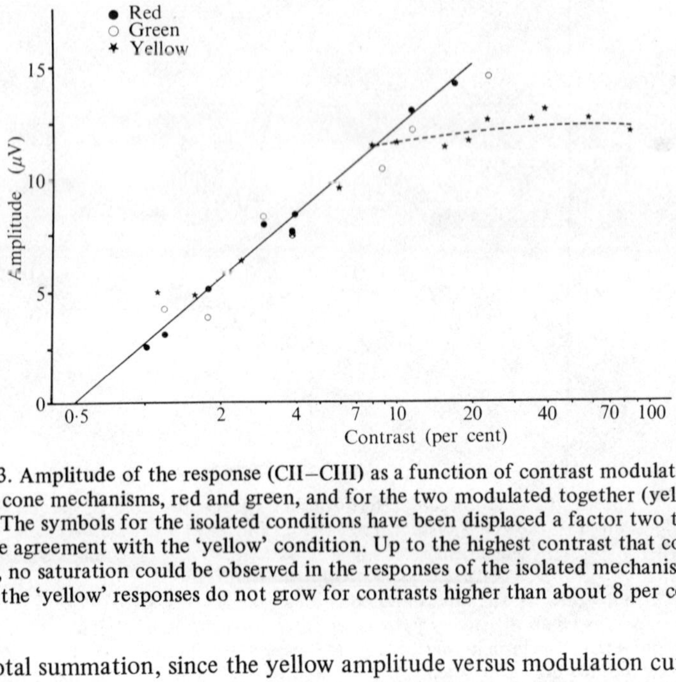

Fig. 2.43. Amplitude of the response (CII–CIII) as a function of contrast modulation for the isolated cone mechanisms, red and green, and for the two modulated together (yellow condition). The symbols for the isolated conditions have been displaced a factor two to the left to show the agreement with the 'yellow' condition. Up to the highest contrast that could be reached, no saturation could be observed in the responses of the isolated mechanisms whereas the 'yellow' responses do not grow for contrasts higher than about 8 per cent.

to be total summation, since the yellow amplitude versus modulation curve resembles the curves obtained in the isolated situation when the isolated curves are displaced by a factor of two along the modulation axis. These results seem to indicate that (a) a single contrast-evoking mechanism receives inputs from both long-wavelength systems and (b) the saturation of the white responses would be but a reflection of some form of interaction between the red and green cone systems. Regan (1970*b*) observed a similar saturation behaviour for the medium-frequency luminance response, which suggests that the pattern CII and the medium frequency response have a common origin.

It was observed that in the white-light situation the amplitude of the contrast VEP reduces when a contrast offset is added to the pattern being presented (Spekreijse *et al.* 1973). For an initial contrast of 10 per cent the appearance response is already much depressed and is almost absent for 20 per cent steady contrast. If a similar manipulation is performed in the isolated-cone situation, the results presented in Fig. 2.44 are obtained. A surprising fact emerges in this

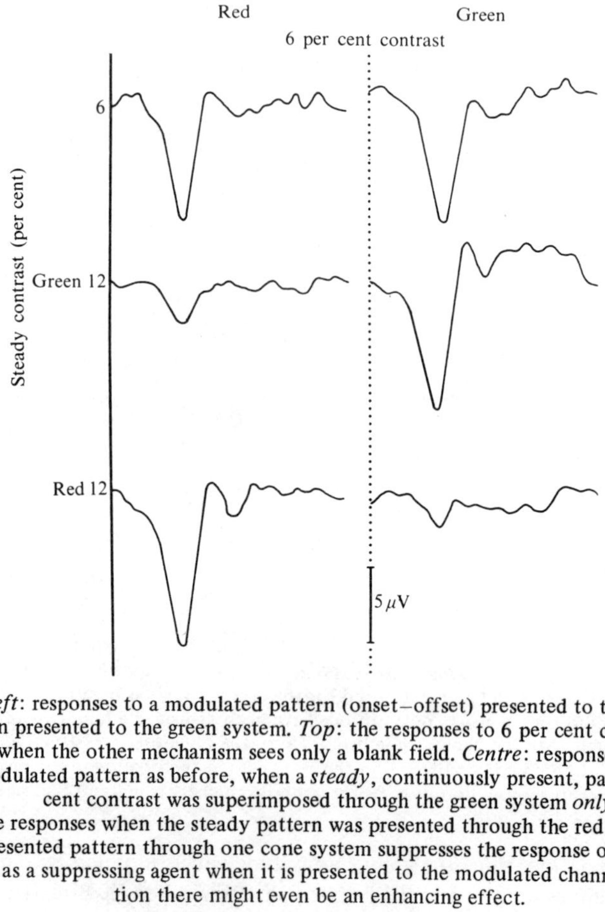

Fig. 2.44. *Left*: responses to a modulated pattern (onset–offset) presented to the red system; *right*: pattern presented to the green system. *Top*: the responses to 6 per cent contrast modulation when the other mechanism sees only a blank field. *Centre*: responses obtained, to the same modulated pattern as before, when a *steady*, continuously present, pattern of 12 per cent contrast was superimposed through the green system *only*.
Bottom: The responses when the steady pattern was presented through the red system. A continuously presented pattern through one cone system suppresses the response of the *other*, but does not act as a suppressing agent when it is presented to the modulated channel. In this situation there might even be an enhancing effect.

experiment: a steady contrast of 12 per cent within the cone system being modulated *is not* effective in suppressing the appearance response. On the other hand, when the steady pattern is presented to the other cone system the response diminishes in the same way as already described for the white-light condition. This result suggests that saturation is due to interaction between colour-coded channels at the stage of the contrast mechanism. Whenever the contrast within one of the channels exceeds a certain level (in the example of Fig. 2.44 this level is about 10 per cent), then the two inputs start to compete with each other. Although the above results seem to point to the existence of a single cortical contrast mechanism which can be reached by either cone system and which 'latches' to the colour-channel, there is still the possibility that each colour channel possesses a contrast element which, when stimulated above a certain level, would block the contrast system of the other cone channel.

To test this possibility the following experiment was carried out. An onset–offset pattern was presented in counterphase to both the red and the green system, i.e. the pattern was first presented during 250 ms through the red system whereas the green system 'perceived' an homogeneous field, and during the subsequent 250 ms the situation was reversed. As can be seen in Fig. 2.45 the responses obtained in

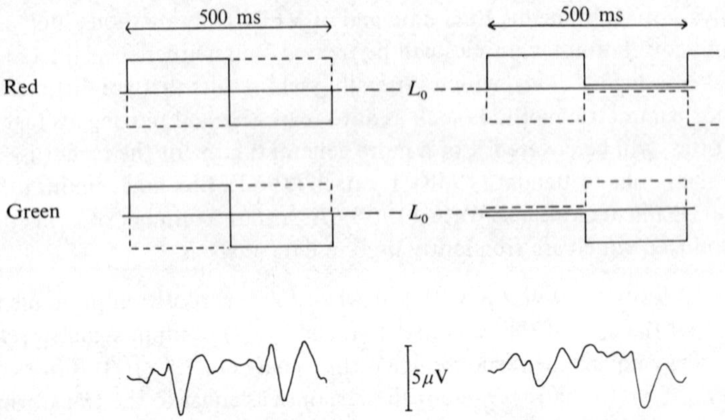

Fig. 2.45. The upper two rows depict the way the two cone mechanisms, red and green, were stimulated. *Left*: pattern was presented to both simultaneously, and with the same contrast, so that a yellow pattern was seen which reversed in contrast every 250 ms. *Right*: the pattern was presented first to the red cone system, while the green cone system saw a blank field, for 250 ms; this situation is reversed in the next 250 ms period: the red system saw a blank field, while the green saw a pattern of the same contrast as the red saw before. The last row shows that the respective responses are rather similar between each other and different from those obtained when stimulating each system independently in the onset–offset condition (cf. Fig. 2.42).

this situation do not differ from those to yellow pattern reversal where the appearance components are much reduced. These results seem to rule out the possibility of two contrast mechanisms, one for each long-wavelength cone system, switching each other off, since in the above experiments the two contrast inputs were never simultaneously present.

Conclusion

On the basis of the experiments described above, we can advance the hypothesis that contrast-appearance VEPs are generated by a single cortical contrast mechanism which can be independently reached by either of the long-wavelength cone channels, and that once one of these inputs attains a certain value, the contrast mechanism effectively blocks the input of the other cone system. It should be realized, however, that this model is restricted to the CII appearance component which according to Jeffreys is associated with the presence of sharp contours in the pattern (cf. Jeffreys, Chapter 6 of this book). Since the behaviour of the other components in the contrast VEPs was not studied, we cannot rule out the possibility that they may be generated within the various cone channels.

Analysis of VEPs

Introduction

In this section a survey will be given of some techniques that are commonly used for the analysis of spontaneous EEG data and of VEPs. Only methods such as averaging and correlation techniques will be treated, and neither special techniques such as level-crossing methods, which generally yield results that are difficult to interpret, nor parametric methods such as auto-regressive and moving-average approximations, will be covered. For a more general treatment the reader is referred to the books of Bendat (1958), Deutsch (1962), Box and Jenkins (1970), Gibson (1963), and Jenkins and Watts (1968). As a start a number of concepts will be introduced which are frequently used in data analysis.

Linear system. A system is said to be linear when the superposition principle holds. This means that the sum of the responses $y_1(t)$ and $y_2(t)$ to input signals $x_1(t)$ and $x_2(t)$ respectively equals the response when the signal $(x_1(t) + x_2(t))$ is presented to the system. If we formally represent the response as equal to the transformation $T(x)$ on the input $x(t)$ it holds that $T(x_1 + x_2) = T(x_1) + T(x_2)$. An important property of a linear system is that the response to a sine-wave input signal is also a sine wave of the same frequency, but which in general has different amplitude and phase.

The response of a linear system to an impulse, a so-called δ-function, is the *impulse response* $h(t)$ of the system. For a linear system the relation between the output signal $y(t)$ and the input signal $x(t)$ is completely specified by

$$y(t) = \int_0^\infty h(\tau)\, x(t-\tau)\mathrm{d}\tau .$$

This formula can be understood if we imagine that the signal $x(t)$ is built up from an infinite series of δ-functions and then apply the superposition principle. The Fourier transform of the impulse response is called the *transfer function* $H(\mathrm{j}\omega)$ of the system:

$$H(\mathrm{j}\omega) = \int_0^\infty h(t)\, \mathrm{e}^{-\mathrm{j}\omega t}\mathrm{d}t = |H(\mathrm{j}\omega)|\, \mathrm{e}^{-\mathrm{j}\phi(\omega)} .$$

The amplitude characteristic is given by $|H(j\omega)|$ and the phase characteristic by $\phi(\omega)$.

Nonlinear system. All systems that do not fulfil the superposition principle are called nonlinear. No general techniques exist for the analysis of these systems. Some 'tailored' techniques which have been successfully applied in the analysis of the VEP system will be described later.

A simple example of a nonlinear system is a half-wave linear rectifier in which the positive input signals are not changed while negative inputs become zero. To a sine-wave input $x(t) = A \sin \omega t$ the output signal $y(t)$ is a half sine wave, which can be described by a series of harmonics:

$$y(t) = \frac{A}{\pi} + \frac{A}{2} \sin \omega t - \frac{2A}{\pi} \sum_{k=1}^{\infty} \frac{\cos(2k\omega t)}{(2k-1)(2k+1)} . \qquad (2.2)$$

Stochastic signal. A signal is called stochastic when the amplitude sample at time t_0 cannot be predicted with certainty from the amplitude sample at another moment $(t_0 - \tau)$. For relatively small values of τ the amplitude can only be predicted to fall within a certain range with a certain probability. As soon as the probability equals zero then two samples do not bear any relation to each other and are called independent. Stochastic signals can be characterized by their statistical properties, such as the mean and the variance of the amplitude distribution of the signal. An example of a stochastic signal is the spontaneous EEG. The narrower the bandwidth of the signal (e.g. alpha activity), the longer the time before subsequent samples become independent.

Stationarity. When the statistical properties of signals are time-invariant then these signals are said to be stationary. In general an EEG signal is not stationary. However, if two samples of EEG signals do not differ in statistical sense, they can be treated as if the concept of stationarity holds. The remaining part of this chapter will be mainly restricted to the analysis of stationary signals.

Analysis techniques

Since the VEPs to light stimulation are generally small compared to the background EEG (poor signal-to-noise ratio), the stimulus is repetitively presented and the EEG is averaged. For flashes or periodic stimuli two methods for detecting the response are commonly used: superposition by photography or pen-writing and averaging by digital or analog methods.

Superposition. In this technique, introduced by Dawson (1951), the EEG signal is fed into an oscilloscope. The time-base is triggered at the same time or shortly before the presentation of the stimulus and the trace is photographed. By superposing many traces on the same photograph, the amplitude distribution of the EP is obtained. The highest density on the photograph occurs at the points where the amplitude distribution of the EP has a maximum. When the amplitude distribution is asymmetric, the EP obtained will be different from the average EP. Apart from the clumsiness of this method, it is not useful when the signal-to-noise ratio is small. The availability of commercial averagers and computers has superseded this technique, although it can give in a simple way an impression about the variability of EPs.

Averaging. This data-processing technique achieves an increase in signal-to-noise ratio by serially adding repetitive signals. The addition cycle is initiated by a synchronizing signal that is time locked to the stimulus. The coherent portions of the responses (phase locked to the stimulus) reinforce each other. Only components which fit an integer number of periods in the interval between two successive trigger pulses are enhanced. The non-coherent response or noise adds with random phase and therefore tends to cancel out. This procedure is equivalent to passing the signal through a filter with amplitude characteristic $|\sin N\nu/N \sin \nu|$, where N is the number of times the signal is averaged and $\nu = \pi T/t$, where T is the time-interval between two successive trigger pulses (sweep time). For large N the bandwidth of the equivalent filter around each harmonic is $0{\cdot}85/NT$ (Fig. 2.46).

It should be stressed that the average EP represents only the coherent part of the evoked activity. The existence of non-coherent evoked activity can be disclosed

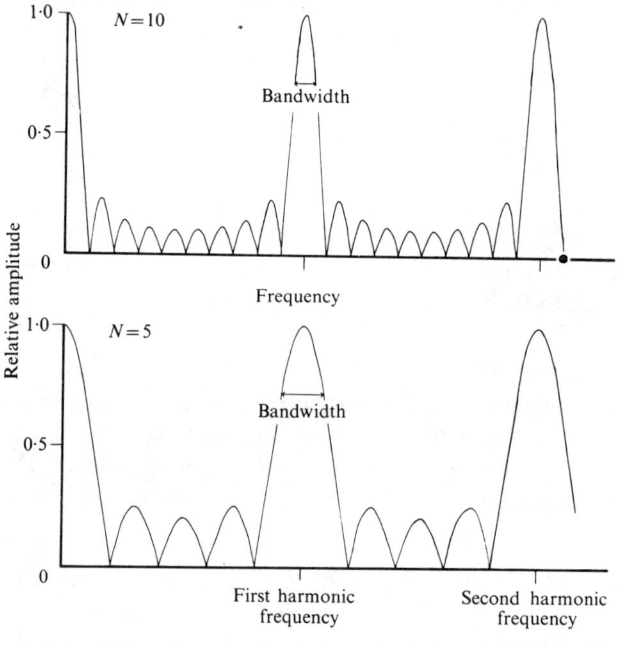

Fig. 2.46. The equivalent filter of an averager in the case where a signal is averaged 10 times (*top*) or 5 times (*bottom*). The peaks are situated at multiples of the frequency of the trigger pulses initiating a sweep.

by comparing the average EP with the auto-spectrum of the EEG signal. In the case where the latency of the response is not constant, the average EP will be smaller than measured in the auto-spectrum. This reduction is greater at higher frequencies. If, for example, the delay fluctuates about 20 ms, the 1 Hz response will scarcely be influenced, whereas the response above 50 Hz will almost disappear (see Harris and Woody 1969). If on the other hand it is the amplitude of the EP which fluctuates, then the average amplitude will be correct, but the variance (auto-spectrum) will be increased irrespective of stimulus frequency.

For a class of frequently used periodic stimuli (such as sinusoidal, triangular, and square waves) it is possible to separate the even harmonics from the total response by triggering the averager at all zero-crossings of the stimulus. The even harmonics are added in phase, while the odd harmonics are added in counterphase. Other harmonics can be suppressed by choosing other trigger levels.

Variance of the average response. When a signal $x(t)$ is averaged N times its average will be

$$x_N(t) = \frac{1}{N} \sum_{k=1}^{N} x_k(t)$$

and the variance of the average equals

$$\frac{1}{N-1}\left[\frac{1}{N}\sum_{k=1}^{N} x_k^2(t) - \{x_N(t)\}^2\right].$$

When the spontaneous activity has a power of σ^2, and the subsequent samples are independent, then for small signal-to-noise ratios the variance of the average response approximates for large N to σ^2/N. In the case where the noise in the subsequent samples is dependent, then the spectrum of the noise will be reflected in the variance of the response.

The latter becomes important when the background EEG is dominated by alpha activity. In this situation the auto-correlation function can be described by

$$R_{xx}(\tau) = \sigma^2 e^{-\beta|\tau|}\cos(2\pi\upsilon_0\tau),$$

where υ_0 is the mean frequency of the alpha rhythm and β/π the bandwidth. This gives for the variance of the average response:

$$\frac{\sigma_x^2}{N}\left\{\frac{1-e^{-2\beta T}}{1-2e^{-\beta T}\cos(2\pi\upsilon_0 T)+e^{-2\beta T}}\right\}.$$

The square root of this variance (standard deviation) is depicted in Fig. 2.47 as a function of $1/T$, i.e. the frequency at which the EEG is averaged. This figure shows that above $1{\cdot}7\upsilon_0$ Hz the standard deviation is about 20 per cent of the value one would expect for independent noise. When the same standard deviation is desired for both υ_0 Hz and $2{\cdot}5\upsilon_0$ Hz responses, the number of sweeps at υ_0 Hz must be 200 times the number at $2{\cdot}5\upsilon_0$ Hz. It should be noted that this requires

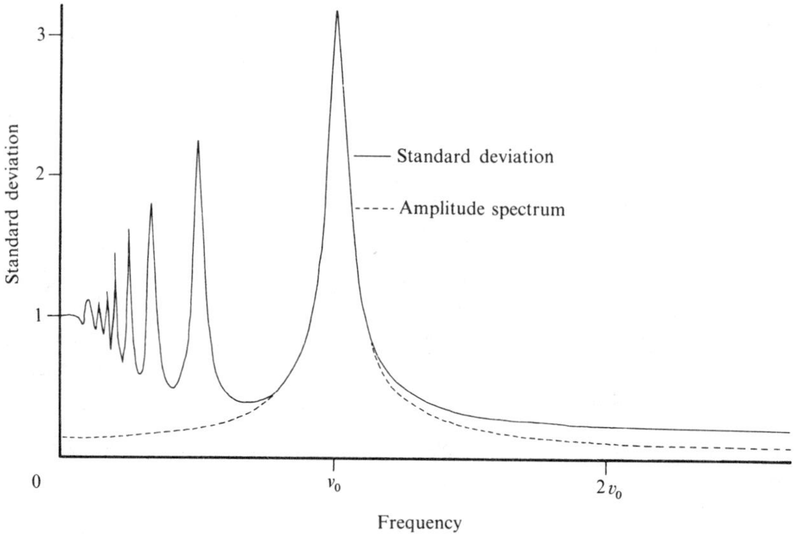

Fig. 2.47. Standard deviation of the average response as a function of the frequency the EEG record is averaged. The EEG record is assumed to consist of a weak VEP of appropriate frequency buried in alpha activity with a peak frequency ν_0 and an amplitude spectrum with a quantity factor of 5π indicated by the dashed line. The peaks in the standard deviation coincide with the subharmonics of the alpha frequency.

a total EEG record time for the υ_0 Hz response of 500 times that of the $2{\cdot}5\upsilon_0$ Hz response.

Lock-in technique. With this instrument a single harmonic of a response to a periodic stimulus is enhanced, while the other harmonics are suppressed. The shape of the amplitude characteristic of the equivalent filter around the selected harmonic (generally the first or the second) is approximately

$$\frac{\nu}{u^2 + \nu^2}\left(\frac{u}{\nu}e^{-\nu}\sin u - e^{-\nu}\cos u + 1\right)$$

where $u = 2\pi\Delta\upsilon T$, $\Delta\upsilon$ is the difference between a frequency in the output signal, and the selected harmonic, T is the duration of the record, and $\nu = T/RC$, where RC is the time-constant of the lock-in amplifier. In Fig. 2.48 the bandwidth of the equivalent filter is depicted as a function of record length. For $T < RC$ the bandwidth is proportional to $1/T$. As T becomes greater the signal leaks away over the integrator of the lock-in amplifier. Because of this leakage the bandwidth of the equivalent filter has a lower limit of $0{\cdot}2/RC$ Hz. In an averager no signal leakage occurs, so that the bandwidth of the average response becomes narrower in proportion to $1/T$.

It can be seen from Fig. 2.48 that the optimal choice of integration time and record length lies near the point where the product of bandwidth and RC time is

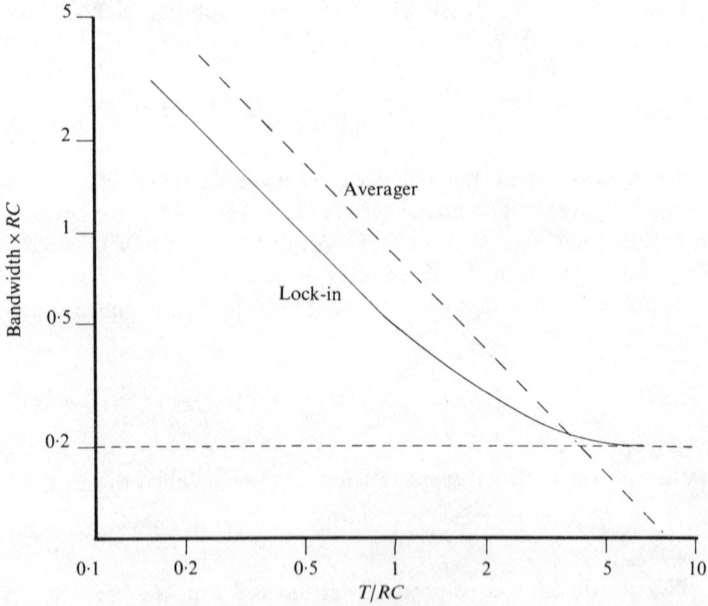

Fig. 2.48. Comparison of the bandwidths of the filtering achieved by analysing a record with length T with either a lock-in amplifier or an averager. RC represents the time-constant of the lock-in amplifier. For the averager the RC term has to be omitted along the axes.

0·3, and the record length is twice the RC time. Thus to obtain a bandwidth of 0·1 Hz, the optimal choice of the integration time is 3 s and of the record length is 6 s. For a bandwidth of 0·002 Hz the values are 150 s and 5 min respectively.

Correlation analysis. When an EEG signal is analysed by visual inspection the signal is conventionally divided into different frequency bands, such as the 8–13 Hz (α-band) and the 13–40 Hz (β-band), and the mean amplitude of the signal in each band is estimated. This analysis can also be performed by a battery of commercially available selective filters, each tuned to one of the frequency bands of interest. When sufficient filters are available, their outputs form an estimate of the power spectrum of the EEG. However, power spectra (*auto-spectra*) are preferably calculated by means of a digital computer, since the bandwidths and the central frequencies of the filters can be changed easily. This can be accomplished either directly (fast Fourier transform) or by taking the Fourier transform of the auto-correlation function of the EEG signal.

The definition of the *auto-correlation function* is

$$R_{xx}(\tau) = \lim_{T \to \infty} \frac{1}{2T} \int_{-T}^{T} \{x(t) - \overline{x(t)}\}\{x(t-\tau) - \overline{x(t)}\}\mathrm{d}t.$$

This expression simplifies for signals with zero mean amplitude such as is usually the case in EEG studies, to

$$R_{xx}(\tau) = \lim_{T\to\infty} \frac{1}{2T} \int_{-T}^{+T} x(t)\, x(t-\tau)\, \mathrm{d}t.$$

For $\tau = 0$, this function equals the variance (power) of the signal. Whereas for stochastic signals $R_{xx}(\tau)$ will approach zero for large values of τ, for periodic signals this function will also be periodic, i.e. $R_{xx}(\tau) = R_{xx}(\tau + kT)$, where k is an integer and T the period of the signal.

The *cross-correlation function* of two signals $x(t)$ and $y(t)$ is similarly defined as

$$R_{yx}(\tau) = \lim_{T\to\infty} \frac{1}{2T} \int_{-T}^{T} \{y(t) - \overline{y(t)}\}\, \{x(t-\tau) - \overline{x(t)}\}\, \mathrm{d}t.$$

The Fourier transform of the cross-correlation function is called the *cross-spectrum*,

$$S_{yx}(\omega) = \int_{-\infty}^{\infty} R_{yx}(\tau)\, \mathrm{e}^{-\mathrm{j}\omega t} \mathrm{d}t = |S_{yx}(\omega)|\, \mathrm{e}^{-\mathrm{j}\phi(\omega)},$$

where $|S_{yx}(\omega)|$ is called the cross-power spectrum and $\phi(\omega)$ the phase spectrum. The phase spectrum gives, as a function of frequency, the average phase difference between two signals in a narrow frequency band. When the phase difference is constant the cross-power spectrum will have a large value compared to the values of the auto-spectra of the signals. When the phase difference fluctuates randomly the cross-power spectrum tends towards zero.

When $y(t)$ is the output signal of a linear system with an impulse response $h(t)$ to an input signal $x(t)$ with zero mean, the cross-correlation function is

$$R_{yx}(\tau) = \lim_{T\to\infty} \frac{1}{2T} \int_{-T}^{T} \int_{0}^{\infty} h(\tau_1) x(t-\tau_1) x(t-\tau)\, \mathrm{d}\tau_1 \mathrm{d}t$$

$$= \int_{0}^{\infty} h(\tau_1)\, R_{xx}(\tau - \tau_1)\, \mathrm{d}\tau_1.$$

Fourier transformation of both sides gives $S_{yx}(\omega) = H(\mathrm{j}\omega)\, S_{xx}(\omega)$. Thus the transfer function of a linear system can be found by calculating the auto-spectrum of the input signal and the cross-spectrum between the output and input signals,

$$H(\mathrm{j}\omega) = \frac{S_{yx}(\omega)}{S_{xx}(\omega)}.$$

Using this formula the transfer function at a certain frequency can be estimated if the input signal $x(t)$ contains frequencies in that range. Similar computation gives for the auto-spectrum of $y(t)$: $S_{yy}(\omega) = |H(\mathrm{j}\omega)|^2\, S_{xx}(\omega)$. It should be realized that in this way only can the amplitude characteristic of the system be determined.

Nonlinear systems analysis

Sinusoidal stimulation. The fact that the VEP to sinusoidally modulated light contains higher harmonics indicates directly that the human VEP system is non-linear. Spekreijse (1966) observed that apart from the fundamental component, mainly even harmonics were present in the VEP to homogeneous field stimulation. Since the amplitudes of these harmonics were proportional to the amplitude of the sinusoidal stimulus, it was concluded that the nonlinearity has the nature of an asymmetric linear rectifier (see eqn (2.2)). By developing a 'linearizing' technique, Spekreijse (1966) was able to split up the VEP system into linear and nonlinear processes and to determine their sequence and properties. Such a sequential analysis could not have been carried out if the VEP system had been linear.

The method of linearizing can be explained by referring to Fig. 2.49. When the input signal to a half-wave linear rectifier is a sine wave, the output signal consists of the positive halves of the sine wave. Noise with a symmetric amplitude

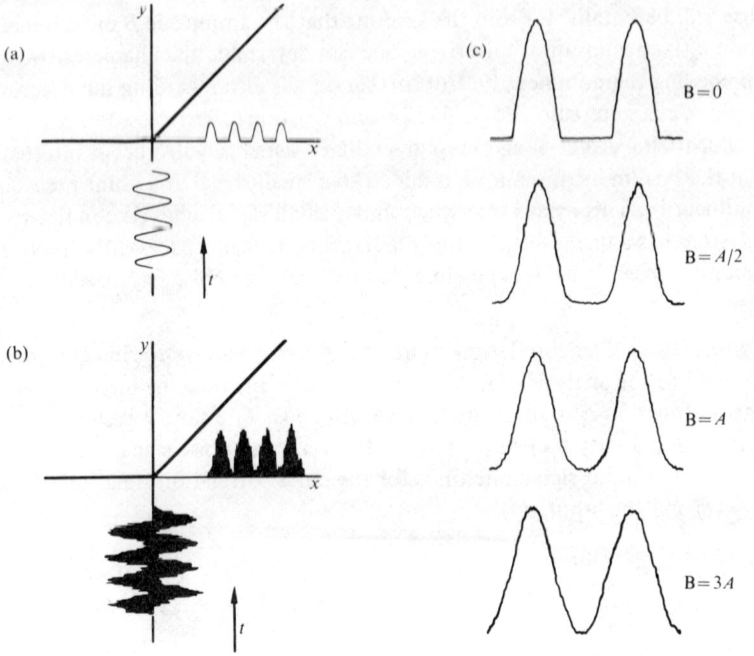

Fig. 2.49. The response of a linear half-wave rectifier for a sine-wave input signal (a) and for a sine wave with added noise (b). (c) the linearizing effect of a sine-wave auxiliary signal (*B* sin *βt*) added to a sine-wave stimulus (*A* sin *αt*). These output signals of a half-wave linear rectifier are averaged with a CAT, whose sweep is triggered by sine-wave stimulus (*A* sin *αt*). The upper figure shows the familiar half-wave rectified sine wave, obtained without adding an auxiliary signal, i.e. $B = 0$. With increasing amplitude *B* the distortion in the response reduces, until for $B = 2A$ an almost pure sinusoid is obtained (bottom figure). Comparison of the top and bottom figures shows that the amplitude of the fundamental component in the response is not affected by the auxiliary signal. This is characteristic for a half-wave linear rectifier.

distribution added to the sinusoidal stimulus acts as a carrier signal, whose effect is, on the average, to shift the amplitude domain of the sine wave to both sides of the break-point in the rectifier. The sine wave is then, on the average, half of the time in the linear region of the rectifier. In this way the break-point can be completely masked when a sufficiently small signal-to-noise ratio is present, and a sinusoidal response is obtained. The masking property also holds for other auxiliary signals, like a sine wave with a different frequency as can be seen in in the left column of Fig. 2.16.

If the nonlinearity is preceded by a linear process, then by using an auxiliary sine wave $B \sin \omega' t$ added to the sinusoidal stimulus $A \sin \omega t$ (where $\omega \neq \omega'$) it is possible to determine the attenuation of this linear process. This analysis is based on the fact that the incoming signal to the nonlinearity will still consist of two sine waves but with amplitudes A^* and B^*. Suppose that the linear process before the nonlinearity has a high-frequency cut-off at $\omega < \omega'$. Then, for increasing frequencies ω', the amplitude B^* will be progressively reduced and a more distorted response will be obtained. From the amount that the amplitude B must be increased to obtain a fixed amount of linearizing one can determine the characteristic of the filter preceding the nonlinearity. For further details also regarding the determination of the phase characteristic, see Spekreijse and Oosting (1970).

The linearizing effect of an external auxiliary signal can also occur internally when in the system intrinsic noise is added to a small signal at a point preceding the nonlinearity. This means that when under small-signal analysis conditions a noisy system has a linear output, this observation does not necessarily imply that the system is linear, since it is possible that the intrinsic noise has masked the nonlinearity.

Noise stimulation. The correlation technique described above for linear systems can be extended to the analysis of nonlinear systems by introducing higher-order correlation functions. To illustrate this we will consider a simple system consisting of a static nonlinearity $f(x) = a_1 x + a_2 x^2$. If a Gaussian-noise signal $x(t)$ (with zero mean) is used as input signal one finds for the cross-correlation function of the output $y(t)$ and the input $x(t)$

$$R_{yx}(\tau) = \lim_{T \to \infty} \frac{1}{2T} \int_{-T}^{T} [a_1 x(t) + a_2\{x^2(t) - \overline{x^2(t)}\}]\, x(t-\tau)\, \mathrm{d}t.$$

Thus

$$R_{yx}(\tau) = \lim_{T \to \infty} \frac{1}{2T} \int_{-T}^{T} a_1 x(t) x(t-\tau)\, \mathrm{d}t = a_1\, R_{xx}(\tau).$$

This cross-correlation function represents only the linear term of the function $f(x)$; the quadratic information is lost. This result holds for all input signals with a symmetric amplitude distribution. In contrast to this the auto-correlation function of $y(t)$ contains both the linear and quadratic terms,

$$R_{yy}(\tau) = \lim_{T \to \infty} \frac{1}{2T} \int_{-T}^{T} [a_1 x(t) + a_2\{x^2(t) - \overline{x^2(t)}\}]$$

$$= [a_1 x(t-\tau) + a_2\{x^2(t-\tau) - \overline{x^2(t)}\}]\ \mathrm{d}t$$

Thus for a Gaussian input $x(t)$,

$$R_{yy}(\tau) = a_1^2 R_{xx}(\tau) + 2a_2^2 R_{xx}^2(\tau).$$

In the case of a noise-free system both correlation functions can be computed to estimate the form of the nonlinearity.

When a system is intrinsically noisy, the auto-correlation function of the intrinsic noise will be added to the auto-correlation function of the 'response'. On the other hand the cross-correlation function is not influenced by the internal noise, only its variance. Thus in this situation it is difficult to determine the form of the nonlinearity from the auto-correlation function of the output signal.

In the specific case of the VEP system, the response to a wide-band noise modulated light consists of a small signal in a large background of EEG activity: the amplitude of the response is typically about 10 per cent of the amplitude of the background activity, which gives a contribution of about 1 per cent to the output auto-correlation function. Thus the auto-correlation function of $y(t)$ cannot be used with reliability to estimate the nonlinearity. Only cross-correlation functions can be computed with a sufficient accuracy.

To obtain information about the even terms of the nonlinearity one can introduce the cross-bicorrelation function,

$$R_{yxx}(\tau_1, \tau_2) = \lim_{T \to \infty} \frac{1}{2T} \int_{-T}^{T} \{y(t) - \overline{y(t)}\}\, x(t-\tau_1)\, x(t-\tau_2)\ \mathrm{d}t.$$

For the above-mentioned example $f(x) = a_1 x + a_2 x^2$ this function becomes for a Gaussian input $x(t)$: $2a_2 R_{xx}(\tau_1) R_{xx}(\tau_2)$. Only the quadratic term contributes to the cross-bicorrelation function. In general for an input signal with a symmetric amplitude distribution the odd terms of a nonlinearity contribute to the cross-correlation function and the even terms to the cross-bicorrelation function. Both functions give therefore independent information about a nonlinearity.

Sequential analysis. In this section it will be shown how a system consisting of two linear elements with impulse responses $h_1(\tau)$ and $h_2(\tau)$, linked by a zero-memory nonlinearity $f(v)$, can be analysed by means of the correlation technique Fig. 2.50).

Consider a Gaussian-noise input signal $x(t)$ with auto-correlation function $R_{xx}(\tau)$ and auto-spectrum $S_{xx}(\omega)$. Then, because the first element is linear, the input signal $v(t)$ to the nonlinear element,

$$v(t) = \int_0^{\infty} h_1(\tau_1)\, x(t-\tau_1)\ \mathrm{d}\tau_1,$$

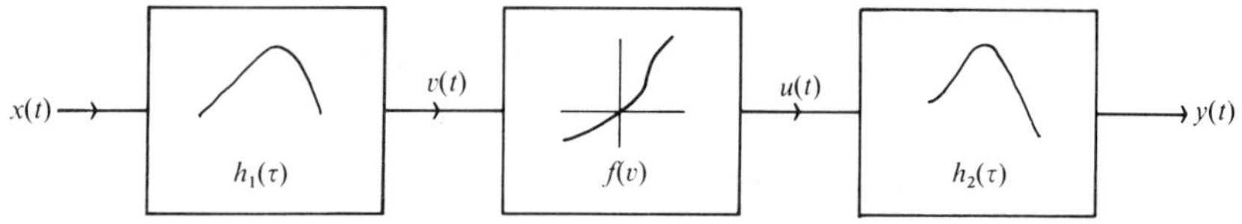

Fig. 2.50. A sequential system consisting of two linear elements with impulse functions $h_1(\tau)$ and $h_2(\tau)$ respectively, which are linked by a single-valued zero-memory nonlinearity $u = f(u)$.

also has a Gaussian amplitude distribution. The input to the second linear element will be

$$u(t) = f\{v(t)\} = f\left\{\int_0^\infty h_1(\tau_1)\,x(t-\tau_1)\,\mathrm{d}\tau_1\right\}$$

and its output equals

$$y(t) = \int_0^\infty h_2(\tau_2)\,u(t-\tau_2)\,\mathrm{d}\tau_2.$$

Thus

$$y(t) = \int_0^\infty h_2(\tau_2)\,f\left\{\int_0^\infty h_1(\tau_1)\,x(t-\tau_1-\tau_2)\,\mathrm{d}\tau_1\right\}\mathrm{d}\tau_2.$$

Because the input signal of the nonlinearity has a Gaussian amplitude distribution the Price's theorem (1958) can be used. This theorem states that $R_{ux}(\tau) = C_1 R_{vx}(\tau)$, where

$$C_1 = \int_{-\infty}^{\infty} \frac{\mathrm{d}f(v)}{\mathrm{d}v}\,p(v)\,\mathrm{d}v$$

and the Gaussian amplitude distribution of $v(t)$,

$$p(v) = \frac{1}{\sigma_v\sqrt{2\pi}}\exp\left(-v^2/2\sigma_v^2\right),$$

where

$$\sigma_v^2 = \frac{1}{2\pi}\int_{-\infty}^{\infty} |H_1(\mathrm{j}\omega)|^2 S_{xx}(\omega)\,\mathrm{d}\omega.$$

Because $p(v)$ is an even function, only the odd terms of $f(v)$ contribute to the cross-correlation function.

For the cross-correlation function of $y(t)$ and $x(t)$ one finds

$$R_{yx}(\tau) = C_1 \int_0^\infty\int_0^\infty h_2(\tau_2)\,h_1(\tau_1) R_{xx}(\tau-\tau_1-\tau_2)\,\mathrm{d}\tau_1\,\mathrm{d}\tau_2$$

and for the cross-spectrum

$$S_{yx}(\omega) = C_1 S_{xx}(\omega)\,H_1(\mathrm{j}\omega)\,H_2(\mathrm{j}\omega).$$

Application of Price's theorem gives for the cross-bicorrelation function of $u(t)$ and $x(t)$:

$$R_{uxx}(\tau_1, \tau_2) = C_2 R_{vx}(\tau_1) R_{vx}(\tau_2)$$

where

$$C_2 = \int_{-\infty}^{\infty} \frac{d^2 f(v)}{dv^2} p(v) \, dv.$$

Only the even terms of $f(v)$ contribute to the cross-bicorrelation function. The cross-bicorrelation function of $y(t)$ and $x(t)$ is

$$R_{yxx}(\tau_1, \tau_2)$$

$$= C_2 \int_0^{\infty}\int_0^{\infty}\int_0^{\infty} h_2(\tau) h_1(\tau_4) h_1(\tau_5) R_{xx}(\tau_1 - \tau - \tau_4) R_{xx}(\tau_2 - \tau - \tau_5) \, d\tau d\tau_4 d\tau_5$$

and the corresponding cross-bispectrum

$$S_{yxx}(\omega_1, \omega_2) = \iint_{-\infty}^{\infty} R_{yxx}(\tau_1, \tau_2) \exp\{-j(\omega_1\tau_1 + \omega_2\tau_2)\} \, d\tau_1 \, d\tau_2$$

$$= C_2 S_{xx}(\omega_1) S_{xx}(\omega_2) H_2\{j(\omega_1 + \omega_2)\} H_1(j\omega_1) H_1(j\omega_2).$$

From the two spectra one can calculate the amplitude spectrum of the linear elements,

$$|H_1(j\omega)| = \frac{C_1 \, |S_{yxx}(-\omega/2, \omega)|}{C_2 \, |S_{yx}(\omega/2) S_{xx}(\omega)|}$$

and

$$|H_2(j\omega)| = \frac{C_2 |S_{yx}(\omega) S_{yx}(\omega/2)|}{C_1^2 |S_{yxx}(-\omega/2, \omega)|}$$

In this way the cross-correlation and cross-bicorrelation functions of the output and input signals can be used to determine the transfer characteristics of the linear elements before and after the nonlinearity. By varying the amplitude of the input noise the form of the nonlinearity can also be estimated (Reits 1975).

Triggered correlation. The correlation technique has the disadvantage that a general-purpose computer is required to carry out the calculations. It has been shown, however, by De Boer and Kuyper (1968) that for a linear system the input–output cross-correlation function can also be computed by means of an averager. In the following paragraph this technique will be extended to analyse systems which contain a static nonlinearity like the one depicted in Fig. 2.50.

The triggered correlation function is defined as a function obtained by averaging one signal on the synchronization or trigger pulses generated by another or the same signal. In the following we restrict ourselves to the calculation of the triggered correlation function obtained by averaging the output signal $y(t)$ on synchronization pulses generated whenever the Gaussian noise stimulus $x(t)$ crosses a pre-set amplitude level x_a. De Boer and Kuyper (1968) have shown that this procedure results for a linear system in a function which is proportional to the true cross-correlation function. For the nonlinear system of Fig. 2.50 the analysis is as follows.

Since the input signal $v(t)$ of the nonlinearity is a Gaussian signal, the expected value of $u(t)$ is

$$\langle u(t) | \, x(0) = x_a \rangle = \int_{-\infty}^{\infty} \frac{f(v) p_2(v, x_a) \, dv}{p_1(x_a)} ,$$

where $p_1(x)$ and $p_2(v, x)$ are the Gaussian univariate and bivariate amplitude distributions. For $f(v) = a_1 v + a_2 v^2$ one finds

$$\langle u(t) | x(0) = x_a \rangle = a_2 \sigma_v^2 + a_1 \sigma_v \rho_{vx}(t) \frac{x_a}{\sigma_x} + a_2 \sigma_v^2 \rho_{vx}^2(t) \left(\frac{x_a^2}{\sigma_x^2} - 1 \right) ,$$

where

$$\rho_{vx}(t) = \frac{R_{vx}(t)}{\sigma_x \sigma_v}$$

is the normalized cross-correlation function of the signals $x(t)$ and $v(t)$.

Triggering at the level $-x_a$ gives

$$\langle u(t) | x(0) = -x_a \rangle = a_2 \sigma_v^2 - a_1 \sigma_v \rho_{vx}(t) \frac{x_a}{\sigma_x} + a_2 \sigma_v^2 \rho_{vx}^2(t) \left(\frac{x_a^2}{\sigma_x^2} - 1 \right) .$$

By adding and subtracting these two triggered correlation functions, one can separate the even and the odd terms of the nonlinearity,

$$\langle u(t) | x(0) = x_a \rangle - \langle u(t) | x(0) = -x_a \rangle = 2 a_1 \sigma_v \rho_{vx}(t) \frac{x_a}{\sigma_x} ,$$

and $$\langle u(t) | x(0) = x_a \rangle + \langle u(t) | x(0) = -x_a \rangle = 2 a_2 \sigma_v^2 \left\{ 1 + \rho_{vx}^2(t) \left(\frac{x_a^2}{\sigma_x^2} - 1 \right) \right\} .$$

An expression which is proportional to the true cross-correlation function can also be determined directly by choosing $x_a = \sigma_x$, and the bicorrelation function by taking $x_a = 0$. In these two situations longer recording durations are generally required to obtain the same accuracy as with the adding/subtracting method.
The expected value of the output $y(t)$ of the second linear element is

$$\langle y(t) | x(0) = x_a \rangle = \int_0^{\infty} h_2(\tau) \langle u(t - \tau) | x(0) = x_a \rangle \, d\tau .$$

Taking the Fourier transforms of

$$\langle y(t) | x(0) = x_a \rangle - \langle y(t) | x(0) = -x_a \rangle$$

and

$$\langle y(t) | x(0) = x_a \rangle + \langle y(t) | x(0) = -x_a \rangle$$

one finds expressions that are proportional respectively to

$$H_2(\mathrm{j}\omega)\, S_{vx}(\mathrm{j}\omega),$$

and

$$A\,\delta(\omega) + H_2(\mathrm{j}\omega) \int_{-\infty}^{\infty} S_{vx}(\mathrm{j}z) S_{vx}\{\mathrm{j}(\omega - z)\}\, \mathrm{d}z,$$

where $S_{vx}(\mathrm{j}\omega) = H_1(\mathrm{j}\omega) S_{xx}(\omega)$ and A is a constant. The transfer functions of the linear elements combine in different ways in these two Fourier transforms, so $H_1(\mathrm{j}\omega)$ and $H_2(\mathrm{j}\omega)$ can be estimated. This type of analysis can be extended to systems containing a nonlinearity with terms up to the fourth power. This turns out not to restrict the applicability of the triggered correlation technique seriously since in biological systems the higher-order terms are generally small due to intrinsic noise (intrinsic linearizing) and saturation.

Acknowledgements

We are grateful to Drs. T. J. T. P. van den Berg, G. Dagnelie, A. Duwaer, and N. A. M. Schellart for providing material and helpful suggestions. Much of the research reported in this chapter was made possible by grants from the Netherlands Organization for the Advancement of Pure Research (ZWO) and by the Organization for Health Research (TNO), The Hague.

3. A versatile television pattern generator for visual evoked potentials

G. B. ARDEN, D. J. FAULKNER, and C. MAIR

Department of Visual Science, Institute of Ophthalmology and *Electrodiagnostic Clinic, Moorfields Eye Hospital, London*

Introduction

This chapter describes a television system for eliciting evoked potentials. This system has greater versatility, and potential for development, than any system so far described. We present data which show that the system works well in spite of the limitations inherent in the use of television techniques.

VEPs evoked by flashes of light contain nonspecific components. However, those generated by patterns are specific to the visual cortex and correlate well with psychophysical and single-cell findings: thus in principle they can be used for detailed analysis. The generation of a pattern VEP implies that the contrast of the retinal image is changed without overall change in mean luminance. Gratings of various forms have been used, and of these, the largest VEPs are elicited by checkerboards. A sudden change in contrast – the onset or offset of the checkerboard, or its phase inversion (contrast reversal) – is the effective stimulus for the VEP.

Various devices have been built to produce stimuli of these types. The patterns are produced optically, using semi-silvered mirrors, polaroid, or photographic transparencies, and movement is produced mechanically, by vibrators, galvanometer motors, or rotating wheels. With these devices, there are problems of alignment; patterns cannot be made to appear and disappear as well as reverse in contrast; it is difficult to change patterns rapidly; and it is frequently impossible to use stimuli of low contrast (see Chapter 1 of this book).

Van der Tweel and Spekreijse (1969) have produced an elegant optical technique using semi-silvered mirrors and an optical train, which allows the production of low-contrast patterns which can either appear or phase invert. Unfortunately, this system is not suitable for clinical work; the display is small; cooperative subjects are required; the mirrors are delicate and difficult to construct; and the stimulus cannot be changed easily.

In clinical work, it is necessary to stimulate various parts of the visual field and to select rapidly the appropriate stimulus. For these reasons, a fully electronic

Visual evoked potentials in man: new developments (ed. J. E. Desmedt), pp. 90–109. Clarendon Press, Oxford 1977.

system is required. Sine-wave gratings have been produced on oscilloscope screens for VEP experiments (Campbell and Robson 1968) but for a checkerboard the bandwidth of the processing system must be much higher, and unless large expensive display tubes are used there is a severe limitation on the number of squares which can be produced on the screen. The overall luminance is very low compared with the mirror system. However, displays with electromagnetic deflection systems are much brighter and larger. It is therefore natural to use such a system to display patterns, and the most readily available and cheapest is the TV monitor.

There are certain limitations in using a TV system. The relatively low repetition rate of the TV frame limits the temporal frequency response. Precise control of contrast ratio is limited by phosphor nonlinearity and, at low contrasts, by system noise. The system bandwidth determines the spatial frequency cut-off. In these latter respects, TV pictures are inferior to photographs. Thus it is difficult to predict whether standard TV techniques can produce patterns capable of testing the performance of the visual system.

On the other hand, significant advantages follow from the use of TV techniques: the price of the system is reduced compared to a large-screen oscilloscope display; it is possible to produce coloured stimuli; split-screen techniques facilitate field tests; programme material – either broadcast or derived from video recorders – can be mixed with the patterned stimuli. The latter is of special importance in clinical applications since the additional material serves to attract and to hold the patients' attention. Plate 3.1 (see between pp. 418–19) shows typical displays obtained with this system.

This chapter is concerned with one clinically acceptable form of a TV pattern generator. We include some data on normal and abnormal eyes to illustrate the versatility of the device.

Description of system

Specifications

We have produced a pattern generator using standard TV techniques. This method is extremely versatile, the prototype producing displays with the following specifications:

Patterns: square-wave gratings (horizontal or vertical); checkerboards.

Spatial frequency: choice of four.

Stimulus: square-wave contrast reversal or appearance–disappearance about a mean luminance level.

Temporal frequency: choice of twelve internal rates, or external triggering.

Contrast ratio: choice of six values, down to 2 per cent nominal.

Display modes:

1. Independent control of temporal frequency in four modes: (a) full screen, (b) left and right halves, (c) top and bottom halves, (d) quadrants.

2. Independent control of contrast in left and right halves of the screen (modes (b) and (d) above).
3. Blanking of pattern in central strip – variable width controlled by a front-panel potentiometer.

All these patterns can be mixed with any picture signal.

The mean luminance of the display does not change when the contrast of the patterns is changed, or when the patterns themselves are altered.

Our system typically stimulates $14^\circ \times 10^\circ$ of retina, provides square-edge subtenses between $6'$ and $48'$ of arc at a viewing distance of 1·5 m, and reversal rates of 1–20 Hz. Mean luminance is typically 100 cd m^{-2}.

General

A TV picture is produced by displaying a series of frames, each of which consists of horizontal lines written sequentially from top to bottom of the screen. Each line is preceded by a synchronizing line trigger pulse, and each frame by a longer frame (or field) trigger pulse. Between successive lines, and successive frames, the picture information is 'blanked' to allow the insertion of the trigger pulses and additional information (e.g. colour control). In the United Kingdom there are 625 lines in a frame, and 50 frames in a second. Other standards exist but frame rate is usually related to local mains frequency.*

The combination of triggers and picture information is known as a composite video signal, and a demodulated broadcast signal is of this form. For studio work trigger pulses and blanking periods are produced by a synchronizing pulse generator (S.P.G.). In order to mix composite video signals from more than one source the trigger pulses on each signal must be coincident; this locking of a local S.P.G. to a remote signal (e.g. broadcasts) is achieved with a 'gen-lock' unit. Both of these units are standard TV studio equipment.

Fig. 3.1 shows a block diagram of our system. The picture signal (composite video) may be derived from either a video recorder or broadcast programmes. Trigger and blanking pulses from a local S.P.G., gen-locked to the picture signal, drive the pattern generator. The output of the pattern generator is a composite video signal which can be mixed with the picture signal for display on a TV monitor. A number of standard TV techniques can now be used to modify the display, since the pattern has been produced as a composite video signal. In particular, the screen can be split, portions of it blanked, and colour information introduced (e.g. changes in grey levels can be transformed into arbitrary changes of hue).

Of course, picture information is not necessary to the operation of the system: one can then dispense with the gen-lock unit. The quality of the display pattern is limited by the TV monitor employed: high-quality black and white monitors can resolve high spatial frequencies, whilst the use of three physically separated

* This is a simplified description of television operation; Towers (1967) gives a more complete account.

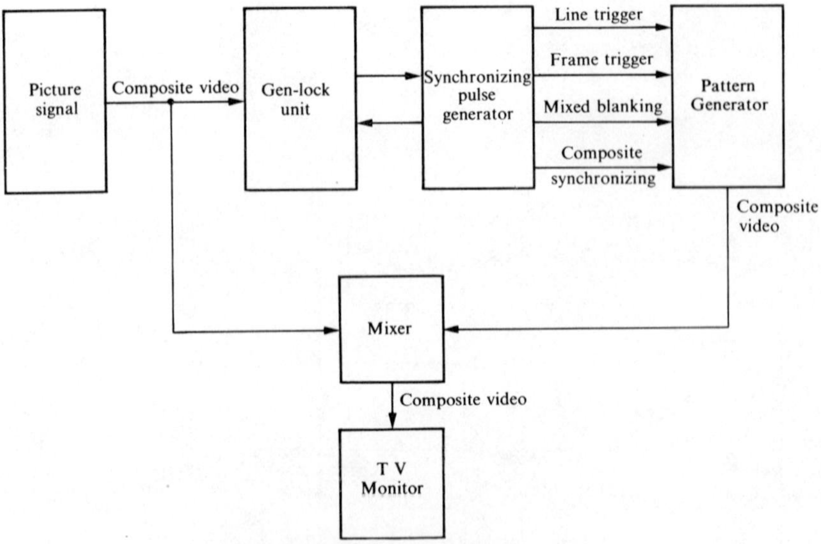

Fig. 3.1. Block diagram of TV system.

phosphors in adjacent screen areas limits the spatial resolution of colour monitors. The results described below were obtained using cheap colour monitors, modified from domestic TV receivers, which employ 'shadowmask' tubes.

Electronic techniques for pattern production

A simplified block diagram of the pattern generator is shown in Fig. 3.2. The horizontal oscillator produces high-frequency square waves. These are gated by each line pulse from the S.P.G., to ensure phase coherence from line to line. This signal alone produces a static vertical square-wave grating. The vertical line counter inverts the video signal after a pre-selected number of lines, and is reset by frame pulses from the S.P.G. to ensure phase coherence from frame to frame. This signal alone produces a static horizontal square-wave grating. Combining signals from these two sources in the first exclusive-OR gate produces a static checkerboard pattern. Spatial frequency is controlled by a two-channel data selector, ganged to produce a square display. In practice, the counters run continuously and gratings are produced by inhibiting one or other half of the data selector.

The temporal-frequency generator produces square waves. If contrast reversal is selected, these square waves invert the pattern signal in the second exclusive-OR gate; if onset–offset is selected, the positive level of these square waves acts as a blanking signal for the pattern. The temporal frequency generator is fed with transistor–transistor logic (T.T.L.) line and frame pulses which enable it to allocate independent temporal frequencies to the quadrants of the display. The unit also provides additional blanking pulses for the 'centre-off' facility, and trigger pulses for averagers. It can, moreover, be driven from external oscillators.

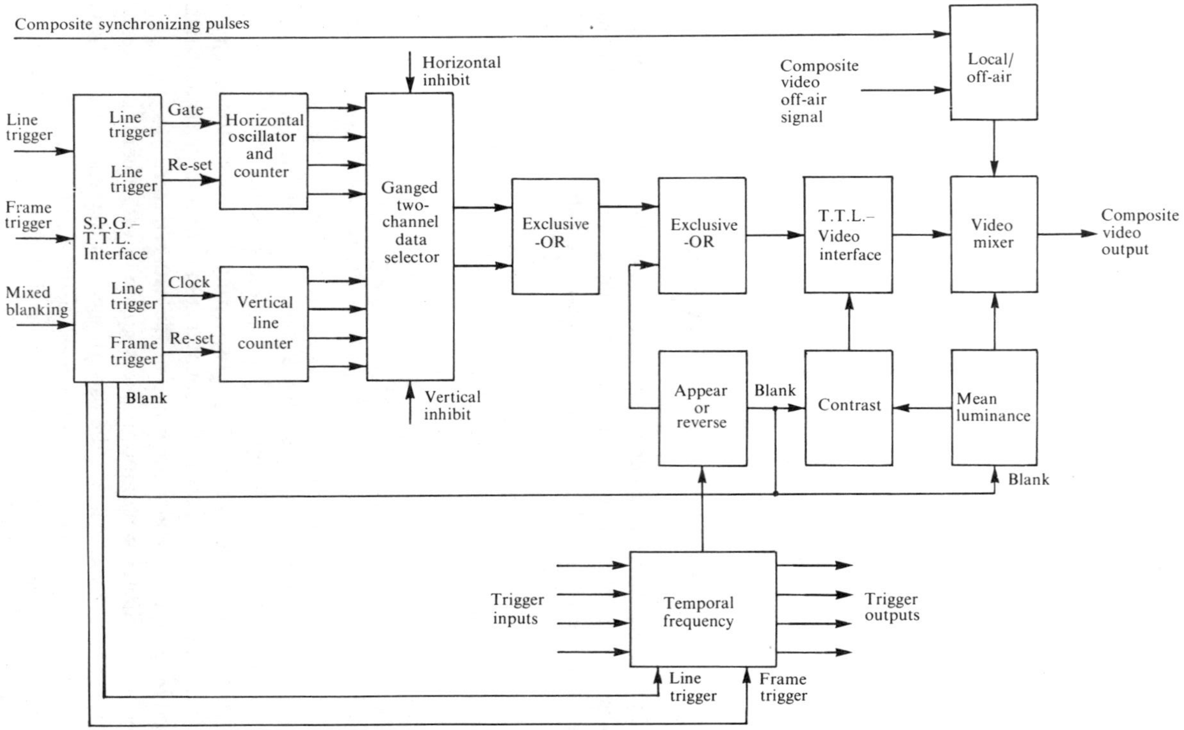

Fig. 3.2. Block diagram of TV pattern generator.

The functions described above are realized with T.T.L. circuitry. An interface translates the T.T.L. signal into a video signal, the amplitude of which is controlled to alter the contrast of the display. The mean d.c. level of the video signal is defined by the same reference voltage as is used to define the amplitude of the 100 per cent contrast ratio square wave so that luminance and contrast may be controlled independently. Blanking from the S.P.G. and temporal-frequency generator is also introduced at this point, as is the selection of the contrast in the left and right halves of the display. For a pattern-only display the video signal from the interface is mixed with composite synchronizing pulses (i.e. line and frame) from the S.P.G. If a picture signal is selected the pattern is mixed with off-air material, which already contains the required synchronizing pulses. This system can be realized in a number of ways, but all involve the use of fast logic circuits, with the attendant problems of breakthrough of switching transients.

Recording and display

VEPs were recorded using surface silver–silver chloride EEG electrodes, placed according to the International 10–20 system (Jasper 1958). The active electrode was O_Z (10 per cent above inion) the reference electrode C_Z (vertex), and P_Z (midway between active and reference) was grounded. Inter-electrode resistances were measured and kept below 5 kΩ. An S.L.E. EEG machine was used to amplify the signal and monitor the output. The time-constant was 300 ms, and the frequency response 3 dB down at 25 Hz. A CAT 400 C was used to average the VEPs. Sweep times of 250 ms or 500 ms were employed. Between 50 and 150 repetitions were averaged. Positive-going signals at the active electrode are shown by an upward deflection on the traces, which were written out on an X–Y recorder. Onset and offset waves were recorded separated by selecting the appropriate trigger polarity from the pattern generator. In a few early experiments (Figs. 3.3–3.6) a Medelec polygraph was used for amplification, recording, and display.

Results and discussion

In this section we present data illustrating the performance of the system, and examine the limitations imposed by the use of TV techniques.

Spatial frequency

Fig. 3.3 shows amplitude of pattern-reversal VEP as a function of square size. A square-edge subtense of 20′ produced maximum response. Regan (1972*a*) found that for high-definition stimuli a square-edge subtense of 10′ gave maximum response; moderate defocusing shifted the optimum size towards larger subtenses. Our findings are in agreement with his since the televisions we employed were domestic-quality colour monitors which did not give high-definition images.

Preliminary results using black and white monitors showed that a 10′ square edge subtense gave maximal response, further supporting Regan's findings. In

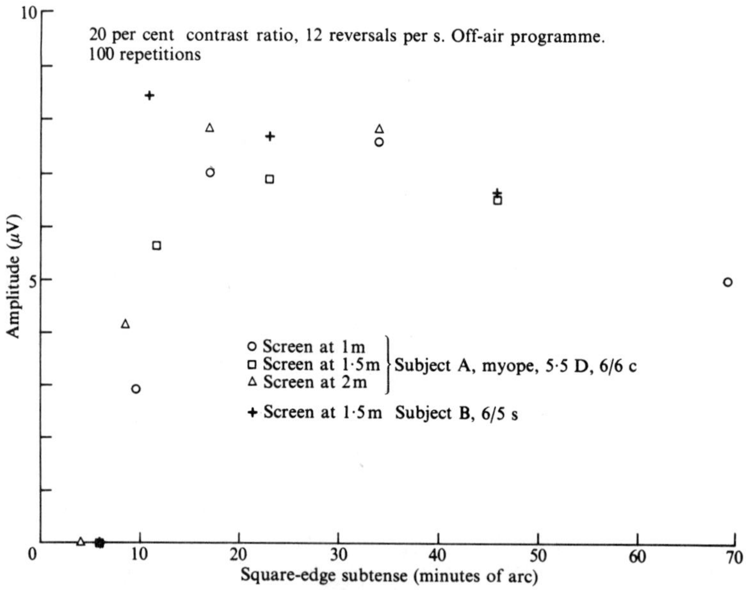

Fig. 3.3. The effect of square-edge subtense on VEP amplitude.

previously reported clinical and experimental work, however, squares of edge subtense between 30′ and 1° have been employed.

Contrast ratios

Fig. 3.4 shows the relation between VEP amplitude and contrast ratio. Contrast

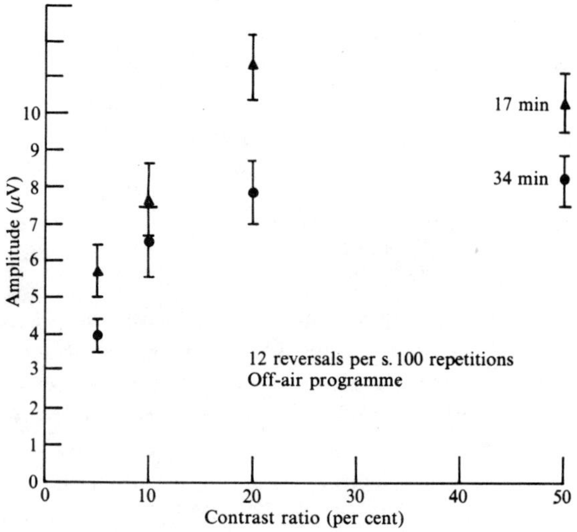

Fig. 3.4. Effect of contrast ratio on VEP amplitude, for two square-edge subtenses.

ratios of more than 20 per cent produce submaximal responses, and in some individuals there is a marked decrease at higher contrasts (Fig. 3.10): No VEPs were obtained with 2 per cent contrast.* It should be remembered that this is a nominal figure: combined with the varying contrast of the coloured off-air signal, a 2 per cent contrast checkerboard is scarcely visible. In our experience, the 20 per cent contrast ratio produces a square pattern which does not obscure the off-air signal, whilst 50 per cent contrast makes viewing difficult.

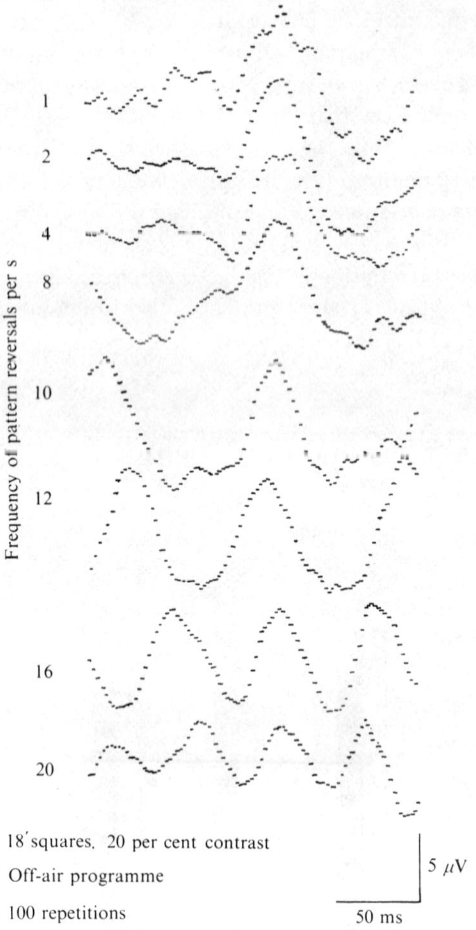

Fig. 3.5. VEP waveforms as a function of pattern-reversal rate over the range provided by the pattern generator.

*Long averaging sequences were avoided – 150 sweeps being the maximum employed – since they are unacceptable in clinical work. Very low-contrast VEPs can be obtained (Campbell and Kulikowski 1972), but only with very cooperative subjects.

Temporal frequency

Fig. 3.5 shows the VEPs elicited by a reversing checkerboard, in which the frequency of reversal varies over the full range of the temporal frequency generator. The amplitude of the VEP is only significantly reduced at a repetition rate of 20 Hz:* this reduction has been reported previously for other systems, and we conclude that this is a function of the visual system and that the TV frame rate has not imposed restrictions on the response.

Most VEPs are recorded at low repetition rates (transient VEPs), or at a rate which produces a maximal VEP (steady-state VEPs). The latter (see Fig. 3.5 at 10, 12 reversals per s) are considerably simpler in waveform and offer advantages for clinical purposes. The transition from transient to steady state is well illustrated by Fig. 3.5. It is noteworthy that the major peak of the VEP is unaffected by alteration in frequency within the range investigated, both for amplitude and time-to-peak. This finding implies a genuine time-delay between stimulus and response. This imposes severe restrictions (i.e. linear phase response over several octaves) on any description of the visual system based on phase-shifting networks.

Note that the sweep duration in Fig. 3.5 is 200 ms, and therefore that later VEP components are not visible. The effect of these late components on the first wave of the steady-state VEP is discussed below.

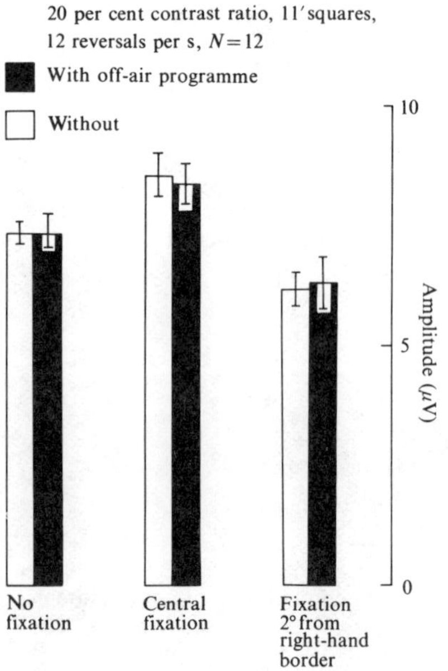

Fig. 3.6. The effect of off-air programmes and fixation on pattern-reversal VEP amplitude.

* Following common use, we write 'Hz' implying reversals (or onsets) per second.

Effect of off-air stimulus

In VEPs produced by pattern reversals, the off-air stimulus has almost no affect. Fig. 3.6 is a histogram showing this gratifying result. It can be seen that the amplitudes of the responses vary depending upon the fixation, but in the three cases illustrated (no fixation, fixation at the centre, and fixation 20° from the side of the screen) the off-air programme has no significant effect. With no fixation target a subject could comfortably watch the off-air programme without altering the recorded VEP. It seems possible that movements of the eyes about the screen centre reduce the size of the VEP, compared to maintained fixation, by altering the temporal dispersion of the response. Most of the VEP is generated by foveal and peri-foveal retina, so that even when fixation is maintained at a point 2° from the screen edge, sizeable VEPs are produced. These findings demonstrate that good full-field responses can be obtained with no fixation target, which is of importance if the device is to be used with patients or untrained subjects.

Appearance and disappearance responses are affected by the off-air programme. In some subjects, the VEP amplitude is reduced (by as much as half) by the presence of off-air material. In other subjects, the peak amplitude is not greatly affected, but the waveform of the response is changed.

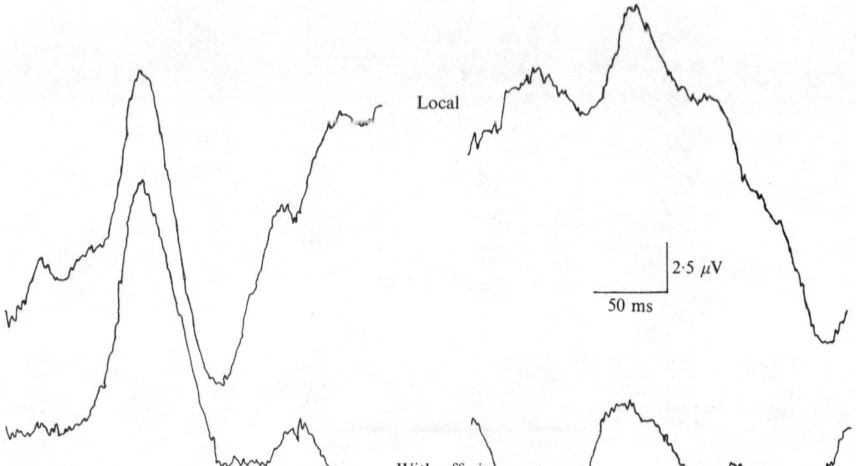

Fig. 3.7. The effect of off-air programme on the waveform of appearance and disappearance VEPs. Binocular viewing, contrast ratio 20 per cent, square-edge subtense 46′, 50 repetitions.

Fig. 3.7 demonstrates the effect of off-air signal on onset and offset VEPs. The large, slow positive onset wave (peak time ~ 250 ms) and the corresponding negative offset wave are selectively reduced. The direction of the subject's attention to the programme appears to be responsible for this modification of the response. This attenuation of the late VEP components also seems to happen in steady-state VEPs (see Fig. 3.5), where the resulting response is near sinusoidal.

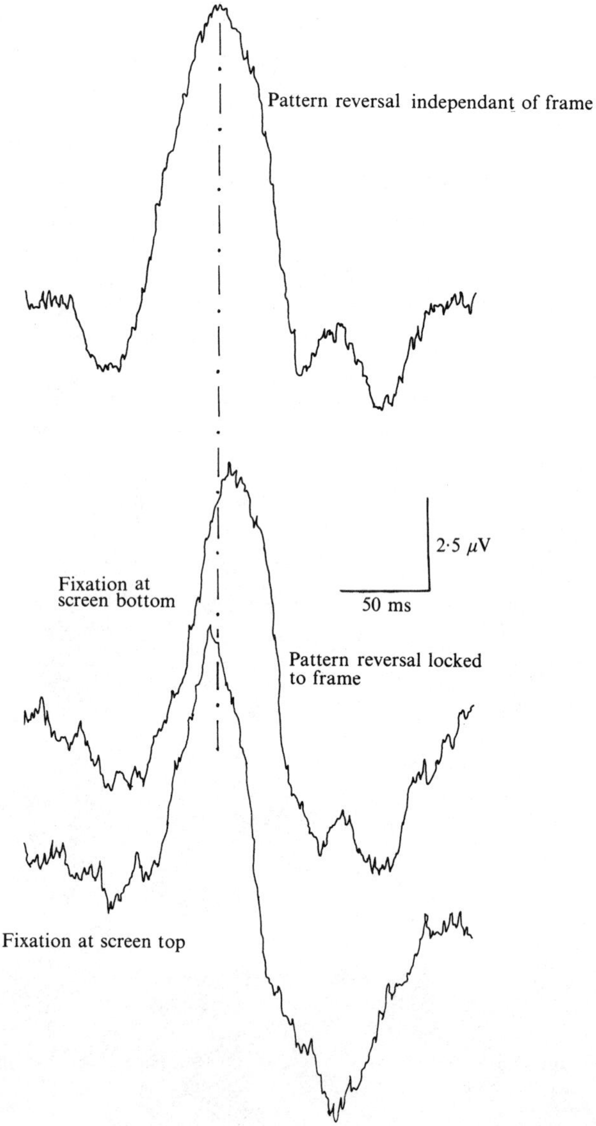

Fig. 3.8. The effect of frame locking the stimulus on the VEP. Pattern reversal rate 2 Hz. Monocular viewing, contrast ratio 50 per cent square subtense 46′, 50 repetitions. No off-air programme. The vertical line shows the displacement of the time to peak of the lower traces with respect to the uppermost trace.

Time to peak

Clinically, the most important use of VEPs is to diagnose demyelinization in the optic nerve which causes a delay in the time to peak of the VEP. In our system, the pattern change is produced by a free-running oscillator, and the pattern could therefore reverse at the moment when the raster of the TV had just passed that point on the tube face which marked the peripheral limit on the retina from which VEPs could be produced. Thus, most of an entire frame would have to elapse before the spot returned to re-illuminate that retinal region which produces the VEP. The lower traces in Fig. 3.8 demonstrate that this effect occurs while the top trace shows that this uncertainty can be removed.

In this experiment the screen was masked, leaving a strip 10 cm high, which was fixated centrally. Two types of recording were made: in the first, the reversal rate was independent of the frame; while in the second it was locked to the frame. Records were made with the mask exposing a strip at the top or bottom of the screen. For the first type of recording, the position of the strip was immaterial. However, for frame-locked recording, the time-delay depended upon the position of the strip, as illustrated. The difference between the mean times to peak, $13{\cdot}4 \pm 1{\cdot}0$ ms ($N = 20$), is exactly the time taken for the raster to write from the top strip to the bottom strip. The time to peak of the frame-independent recording is midway between those of the two frame-locked recordings. Note also, the unlocked response is less 'sharp' than the frame-locked responses. Both these effects are caused by the 'jitter' introduced into the stimulus by de-synchronizing the reversal rate from the frame rate. If the number of repetitions averaged is large, it can be assumed that the 'jitter' is random. Using a 125 ms averaging period, 400-point averaging and 100 repetitions, the standard deviation of repeated time-to-peak measurements is 1·8 ms. Thus time to peak can be measured precisely without frame-locking.

The use of frame-independent reversals is to be preferred, since it removes the need for fixation. There are further advantages: spurious averaging due to rhythmic variations in the stimulus is reduced and mains-locked artifacts are rejected by the averager, whereas frame-locking implies mains-locking.

The measurement of time to peak was undertaken with a normal population. The results are shown in the histograms of Fig. 3.9. The pattern-reversal time to peak is unaffected by the presence of an off-air signal, and the results obtained, when corrected for the average delay between the trigger pulse and the raster reaching the screen centre – a half-frame period, 10 ms – are consistent with those reported by Halliday *et al.* (1972), after deducting the 20 ms delay introduced by their pen-motor system.

The correspondence between our system and a commercially available projector/pen-motor system was checked in one subject under near-identical conditions, and the results are shown in Fig. 3.10. The TV monitor evoked larger responses than the other system, especially when the contrast ratio was reduced.

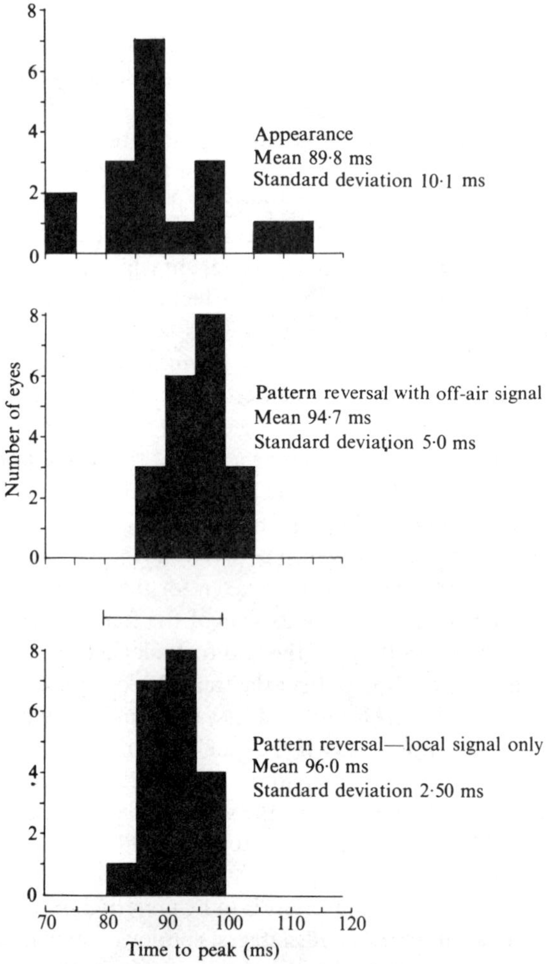

Fig. 3.9. Time to peak of VEPs of normal subjects under conditions indicated. The horizontal bar above the lowest histogram shows the corrected range of times to peak obtained by Halliday *et al.* (1972).

The estimate of time to peak was identical after subtracting the half-frame period of delay inherent in the TV system.

Additionally, the equipment has been used to estimate time to peak of responses in patients with retrobulbar neuritis. Results similar to those previously described, by ourselves and other workers, have been obtained.

Two new points are worth reporting in this context.
First, although, commonly, transient VEPs are used to obtain a time to peak measurement, it is also possible to use steady-state VEPs (see Fig. 3.5). Under these circumstances, it was found that the amplitude decayed more rapidly with

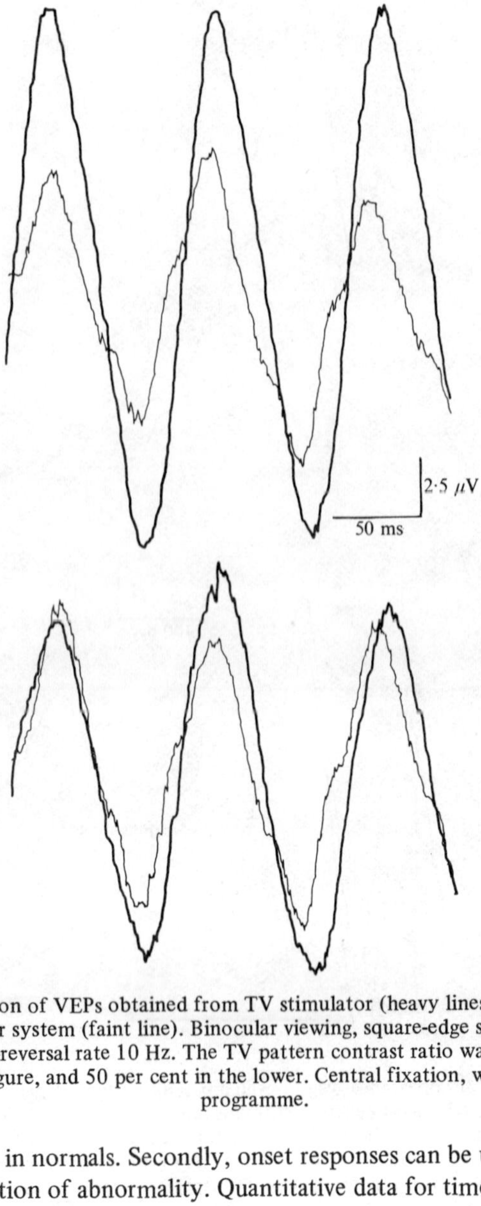

Fig. 3.10. Comparison of VEPs obtained from TV stimulator (heavy lines) and a commercial projector/pen-motor system (faint line). Binocular viewing, square-edge subtense 24′, 100 repetitions. Pattern-reversal rate 10 Hz. The TV pattern contrast ratio was 20 per cent in the upper part of the figure, and 50 per cent in the lower. Central fixation, without off-air programme.

reversal rate than in normals. Secondly, onset responses can be used to obtain a qualitative indication of abnormality. Quantitative data for time to peak of onset responses without off-air signal is shown in Fig. 3.9 for normal subjects. The standard deviation is four times that for pattern reversals, under the same conditions, and although in cases of optic nerve demyelinization there are delays in the time to peak of appearance responses (Fig. 3.11), pattern reversals will give more accurate measurements. On the other hand, the responses in Fig. 3.11

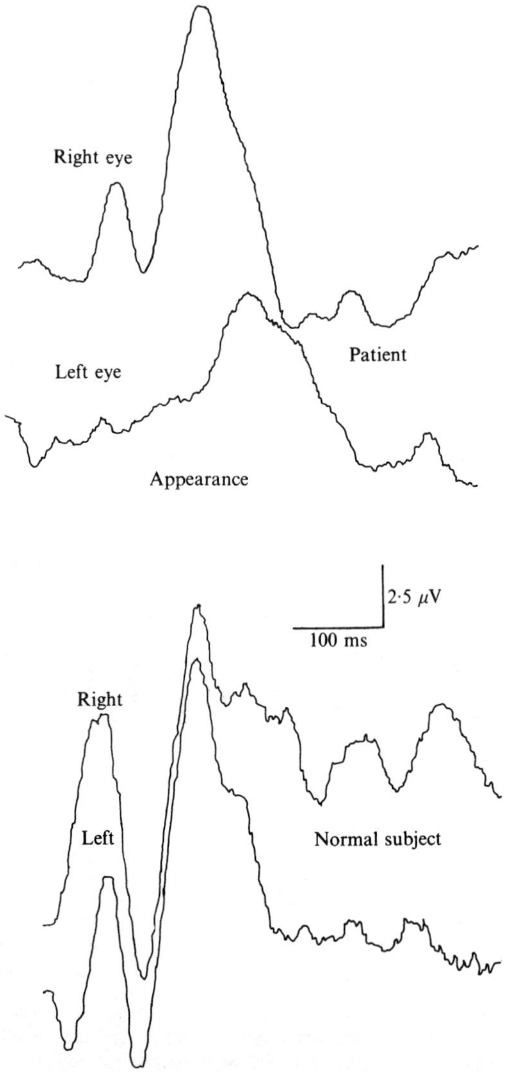

Fig. 3.11. Comparison of appearance responses in a patient with multiple sclerosis with a normal subject. Contrast ratio 50 per cent, stimulus rate 1 Hz, 100 repetitions. No off-air signal, square-edge subtense 46′. The patient was a female aged 45, history 9 years, beginning with one acute attack of retrobulbar neuritis in her left eye. Present visual acuity, right 6/9, left 6/18. No scotomata demonstrable. Multiple long tract and cerebellar signs.

illustrate the grossly abnormal waveforms obtained in this condition. The response is dispersed in time, and the initial peak is selectively depressed. This result, to be reported in detail elsewhere, indicates that changes in the VEP may be mediated by the selective loss of rapidly conducting fibres in the optic pathway.

Centre-off

Fig. 3.12 shows that when VEPs are evoked by pattern reversal and a progressively larger area of the central field is blanked, the response amplitude shows a corresponding decline. This confirms previous work which has shown that peripheral retina produces little of the VEP. If smaller squares are used, the reduction of VEP amplitude with blanking is enhanced.

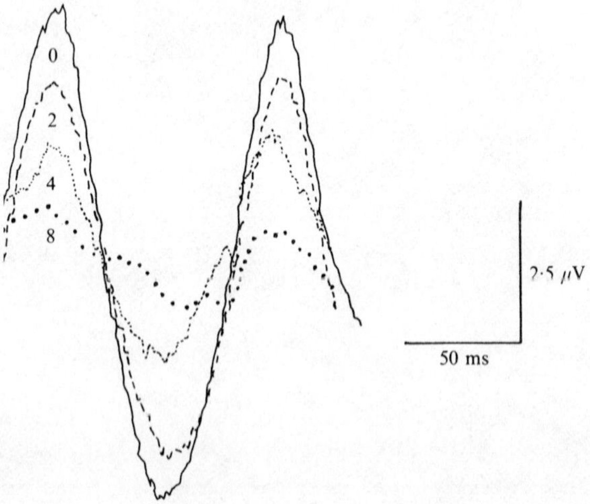

Fig. 3.12. Effect of blanking the pattern in the centre of the screen on VEP amplitude. Central fixation, reversal rate 10 Hz, 50 per cent contrast ratio, no off-air signal, square-edge subtense 46′. The numbers indicate the angular subtense, in degrees, of the vertical strip blanked.

Quadrantic and half-field stimulation

Fig. 3.13 shows VEPs obtained from four simultaneous independent stimuli which occupy the quadrants of the screen. The subject viewed monocularly and fixated centrally. The responses are distinguishable because the reversal in each quadrant were independently controlled. In this experiment, the responses were recorded consecutively, due to the limitations of the averager employed; with four independent asynchronous averager channels, these four responses could be obtained simultaneously from one set of electrodes. Note that the responses differ in size and that the average amplitude is less than in other figures.

Fig. 3.14 shows responses to left and right half-fields. In this figure, reversal rate of the half field being tested was 10 Hz while the fellow half-field was stimulated at 9 Hz. The third trace shows the full-field response at a reversal rate of 10 Hz. On the simplest linear theory, the response would be the sum of the two half-field responses. In practice it is larger, suggesting interactions between the two half-fields.

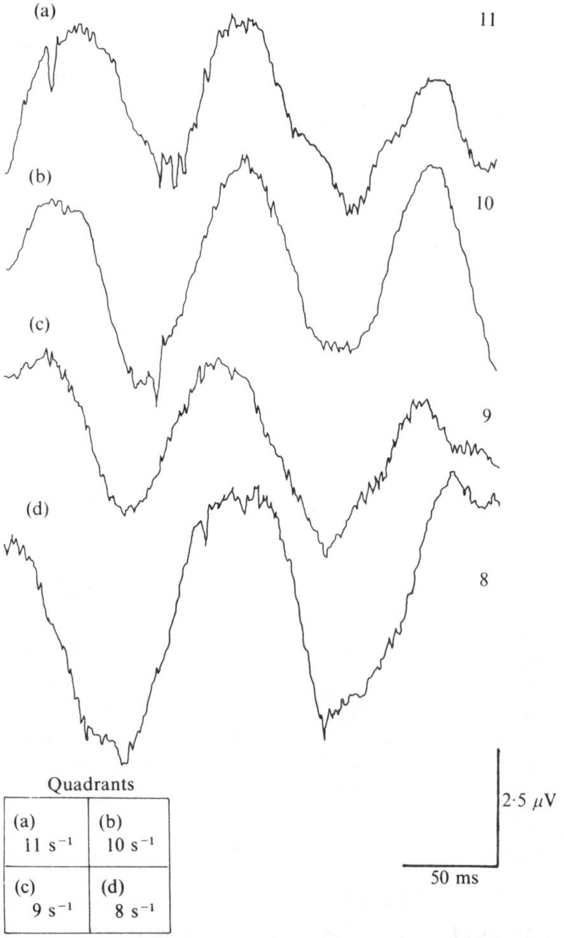

Fig. 3.13. Records obtained with quadrantic stimulation. The inset shows the rates of pattern reversal in the respective quadrants. Central fixation with the right eye. Square subtense 46′. Contrast 50 per cent. No off-air signal.

Fig. 3.15 shows that the split-field technique is clinically useful. The patient suffered a blackout and following this an altitudinal field defect developed, as demonstrated by the fields measured on a Goldmann perimeter. The field defect was unilateral, and the responses from the fellow eye were used for comparison. Whole field, and upper and lower half-fields were tested with a reversal rate of 7 Hz. Note that even in the unaffected eye, upper and lower half-fields do not produce similar responses. No significant response is elicited from the lower half-field of the affected eye, consistent with the loss of visual field. Thus even in a patient with considerable loss of field and visual acuity, fixation is sufficient for VEP field testing.

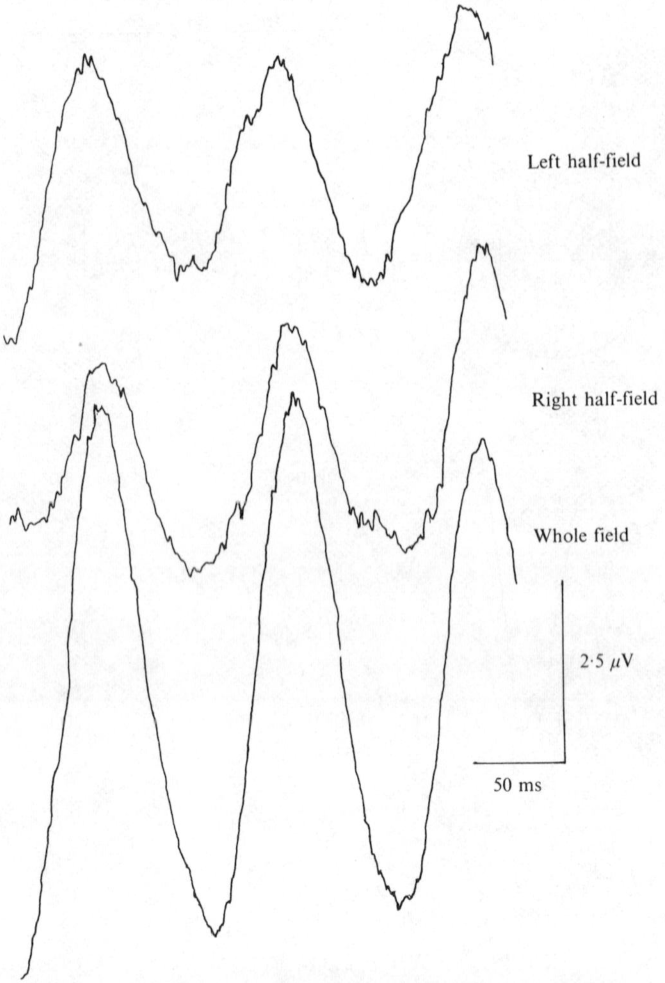

Fig. 3.14. Comparison of whole-field and half-field stimulation. Square-edge subtense 46′, 20 per cent contrast ratio, central fixation, left eye. Reversal rate of whole field, or of the half-field being tested was 10 Hz, while the fellow half-field was stimulated at 9 Hz.

General appraisal

After 6 months of clinical trials, based on three models of the pattern generator, we are satisfied that our TV system is extremely reliable and that the results obtained are meaningful and repeatable. In view of the favourable reactions to the stimulators from technicians and patients, our earlier polaroid apparatus has been abandoned. The virtues of the new system are most evident in testing difficult patients. The familiarity of the TV screen is reassuring, and the broadcast material (complete with sound) is both compelling and relaxing.

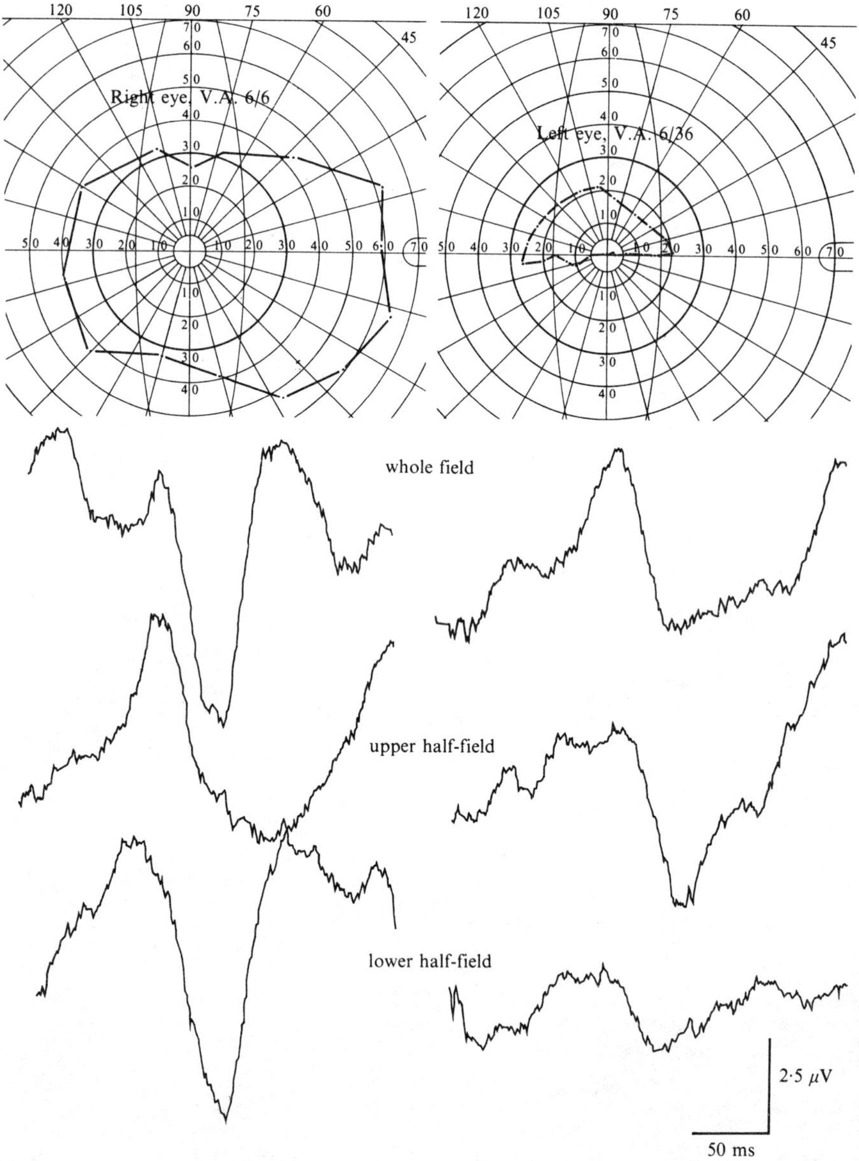

Fig. 3.15. VEPs from a patient with an altitudinal field defect. The records above are copies of fields obtained with a Goldmann perimeter. Pattern-reversal rate 7 Hz, 20 per cent contrast ratio, square-edge subtense 46′, no off-air signal. The half-field not being tested was stimulated at 4 Hz. The patient attempted to fix the horizontal border between the two half-fields. Vision deteriorated over a few days, following transient loss of consciousness.

Some of the new facilities offered by our pattern generator were designed to fulfil known needs: e.g. quadrantic displays can be used to detect abnormal VEPs in patients with ocular hypertension, who may go on to develop glaucomatous field defects; half-field displays should enable hononymous and bi-temporal hemianopias to be as easily characterized as altitudinal field defects; the use of small squares and low contrast ratios enables us to provide better estimates of visual acuity. The inclusion of other facilities was more speculative, but is yielding interesting preliminary results. The relative complexity of the appearance and disappearance responses may enable more subtle analysis of complex visual functions. Independent control of contrast can provide a convenient measure of the depth of suppression in amblyopia, and interactions in binocular vision.

Looking further to the future, the basic TV system can be expanded for other uses. Colour vision can be tested, both by the production of checkerboards in which colour contrast reversals occur, for VEP tests, and by quantifying colour-matching anomalies. Both these tests can be implemented by the addition of standard studio equipment to the basic pattern generator. More complex stimuli, such as those required in psychological research, can also be produced, and the all-electronic design of the system will permit parameter control by computer program.

Acknowledgements

We would like to thank Dr. U. B. Sheorey for helpful discussions and assistance with some of the experiments, and Mr. J. Chalker and Dr. J. Cook for assistance in construction of equipment, and Ms. C. Szymonowicz for technical assistance. The equipment described in this Chapter is available from Medelec Ltd.

This work was assisted by an MRC grant.

4. Fourier analysis of evoked potentials; some methods based on Fourier analysis

D. REGAN

Department of Communication, University of Keele

Transient and steady-state VEPs

Although averaged transient VEPs are much the more familiar, there is a growing body of reports that deal with steady-state VEPs. It should be said right away that, in practice, each approach has its own special advantages and disadvantages. Also, transient and steady-state VEPs offer complementary insights into brain function.

The term 'steady-state' was originally introduced into EP analysis by analogy with electrical-engineering usage (Regan 1966*a*). The distinction between steady-state VEPs and transient VEPs can be understood as follows. When a system (e.g. a circuit) receives an input (e.g. a pulse or step) the system gives an initial response that dies away, maybe quite quickly. This disturbance is the system's 'transient' response. An important way of describing the system's behaviour is by plotting the amplitude of the transient response versus time.

In contrast, when the same system is fed with a long train of repetitive stimuli (e.g. a long train of sine waves) and given time to settle down, the output of the system becomes a long train of identical repetitive waveforms (steady-state response). The system can now be described in terms of two graphs, namely (1) response amplitude/input amplitude versus input frequency, and (2) response phase versus input frequency.*

For a simple linear system the two descriptions (transient and steady-state) are exactly equivalent. However for a nonlinear system the two descriptions may give different, complementary information. Since those brain functions that underlie VEPs are very nonlinear in several ways, it is not surprising that transient and steady-state VEPs should provide different insights into brain function. For example, steady-state VEPs do not seem much affected by attention, though this is a well-documented effect for transient VEPs. Transient and steady-state VEPs also seem to reveal different features of demyelinating disease (Regan, Milner, and

Visual evoked potentials in man: new developments (ed. J. E. Desmedt), pp. 110–17. Clarendon Press, Oxford 1977.

*For a linear system the response waveform is a sine wave, and only two graphs are required to describe the system. For a nonlinear system, the output waveform may not be a sine wave, but it is equivalent to the sum of several sine waves (harmonics), in which case at least one pair of graphs is needed for each harmonic.

Heron, Chapter 29 of this book). It may often pay to use both approaches together. *Fourier analysis is appropriate with rapidly repetitive stimulation, whereas averaging is appropriate for transient VEPs.* The most familiar way of handling transient VEPs is to average, display in terms of amplitude versus time, and then analyse the waveform into several components on the basis of time (latency). On the other hand, a long train of rapidly repeated stimuli gives a long train of similar VEP waveforms, none of which can be related to a particular stimulus cycle. Therefore analysis in terms of time is not appropriate. However if certain conditions are met (see below), any repetitive waveform of frequency F Hz can be completely described as the sum of several sine waves called harmonics. Their frequencies are F, $2F$, $3F$, $4F$ etc. Thus, in one way harmonic components are to steady-state VEPs what 'components' are to transient VEPs. A Fourier analyser automatically splits up the VEP waveform into its constituent harmonic components and describes each component by specifying its amplitude and phase.

If the stimulus-repetition frequency is sufficiently high in relation to the frequency response of the sensory system being studied, then only a few harmonics may suffice to give an approximate description of the VEP. For example, flicker frequencies exceeding 7 Hz or so elicit VEPs that can be adequately described by four harmonics and often by only two harmonics (Regan 1968*a*); pattern-reversal frequencies exceeding 5 Hz or so give VEPs that can usually be adequately described by two harmonics (Regan 1973*a*). Thus, by using rapidly repetitive stimulation of F Hz the experimenter forces the VEP entirely into a few narrow frequency bands centred on F Hz, $2F$ Hz, etc. Since, for carefully controlled stimulation, a Fourier analyser whose bandpass is as narrow as 0·001 Hz can record a similar VEP amplitude to that recorded by a wide-bandwidth averager (Regan 1970*a*, 1972*b*, p. 256), VEP power may be restricted to very narrow frequency bands not much wider than 0·001 Hz.

Conditions for validity of Fourier analysis method

One of the conditions that must be met if Fourier analysis is to be an appropriate or even a valid means of analysing VEPs is that an unvarying repetitive stimulus must give a repetitive VEP waveform whose phase and amplitude remain constant from moment to moment. It should be noted that the steady-state condition is not established until some time has elapsed after the onset of repetitive stimulation (Tweel 1964; Regan 1966*a*). By using one form of Fourier analyser this 'stationarity' of the response can be experimentally checked, since the analyser outputs VEP amplitude and phase in the form of a 'running average'. Fig. 4.1(b) illustrates the running-average output. By careful stimulus control, the moment-to-moment values of VEP latency can be held constant to about ± 1 ms in 100 ms and amplitude to better than ±6 per cent over some minutes (Regan 1966*a*, 1972*b*). Conversely, the running-average display makes any deficiencies in stimulus control very evident (e.g. variations of the eye's fixation or accommodation).

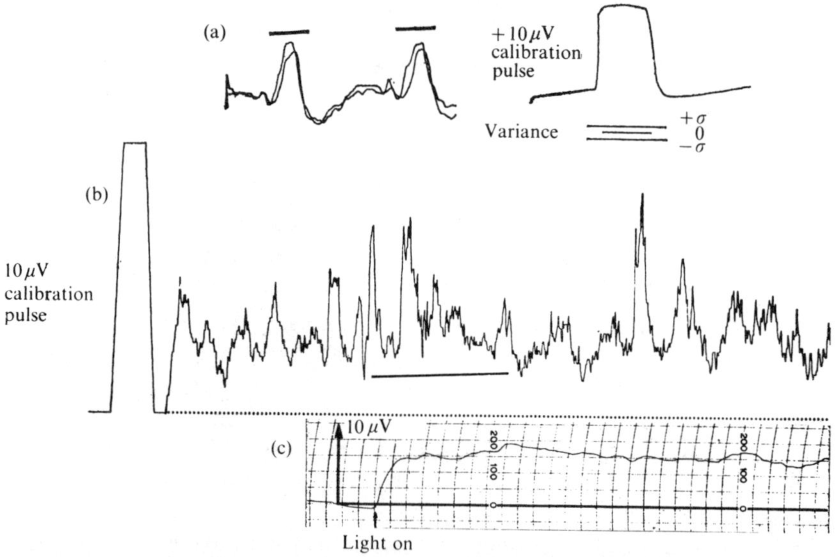

Fig. 4.1. (a) VEP recorded while the subject viewed a 4° pattern of 13′ checks that reversed 6 times per s. Average of 200 sweeps. Trace length, 311 ms. Two traces are shown but a better impression of variability is given by the standard deviation of mean amplitude. Note that about one third of all averages would fall outside even these limits. Positivity records upwards.

(b) and (c) Effect of bandwidth of recording apparatus on apparent variability of VEPs. (b), running average of summed VEP. A digital computer integrated the EEG for a 50 ms period centred on a latency of 90 ms after each stimulus. The integration period is shown by black bars above averages in (a). A running average was formed of a block of 16 successive responses. The system's response time is shown by calibration with a square 10 μV pulse. (c) Running average of VEP analysed by the analog Fourier analyser. The stimulus conditions and subject were as in (a). The moment-to-moment variability is very small, much less than in (a), showing that most of the variability in (a) was not due to the VEP but to noise passing through the wider-bandwidth analysing apparatus. The recording period was 320 s in (a) and 430 s in (b). The computer program used to obtain records was written by J. Axford (b) and (c) (from Regan (1972)).

Advantages of Fourier analysis compared with straightforward averaging

1. When rapidly repetitive stimulation is used, the resulting averaged VEP waveform may be uninterpretable (or almost so) since it is made up of, for example, two or more harmonic components whose properties are quite different (Regan 1970*a*, and see Regan, Fig. 11.9 of this book).

Two such components add to give an averaged waveform whose shape and peak-to-peak amplitude depends on the phase difference between the two components. Since this relative phase may be arbitrary, the amplitude and shape of the resulting averaged waveform may have little meaning. For the same reason, the latency to peak of the averaged waveform may also be meaningless. Furthermore, one harmonic may be masked by another larger (but possibly less interesting) harmonic. In general, therefore, measurements of the amplitudes and atencies of averaged steady-state VEP waveforms have little value unless VEP hanges are very large.

However, in some situations the average waveform may be approximately nusoidal, and useful estimates of phase and amplitude may be obtained (Van der 'weel and Lunel 1965). Again, waveforms may approximate sine waves when timulus frequency is sufficiently high since the high-frequency attenuation of the rain itself ensures a sine wave response. It is unnecessarily restricting, though, and ıay even give misleading results to confine measurements to high-stimulus requencies. This is because steady-state VEPs of low frequency can have quite ifferent properties to high-frequency VEPs (Regan, Chapter 11 of this book).

In contrast, EP interpretation may be straightforward when a Fourier analyser s used instead of an averager. The Fourier analyser isolates and separately neasures the different harmonic components so that their different properties can asily be distinguished. Fig. 1 in Regan (1970*a*) illustrates this point (see also Regan, Chapter 11 of this book). With ordinary care, and providing signal-to-noise atio is reasonable, latency can be measured to an accuracy of roughly 4 ms tandard deviation (Regan 1966*a*) (though latency *differences* can be measured to vithin 1 ms (Regan 1970*a*)). Given reasonable signal-to-noise, amplitude can be neasured to about 10–20 per cent standard deviation (Regan 1968*a*, 1970*a*). This recision compares favourably with the everyday precision of measuring averaged ransient VEPs.

2. A second advantage of Fourier analysis is that the 'running-average' presentation of VEP data can provide feedback to the experimenter so that when ıe changes the stimulus he knows almost immediately how the VEP is affected (Regan 1966*a*, 1968*b*, 1973*b*). Additionally, it is the running-average output of lata that makes possible the methods based on Fourier analysis described in the next section.

3. A Fourier analyser can often record a VEP in much less time than an averager.

4. A Fourier analyser can measure smaller signals with precision (e.g. 0·2 μV in 50 μV of noise within a 30 s recording period (Regan 1970*a*, Fig. 3)).

5. A Fourier analyser is less disturbed by certain kinds of noise (e.g. alpha activity). This is because the stimulus-repetition frequency (F Hz) can be chosen so that all harmonics (F Hz, $2F$ Hz, etc.) are more than about 1 Hz removed from the alpha frequency. The narrow bandwidth of the analyser then renders it almost immune to alpha noise (Fig. 4.1 (b) and (c); Regan 1966*a*, 1973*a*).

6. The relation between spontaneous EEG activity and the steady-state VEP can be investigated moment by moment. For example, it is not difficult to investigate whether the occurrence of a burst of alpha activity causes the VEP amplitude to change momentarily (Regan 1966*a*).

Disadvantages of Fourier analysis

1. A Fourier analyser is not appropriate for recording transient VEPs.

2. The reason that a Fourier analyser can be faster than an averager is that it 'sees' less information than an averager. In other words it exchanges bandwidth for speed. This carries the danger that a Fourier analyser, operated alone, might be blind to important information.

(Information missed by a Fourier analyser might be either stimulus locked, or not locked to the stimulus. Stimulus-locked VEP components might be located at harmonic frequencies other than that to which the Fourier analyser is set. This possibility can be guarded against by using an averager in parallel with a Fourier analyser; a practical procedure is to rely on an averager for coarse scans, reserving the Fourier analyser for precise quantitative measurements.

Information not locked to the stimulus would be missed by both averager and Fourier analyser but could be picked up by a method that examined a broad frequency range. This can be done in a number of ways. For example, banks of narrow-band filters have long been used to carry out such a wide-ranging (but necessarily coarse) analysis of the EEG. Alternatively a small digital computer using the fast Fourier transform would serve this purpose. It should be noted however that these methods give amplitude information only and do not indicate whether the stimulus organizes the relative phasing of EEG frequency components. There is in any case little evidence so far available that repetitive visual stimuli have any consistent effect on EEG power at other than harmonic frequencies (apart from some reduction of alpha activity).)

3. Latency cannot be measured unequivocally by recording the VEP for a single stimulus frequency, since EP phase can be markedly affected by factors other than latency. In other words the simple equation $\tau = \theta/360F$ (where τ = latency, θ = phase, and F = frequency) is not generally valid for EPs.*

A better estimate can be obtained by plotting VEP phase versus frequency over a range of frequencies. If the plot is a straight line the 'apparent latency' (Regan 1966*a*) can be calculated from its slope as follows: $\tau' = \text{slope}/360$ (where τ' = apparent latency and slope is in degrees per Hz). However, it should be noted that this apparent latency is not necessarily the same as the real delay (Regan 1972, p. 77).

Methods based on Fourier analysis

The multiple-stimulus method

The very narrow bandwidth of a Fourier analyser is the basis of the 'multiple-stimulus' method (Regan and Cartwright 1970; Cartwright and Regan 1974). In one variant of this method several (e.g. four) different retinal sites are stimulated at slightly different frequencies (F_1, F_2, F_3, and F_4 Hz). The frequencies are so

*For example, curvature of the amplitude versus frequency plot affects phase. Also, a plot of phase versus frequency can be shifted bodily without affecting either latency or the amplitude versus frequency plot (see Regan, Milner and Heron, Chapter 29 of this book). Though this is difficult to explain, it clearly invalidates the simple $\tau = \theta/360F$ equation.

close (e.g. 0·15 Hz apart) that they are identical so far as the VEP is concerned. The EEG is analysed by four parallel Fourier analysers, one locked to F_1 Hz another to F_2 Hz, and so on. The Fourier analysers can easily separate the four stimulus frequencies. In this way four different VEPs are simultaneously recorded from each electrode derivation.

A second variant of the multiple-stimulus method is to superpose on the same retinal site several (e.g. three) stimuli, identical in all respects except that their repetition frequencies differ. For example, three patches of light, one modulated at F_1 Hz, one at F_2 Hz, and one at F_3 Hz may be superposed on the same retinal area. Again the various VEPs may be simultaneously recorded by several (here three) Fourier analysers operating in parallel. VEP latency can be estimated from the three values of VEP phase.

The major advantage of the multiple stimulus method is that the *relationships* between the several VEPs can be measured more precisely, more quickly, and with less disturbance from VEP variability than when the VEPs are measured separately. The explanation for this empirical finding seems to be that to a large extent the simultaneously recorded VEPs vary together (Regan and Cartwright 1970).

This method is not restricted to visual work; in principle it is applicable to auditory and somato-sensory EP recording and to multiple-modality studies.

Averaging graphs rather than averaging points

The aim of many VEP experiments is to obtain a graph – e.g. a plot of VEP amplitude versus the size of checks in a checkerboard stimulus pattern. Such a graph is usually obtained by separately averaging VEPs for each of several stimulus check sizes. A curve through these separate points gives the required graph. There is an alternative way of obtaining the required VEP graph considerably more rapidly and precisely, and with less disturbance from certain types of noise than the method described above. If the experimenter is more interested in the shape of the graph than in absolute VEP measurements (as he often is), then he may prefer this alternative method, in which he rapidly samples the whole graph, repeats this procedure several times, then averages the samples. The application of this method to rapidly obtaining a graph of VEP amplitude versus stimulus check size for an amblyopic eye is discussed in Regan (Chapter 24 of this book). This method offers a means of more rapidly and precisely determining the shapes of graphs of VEP amplitude or phase versus a wide range of visual and other stimulus parameters.

VEP feed-back

The Fourier analyser enables a subject to be placed inside a feed-back loop so that his VEPs directly control the stimulus (Regan 1975*b*).

The stimulus can be controlled in a graded or continuous manner by virtue of the running-average output of VEP data. Compared with conventional methods this technique has the advantage of speed. Since a short recording procedure minimizes the effects both of VEP variability and of progressive changes in the VEP, this method has the further advantage of improved precision.

One application of VEP feed-back is to obtain directly the sensitivity of the VEP to a given stimulus. The force of this point is that VEP sensitivity is often more informative than VEP amplitude. In the feed-back procedure the experimenter chooses a criterion level for the VEP (e.g. 3 μV) and sets the feed-back device to this value, whereupon the VEP automatically controls the stimulus so as to maintainVEP amplitude constant at 3 μV. An example of this technique described in Regan (Fig. 11.7 of this book) is the measurement of action spectra for the red and green channels of pattern vision. The feed-back method is particularly speedy in this application. Each point in Fig. 11.8 (this book, p. 242) was measured in roughly 1 min using feed-back. About 10–20 min was needed for one point when the conventional method was used of first plotting graphs of VEP amplitude versus stimulus intensity, then reading from the graphs the stimulus intensity that gave the criterion response. In this example the 10–20-fold reduction in experimental duration meant that an action spectrum could be measured in a single experimental session rather than over several days. This gave usefully increased precision.

In principle the VEP feed-back method offers improvements in speed and precision when determining VEP sensitivity to a wide range of visual and other stimulus parameters.

Practical devices

Digital computers have been used to Fourier analyse the EEG in many laboratories. On the other hand, a practical analog Fourier analyser can be used independently of a digital computer, is simple to construct, and is much cheaper than an averager (e.g. Regan 1966*a*). A version that uses more recently available components is illustrated in Fig. 4.2. An effective and cheap analyser requires only the amplifier A, the multipliers M, the filters F_1, F_2, and a two-channel recording device (not shown). This recorder, for example a two-pen recording potentiometer, is fed by

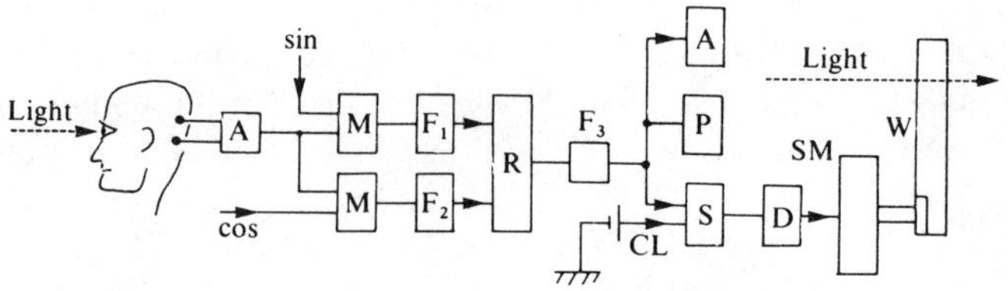

Fig. 4.2. Simple Fourier analyser and apparatus for VEP feed-back. A, EEG amplifier; M, multiplier (e.g. Burr Brown model 4097/25); F_1, F_2, F_3, low-pass filters (e.g. three-stage passive filters with time-constant adjustable in six steps between about 0·1 s and 3 s per stage); R, device for computing $(x^2 + y^2)$ where x and y are its inputs (e.g. Teledyne Philbrick model 4352); A, averager; P, recording potentiometer; S, summing amplifier; D, servomotor drive unit; SM, servomotor; W, neutral density wedge.

the outputs of F_1 and F_2. The sine and cosine waves are conveniently supplied from a two-phase oscillator that also drives the stimulator. If second-harmonic analysis is required, a frequency divider can be interposed between the oscillator and stimulator.

The multipliers should be supplied with multiturn potentiometers for all trims and are best mounted in a draught-proof box in order to minimize temperature drift. It is advisable to allow the multipliers to warm up for 10 min or so and then zero them before any experiment.

Fig. 4.2 also shows how this basic analyser can be extended so as to give a direct indication of EP amplitude. In this arrangement filters F_1 and F_2 feed module R whose output is filtered by F_3 before passing to recording potentiometer P. The choice of filter time constants between F_3 and (F_1, F_2) is important. If (F_1, F_2) is larger, then the multiplier's noise output is comparatively small, but the analyser records a spurious amplitude change when signal phase is abruptly changed. This artifact is comparatively small when most of the filtering is done by F_3, but then the multiplier's noise level is comparatively high. The filter time-constants must be selected empirically, on the basis of the signal-to-noise level and whether signal phase is likely to change appreciably during a recording. The basic Fourier analyser described above is considerably more resistant to noise and can measure smaller VEPs than when the module R is added. This is because the basic analyser can use VEP phase and the constancy of VEP phase to recognize and distinguish VEP from noise.

The whole of Fig. 4.2 gives one example of the way in which VEP amplitude can control the stimulus (VEP feed-back mode). The output of F_3 is proportional to VEP amplitude. This is compared with a pre-set reference voltage CL in the summing amplifier S. If VEP amplitude is greater than the criterion level CL, then the output of S is (say) positive and the servomotor SM drives the neutral density wedge W so as to decrease stimulus intensity. On the other hand, if VEP amplitude is less than the criterion level, then the output of S is negative and the servomotor drives the wedge in the opposite direction so as to increase stimulus intensity.

Part 2 Visual evoked potentials to pattern, colour, and saccadic eye movements in normal man

5. The topography of the pattern-evoked potential

A. M. HALLIDAY, G. BARRETT, E. HALLIDAY, and W. F. MICHAEL
Institute of Neurology, National Hospital, London

The potential field of the occipital response to a pattern stimulus varies significantly according to the part of the visual field stimulated. For instance, using an ear reference, there is a striking reversal of polarity of at least one major component at about 100 ms, comparing the upper and lower field responses (Figs. 5.1 and 5.2, upper records). There are also important differences in the distribution and polarity of the voltage field in the sagittal and trans-occipital planes, not only between upper and lower field stimulation, but between stimulation of the left and right half fields and their constituent octants. This is equally true of the responses to pattern reversal (Halliday and Michael 1970, 1972; Michael and Halliday 1971; Halliday 1972*a*) and pattern onset (Jeffreys 1969, 1971*b*; Lesèvre 1973; Lesèvre and Rémond 1972). All these studies employed a black-and-white checkerboard stimulus. The similarity of the polarity reversal between upper and lower field responses for pattern onset and pattern reversal is all the more striking because the corresponding components have opposite polarities for these two types of pattern response, even when the same area of retina is being stimulated. For lower-field stimuli, for instance, there is a prominent surface negative wave at about 100 ms in the response to pattern onset, and a surface positive wave at the same latency in the response to pattern reversal. These components appear with reversed polarity following upper-field stimuli.

Studies of the potential field on the head ideally demand simultaneous recording and averaging from a large number of electrodes. Not only the electrode placement but also the use of monopolar or bipolar modes and the choice of reference significantly affect the outcome. Common to all three studies cited is the use of an ear reference for monopolar recording, although the study by Lesèvre and Rémond has been mainly concerned with the potential gradient recorded from two bipolar chains of electrodes, one arranged longitudinally along the midline and the other placed transversely across the occipital region.

Michael and Halliday (1971) have shown conclusively, however, that the ear reference is far from indifferent in recording the pattern evoked response. Moreover, it affects differentially the responses from upper and lower fields. Changing from

Visual evoked potentials in man: new developments (ed. J. E. Desmedt), pp. 121–133. Clarendon Press, Oxford 1977.

an ear reference (upper records) to a mid-frontal reference (lower records) has little effect on the lower-field response (Fig. 5.1), but profoundly alters both the polarity and distribution of the response to upper-field stimulation (Fig. 5.2).

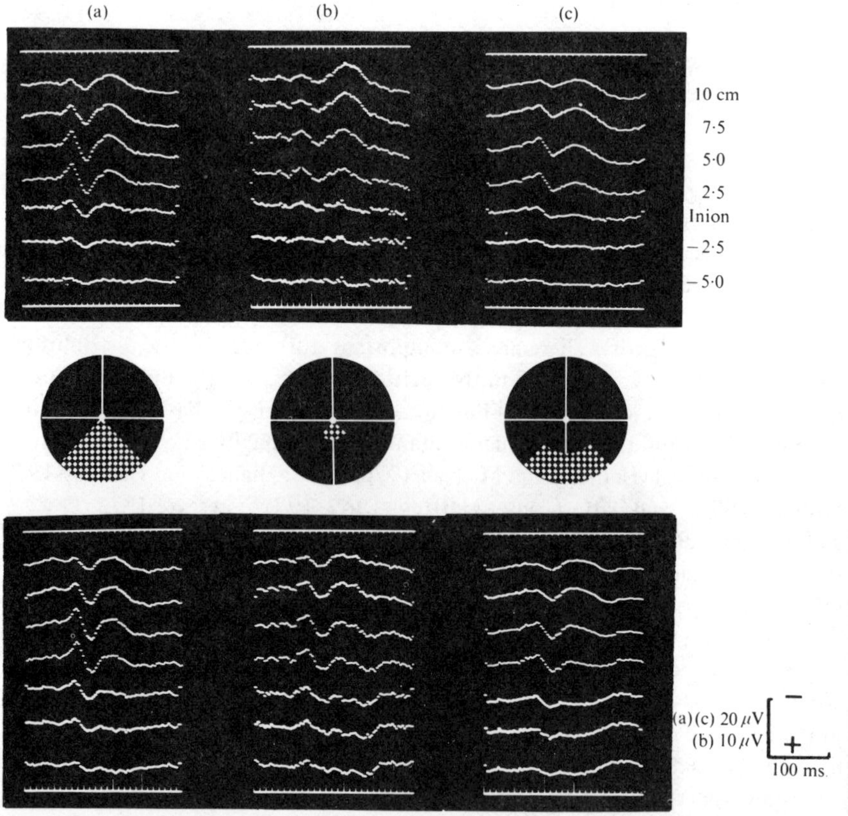

Fig. 5.1. Responses to a reversing checkerboard stimulus of 50′ squares presented in different segments of the lower visual field. (a) from 0° to 8° out from the fixation point; (b) for the central 2°; (c) from 4° to 8° out from the fixation point. The stimulus is confined to the two octants of the field immediately adjoining the lower vertical meridian. The *upper* three records are recorded with a two-ear reference and the *lower* three records with a mid-frontal reference. Recordings are for a chain of midline electrodes whose distances above and below the inion are shown on the right as plus and minus figures. Note that the records for the central stimulus are at twice the gain. Only minimal differences are found between the recordings with the two references. Compare the responses to upper field stimuli recorded in the same way in Fig. 5.2. (From Michael and Halliday 1971.)

Similar changes are to be seen in the group data obtained from seven healthy individuals (Figs. 5.3 and 5.4). This demonstrates that the upper- and lower-field generators are spatially distinct and quite widely separated. The evidence suggests that both the position and the orientation of the generator areas are important.

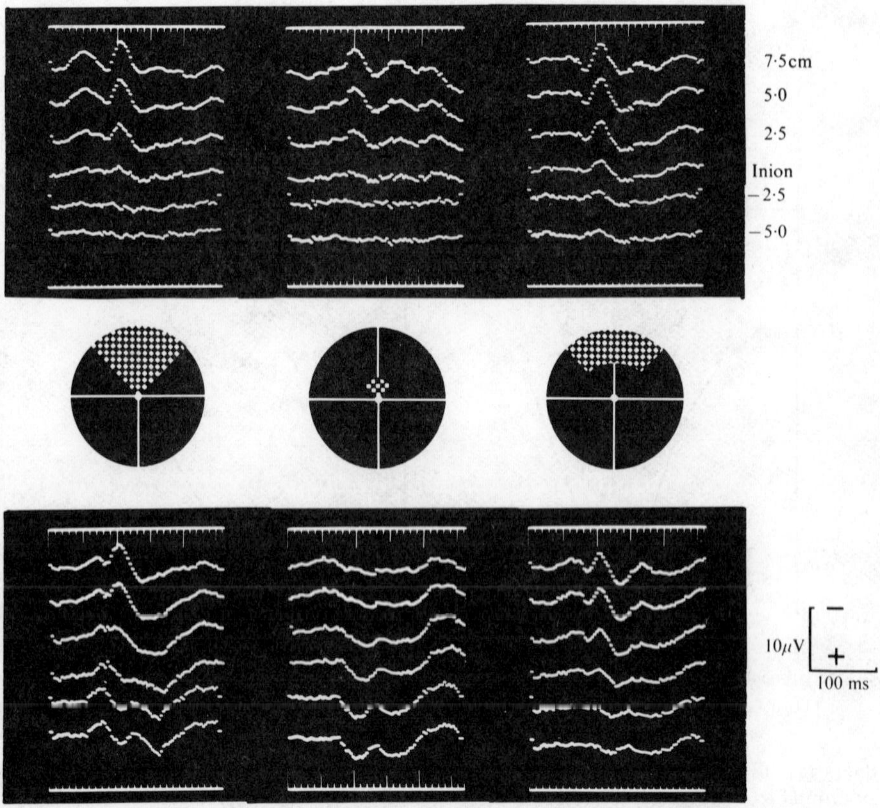

Fig. 5.2. Responses to upper-field stimuli recorded with a two-ear (*above*) and a mid-frontal reference (*below*) from the same subject as in Fig. 5.1. Note the polarity reversal of the prominent component at 100 ms compared with the lower-field response shown in Fig. 5.1. There is also a marked difference in the response to the full 8° stimulus with the change of reference electrode. This difference seems to depend largely on the response to the central 2° of the visual field. (From Michael and Halliday 1971.)

Attempts have been made to relate the changes observed in the occipital field when stimulating different areas of the retina to the known retinotopic projections on striate and extrastriate cortex (Jeffreys 1969, 1971*b*, 1972; Jeffreys and Axford 1972*a*, 1972*b*; Halliday and Michael 1970, 1972; Michael and Halliday 1971; Halliday 1972*a*). Fig. 5.5 illustrates the general arrangement of the cortical generator areas suggested by Michael and Halliday (1971) to account for the responses shown in Figs. 5.1–5.4.

Factors relating the occipital response and pattern stimulation in different parts of the visual field

The effectiveness of a pattern stimulus presented in different parts of the visual field in producing an occipital response depends on a number of major factors

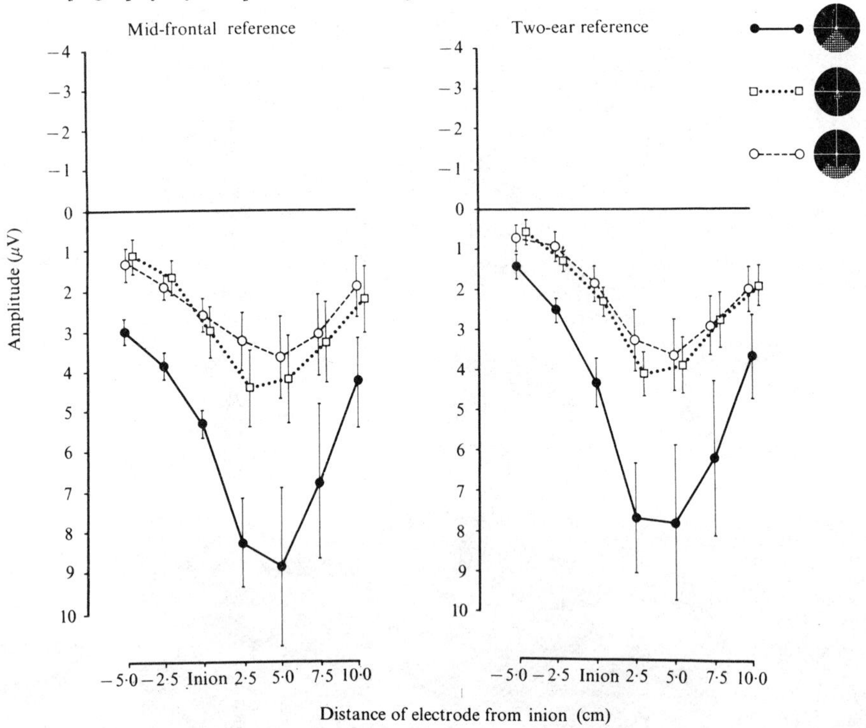

Fig. 5.3. Mean potentials ± standard error for a group of seven subjects to the same lower field stimuli as in Fig. 5.1 at each of the midline chain of occipital electrodes. Recordings with a mid-frontal reference (*left*) differ little from those with a two-ear reference (*right*). (From Michael and Halliday 1971.)

operating at retinal and central levels. In the retina, the effectiveness of the pattern itself varies significantly with *retinal eccentricity*, so that it is not sufficient to consider only the mean intensity, contrast level, and the total area of the visual field stimulated in order to assess the comparability or equivalence of two stimuli. Early investigations suggested that the pattern response came exclusively from the central 2–3° of the visual field and that a checkerboard whose individual squares subtended between 10′ and 20′ produced the largest response (Spekreijse 1966; Rietveld *et al.* 1967; Regan 1972*b*; Regan and Richards 1973). Michael and Halliday (1971) demonstrated, however, that pattern responses can readily be produced by stimulation of the retinal areas between 4° and 8° out from the fixation point with a checkerboard of 50′ squares (Figs. 5.1 and 5.2, right-hand records). Harter (1971*b*) using flash-presented patterns, found that the most effective check size increased progressively with increasing retinal eccentricity, and other studies have since confirmed that larger check sizes produce their maximal response when the stimulus extends out to more peripheral areas of the field (Behrman *et al.* 1972; Lesèvre 1973; Halliday and Mushin, unpublished). This

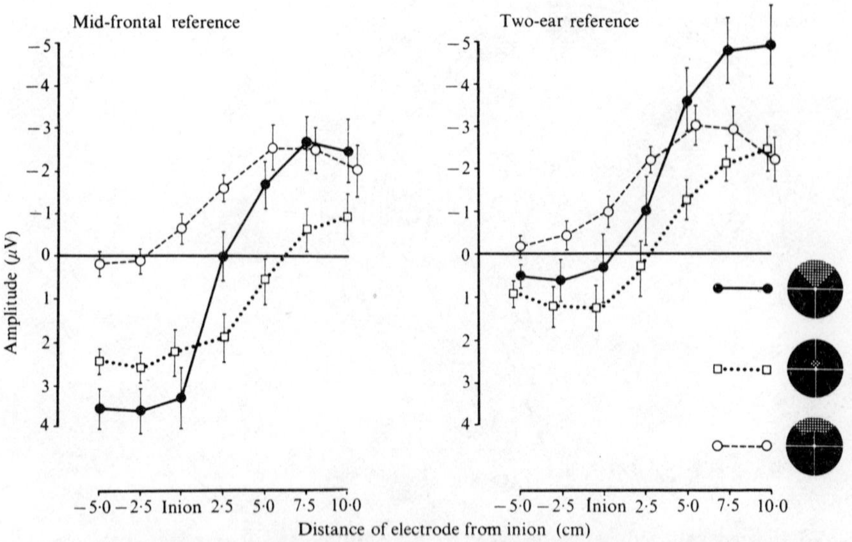

Fig. 5.4. Mean potentials ± standard error for the same group of subjects to the same upper-field stimuli as in Fig. 5.2. A change from the two-ear (*right*) to the mid-frontal (*left*) reference introduces a positive shift of several microvolts for the full 8° and central 2° stimuli. There is no comparable shift in response to the peripheral 4–8° stimulus. (From Michael and Halliday 1971.)

important difference in optimal check size with eccentricity is no doubt related to the increasing mean size of the receptive fields of the retinal units with increasing distance from the fovea.

Quite apart from the matching of the size of the pattern elements to the mean size of the receptive fields of the retinal units, a further important factor relating the effectiveness of the pattern stimulus and eccentricity at retinal level is the concentration of '*sustained*' *retinal units*, sensitive to steady pattern stimulation, in the central areas of the retina, in contrast to the '*transient*' *movement detectors*, which predominate in more peripheral parts of the retina. These two populations of receptors have been clearly demonstrated in the retina of the cat and monkey (Enroth-Cugell and Robson 1966; Gouras 1968; Cleland, Dubin, and Levick 1971; Fukada 1971; Ikeda and Wright 1972*b*) and there is good psychophysical evidence for the existence of two similar classes of detectors in the human visual system (Van Nes, Koenderick, Nas, and Bouman 1967; Keesey 1972; Tolhurst 1973; Kulikowski and Tolhurst 1973; King-Smith and Kulikowski 1973). The relative contribution of these two types of receptors to the occipital response may explain some of the observed differences and interactions between contour-related and luminance-related elements of the VEP. There are, for instance, relatively minor differences in the form of the occipital response to an unpatterned flash stimulus presented in the upper and lower half-fields and quadrants in central vision (Rietveld, Tordoir, Hagenouw, and van Dongen 1965; Halliday and Wilson, un-

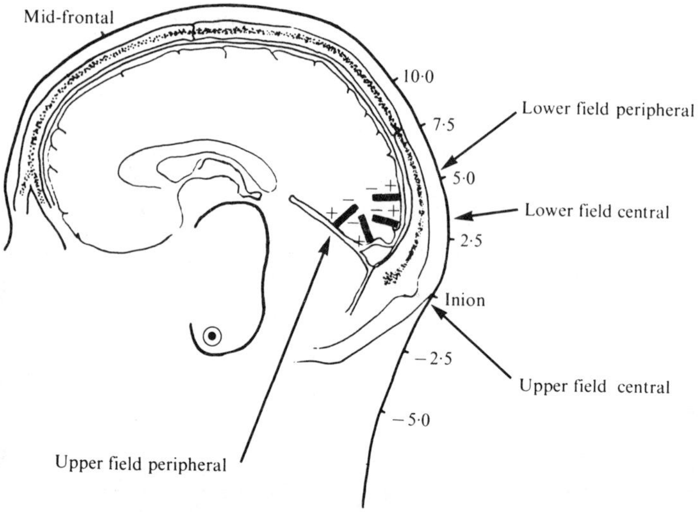

Fig. 5.5. Diagrammatic representation of the relative positions and orientations of the hypothetical dipoles representing the central and peripheral parts of the upper and lower visual field. Note that the peripheral and central lower field dipoles (at 3 and 4 o'clock) are nearly parallel and optimally placed to produce a surface positivity at the occipital electrode with either a two-ear or mid-frontal reference. The central and peripheral upper field dipoles (at 5 and 8 o'clock respectively) are oriented almost at right-angles to each other. These suggested orientations would explain the surface positivity recorded at lower occipital electrodes in response to the central upper-field stimulus when using a mid-frontal reference, which changes to a surface negativity recorded at upper occipital electrodes when a two-ear reference is used. They would also account for the surface negativity recorded at upper electrodes with either the two-ear or mid-frontal reference in response to the peripheral upper-field stimulus. (From Michael and Halliday 1971.)

published) in contrast to the striking polarity reversals seen with checkerboard stimulation. There is also the interesting interaction between the *sharpness of focus* of pattern visual stimuli and the *size of the elements* of the pattern, noted for flash-presented pattern stimuli by Harter and White (1968). The VEP to patterns of small checks is greatly attenuated by even slight blurring of the image, whereas the VEP to larger check sizes is relatively insensitive to de-focusing. This effect is independent of the brightness of the pattern (Regan and Richards 1973). This, together with the earlier observation of Spekreijse (1966) that with small checks, a pattern-reversal stimulus could be rendered ineffective by superimposing a steadily presented outline of the edges, suggests that for small checks the pattern VEP depends on edge detectors whereas for larger checks it depends partly on detectors of areas of varying luminance.

In addition to these factors modifying the effectiveness of a pattern stimulus in different parts of the visual field at purely retinal level, there are further factors concerned with the *retino-cortical pathways.* The mapping of the visual field in the striate cortex includes an important *magnification factor*, providing for a much larger cortical generator area for the foveal and parafoveal projection than for more peripheral areas (Daniel and Whitteridge 1961; Cowey 1964, 1973). In the monkey striate cortex there is a more than ten-fold reduction in the area of cortex representing a corresponding area of the retina by 15° out from the fovea (Daniel and Whitteridge 1961). Cowey (1973) has used the data provided by Brindley and Lewin (1968) on a blind patient with a stimulating prosthesis implanted over the left striate cortex to obtain comparable data on the magnification factor in man. There were no phosphenes produced at the fovea itself, but in the parafovea the magnification factor was 5 mm per degree, and this declined ten-fold to 0·5 mm per degree at an eccentricity of 20–30°. This suggests that the human and monkey magnification factors are surprisingly similar. The monkey data showed that the change in the magnification factor with eccentricity was similar in all directions (i.e. along all the radii). This implies that the area of field stimulated has to be increased as a function of increasing eccentricity if the same 'area' of cortical generators is to be activated.

A third set of factors concerns the *cortical generators* themselves. The anatomical relation of the cortical projection areas to the recording electrodes on the scalp is complex. The detailed mapping of the contralateral visual field on the striate cortex is fairly well established (Holmes 1918, 1945; Spalding 1952; Teuber, Battersby, and Bender 1960; Brindley and Lewin 1968) but the complicated infolding of the cortical sulci is subject to a large degree of individual variability (Polyak 1957). Moreover, the retinotopic projections to extrastriate areas can be inferred only by analogy with the studies in animals (Talbot and Marshall 1941; Talbot 1942; Daniel and Whitteridge 1961; Myers 1962; Hubel and Wiesel 1962, 1965, 1967, 1968; Bilge, Seneviratne, and Whitteridge 1963; Bilge, Bingle, Seneviratne, and Whitteridge 1967; Cowey 1964; Cragg 1969; Zeki 1969). Not only the position of the cortical generators, but also their orientation, is critical in determining the field picked up by the scalp electrode (Shaw and Roth 1955; Vaughan 1969; Michael and Halliday 1971).

Spatio-temporal mapping of the occipital response

Previous methods of studying the spatio-temporal pattern of the occipital VEP have relied either on measuring the amplitude distribution of identified 'components' along the sagittal or trans-occipital planes (e.g. Halliday and Michael 1970; Halliday 1972*a*; Jeffreys and Axford 1972*a*, 1972*b*) or on constructing isopotential contour maps by extrapolation from the data obtained from an array of many scalp electrodes. The isopotential maps have either been plotted on drawings of the head itself (Vaughan 1969; Nakamura and Biersdorf 1971; Biersdorf and Nakamura 1971; Kooi, Yamada, and Marshall 1973) or have been presented in terms of the sagittal or trans-occipital voltage gradients against time (Lesèvre and Rémond 1972, Lesèvre 1973). An alternative method has recently been developed in our laboratory, which avoids the need for extrapolation, with the attendant dangers of aliasing, and presents the voltage field recorded from an array of occipital electrodes of any desired montage as a three-dimentional lattice displayed on an oscilloscope screen (Barrett, Halliday, Halliday, and Michael 1974). The display is generated from the raw VEP data by a computer program written for the PDP-12.

In the original study, a montage of 13 monopolar occipital electrodes (Fig. 5.6), spaced 5 cm apart and referred to a common mid-frontal electrode, is viewed as if

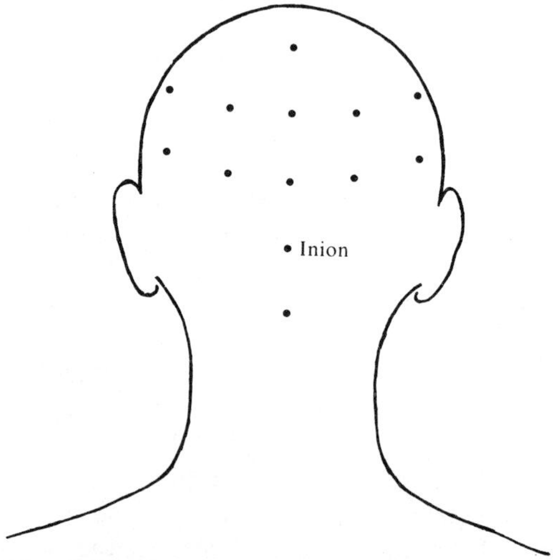

Fig. 5.6. Montage of 13 occipital electrodes used to generate the display of the voltage field over the occiput. Three further channels are used to provide alternative inter-reference recordings, the standard record being monopolar to a common mid-frontal reference. The spacing of the electrodes is 5 cm in both axes.

flattened out onto a horizontal plane (Fig. 5.7(a)). This plane represents zero potential level, and the instantaneous voltage of each electrode is represented by a line drawn vertically upwards or downwards from this plane, the length being proportional to the negative or positive voltage recorded at that point (Fig. 5.7(b)).

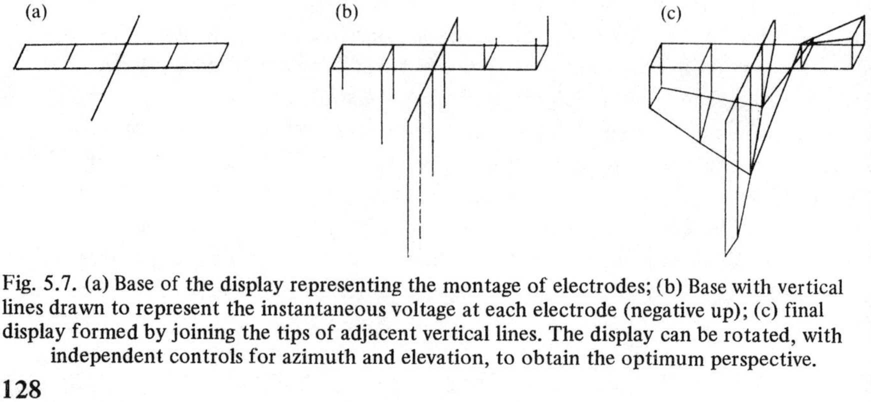

Fig. 5.7. (a) Base of the display representing the montage of electrodes; (b) Base with vertical lines drawn to represent the instantaneous voltage at each electrode (negative up); (c) final display formed by joining the tips of adjacent vertical lines. The display can be rotated, with independent controls for azimuth and elevation, to obtain the optimum perspective.

The tips of the neighbouring lines in the electrode display are joined to form a lattice whose upper and lower surface represents the potential recorded over that part of the head and whose slopes indicate the rate of change of potential (Fig. 5.7(c)). The display brings out the spatial maxima and minima of the voltage distribution and clearly indicates points of voltage reversal and areas of rapid potential change. The rise and fall of the VEP over time can be followed in slow motion by displaying a series of frames corresponding to the input sampling, and these changes can be speeded up or slowed down by altering the frame repetition rate. Alternatively, a single frame can be frozen for detailed examination. The whole display can be rotated to obtain the optimum perspective, separate controls being provided for azimuth and elevation. Permanent records can be plotted out on an $x-y$ plotter as a series of consecutive frames (Fig. 5.8).

Fig. 5.8 shows a representative display of the changes occurring in the spatial distribution of the voltage field over a period of 30 ms, starting 72·5 ms after the reversal of a checkerboard stimulus presented in the left upper vertical octant of the visual field extending from 0° to 8° out from the fixation point. This is a section of the same data which is presented in the form of a conventional 16-channel averaged VEP record in Fig. 5.9. A comparison of the two Figures will show how quite complementary information is brought out by the two methods of display. In the conventional average record (Fig. 5.9) the eye easily picks out prominent wave shapes and 'components' occurring in particular channels, but has difficulty in translating these into a spatial map. The three-dimensional display (Fig. 5.8), on the other hand, is particularly good at bringing out shifts in the spatial distribution of the voltage peaks and their relationship to the zero-potential baseline.

The section of record shown in Fig. 5.8 indicates that 72·5 ms after pattern reversal there is a negative peak maximal in the left-sided and posterior electrodes with little contralateral polarity reversal, which gradually subsides to give way to a voltage field of opposite polarity which is strongly phase reversed across the midline, with a positive peak posteriorly and ipsilaterally to the stimulus and a negative peak contralaterally.

Alternative reference recording

The three last channels in the record shown in Fig. 5.9 are used to record inter-reference potentials. This enables several alternative displays to be computed, representing the records which would have been obtained using either a mid-frontal or an ear reference (either left or right ear singly or the average of the two ears). This information may have great practical importance in some contexts, as the results reported by Michael and Halliday (1971) demonstrated. It can be seen from Fig. 5.9 that there are important elements of the VEP appearing in the inter-reference channels. This implies that the waveforms of the monopolar records from the occipital electrodes will be significantly altered when the reference is changed.

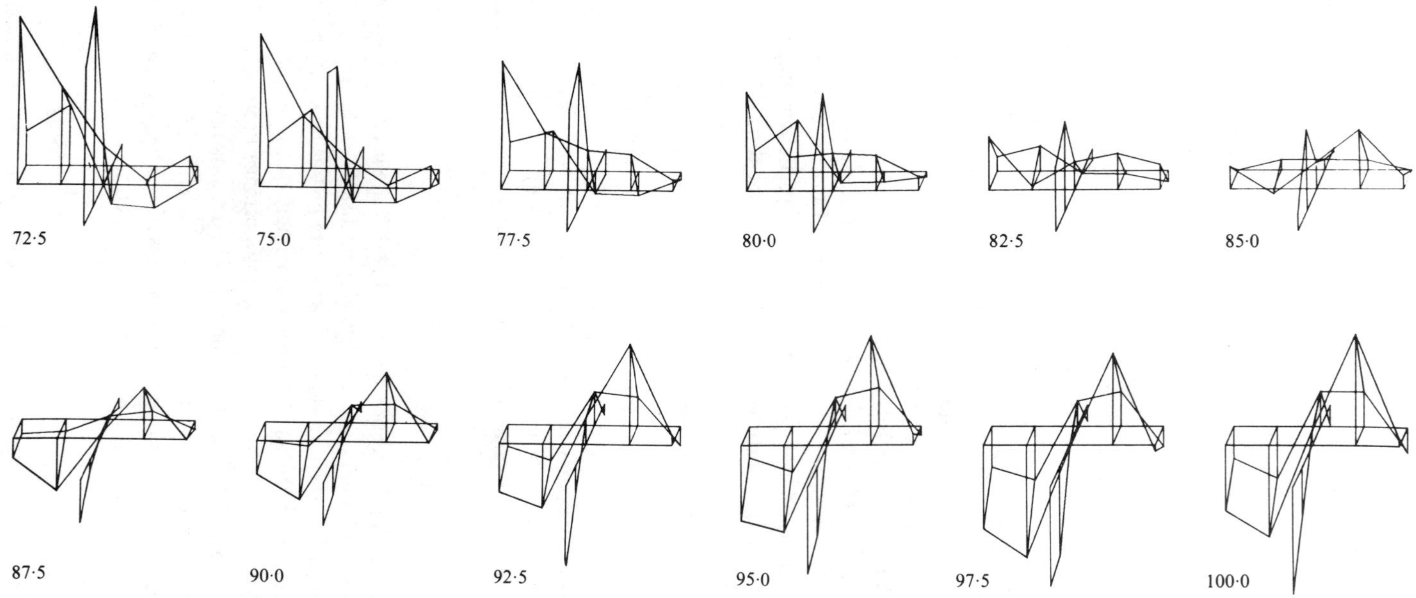

Fig. 5.8. Three-dimensional display of the potential field over the occiput for 12 successive input samples between 72·5 ms and 100 ms. The data is the same as that in the conventional average response record shown in Fig. 5.9. The latency for each sample is indicated in milli-seconds. Electrode montage as in Figs. 5.6 and 5.7(a). For explanation see text.

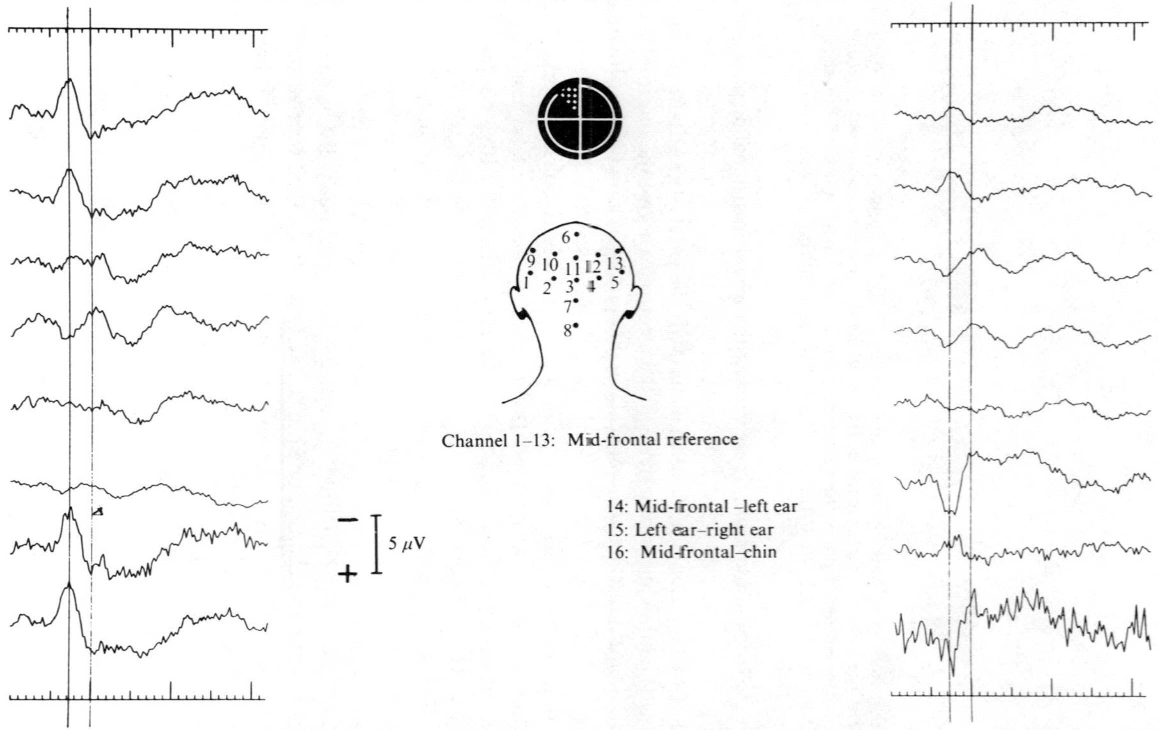

Fig. 5.9. Conventional 16-channel VEP record of the averaged response to 200 pattern reversals for a checkerboard stimulus presented in the left upper vertical octant. The first 13 channels are monopolar records to a common mid-frontal reference. The last three channels provide inter-reference recordings and enable alternative reference records to be computed. The two vertical lines are drawn at latencies of 72·5 ms and 100 ms and indicate the duration of the record of the three-dimensional voltage field shown in Fig. 5.8.

Responses from different octants of the visual field

The changes in the field of the occipital response at a latency of 100 ms with stimulation of eight different octants of the visual field for the segment from 0–8° out from the fixation point is shown for one subject in Fig. 5.10. In this

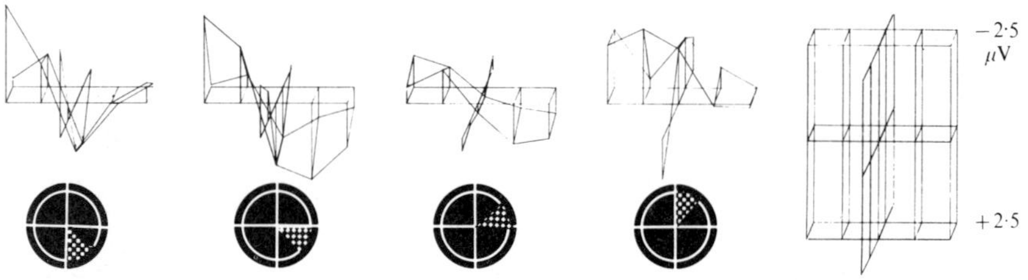

Fig. 5.10. The distribution of the occipital potential field at 100 ms following pattern reversal of a checkerboard presented in each octant of the visual field. The responses are averaged in one subject for 200 reversals of the pattern stimulus. The checkerboard was made up of 50′ squares and extended from 0° to 8° out from the fixation point. For explanation see text.

record which is that for a mid-frontal reference, the three-dimensional display confirms that pattern-reversal stimulation of the upper vertical octant produces a phase reversal of voltage along the sagittal plane with the greatest positivity at the electrode below the inion and a negativity at the electrodes above the inion. Conversely, stimulation of the lower vertical octants produces a midline positivity above the inion. This is in line with the earlier result (Michael and Halliday, 1971).

The three-dimensional display also brings out very clearly the phase reversal across the midline associated with stimulation of the upper horizontal octants. Stimulation of the upper vertical octant is associated particularly with a contralateral negativity. This may or may not be accompanied by an ipsilateral positivity (compare left and right upper vertical octants in Fig. 5.10). In the response from the upper horizontal octants there is an ipsilateral positivity with a rather well lateralized maximum, associated with a contralateral negativity. In the response from the lower horizontal octants the ipsilateral positivity begins to spread towards the midline channels, and in the response from the lower vertical octants the positivity is definitely maximal in the midline. It is to be noted that corresponding octants in the left and right half-fields do not always produce responses of complementary pattern. This is particularly marked for the upper vertical octants. Jeffreys and Axford (1972*a, b*) noted comparable anomalies in the pattern-onset response. Their results also stress the inter-subject variability which has also been a feature of our own findings. Some of these differences may well be related to the anatomical variability of the cortical generator areas.

An important outcome of this analysis is that an ipsilateral positivity is typical for stimulation of a large part of the half-field centred on the horizontal meridian. It is only for stimuli near the lower vertical octant that the maximal positivity tends to be in the midline or even slightly contralateral. This finding, which appears at first sight somewhat paradoxical in view of the known projection of each half-field to the contralateral hemisphere, may imply that much of the VEP arises from the cortical generator areas of the medial surface of the occipital lobe, rather than on the convexity. Further, for the upper field responses the positivity has a very much more posterior and inferior location, being maximal at the electrodes below the inion. This no doubt reflects the fact that the retinotopic projection on to the cortical visual areas is inverted, with the upper field represented below the lower field. The more posterior distribution of the area of maximal potential for upper field responses has also been reported for the pattern-onset response (Lesèvre 1972; Lesèvre and Rémond 1972). This applies both to their 'component 1' and 'component 2', the former being a surface positivity for lower field stimulation and a negativity for upper field stimulation with a mean latency of 90 ms, while the latter has the opposite polarity and a mean latency of 118 ms. Jeffreys and Axford (1972*b*) find a more anterior distribution for the upper field response, but the results reported by Halliday and Michael (1970) strongly suggest that this is an artifact of the use of an ear reference recording, and the alternative chin reference which they reported using would be expected to give the same result, a point which is well illustrated by the general similarity of channels 14 and 16 in Fig. 5.9.

6. The physiological significance of pattern visual evoked potentials

D. JEFFREYS
Department of Communication, University of Keele.

The scalp-recorded potentials evoked by any form of transient visual stimulus are composite in nature, containing contributions from several different cortical regions and/or processes. Since the various contributions to these VEPs often overlap in time, studies limited to measurements of the individual peaks of their polyphasic waveforms must be of uncertain physiological significance. If these surface VEPs are to provide meaningful information about underlying cortical activity it is first necessary to identify their constituent (anatomically and/or physiologically defined) components.

This chapter describes how appropriate experimental techniques can be used to identify and distinguish the various contributions from different anatomical regions and from distinct cortical processes to pattern VEPs. The choice of a patterned rather than an unpatterned stimulus was based mainly on the neurophysiological findings (e.g. Hubel and Wiesel 1962, 1965, 1968) that, at least for cats and monkeys, the majority of neurones in the visual cortex are sensitive to 'contoured' visual stimuli and relatively insensitive to overall luminance changes. The reasons for the particular choice of patterned stimulus – a brief (25 ms) presentation of a high-contrast pattern at constant luminance – are made apparent later in the chapter.

The chapter is divided into three main sections. The first section describes methods and results of the 'component analysis' of these pattern VEPs whereby the various pattern- and non-pattern-related contributions are identified and distinguished. It also shows how the different pattern-related components can often be effectively isolated, thus allowing the study of their individual properties. The second section describes how such studies of various characteristics of the individual pattern-related components can be used to provide clues both to the likely sites of origin of these components within the visual cortex and to the nature of the cortical processes involved in their production. The third section compares these pattern VEPs with those produced by other commonly used forms of pattern presentation and shows how the very different forms of these pattern VEPs can largely be explained in terms of the basic properties established for the individual pattern-related components.

Visual evoked potentials in man: new developments (ed. J. E. Desmedt), pp. 134–167. Clarendon Press, Oxford 1977.

Component analysis of VEPs obtained to brief pattern presentation

Jeffreys and Axford (1972*a*, *b*) showed that pattern-related components of anatomically separate origin can readily be identified in these VEPs by studying the influence of the *retinal location* of the stimulus pattern on their *surface distributions*. In these studies they were thus able to identify two distinct components related to pattern onset: CI and CII, in the initial portion (0–120 ms) of these VEPs. A subsequent pattern-related component was often evident but was not studied in detail at that time, as the later portions of these VEPs, being more variable in form and obviously composite in nature, were less suitable for the simple form of analysis used, namely plotting of amplitude distributions of VEP samples of pre-set duration and latency with respect to a common 'pre-response' (0–40 ms) baseline.

This section describes the results of further experiments designed to study in more detail the composition of these pattern VEPs in several subjects, and in particular to study the characteristics of the later pattern-related component CIII, in relation to CI and CII. In these experiments the various pattern- and non-pattern-related contributions to these composite VEPs were identified from comparative studies of the surface distribution characteristics of the VEPs obtained to the test pattern and those obtained in several control runs using stimuli which were known to influence selectively either pattern- or non-pattern-related components.

Methods

The basic stimulus consisted of a 25 ms-duration binocular presentation of a high-contrast pattern in place of an otherwise continuously illuminated, centrally fixed blank field. This was produced by alternately switching two fields, one patterned (test) and the other blank (reference), of a four-field tachistoscope (cf. Chapter 1 of this book). The test pattern was a regular array of isolated squares of 15′ (3 mm) square side and separation, viewed at 75 cm, and presented aperiodically (mean interval of 600 ms). The pattern was presented in turn to each quadrant, half- and full-field. The unpatterned region of the circular (10°; 12 cm) stimulus field was kept at constant luminance of about 1·8 log ft-L, and a third tachistoscope field was used to provide a small, steady surround field of the same luminance.

The following *control stimuli* were used in addition to the test pattern for each subject. 1. An overall luminance change in the appropriate region of the test field, produced by replacing the stimulus pattern by a 50 per cent neutral filter. This luminance change, which was greater than that occurring in the patterned regions of the test field, was shown by control tests to produce very similar VEPs to those produced by the fully defocused pattern. 2. A square-wave profile grid pattern of 3 mm stripe width. 3. The test pattern with thin (0·1 mm) outlines of the squares continuously present in the stimulus field. (In this case, the blank reference field was replaced by a pattern of square outlines.) The reasons for using control stimuli 2 and 3 are made apparent in the next section of this chapter. The VEPs obtained to the test pattern with and without the steady outlines were recorded for different pattern durations in three subjects to help identify components related to pattern offset in these short-duration pattern VEPs. In addition to the test pattern and various control-run VEPs, the full-field and half-field VEPs obtained to flash-presentation of the blank test field were also recorded in each subject.

The recording techniques are basically similar to those described by Jeffreys and Axford (1972*a*) but in this case the data were analysed by visual inspection of the averaged VEP waveforms. The EEG signals were simultaneously recorded from two orthogonal rows of 6 'vertical' (midline) and 7 'horizontal' electrodes (Ag–AgCl discs attached by collodion) to a common 'linked-earlobe' reference: lowest midline electrode at inion; the central horizontal electrode on the midline 5 cm above inion; and an electrode separation of 2·5 cm. The EEG signals were amplified by a Beckman 'TC' 16-channel recorder (time-constant 0.3 s.; high-frequency cut-off 50 Hz), recorded on a Thermionic Instruments 14-channel 0·3 s.; high-frequency cut-of subsequently averaged (45 samples) over a 500 ms post-stimulus period by a CAT 400 B. The VEPs to at least two identical runs were computed in every case. Six adult members of this department acted as subjects.

Results

Components related to pattern onset. Three distinct components related to pattern onset: CI, CII and CIII, of different surface distribution characteristics, have been identified in these pattern VEPs for all subjects. The peak *latencies* of these individual components are similar for each subject and do not appear to vary much with either the electrode position or for the different retinal locations used in these experiments. Under these conditions, they are about 75 ms, 100 ms, and 150 ms, respectively. However, the form and polarity of the *amplitude* distributions of these components are dependent on retinal location (Fig. 6.1). Also, there is an additive relationship for the amplitude distributions of the individual components of the different quadrant VEPs, i.e. the component distributions for a given half-field or full-field VEP are the sum of those of the constituent quadrant VEPs. Jeffreys and Axford (1972*a*, *b*) showed that this additive relationship also holds for separate sectors and annular regions within a single quadrant. They also found that there are different foveal and extrafoveal contributions to these components, CI usually containing a greater relative extrafoveal contribution than CII and CIII.

These and the previous experiments (Jeffreys and Axford 1972*a*, *b*) have shown that although the detailed form of the individual component distributions varies from subject to subject, certain basic features are common to the VEPs obtained for the majority of subjects.

1. There is a reversal of the polarity of each component in the VEPs obtained to upper and to lower half-field stimulation (Fig. 6.1(a)). For the lower half-field responses the polarities of CI, CII, and CIII are generally positive, negative, and positive, respectively. (See also Lesèvre and Rémond 1972; Spekreijse and Estevez 1972; Spekreijse *et al.* 1973).

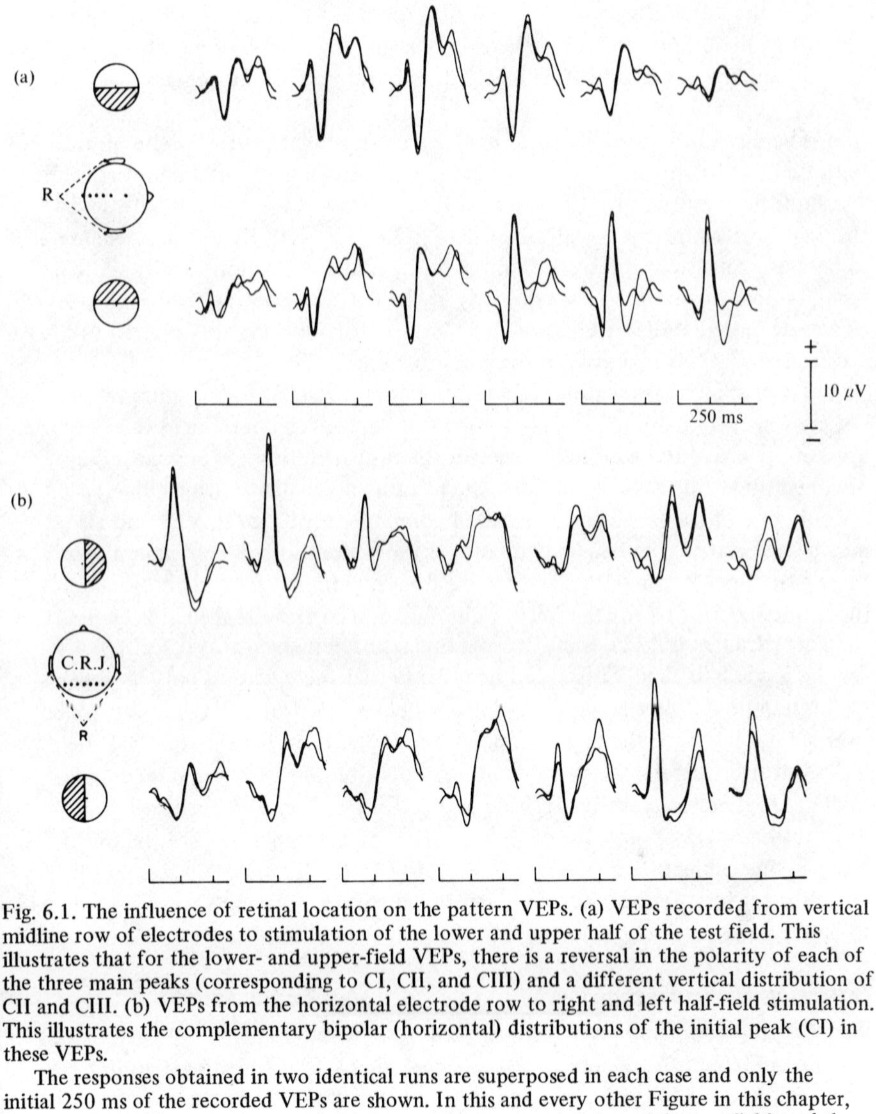

Fig. 6.1. The influence of retinal location on the pattern VEPs. (a) VEPs recorded from vertical midline row of electrodes to stimulation of the lower and upper half of the test field. This illustrates that for the lower- and upper-field VEPs, there is a reversal in the polarity of each of the three main peaks (corresponding to CI, CII, and CIII) and a different vertical distribution of CII and CIII. (b) VEPs from the horizontal electrode row to right and left half-field stimulation. This illustrates the complementary bipolar (horizontal) distributions of the initial peak (CI) in these VEPs.

The responses obtained in two identical runs are superposed in each case and only the initial 250 ms of the recorded VEPs are shown. In this and every other Figure in this chapter, the cross-hatched area within the circle denotes the patterned region of the test field, and the VEPs are laid out according to the electrode positions indicated in the diagram.

2. There is a consistent difference in the shape as well as in the polarity of the upper- and lower-field vertical distributions of CII and CIII (but not CI). The lower half-field distributions have a more symmetrical form of distribution and, with a common earlobe reference, are more posteriorly located than those of the upper half-field (Jeffreys 1971) (Fig. 6.1(a)).

3. For the left and right half-field VEPs, the horizontal distributions of CI, but not of CII, are bipolar in form, reversing polarity near the midline. These complementary left and right half-field distributions of CI are generally asymmetric (Fig. 6.1 (b)).

4. The distributions of CIII are generally more similar (but opposite in polarity) to those of CII than CI. In some cases almost identical horizontal and vertical distributions are found for CII and CIII for the lower quadrant and half-field VEPs, although this is not true for all subjects (e.g. Fig. 6.15(a)). By contrast, there appear to be more consistent differences in the horizontal distributions of CII and CIII for the upper quadrant VEPs, especially at the extreme contralateral electrodes. However, more detailed studies of their surface distributions are required to clarify the relationship between these components.

These characteristic features of the components related to pattern onset are not seen in every case. In fact, for some subjects, a given component can have the opposite polarity and a quite different form of distribution to those generally obtained under the same conditions. Such 'anomalous' distributions may occur for only one of the three pattern-related components of a given VEP and also may be associated with single quadrants of the stimulus field. For example, in these experiments, the only clearly anomalous quadrant VEP distributions were those obtained for Cl for the lower right quadrant of the visual field in two of the subjects (R. Q. and I. C.). In both cases this resulted in a *negative* CI distribution for the lower half-field VEPs (see Fig. 6.2), so that there was no polarity reversal of this component in the upper- and lower-field VEPs. In these two cases, moreover, CI did not have the typical bipolar horizontal form for the right half-field VEPs but had instead a negative monopolar distribution with a maximum near the midline. In a previous study (Jeffreys and Axford 1972*a*, *b*) anomalous distributions were observed for CII (and CIII) for the upper but not the lower-field VEPs in one subject (S. H.).

The most inter-individually consistent of these pattern-related components seems to be the negative CII component of the lower-field VEPs.

Pattern-offset-related contributions to the brief presentation VEPs

With the short-duration presentations used in these experiments the pattern VEPs contain contributions related to the offset of the pattern which overlap in time with the onset-related components CII and CIII. By increasing the duration it has been found that the most consistent features of these offset-related potentials are positive and negative peaks at about 110 ms and 150 ms, respectively, which in many cases are preceded by a component corresponding in characteristics to CI. Since these main offset-related peaks have quite different properties from those of CII and CIII, it is possible to distinguish between the onset- and offset-related contributions to the short presentation VEPs by changing stimulus parameters which selectively influence these components. For example, in contrast to CII and CIII, the main offset-related peaks vary less with retinal location and are less

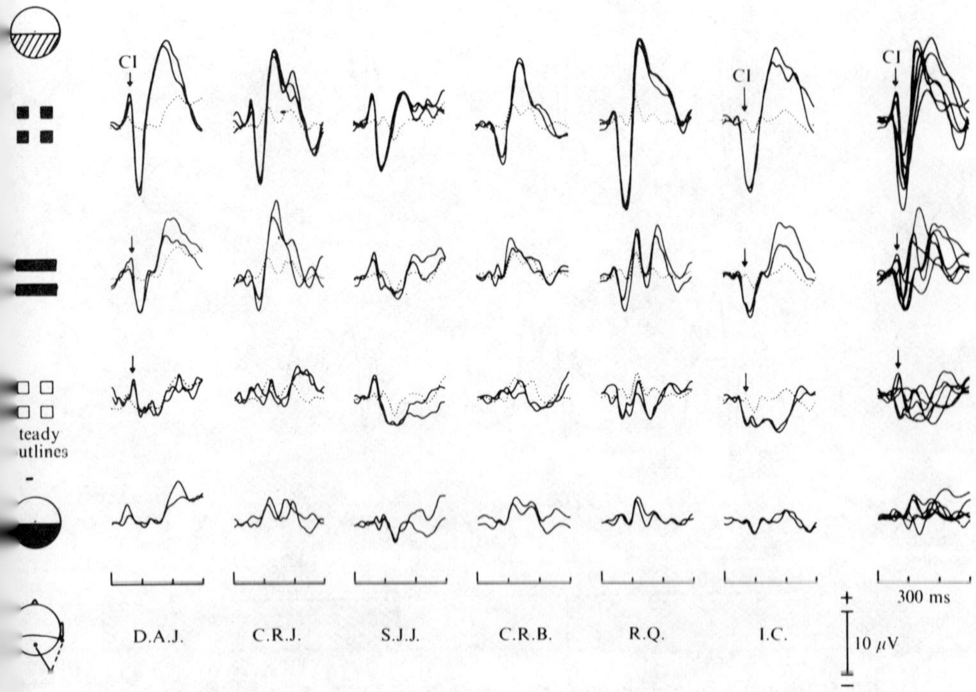

Fig. 6.2. Comparison of lower half-field VEPs obtained to the test pattern and to the control stimuli. VEPs from midline electrode (5 cm above inion) for each of the six subjects to (a) test pattern of isolated squares; (b) horizontal grid pattern; (c) test pattern in presence of steady outlines of the squares; (d) (and dotted traces in (a), (b), and (c)) overall luminance change (50 per cent filter). The corresponding (mean) VEP waveforms for each subject are superposed on the right of the figure.

The luminance-change VEPs in (d) are very small compared to the test pattern VEPs in (a) in each case. A negative peak at about 100 ms (CII) and a positive peak at about 150 ms (CIII) are prominent in each test-pattern VEP. These have smaller amplitudes in the grid pattern VEPs in (b) and are absent from both the 'steady-outline' VEPs in (c) and the luminance-change responses in (d). However, whereas the initial peak (CI) of the test-pattern VEPs is clearly positive for three subjects, it is negative in two cases (R.Q. and I.C.), where it combines with the succeeding negative CII component to form an apparently single broad negative peak. The negative CI contribution to this composite peak is apparent in the VEPs in (c) obtained with the steady outlines, which selectively attenuate CII (and CIII) but not CI.

influenced by the presence of steady outlines of the test-pattern elements (see Fig. 6.13). Thus the offset-related contributions can often be identified by comparing the forms and distributions of the VEPs obtained at different durations with and without the presence of steady outlines.

Such experiments have shown that the offset-related contributions to these 25 ms VEPs vary from subject to subject (Fig. 6.3), but in most cases appear to be relatively small compared with the onset-related components.

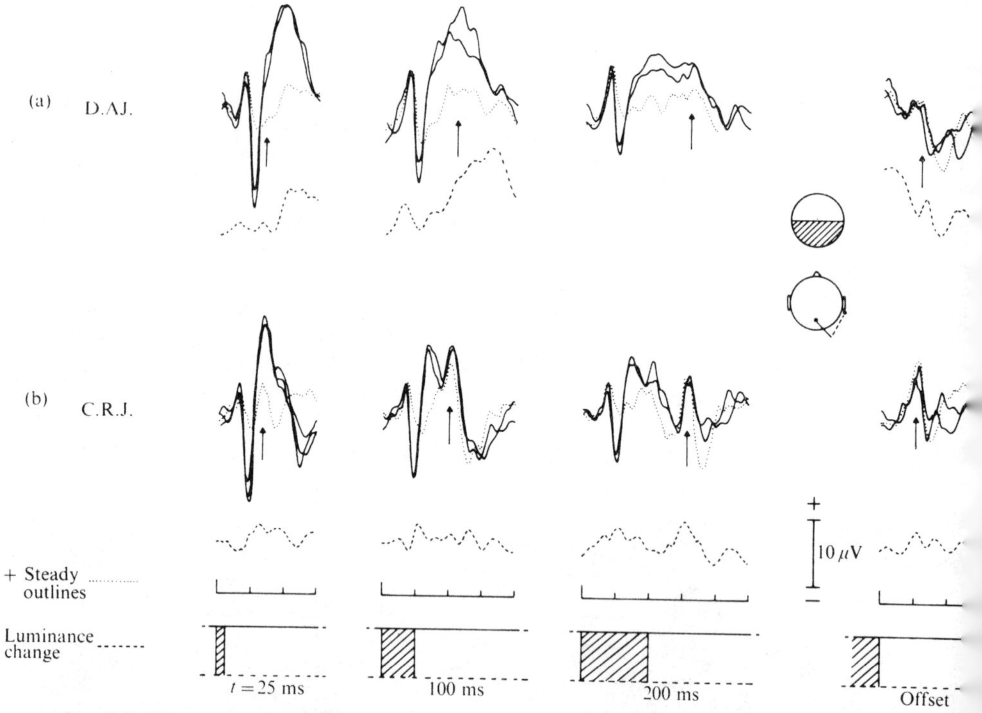

Fig. 6.3. Offset-related contributions to the lower half-field VEPs. VEPs recorded from midline electrode (5 cm above inion) in two subjects (a) D.A.J., and (b) C.R.J., to the onset of the test pattern for durations of 25 ms, 100 ms, and 200 ms; and to the offset of the 300 ms presentation of the same pattern. The (mean) VEPs obtained to the test pattern in presence of steady outlines are indicated by the dotted traces, and those to luminance changes by the dashed traces.

The most prominent component in the offset VEPs is a positive peak at about 120 ms latency (arrow) which is not greatly influenced by the steady outlines. Thus the 'steady-outline' VEPs in each case provide an inducation of the contribution of this component to the VEPs at short durations. In (b) this component clearly has a large amplitude in the 100 ms and 200 ms VEPs and although this is reduced in the 25 ms response, it still appears to contribute significantly to the third (positive) peak of this response. By contrast, there is very little evidence of any substantial contributions from this or any other offset-related component to the 25 ms VEP for subject D.A.J. in (a).

Non-pattern-related contributions to the pattern VEPs

In most cases, the non-pattern-related contributions to the initial portion (0–150 ms) of these pattern VEPs (as indicated by the unpatterned control runs) are relatively small, although the exact degree and form of these contributions vary from subject to subject (e.g. Figs. 6.1–6.3). Thus, the small overall luminance change associated with this method of pattern presentation does not contribute significantly to these pattern VEPs for most subjects. In some cases, however (e.g. subject D.A.J. in Fig. 6.4(b)), positive and negative peaks of about 100 ms and 150 ms latency, respectively, are evident in the VEPs obtained to the overall ıminance change. These are probably luminance-dependent as they correspond) components of similar characteristics but greater amplitude in the flash VEPs Fig. 6.4(c)).

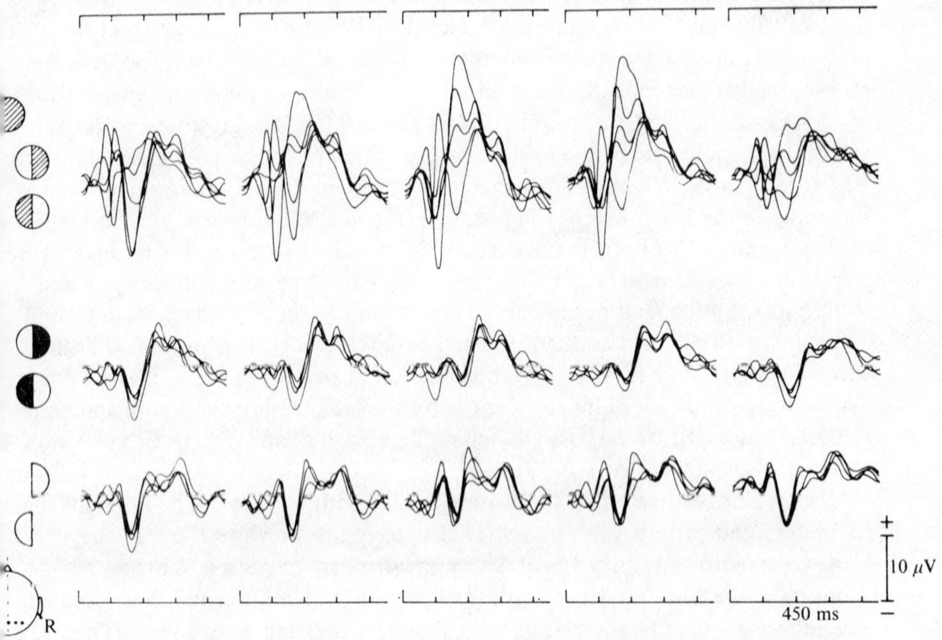

'ig. 6.4. Influence of retinal location on pattern- and non-pattern-related VEP components. uperposed (mean) waveforms of VEPs recorded from central five horizontal-row electrodes in ubject D.A.J. to stimulation of each half-field (and the full field in (a)) by (a) the test pattern; b) luminance change (100 per cent); and (c) flash-presentation of blank field. This shows learly that whereas the polarity of the major components in the 40–200 ms portion of the est-pattern VEPs in (a) is very dependent on retinal location, the polarity of main peaks in the uminance-change and flash VEPs is invariant. The earlier peaks (< 100 ms) of these responses how greater variation with retinal location. There is a close similarity in the form and distribution of the later (200–450 ms) portions of the pattern and luminance-change VEPs.

In general, the greatest non-pattern-related contribution is to the later portion of these pattern VEPs. For example, in Fig. 6.4, a later positive complex with peaks at about 200 ms and 300 ms is clearly seen in both pattern- and luminance-change VEPs. This has a more anterior distribution than the earlier non-pattern-related peaks with a maximum near the vertex, and can be shown to be non-stimulus-specific.

ndependence of pattern- and non-pattern-related (and flash VEP) components

A most significant finding in these experiments has been that, in marked contrast to the pattern-onset-related components, the main non-pattern-related components and those of the flash (blank field) VEPs are relatively uninfluenced by retinal location (Fig. 6.4). Furthermore, they do not show an additive relationship for stimulation of the different quadrant or half-fields. (In some subjects, early (< 100 ms) components of the flash VEPs appeared to show a greater dependence on retinal location but under these experimental conditions these were too small for detailed study (see Nakamura and Biersdorf 1971).) This suggests that the main pattern- and non-pattern-related components have basically different sources and there is further evidence to suggest that these sources are essentially independent of each other. In Fig. 6.5, for example, for the case of flash-presented patterned and blank stimulus fields, the form and distribution of the basic (blank field) flash VEPs are changed in completely different ways when the pattern is moved from the upper to the lower half of the test field (Fig. 6.5(a)). However, on subtraction of the blank-field VEPs from the pattern VEPs in the two cases, it is found that the resulting waveforms (Fig. 6.5(b)) are composed of peaks whose polarity and surface distribution (but not latencies) correspond to those of the pattern-related components obtained at constant luminance (Fig. 6.5(c)). This suggests that the observed changes produced by the introduction of pattern in Fig. 6.5(a) are due mainly to the *addition* of independent pattern-related components corresponding to CI, CII, and CIII to the basically unmodified flash (blank field) VEPs (Jeffreys 1968; MacKay and Jeffreys 1973).

These results indicate that the pattern-related components can be isolated from flash-presented pattern VEPs by subtraction techniques (White 1969; Kinney, McKay, Mensch, and Luina 1972). However, there are obvious advantages in choosing a constant-luminance method of pattern presentation and thus avoiding any unnecessary contamination by large luminance-related components. The apparent independence of the pattern- and non-pattern-related components seems to justify the use in these experiments of equivalent unpatterned control runs to assess the non-pattern-related contributions to these pattern VEPs.

Selective enhancement of individual pattern-related components

The identification of the various pattern- and non-pattern-related contributions to these pattern VEPs has emphasized the complex and composite nature of these responses. Since the major pattern-related components originate in anatomically distinct regions of the visual cortex, any analysis of these VEPs must treat the properties of these components separately, as peak-to-peak or other overall measures will have dubious significance. However, the study of the individual pattern-onset-related components in a given pattern VEP is hampered not only by the presence of the various pattern-offset and non-pattern-related components but also because these successive components overlap in time, making the apparent amplitude and latency of a given onset-related component depend on the relative polarity and amplitude of the preceding and/or succeeding components (e.g. Shagass 1972). There is, in addition, the general problem of the choice of a satisfactory baseline for any quantitative measure of individual VEP components.

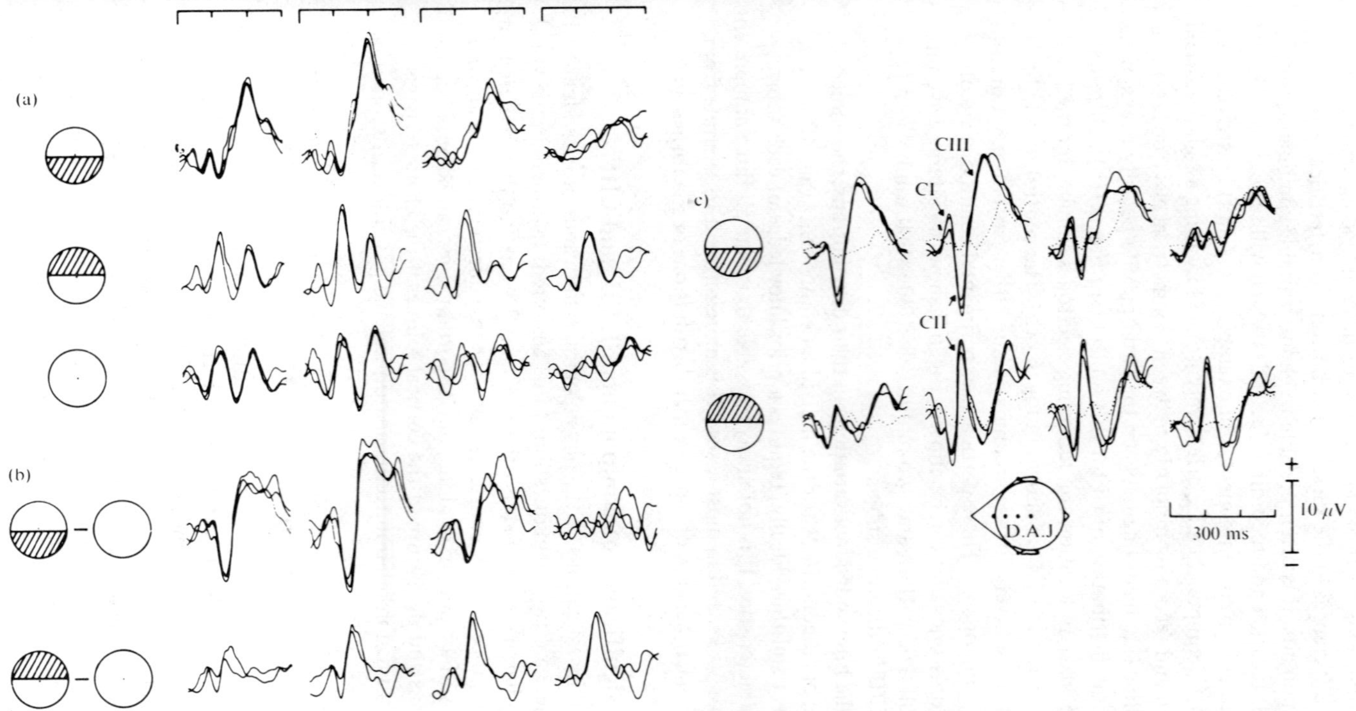

Fig. 6.5. Independence of pattern-related and flash VEP components. (a) VEPs recorded from four vertical (midline) electrodes, 0 cm, 5 cm, 10 cm, and 15 cm above inion, to flash-presentation of the test pattern in the lower and upper half-field and of the full blank field. (b) Waveforms obtained to subtraction of the blank field VEPs from the lower and upper half-field pattern VEPs shown in (a). (c) VEPs recorded from the same electrodes to the lower and upper half-field presentation of the same pattern at constant luminance.

The polarities and distributions of the main peaks of the subtracted flash VEPs are clearly similar to those of the major peaks (corresponding to CI, CII, and CIII) of the corresponding constant-luminance VEPs. The subtracted response peaks, in (b) however, have longer latencies than those of the pattern VEPs shown in (c).

These problems can be overcome to a great extent by choosing appropriate experimental conditions for the study of each of these individual components. Because of the differences in the surface distribution characteristics of the individual components, it is often possible to choose suitable combinations of pattern (retinal) location and recording electrodes which will selectively enhance the amplitude of any given component. For example, Fig. 6.6(a) illustrates how, for subject D.A.J., component CI is effectively isolated by using a right half-field stimulus pattern and recording bipolarly between symmetrical electrodes on either side of the midline (i.e. recording between the two opposite polarity peaks of the bipolar horizontal distribution of CI for this subject (see Fig. 6.1(b)). Different combinations of pattern location and recording electrodes suitable for the enhancement of CII and CIII are shown in Fig. 6.6(b). The control runs in both cases show that there is very little contamination by either pattern-offset or non-pattern-related components. These particular experimental conditions are of course not the only ones that can be chosen; Fig. 6.7 shows an alternative combination of a full-field pattern and two midline electrodes that can be used to study CII and CIII in the same subject.

Because of the inter-individual variations in their distributions, the choice of optimal experimental conditions for the individual components can differ from subject to subject and thus, ideally, requires a prior knowledge of each subject's distribution characteristics. It is not always possible to isolate all three components in every subject's VEPs, and in most cases CII is more difficult to separate from CIII than CI from CII because of more similar distributions of the former pair.

Physiological significance of components CI, CII, and CIII

In these, as in all investigations of the physiological significance of individual VEP components, there are two main questions to be answered: (a) where in the visual cortex do the individual components originate? and (b) what do they represent in terms of cortical processes? Of course, neither of these questions can be answered from studies of surface potentials alone, but important clues can be obtained to both the locations and the nature of the cortical sources if the characteristics of these VEPs are studied in relation to the anatomical and physiological properties of the visual cortex.

Location of the sources of CI, CII, and CIII

The observed differences in the surface distribution characteristics of CI, CII, and CIII and in their relationship to retinal location are presumably due to topographical variations of the various retinotopically organized cortical regions involved in their production. Given sufficient information on the general layout and retinotopic organization of the different regions of the human visual cortex, it is possible to predict the actual locations of individual component sources by relating the basic features of the observed surface potential distributions to those of volume

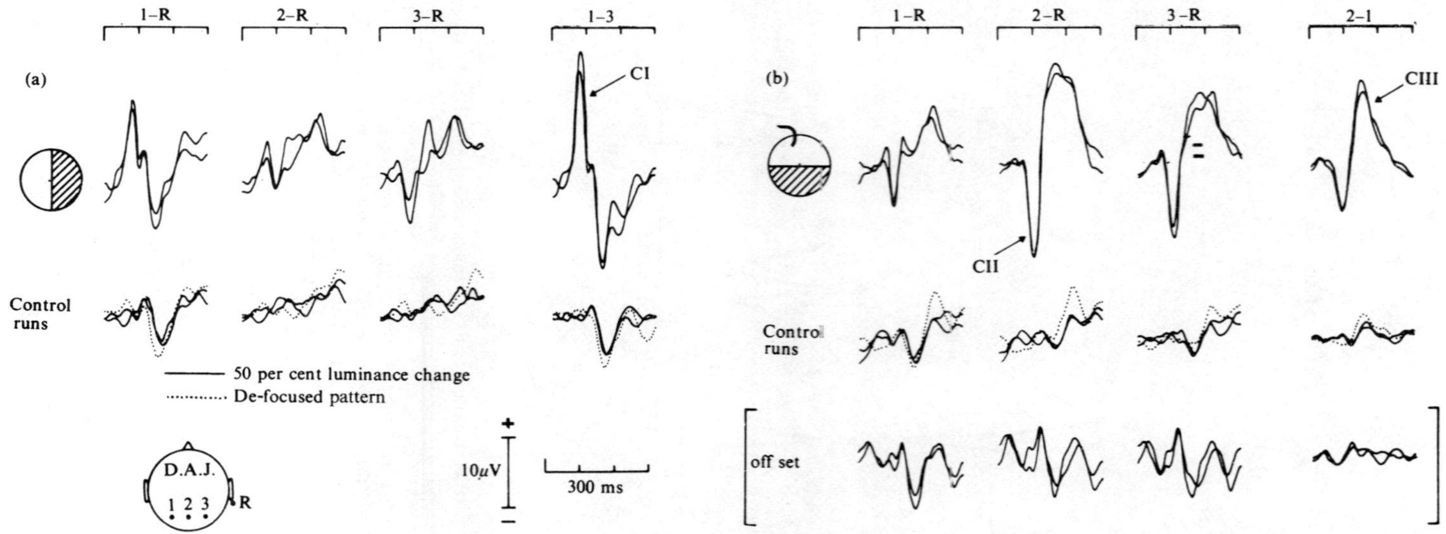

Fig. 6.6. Choice of optimal experimental conditions to enhance individual VEP components selectively. (a) CI. Right half-field recorded from three electrodes 1–3, on the midline and 6 cm to either side, to a common reference, (right earlobe) 1–R, 2–R, and 3–R, and bipolarly between the two extreme electrodes 1 and 3, 1–3, to the test pattern (upper traces) and to unpatterned control runs.

The positions of electrodes 1 and 3 correspond to the (two opposite polarity) peaks of the bipolar horizontal distribution (see Fig. 6.1(b)) of CI. Thus, recording between these electrodes produces a large-amplitude CI component but no significant CII component. The control runs show that there is negligible luminance-related contribution to this portion of the VEP. A succeeding offset-related positive peak is seen at the foot of the CI peak which can, if necessary, be further separated out by slightly increasing the pattern duration.

(b) CII and CIII: lower half-field test-pattern and control VEPs from same three common-reference electrodes as in (a) with, in addition, the VEPs to the offset of the 300 ms pattern presentation. Under these conditions large CII and CIII components are obtained at the mid-line electrode (2). The contamination of CIII by non-pattern- and offset-related contributions can be reduced by recording between electrodes 2 and 1. It is not possible in this case to separate out CII and CIII as effectively as CI and CII are separated in (a).

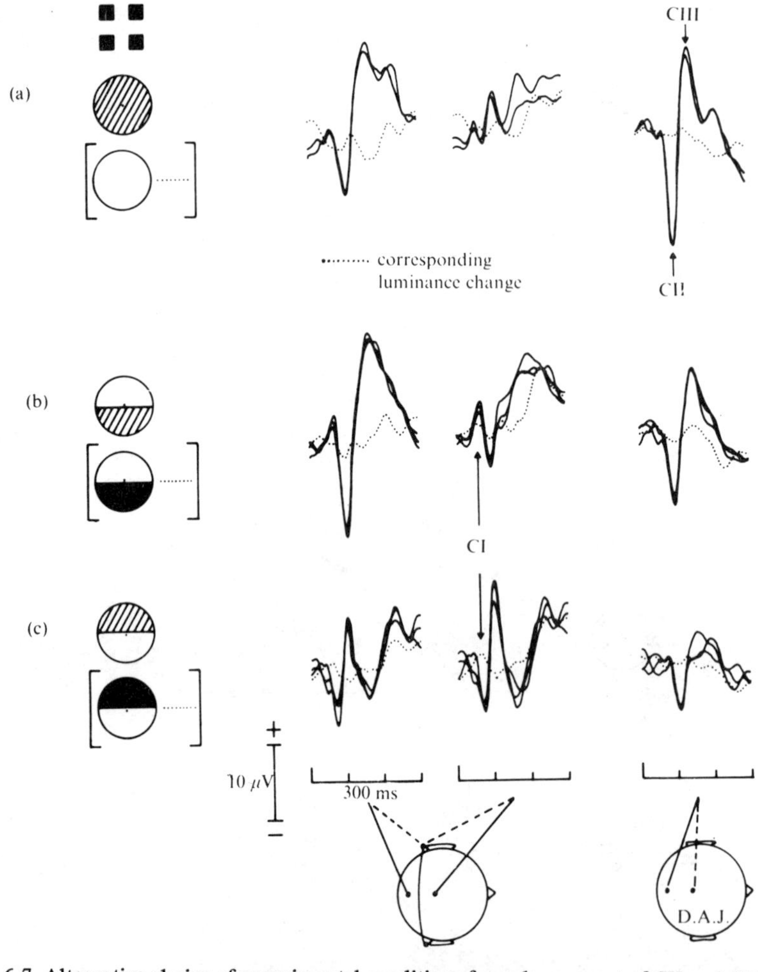

Fig. 6.7. Alternative choice of experimental conditions for enhancement of CII and CIII. VEPs recorded with respect to a common reference (linked earlobes) and bipolarly from two midline electrodes, 2·5 cm and 10 cm above the inion, to (a) full-field, and (b), and (c) lower and upper half-field presentation, respectively, of the test pattern and the corresponding luminance change. Large-amplitude CII and CIII components are obtained in the bipolarly recorded full-field VEPs because of the opposite polarity and different forms of vertical distributions of CII and CIII for the upper and lower half-field VEPs (see Fig. 6.1(a)). By contrast, the CI component in the upper and lower half-field VEPs have more symmetrical (opposite polarity) distributions and thus do not contribute significantly to these full-field VEPs.

conduction models of appropriate geometrical configuration (Jeffreys 1971*a*; Jeffreys and Axford 1972*a*, *b*). It is assumed in such models that the cortical generators of these surface potentials have essentially dipole-like properties.

Jeffreys and Axford (1972*a*, *b*) used such simple dipole models to explain basic qualitative features of the observed distributions of CI and CII, and proposed that CI originates from surface-negative activity in *striate cortex* (area 17) located mainly on the medial surfaces in and around the calcarine fissures, whereas CII is produced by surface-negative activity in *extrastriate cortex* (areas 18 and/or 19) located mainly on the outer surfaces of the occipital lobes. Subsequent studies using a greater number of subjects have provided further support for these results and conclusions. (Note that the proposals of Halliday and Michael (1970) and Michael and Halliday (1971) for the origin of a 100 ms peak of the *pattern-reversal* VEPs in extrastriate cortex are not strictly comparable to those of Jeffreys and Axford (1972*a*, *b*) for the striate and extrastriate cortical origins of C1 and CII, and are discussed in the next section.)

The results of the experiments described in the previous section suggest that CIII, like CII, is also produced in extrastriate cortex but not in identical regions. It has not yet been possible to predict the actual sites of origin of CII and CIII within the extrastriate cortical regions, because of insufficient information on both the detailed distributions of these components and on the layout and organization of the different extrastriate regions of the human visual cortex.

Nature of the sources of CI, CII, and CIII

The three successive components CI, CII, and CIII, obviously reflect changes in the electrical activity of the different cortical regions induced by the presentation of the stimulus pattern. Studies of the stimulus-related characteristics of these individual components can therefore provide information on the properties of the cortical processes in these different regions.

The main results and conclusions of an initial series of experiments designed to investigate the properties of CI, CII, and CIII are reported below. As one of the primary aims of these experiments was to determine the most physiologically informative of the stimulus parameters, the influence of a wide range of parameters on these VEP components has been investigated. Consequently, many of the findings have not yet been investigated in great depth, and relatively few subjects have so far been used. (Only one subject (D.A.J.) has undertaken the whole series of experiments, although each of the main results and conclusions has been verified on at least three subjects.) These experiments have, however, already established some important properties of the sources of these components and have demonstrated distinct differences in the characteristics of the components originating in the different cortical regions.

Variation with contrast and duration. A general feature of these, like most other pattern VEPs, is that for increasing pattern contrast, the VEP amplitude saturates, often at a relatively low contrast level, after an initial steady increase from threshold (Spekreijse 1966; Spekreijse *et al.* 1973). Campbell and Maffei (1970) found that the subsaturation amplitude of the VEPs obtained to 8 Hz alternation of a grid pattern varied linearly with the logarithm of contrast and that the extrapolated zero amplitude correlated with the psychophysical threshold (see also Campbell and Kulikowski 1972). Similar studies of these pattern-onset-related components have shown them to have more complicated contrast-dependent characteristics than the high-frequency responses of Campbell and Maffei (1970) and to be more difficult to quantify, since the variation in contrast produces changes in both latency and duration as well as in amplitude of the individual components. The main findings of these experiments are listed below.

(a) These components show similar subsaturation characteristics for changes of either contrast or duration and seem to obey the contrast equivalent of Bloch's law (Kulikowski 1972). With this tachistoscopic form of pattern presentation it is more convenient to obtain such VEP characteristics to the changes of duration of a high-contrast pattern.

(b) The thresholds (and latencies) and the saturation amplitudes of these VEP components are determined to a large extent by different stimulus parameters. For example in Fig. 6.8, the components of the VEPs obtained to a stimulus pattern of square outlines (Fig. 6.8(b)) have much higher thresholds but similar saturation amplitudes to those obtained to a corresponding pattern of solid squares (Fig. 6.8(a)). It has also been found that VEPs obtained to different forms of stimulus pattern can have similar thresholds (and latencies) but very different saturation amplitudes.

The component thresholds and latencies have been found to be dependent on contrast, duration, overall luminance, and on the spatial density (separation) and dimensions of the pattern elements, but are not greatly influenced by the actual structural details of the pattern elements. The exact dependence of the thresholds on each of these parameters has yet to be established. By contrast, the saturation amplitudes, especially of CII and CIII, are less dependent on contrast and overall luminance and are very dependent on the structural details of the pattern (e.g. Fig. 6.13).

(c) The 'threshold to saturation' characteristics can differ for the individual components in the same pattern VEP. For certain patterns, the later components, especially CIII, build up more rapidly and saturate at a lower contrast or duration level than CI. This is illustrated in Fig. 6.8(a) where, for the VEPs obtained to the solid squares pattern, CIII saturates at a much lower contrast than CI, although there is a less obvious difference in the rise to saturation of these components for the VEPs obtained to the pattern of square outlines (Fig. 6.8(b)).

There are several indications that the observed contrast-dependent properties of CIII, and to a lesser extent CII, parallel the subjective impression of the clarity of the contours (outlines) of the stimulus pattern elements. For example, it has been observed that the level of contrast or duration at which CIII approaches saturation seems to correspond roughly with the level required for the outlines of the pattern elements to be clearly seen throughout the stimulus field. Also, CIII reaches saturation level at lower values of contrast or duration for those stimulus patterns whose outlines are better defined at these low values. This

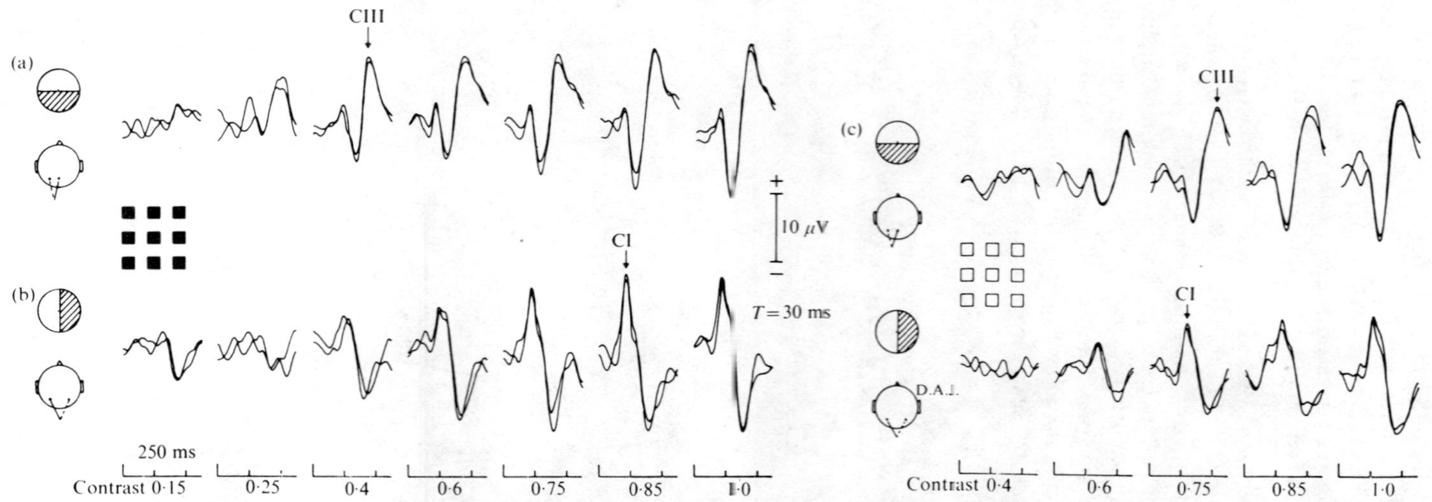

Fig. 6.8. Contrast dependence of the pattern VEPs. VEPs to corresponding stimulus patterns of (a) solid squares, and (b) square outlines, for different contrast values. The square side and separation in each case is 20′, and the outline thickness 2′. The combinations of pattern location and recording electrodes shown are those chosen to enhance CII (and CIII) (upper traces), and CI (lower traces). (Details as in Fig. 6.6).

For the solid squares in (a), there is a more rapid build-up of CIII than of CI (and CII) towards saturation. All components have higher contrast thresholds for the pattern of square outlines (b) than for the solid squares pattern (a), but the final (saturation) amplitudes in the two cases are similar.

could be related to the finding of Spekreijse *et al.* (1973) that 'the [onset] response to a chequerboard with checks exceeding 20′ saturates at a lower contrast than to one with smaller checks.' This behaviour of CIII is in marked contrast to that of CI, whose amplitude can increase substantially when the contrast or duration is increased beyond the level at which the pattern contours become clearly defined.

VEPs to step-changes of contrast. Marked differences in the behaviour of CI and of the later components are also evident in the VEPs obtained to a step-change (a brief increase from a variable resting contrast to the normal high-contrast level and back again) in the stimulus pattern contrast. There is a more rapid attenuation of CII and CIII than of CI as the resting contrast level is increased from zero (blank field) (Fig. 6.9), and there are again indications of an association between the behaviour of CII and CIII and the subjective definition of the outlines of the pattern elements. It appears that once the resting contrast level is raised sufficiently

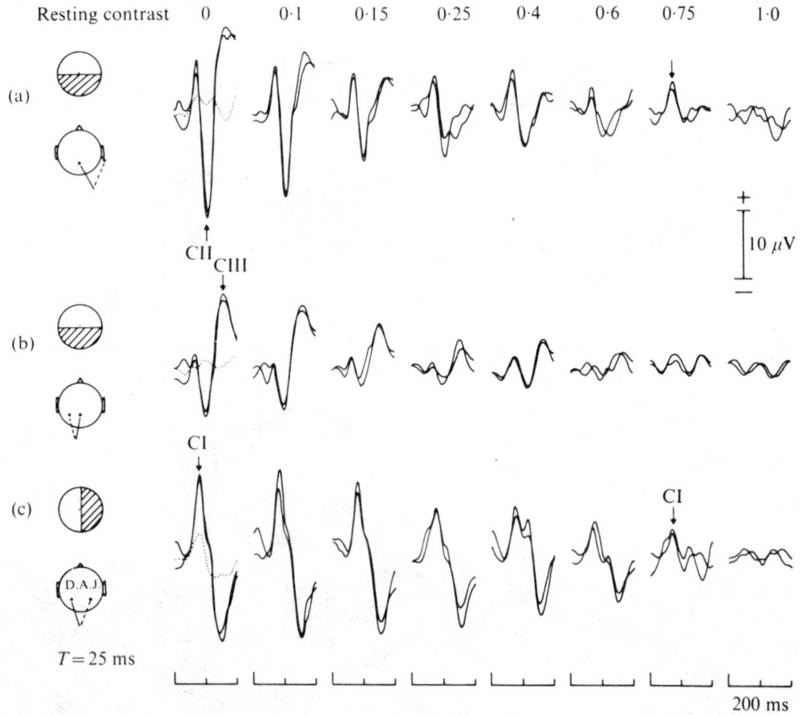

Fig. 6.9. VEPs to step-changes of contrast of the stimulus pattern. VEPs recorded to 25 ms step-increases of contrast of isolated squares pattern (square side and separation 20′) from variable resting contrast to the normal high-contrast level (1·0). The combinations of pattern location and recording electrodes shown in (a), (b), and (c) were chosen to enhance CII, CIII, and CI, respectively. (Details as in Fig. 6.6.)

With increasing resting contrast level, there is a rapid attenuation of CII and CIII in (a) and (b). CI, on the other hand, shows a much more gradual decrease in amplitude over the same range of (resting) contrast values (c).

for the pattern outlines to be clearly seen, i.e. when the stimulus appears solely as a contrast change, CII and CIII are always greatly attenuated but the amplitude of CI can remain relatively large.

Monocular and binocular VEPs. The binocular VEP components have lower thresholds and latencies than the monocular ones but often only slightly greater (saturation) amplitudes. Clear differences in the binocular to monocular amplitude ratio have been observed for the individual components of the same VEPs in some subjects (Harter, Chapter 10 of this book).

Sensitivity to structural details. The amplitudes of these pattern-related components, especially CII and CIII, are very dependent on the structural details of the stimulus pattern but seem independent of the polarity of the contrast of the pattern elements, i.e. similar VEPs are obtained to corresponding patterns whose elements are either lighter or darker than the background (Fig. 6.10). The most striking feature of this structure dependency is the consistent increase in amplitude obtained when patterns of continuous contours are broken up into discontinuous elements (Figs 6.2 and 6.10). No conclusive evidence has yet been obtained to show that either the thresholds or the (saturation) amplitudes of these components are dependent on the orientation of the pattern elements (Maffei and Campbell 1970).

Effects of prolonged pattern presentation. The effects of pattern pre-exposure on these pattern VEPs demonstrate further differences in the properties of the individual components. Comparatively short pre-exposure periods have been found to produce a marked attenuation of CII and CIII but not of CI. This selective attenuation (adaptation) of CII and CIII can occur even for the successive presentations of the stimulus pattern in a conventional averaging run if relatively long pattern durations are used. For example, in Fig. 6.11, components CII and CIII of the 25 ms VEP obtained at an inter-stimulus period (ISP) of 500 ms are much attenuated when the duration is increased to 200 ms, but CII recovers to its original amplitude when the ISP is subsequently increased to 2 s (Fig. 6.11(b)). Similar adaptation effects are observed for a low-contrast pattern (Fig. 6.11(c)). CIII behaves differently from CII under these conditions, and attenuates with increasing ISP for the 25 ms VEPs (Fig. 6.11(a)), although the significance of this has yet to be investigated. (The short-duration stimulus used in these experiments was chosen principally to avoid any such adaptation of these pattern-onset-related components even at short ISPs.)

Preliminary experiments carried out using independently controlled 'adapting' and test patterns have shown that, following pattern pre-exposure, there is an increase of the component thresholds (and latencies) in addition to the eventual attenuation of CII and CIII already described. These adaptation effects appear to be both orientation- and dimension-specific, although the exact degree of such selectivity of the individual components has yet to be established. No adaptation

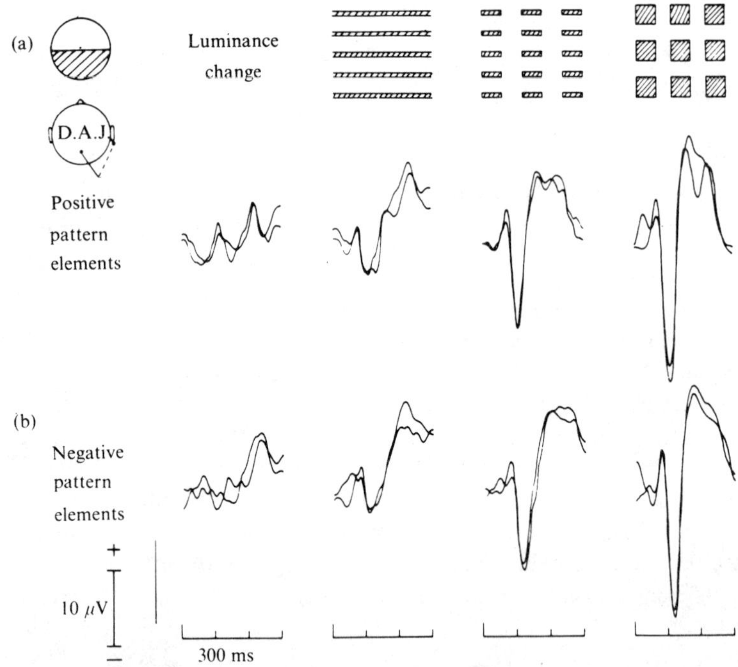

Fig. 6.10. VEPs to pattern of continuous and discontinuous contours. Lower half-field VEPs recorded from midline electrode (5 cm above inion) to patterns whose elements are (a) darker and (b) lighter than the background of the test field. The VEPs in (a) were obtained by the conventional method involving the alternate switching of the test field (positive pattern) and the reference (blank) field of the tachistoscope. For the VEPs in (b), the reference (blank) field was continuously on and only the test field, containing the photographic negative of the required pattern, was switched on and off. The line thickness and separation for both the grid and the short bar pattern were 5′ and 25′, respectively, and the length of the bars 25′. The sides and separation of the squares were 25′ and 45′, respectively. The VEPs obtained to 50 per cent (overall) luminance changes are shown on the left of the figure.

Essentially similar VEPs are obtained to corresponding positive and negative contrast patterns. The amplitudes of CII and CIII are significantly greater for the pattern of short bars than to the grid pattern (continuous parallel straight lines).

effects are evident for components of a given quadrant VEP following pattern pre-exposure in a separate quadrant of the stimulus field. There is at least partial interocular transfer of these adaptation effects.

Role of the contours (outlines) of the stimulus pattern elements. In addition to those already described, there are basic differences between the dependence of CII and CIII and of CI on the contours (outlines) of the pattern elements. For example, these components are selectively influenced by gradual de-focusing of the stimulus pattern, CI being more resistant to de-focusing than either CII or CIII, especially for large-size pattern elements. Thus, for the VEPs obtained to checkerboard patterns of different square size shown in Fig. 6.12, whereas 3

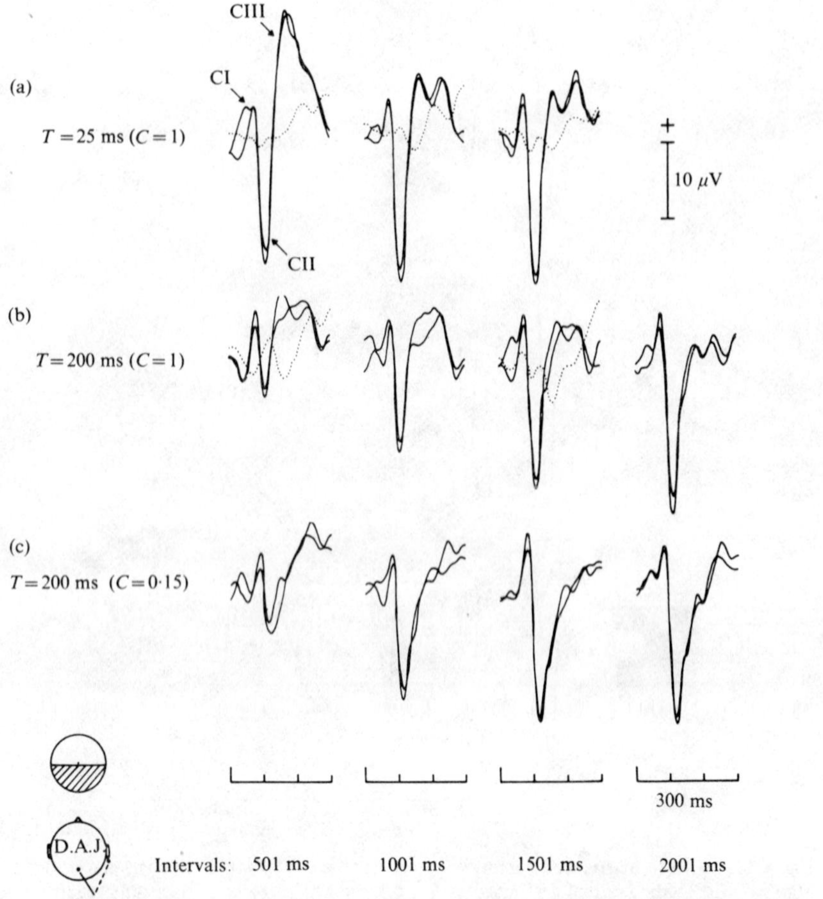

Fig. 6.11. Adaptation of CII and CIII in long-duration (averaged) VEPs. Lower half-field VEPs recorded from midline electrode (5 cm above inion) for (a) 25 ms; (b) 200 ms presentation of a high-contrast (1·0) pattern; and (c) 200 ms presentation of same pattern (isolated squares, 20′ square side and separation) at low contrast (0·15), at intervals of 501, 1001, 1501, and 2001 ms. Overall luminance change (50 per cent) VEPs shown as dotted traces.

There is a marked attenuation of CII and CIII, but not of CI, in the VEPs obtained at 501 ms intervals when the duration is increased from 25 ms to 200 ms (left-hand column). However, CI recovers to its original amplitude with subsequent increase of intervals. (b) The decrease in the amplitude of CIII in the 25 ms VEP with increasing intervals in this case does not appear to occur in all subjects and its significance is not known. Similar changes of components CII and CIII are seen for the low-contrast pattern.

dioptre lenses produce a substantial attenuation of CII and CIII in each case, progressively stronger lenses are required to produce a comparable attenuation of CI for increases in square size. Subjectively, when there is sufficient defocusing to make the outlines of the pattern elements indistinct, CII and CIII are invariably attenuated. By contrast, CI can remain relatively unattenuated in conditions

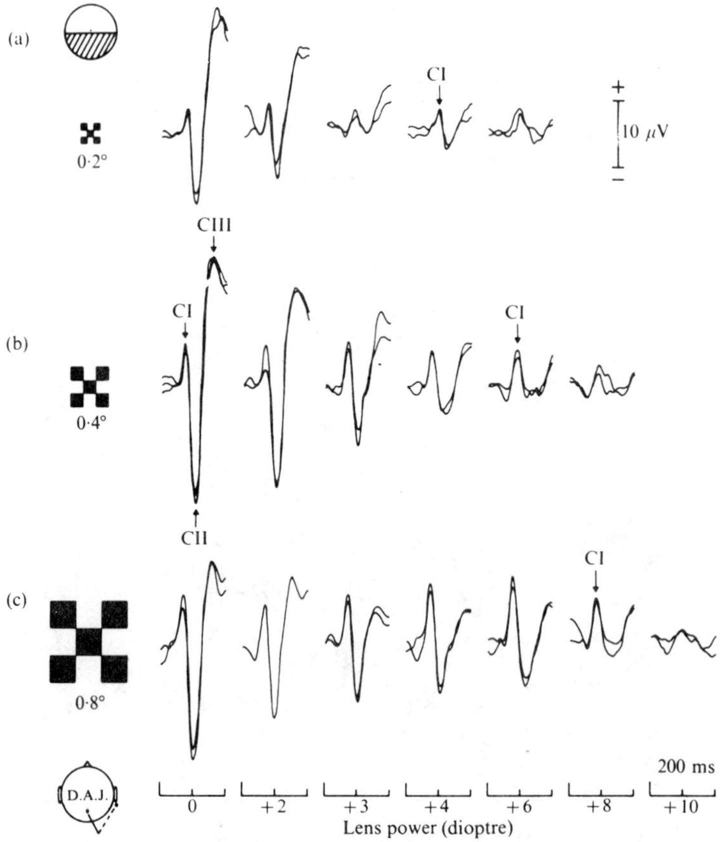

Fig. 6.12. VEPs to de-focused patterns. Lower half-field VEPs from midline electrode (5 cm above inion) to the gradual de-focusing of checkerboard patterns of different square dimensions: (a) 0·2, (b) 0·4, and (c) 0·8° square side. The patterns were de-focused with positive lenses of 2, 3, 4, 6, 8, and 10 dioptres.

There is a more rapid attenuation of CII and CIII than of CI with increased de-focusing. This is most apparent for the large square sizes where lenses of up to 6D or more have apparently little effect on the amplitude of CI.

where the (large-square) pattern appears as an array of very blurred 'contrast' patches, but it disappears when the stimulus field appears uniformly illuminated.

Note that the variations of checkerboard *reversal VEPs* with defocusing described by Regan and Richards (1973), in which moderate blurring increases the VEP amplitudes for large square patterns while attenuating those for small square patterns, is certainly not characteristic of components CII and CIII in these VEPs. They could, however, relate to the observed behaviour of CI which, in Fig. 6.12, shows an apparent increase of amplitude with increasing defocusing of the large square (0·8°). These experiments have not yet been carried out using the optimal conditions needed to isolate CI and therefore it is uncertain whether this is a genuine amplitude increase of CI or an artifact due to the overlap of CI and CII.

The changes induced in these pattern VEPs by the introduction of steady (continuously present) outlines of the stimulus pattern elements also indicates a greater dependence of CII and CIII on the contours of the pattern elements. This is illustrated in Fig. 6.13, which shows the effects of varying duration and ISP on the VEPs obtained to a pattern of isolated squares without and with the steady outlines of the squares. The prominent CII and CIII components seen in the normal lower half-field 25 ms VEPs, which attenuate (adapt) with increasing duration, have virtually disappeared from the responses obtained with the steady outlines (Fig. 6.13(a)). By contrast, the CI component in the VEPs obtained under these particular experimental conditions (chosen for the study of CII) seems uninfluenced either by the effects of adaptation or by the steady outlines. However, when optimal experimental conditions are chosen to isolate CI (Fig. 6.13(b)), this component also shows a similar but relatively smaller reduction and subsequent recovery of amplitude to those observed for CII in Fig. 6.13(a) for these changes of duration and ISP. Furthermore, there is now a definite attenuation of CI when the steady outlines are present although, unlike CII and CIII, it retains a significant residual amplitude in this condition which does not seem to change with these changes of duration and ISPs.

In contrast to CII and CIII, neither of the two main positive offset-related peaks in these VEPs is influenced by the presence of the steady outlines. The earlier peak, seen in the right half-field VEPs (Fig. 6.13(b)) corresponds in latency and distribution to CI, and in this case has a comparable amplitude to that of the residual CI component of the 'steady-outline' VEPs.

Interaction between test- and steady-pattern elements. As shown above, the presence of steady outlines of the discrete elements (squares) in the stimulus pattern produces a substantial attenuation of CII and CIII. This has been found for square sizes up to at least 1°. Further experiments have shown that the alignment of the steady contours and the test-pattern elements is not a necessary requirement for this attenuation, but that their relative linear dimensions seem very important, at least for CII. For example, in Fig. 6.14, whereas both CII and CIII are much attenuated by the steady pattern of short bars or squares (even when displaced), CII seems little affected by an aligned steady pattern of continuous lines (grids). This figure also demonstrates the selective influence of these steady patterns on CII and CIII, as there is a significant (if variable) attenuation of CIII in all cases. These effects seem to differ in several respects from those described by Spekreijse (1966) who found that the *reversal VEPs* to low-contrast checkerboard patterns were almost completely suppressed by the presence of high-contrast fine grid patterns, and that this effect required accurate alignment of the grids and the borders of the squares.

Although in all the examples shown here the steady- and test-pattern elements

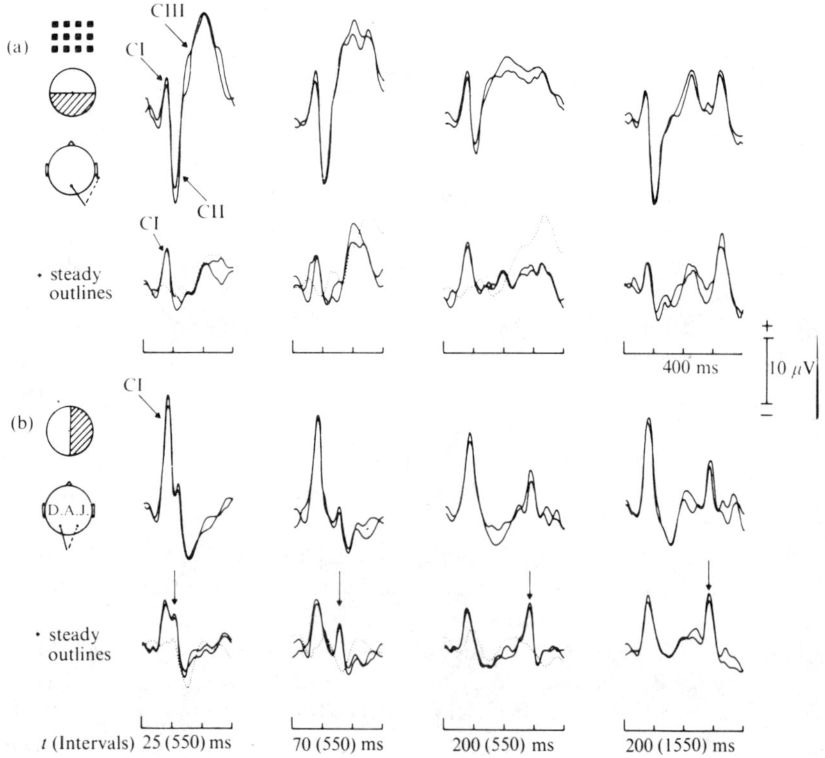

Fig. 6.13. Influence of steady outlines on VEPs for different pattern durations. VEPs to a pattern of isolated squares, without (upper traces) and with (lower traces) (0·5′) steady outlines of the squares at durations of 25 ms, 70 ms, and 200 ms at 550 ms (mean) intervals; and at 200 ms at 1500 ms intervals. The VEPs obtained to corresponding (50 per cent) overall luminance changes are shown as dotted traces. The combinations of pattern location and recording electrodes shown in (a) and (b) were chosen to enhance CII (and CIII) and CI, respectively. (Details as in Fig. 6.6).

Components CII and CIII of the 25 ms lower half-field VEPs in (a) which show similar adaptation effects to those described in Fig. 6.11 for these changes of duration and interval, virtually disappear when the steady outlines are present. By contrast, component CI in these VEPs seems unaffected either by the temporal variations or by the presence of the steady outlines. However, when experimental conditions are chosen to isolate this component (b), CI is then seen both to show similar adaptation effects and to be attenuated by the steady outlines, although to a lesser degree than CII and CIII. There is a residual CI component in the steady-outline VEPs which is apparently uninfluenced by the changes of duration and ISP.

Two offset-related components are seen in these VEPs: a positive 120 ms component seen in the 200 ms lower half-field VEP at the longer interval in (a), and an earlier positive peak (arrow) seen in each of the left half-field VEPs in (b), which corresponds in latency and distribution to CI. In this case, this initial offset-related component has a similar amplitude to the residual CI component of the steady-outline VEPs. Neither of the offset-related components is greatly influenced by the steady outlines.

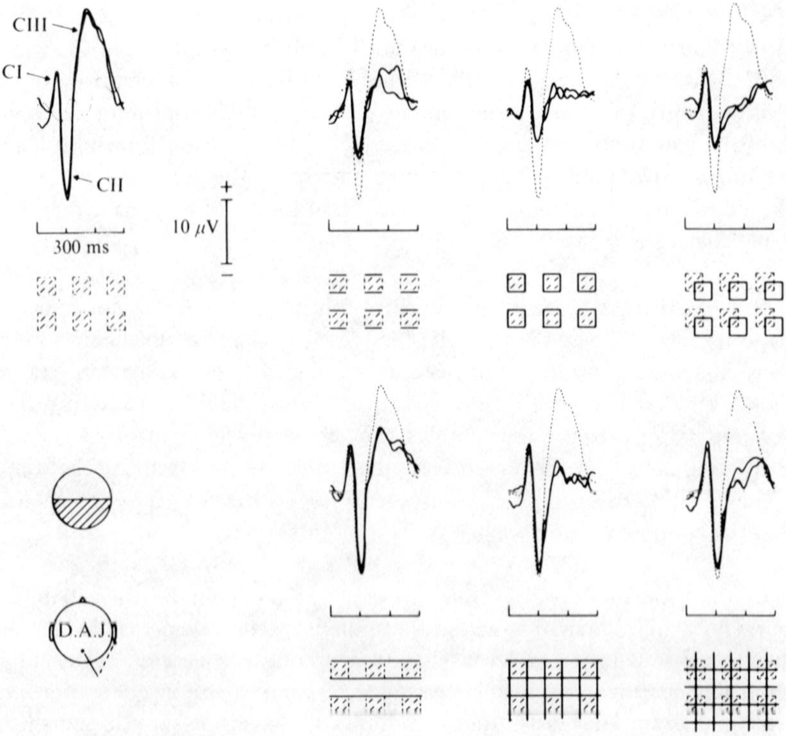

Fig. 6.14. Influence of steady contours on the pattern VEPs. Lower half-field VEPs recorded from midline electrode (5 cm above inion) to the conventional 25 ms presentation of an isolated squares pattern (20′ square side and separation) shown on the upper left of the figure. On the right-hand side are shown the VEPs obtained to the presentation of the same pattern when steady (0·5′ thick) contours are present in the test field. The spatial relationship between the form of the steady contours and the test-pattern squares are as indicated below each VEP.

There is a marked attenuation of both CII and CIII in each of three upper VEPs where the steady-contour dimensions correspond to those of the test-pattern squares. This is true even when the test-pattern squares and the steady (square) outlines are displaced. By contrast, there is little apparent attenuation of CII for steady (continuous) grid patterns (lower traces) even when these are aligned with the borders of the test-pattern squares. Component CIII, however, is still attenuated to varying extents by the grid patterns.

overlap, such interaction effects are also found when these elements are spatially separated. Preliminary experiments have indicated that in such cases the degree of attenuation of CII, at least, is both orientation- and dimension-specific, and for both CII and CIII it decreases with increasing separation of adjacent test and steady pattern elements. Similar interaction effects are observed whether the contrast of the test- and steady-pattern elements has the same or opposite polarity. The precise degree and spatial extent of these interaction effects has yet to be determined, but the range of interaction appears more localized for CII than for CIII. There is at least partial interocular transfer of these effects.

Summary and conclusions

The marked differences in the properties of CI compared with those of CII and CIII indicate that there are two distinct types of cortical processes contributing to these components: (a) 'contrast-specific' mechanisms, which contribute solely to CI, and (b) 'contour-specific' mechanisms, which provide the predominant contributions to CII and CIII but also contribute to CI. The properties so far established for these VEP components suggest that these processes have the following characteristics:

(a) *Contrast-specific processes* are sensitive to pattern stimuli but not to overall luminance changes. They do not require the presence of well-defined contours (outlines) and show a systematic increase of response with increasing contrast from threshold over a relatively wide range of contrast values. Such mechanisms respond to the onset and/or offset of the stimulus; they are relatively unadaptive, and are not greatly influenced by the presence of adjacent (steady) elements in the stimulus field. They seem to be mainly binocularly sensitive. (It has not yet been established whether the contrast-specific portion of CI is orientation specific.)

(b) *Contour-specific processes* respond best to pattern stimuli with well-defined contours (no spatial summation within the stimulus pattern elements) and are less sensitive to the actual contrast level. They respond only to the onset of the stimulus and are highly adaptive, presumably ceasing to respond to prolonged (stationary) pattern stimulation. They are both orientation- and dimension-specific being mainly sensitive to discontinuous contours. They are influenced by adjacent (steady) contours and are binocularly sensitive.

Since CI is thought to originate in striate cortex and CII and CIII in extrastriate cortex (see p. 144), then the contrast-specific mechanisms appear to be confined to the striate cortex, whereas the contour-specific mechanisms predominate in extrastriate regions but are also present to a lesser degree in striate cortex.

Jeffreys and Axford (1972*a*) found that the contributions to these VEP components from separate (sector and annular) regions within individual quadrants of the stimulus field are essentially independent. This indicates that, in common with the 'contour-sensitive' single neurones found in the visual cortex of the cat and monkey (e.g. Hubel and Wiesel, 1962, 1965, 1968), these contrast- and contour-specific VEP sources are sensitive to stimulation within localized regions of the visual field. Moreover, there are several similarities in their basic properties which suggests a possible relationship between these VEP components and populations of such neurones in the human visual cortex. There is already much psychophysical evidence (e.g. Andrews 1965; Campbell and Kulikowski 1966; Blakemore and Campbell 1969; Tolhurst 1972; Nakayama and Roberts 1972) and limited electrophysiological evidence (Marg, Adams, and Rutkin 1968; Maffei and Campbell 1970) to suggest that mechanisms with corresponding properties do exist in the human visual cortex. However, further data are required on the characteristics of these VEP components before accurate comparisons can be made with the known properties of single neurones. Thus, experiments are now under way to study in more detail the dependence of the individual VEP components on parameters such as the spatial configuration, orientation, dimensions, and contrast of the pattern elements, and on their precise orientation and dimension specificity as determined from adaptation (pattern pre-exposure) and lateral interaction (between test- and steady-pattern elements) experiments.

It is interesting that there is relatively little evidence of such clear distinctions in the properties of different classes of neurones in cats and monkeys to compare with those seen between contrast- and contour-specific VEP components in man. However, there have been very few single-unit studies of the influence of those parameters which most clearly differentiate between the two types of VEP sources, namely: contrast, contour definition, and the adaptation effects produced by prolonged stimulation. The VEP results could, however, relate to Wurtz's (1969*b*) findings that single units in the striate cortex of the awake monkey tended to fall into two groups; the first group responded vigorously and with a non-adapting response to a stationary stimulus; the second group responded best to a moving stimulus and gave a rapidly adapting response to a stationary stimulus.

In one of the few studies to specifically investigate the contrast dependency of single units, Maffei and Fiorentini (1973) found that only the *simple cells* in cat consistently showed a linear relationship between the magnitude of their response and the logarithm of the contrast of a sinusoidal grating pattern. Only a small proportion of complex cells in striate cortex showed such a linear relationship and the responses of these cells tended to saturate at relatively low contrast levels. Since simple cells are found exclusively in the striate cortex, and as they show spatial summation within the 'on' and 'off' regions of their location-specific receptive fields, this suggests their possible involvement in the contrast-specific contributions to component CI. Furthermore, Fiorentini and Maffei (1973) have found that the subjective estimate of pattern *contrast* (apparent contrast) shows a similar linear relationship with the logarithm of objective contrast to that found for the simple cells, and also for the amplitude of VEPs obtained to the high-frequency alternation of a sinusoidal grating pattern (Campbell and Maffei 1970).

The properties of the contour-specific mechanisms, on the other hand, make it unlikely that they are at all associated with simple cells, and their sensitivity to discontinuous contours suggests a possible major involvement of hypercomplex-type neurones (Hubel and Wiesel 1965). As mentioned above, there are several indications that these processes are more closely related to aspects of the structure than to the contrast level of the stimulus pattern. They could therefore provide important clues to the nature of the pattern-detection processes in the human visual cortex. For example, the apparent predominance of these (nonlinear) contour-specific processes in extrastriate cortex would seem to argue against a method of pattern detection in these regions based on spatial Fourier analysis techniques (Pollen and Taylor 1974; Campbell 1974), and is more consistent with a 'feature extraction' system (Hubel and Wiesel 1965).

At this stage, any such predictions of relationships between the sources of these VEPs and populations of cortical neurones are, of course, very tentative, and must await the results of more detailed studies. However, the results so far obtained suggest that these pattern-related VEP components are meaningful reflections of underlying physiological mechanisms and thus could provide a useful tool for investigating the cortical pattern-detection processes.

Relationship between the VEPs obtained to brief pattern presentations and to other forms of pattern stimulation

The marked differences in the VEPs produced by brief pattern presentations and those obtained to other forms of presentation of the same pattern are due largely to the highly adaptive properties of the contour-specific components in these VEPs. Because of their rapid attenuation with prolonged stimulation, these contour-specific components are not usually evident in the averaged VEPs obtained in conditions where the stimulus pattern or its outline is present for most of the stimulus cycle.

The relationship between the different types of pattern VEPs can often clarified by using similar component-analysis techniques to those described in the first section of this chapter. Thus, components of common or different cortical origin in the different VEPs can be identified from a comparison of their surface distributions and their relationship to the retinal location of the stimulus pattern. Such studies were carried out in 5 subjects to directly compare the VEPs elicited by brief (25 ms) presentation and to the (300 ms duration) onset, offset, and reversal of the same checkerboard pattern stimulus. The main results and conclusions of these experiments are given below together with a discussion of the relationship of these VEPs with those obtained to some other commonly used patterned stimuli.

Onset, offset, and reversal VEPs

These surface mapping studies showed clearly that there are no components corresponding to either CII or CIII in the offset and reversal VEPs obtained under these conditions. However, a component of similar distribution characteristics to CI (presumably the contrast-specific and relatively unadaptive portion of CI) is often evident in the offset VEPs. This can be seen in Fig. 6.15, which shows the horizontal distributions of each of the lower half-field VEPs for subject D.A.J. The positive and negative peaks at about 100–20 ms and 150 ms latency, respectively, of these offset and reversal VEPs are seen for most of these subjects and seem typical of the responses obtained by other investigators (e.g. Halliday and Michael 1970; Spekreijse *et al.* 1973).

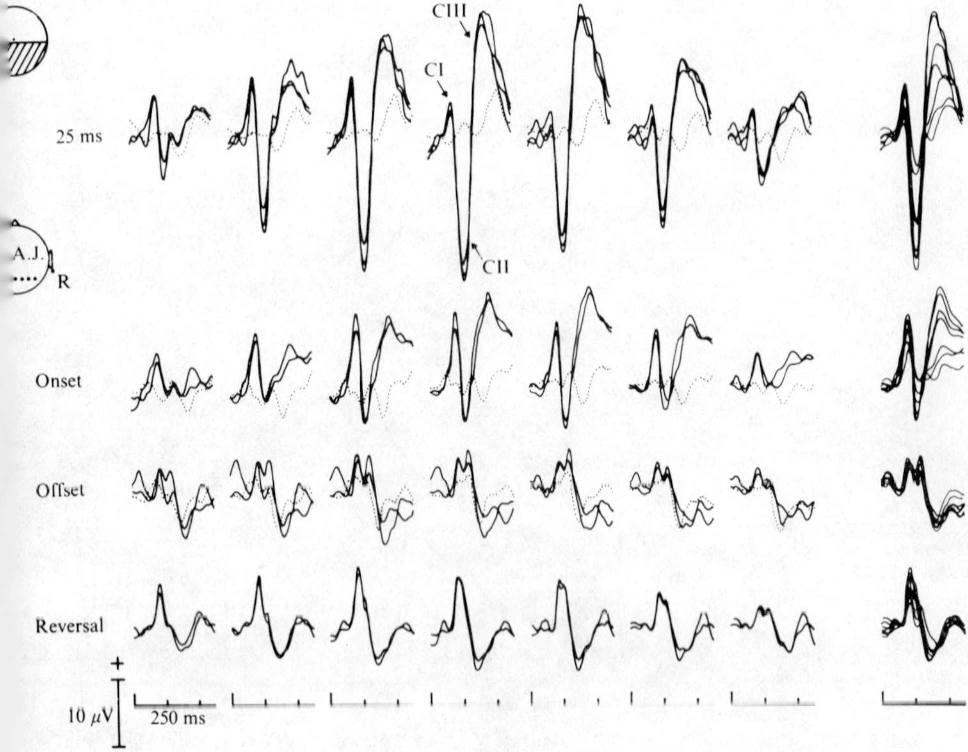

Fig. 6.15. Comparison of 25 ms, onset, offset, and reversal VEPs. Lower half-field VEPs recorded from horizontal row of electrodes to (a) 25 ms presentation, (b) and (c) the onset and offset of a 300 ms presentation, respectively, and (d) the reversal of a 15′ checkerboard pattern. Corresponding (50 per cent) overall luminance-change VEPs are denoted by the dotted traces. The (mean) pattern VEP waveforms recorded at each electrode are superposed on the right of the figure.

No components corresponding in form or distribution to CII and CIII are seen in either the offset or the reversal VEPs, and these components are much reduced in amplitude in the onset VEPs. However, a component corresponding to CI is seen in all these responses. Note that there is an apparent difference in the distribution of CI in the 25 ms and the onset VEPs. This is due to the effects of the overlap of CI with the succeeding large negative CII component in the 25 ms VEP. Since CII is much attenuated in the onset VEPs these give a truer indication of the actual CI distribution. In the offset VEP, the CI component is followed by a second positive 120 ms peak and a negative 150 ms peak. In the reversal VEPs, an apparently single broad positive peak at the midline electrodes can be seen to be made up of the merging of an initial component corresponding to CI and a succeeding positive peak of slightly different distribution. The reversal VEPs also contain a 150 ms negative peak of similar widespread distribution to that of the offset VEPs.

The prominent positive (100–20 ms) peak in these reversal VEPs appears to be composite, containing two overlapping positive peaks of different spatial distributions (Fig. 6.15(d)). The dual nature of this peak is also evident if the contrast of one of the alternating (complementary) checkerboard patterns is

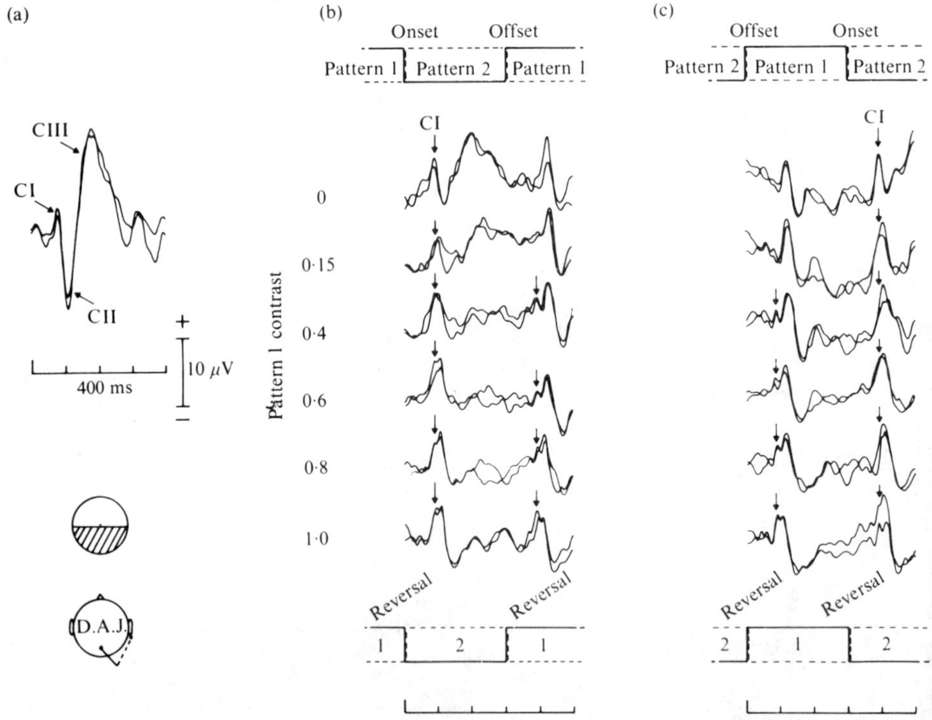

Fig. 6.16. Contributions from onset and offset VEPs to the reversal VEPs. (a) Lower half-field VEPs recorded from midline electrode (5 cm above inion) to conventional 25 ms presentation of 15′ checkerboard pattern. (b) and (c) VEPs obtained to the alternation of the same high-contrast checkerboard with the complementary checkerboard of variable contrast, showing the progressive changes in the VEPs from an initial (b) onset–offset, and (c) offset–onset, through several contrast levels to the final reversal–reversal condition.

The CI component in the onset VEPs (arrowed) and the main positive offset VEP peak can be traced through each of these responses to the reversal VEPs. There appears to be a decrease in the latency of the offset VEP peak with increasing contrast.

varied from zero (blank field) to the normal high contrast level. This is illustrated in Fig. 6.16 which shows the changes produced in the VEP waveshape as the stimulus is changed from an initial onset–offset or offset–onset condition through several (contrast) stages to a final reversal–reversal condition. These results suggest that the two components that make up this composite reversal VEP peak correspond to the CI component of the onset VEP and the main (second) positive peak of the offset VEP. This conclusion is supported by the similarities observed in the distribution characteristics of the early and late portions of this reversal VEP peak with those of CI and of this offset VEP peak, respectively, for all these subjects, including one subject (I.C.) with anomalous CI distributions. Estevez and Spekreijse (1974) have also proposed a similar major offset VEP contribution to the reversal VEPs.

Although some early experiments had suggested a possible similarity in the properties of the main (120 ms) offset VEP peak and of CII (Jeffreys 1972), these experiments have clearly shown that the distribution characteristics of this component (and the later negative 150 ms peak in the offset and reversal VEPs) differ from each of these pattern-onset-related components. In fact, they resemble more closely the main non-pattern-related components in that they vary little with retinal location (Clarke 1973). This is illustrated in Fig. 6.17, which shows that there is no polarity reversal of this component in the VEPs obtained to stimulation of the upper and lower half-fields. These results also indicate that only the CI contribution to these reversal VEPs is very dependent on retinal location – e.g. for the first 4 subjects in Fig. 6.17, the polarity reversal seems to occur only for that portion of the responses corresponding in latency to CI, and furthermore, does not occur at all for the one subject (I.C.) who does not show a polarity reversal of CI in the 25 ms and onset VEPs. These results thus suggest that the main positive offset VEP component (and the negative 150 ms component), which appear to be present also in these reversal VEPs, could be a non-pattern-related component! This might explain the basic differences in the characteristics of this offset VEP component compared to the onset-related components (Spekreijse and Estevez 1972; Spekreijse *et al.* 1973), but does not appear to fit in with Spekreijse's (1966) findings that low-contrast reversal VEPs are completely suppressed by the presence of steady high-contrast outline grids.

The characteristics of the reversal VEPs obtained under these conditions clearly conflict with those reported by Halliday and Michael (1970; Halliday, 1972*b*) for reversal VEPs obtained with a different form of stimulation. They reported that a prominent 100 ms component showed consistent and systematic changes with retinal location and showed a clear polarity reversal for stimulation of the upper and lower field for all subjects. Moreover, they found that this polarity reversal is associated with the vertical but not the horizontal octants of the stimulus field, which thus argued against a striate cortical origin for this component (cf. Halliday, Barrett, Halliday and Michael, Chapter 5 of this book).

Corresponding experiments carried out by the author with three subjects showed no clear evidence of a similar polarity reversal of a corresponding component in these reversal VEPs for either vertical or horizontal octants of the upper and lower field (Fig. 6.18). On the contrary, these experiments provided further evidence both for the presence of a component corresponding to CI in these responses and for its origin in striate cortex. For example, in Fig. 6.18(a), there is a clearer polarity reversal of the CI component in all these VEPs for stimulation of the *horizontal* than for the vertical octants of the upper and lower fields. In addition, there is a larger contralateral amplitude of this component for stimulation of the *vertical* than for the horizontal octants of the right half-field (Fig. 6.18(b)). These results are thus consistent with the proposed model for the striate cortical origin of CI (Jeffreys and Axford 1972*a*).

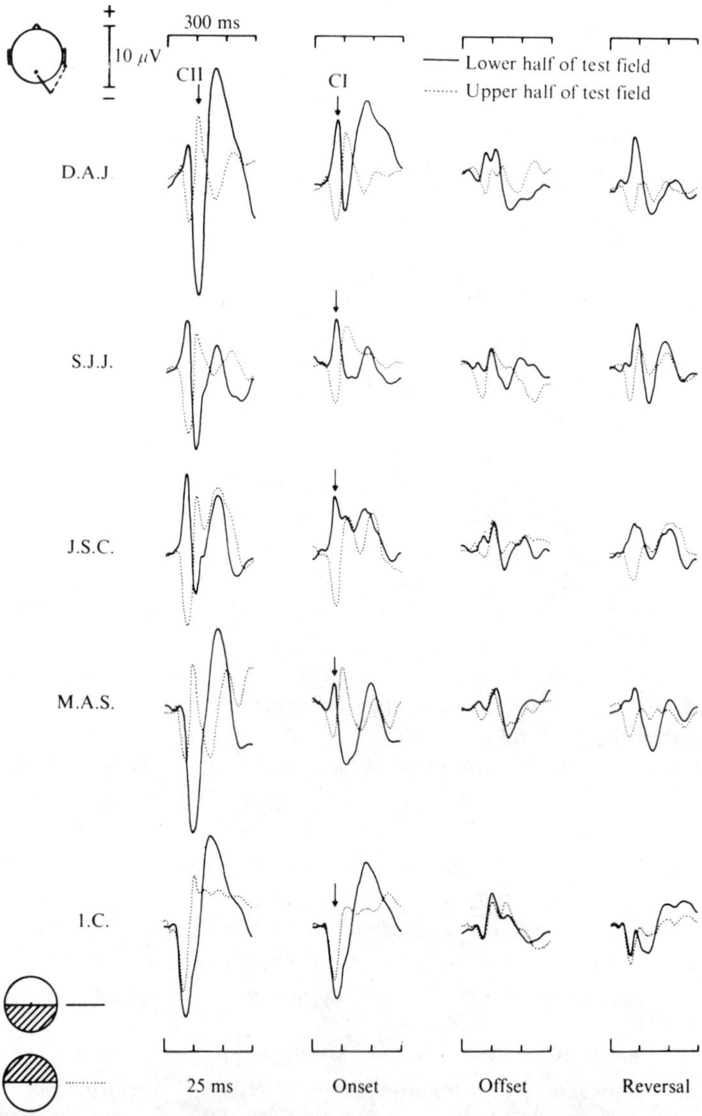

Fig. 6.17. Comparison of the different forms of pattern VEPs for upper and lower field stimulation. VEPs recorded from midline electrode (5 cm above inion) in each of the five subjects to the 25 ms presentation, the onset and offset of a 300 ms presentation, and to the (300 ms) reversal of a checkerboard pattern in the lower and upper half of the test field.

The onset VEPs show that the CI component (arrowed) has opposite polarity for the upper and lower field VEPs in four of these subjects, but has the same (negative) polarity for subject I.C. Corresponding components of smaller amplitude are seen in the offset and reversal VEPs which again have reversed polarity for the upper and lower field responses for four subjects but not for subject I.C. By contrast, there is no clear polarity reversal of the succeeding portions of the offset and reversal VEPs to compare with that seen in the 25 ms VEPs for CII and, in some cases, for CIII. These results thus indicate the presence of a component corresponding to CI but none corresponding to either CII or CIII in these offset or reversal VEPs.

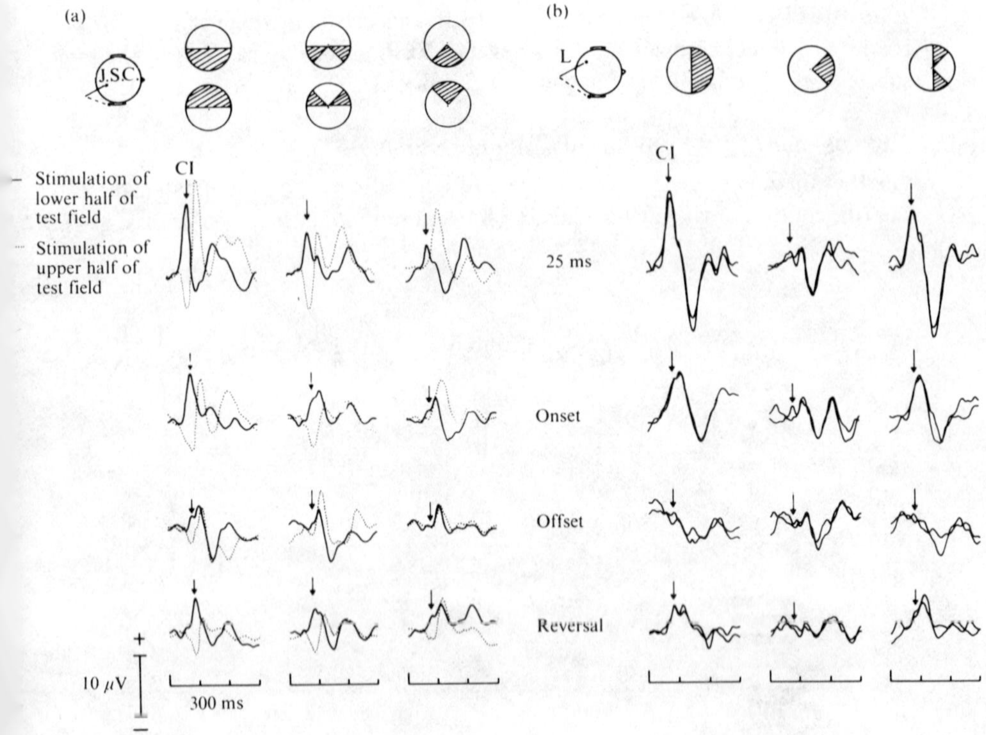

Fig. 6.18. Comparison of the different pattern VEPs for stimulation of the horizontal and vertical octants of the test field. In (a), the VEPs recorded from an electrode 5 cm above the inion and 2·5 cm to the right of the midline to stimulation of the lower and upper half of the test field (by a 0·508 mm (0·02 in) checkerboard pattern) are shown in the left-hand column. The VEPs obtained to stimulation of the two horizontal, and the two vertical octants of the lower and upper field are shown in the middle and right-hand columns, respectively. (b) VEPs recorded from an electrode 5 cm to the left of the midline, and 5 cm above the inion, to the presentation of the right half-field pattern and to the selective stimulation of its horizontal and vertical octants.

In (a), the polarity reversal of CI in the 25 ms and onset VEPs for upper- and lower-field stimulation is clearly associated more with the horizontal than with the vertical octants. This also appears to be the case for the corresponding regions of the offset and reversal VEPs. In (b) the large positive CI component of the 25 ms and onset VEPs, recorded at the contralateral electrode for right half-field stimulation, is clearly associated with the vertical and not the horizontal octants of the field, and this is again true for the corresponding region of the reversal VEPs.

There is therefore no indication in these reversal VEPs of a component corresponding to that which Halliday proposes originates in extrastriate cortex. Moreover, Halliday does not appear to find a component corresponding to CI in the reversal VEPs produced using his slide-projector stimulus (cf. Chapter 1 of this book). This basic conflict in *data* suggests possible differences in the form of the reversal VEPs obtained with the different stimulus methods which can best be resolved by direct comparison of the reversal VEPs in the two cases using the same subjects (cf. Halliday *et al.*, Chapter 5 of this book).

VEPs obtained at high-frequency pattern presentation

Another method of generating pattern VEPs, initially used by Campbell and Maffei (1970), consists of the high-frequency (8 Hz) reversal of a sinusoidal-profile grating

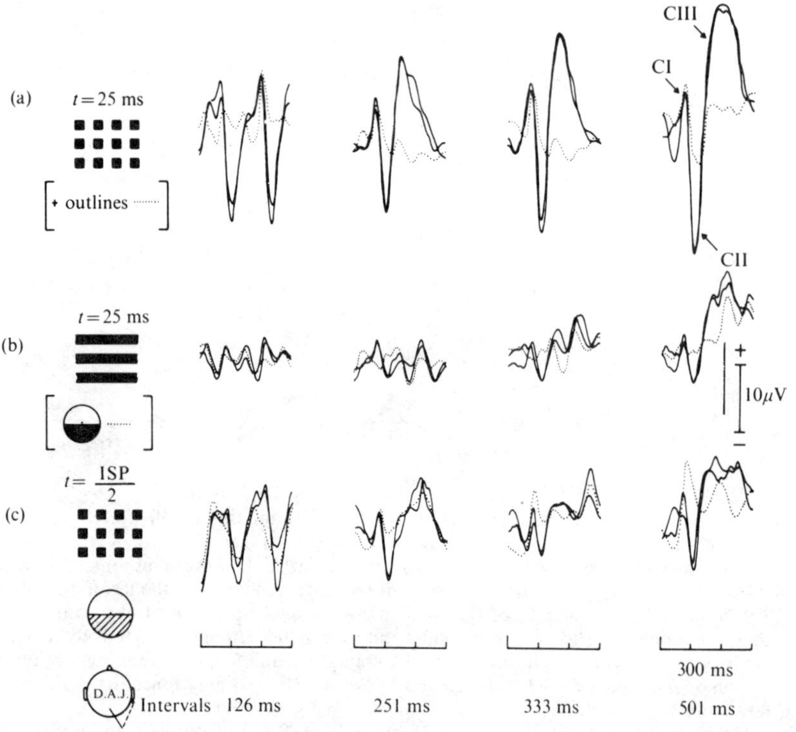

Fig. 6.19. Comparison of low and high temporal frequency pattern VEPs. Lower half-field VEPs recorded from a midline electrode (5 cm above inion) to the presentation of a pattern of isolated squares ((a) and (c)), and (b) a grid pattern, at frequences of 8 Hz, 4 Hz, 3 Hz, and 2 Hz. The duration of presentation is 25 ms in (a) and (b) and equal to half the intervals in (c). Square side and separation and stripe thickness 15′. The dotted traces in (a) and (c) represent the VEPs obtained in the presence of steady outlines of the squares, and those in (b) the overall (50 per cent) luminance-change VEPs.

In (a), the large-amplitude CII and CIII components in the 25 ms VEPs at 2 Hz attenuate with increasing frequency, and although there still appears to be a CII contribution to the 8 Hz responses there is little evidence of any CIII component at these high frequencies. In (b), much smaller CII and CIII components are seen in the 2 Hz grid pattern VEPs, which again attenuate with increasing frequency, and there is no evidence of either of these components in the 8 Hz VEPs. CII and CIII are also reduced in the longer duration VEPs obtained to the squares pattern at 2 Hz in (c). In this case, relatively large amplitude VEPs are obtained at 8 Hz both with and without the steady outlines.

pattern. This stimulus produces a roughly sinusoidal VEP which is easy to quantify but whose composition is obscure. However, the properties already established for both the low-frequency reversal VEPs and for the pattern-onset-related components suggest that these responses are likely to reflect the activity of contrast-specific processes with little if any contour-specific contributions. The author has made no direct studies of these high-frequency reversal VEPs as yet, but Fig. 6.19(b) shows that even with the 25 ms presentation of a (square-wave profile) grating pattern, the relatively small CII and CIII components obtained at low-stimulus frequencies are no longer detectable at 8 Hz, apparently due to the adaptation of these components at the high frequencies.

VEPs to contrast changes

Bodis-Wollner, Hendley, and Kulikowski (1973) have studied the VEPs produced when the contrast of a stationary pattern is modulated about fixed mean levels. Since in this situation the pattern is present continuously, it is again unlikely that these responses contain significant contour-specific contributions and they probably reflect mainly the activity of contrast-specific cortical processes (see Fig. 6.9).

Summary and conclusions

These results have illustrated that different methods of presenting a given stimulus pattern can produce very different pattern VEPs. They have also shown how it is possible, using component-analysis techniques similar to those described in the first section of this chapter, to determine the composition of various forms of pattern VEP and the relationship between these different responses. In particular, they have shown that because of the rapid attenuation of contour-specific components with prolonged stimulation, these prominent components of the VEPs to brief pattern presentations are absent from the responses obtained to a pattern reversal or other forms of stimulation in which the pattern is continuously present. Thus the brief pattern presentation appears to be the most appropriate of the more commonly used methods of pattern stimulation for studies of the underlying cortical processes.

Acknowledgements

I am grateful to Professor D. M. MacKay and Mr. C. R. James for helpful criticism in the preparation of this chapter, and to Mr. P. W. Lynch for technical assistance.

7. Visual evoked potentials as a measure of visibility

J. KULIKOWSKI

Department of Ophthalmic Optics, University of Manchester Institute of Science and Technology

Patterned photic stimuli are much more effective than diffuse flashes of light to activate neurones in the visual cortex of higher mammals (Hubel and Wiesel 1959, 1968). The human visual cortex is also most sensitive to bars of specific orientations (Campbell and Kulikowski 1966), as shown by psychophysical techniques which allow complex perceptual phenomena to be examined since the conscious human subject can give verbal reports about the stimulus. This chapter correlates VEPs with the psychophysical threshold for detection of patterns of bright and dark bars (gratings).

Methods

Stimulus

Grating patterns may be conveniently generated on the face of a television oscilloscope (see Chapter 1 of this book). This allows the grating contrast C to be varied without changing the space-average luminance L_0. The standard definitions of these parameters are

$$C = (L_{max} - L_{min})/(L_{max} + L_{min}), \text{ and } L_0 = \tfrac{1}{2}(L_{max} + L_{min}),$$

where L_{max}, L_{min} are luminances of bright and dark stripes respectively. Gratings usually have a sinusoidal or square-wave luminance profile, both easily generated by modulation of the beam intensity. The number of bars per unit angle (spatial frequency expressed in cycles per degree) can be altered by varying the generator frequency. The stimuli described above can also be generated by optical systems which however often produce difficulty in keeping the space-average luminance constant when changing the other parameters.

Two modes of presentation of a grating stimulus for VEP have been independently developed since 1967.

(a) *'On–off' presentation*: a grating is presented for a certain time and then is replaced by a blank field of the same average luminance; the rate of

Visual evoked potentials in man: new developments (ed. J. E. Desmedt), p. 168–83. Clarendon Press, Oxford 1977.

presentation is rather slow, usually 0·3–1 Hz (Kulikowski and Kozak 1967).

(b) *Contrast reversal*: dark bars of a grating become bright and vice versa; the reversal rate was usually 8–10 Hz (Riggs and Whittle 1967; Cobb, Morton, and Ettlinger 1967; Campbell and Maffei 1970).

Subjects

The subjects were corrected myopes, usually right-handed. For long-lasting experiments only highly motivated subjects could be used. Since 1966 I have served as subject (J.J.K., corrected myope) in all the experiments. Simple control runs were carried out using other subjects (usually other scientists). In most experiments the subject was required to perform certain tasks such as to change the fixation point on the test screen to prevent image-stabilization effects. In addition, just before and after each recording session the subjects were required to set a threshold for contrast, that is at a level at which a given stimulus just ceased to be seen. In a more sophisticated experiment (Campbell and Kulikowski 1971) the subject viewed a grating pattern presented near its contrast threshold. The presentations were classified by the observer as *seen*, *not seen*, or *uncertain*, and the corresponding VEP samples directed to appropriate stores.

Recording equipment

Standard Ag–AgCl cup electrodes were used; the active electrode placed 2·5 cm above the inion (O_z) was referred to the temporal bone (T_4) (International 10–20 electrode convention; Jasper 1958), unless otherwise stated. The ground electrode was placed on the forehead. The scalp potentials were differentially amplified and filtered in order to optimize signal-to-noise ratio and to obtain the most reliable signal for weak stimuli near the contrast threshold. For this reason the low- and high-pass filters (slope 12 dB per octave) were set at corner frequencies usually of 3 Hz and 30 Hz, and sometimes even of 8 Hz and 25 Hz. When responses to long-lasting stimuli were recorded, the lower corner frequency could be reduced to 0·2 Hz. The signals were averaged either with an averager (e.g. Biomac) or with a PDP-8 computer which could also be used to randomize the stimulus presentations. Positivity of the active electrode was recorded downwards. The whole system (amplifiers and averager) was always calibrated before each recording session usually by a 1 μV rectangular pulse of 100 ms.

Description of the VEP

The VEPs to grating stimuli have components which might not be related to those obtained with flashes of light. Moreover the VEP shape depends on the stimulus parameters. For this reason an adequate description of the VEP requires consideration of both the magnitude and the latency of components. Fig. 7.1(a) shows a VEP to a 10 cycles per degree grating of high contrast. The components of this waveform will be referred to as N (negative) or P (positive) followed by the peak

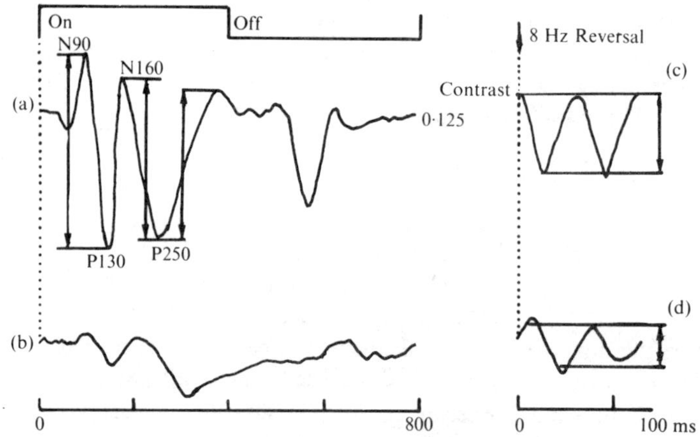

Fig. 7.1. VEP to a 10 cycles per degree grating either presented 'on' and 'off' at a rate of 1·25 Hz ((a) and (b)) or reversed in contrast at a rate of 8 Hz ((c) and (d)). Amplifier bandpass, 0·2–30 Hz ((a) and (b)) and 8–25 Hz ((c) and (d)). Negativity of the active electrode (O_Z) is upward in this and in the subsequent records. The contrast is 0·125 in (a) and (c) and 0·063 in (b) and (d).

latency in milliseconds. The off-components are similar although usually less conspicuous. The following simplifications will be used to specify each latencies shorter than 50 ms will not be considered because of their relatively small size in the pattern VEP; (b) since the latencies of components vary with contrast the mean of the high-contrast latencies will be used to specify each component; (c) for brevity's sake the first two components will be referred to as early waves, whereas the subsequent components will be referred to as late waves.

The relative size of components may be completely changed when the grating contrast is reduced. In Fig. 7.1(b) the early negative N90 is virtually absent whilst P250 is dominant and peaks now at a latency of 320 ms. The continuity between waves in (a) and (b) can be shown when changing contrast in small steps.

The variations in the waveform of the VEP make it sometimes difficult to decide how to measure the magnitudes of all the components. At high contrasts it is relatively easy to measure particular waves from their peaks to the baseline. At contrasts near threshold, however, the baseline is too noisy to be taken as a reference and one has to choose a method of estimation giving the most reliable results. In our present experiments it is the magnitude and not the latency of the VEP which provides the most consistent data. From that pragmatic viewpoint it seems satisfactory to measure peak-to-trough magnitudes (N90–P130 and N160–P250) or for longer durations the peak-to-baseline magnitude of the P250 wave.

It seems that a much simpler analysis of the VEP may be carried out when the grating stimulus is reversed in contrast at a rate of 8 Hz and when the amplifier bandwidth is restricted from 8 Hz to 25 Hz; the waveform is then almost sinusoidal (Fig. 7.1(c)) and the peak-to-trough amplitude can be measured. When the grating contrast is reduced the VEP decreases but still remains practically sinusoidal in spite of some random asymmetry of its waves (Fig. 7.1(d)) (cf. Campbell and Maffei 1970). The position of this sinusoidal VEP waveform should be described by its phase rather than by its latency.

Results and discussion

VEP as a function of suprathreshold contrast

For studying human vision a pattern of bright and dark bars (grating) is more advantageous than a single bar since it will activate many more cortical cells and the scalp VEP is considerably larger. A further advantage of a grating is that it is also used as one of the standard tests of visual resolution.

The principal aim of this work was to determine if a correlation exists between a visual contrast threshold determined by psychophysical methods and one determined by the VEP.

A 2·2 cycles per degree grating was presented to an inexperienced observer for 500 ms at a rate of 0·3 Hz (Fig. 7.2). At the highest contrast (Fig. 7.2(a)) the VEP

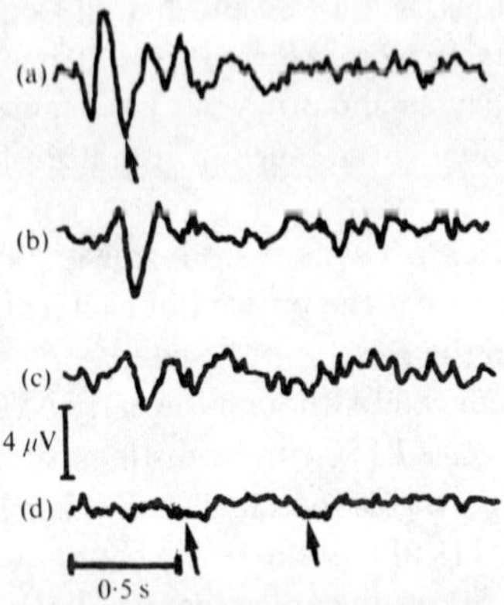

Fig. 7.2. VEP to a 2·2 cycles per degree grating turned on for 0·5 s and followed by a blank screen for 1–3 s. Contrast levels, 0·25 (a); 0·1 (b); 0·03 (c), and 0·01 (d) (contrast threshold). Average luminance of the display screen, 0·7 cd m^{-2}. Samples averaged: 127 in (a) to (c) and 511 in (d). Amplifier bandpass, 0·8–30 Hz. Electrodes: O_Z–C_Z (Jasper 1958) (subject J.P., 33 years, corrected myope). (Modified from Kulikowski and Kozak 1967.)

consists of a prominent early component (P140) followed by components N190 and P280, and smaller off-components (Kulikowski and Kozak 1967). When the contrast of the pattern is reduced the early component becomes more attenuated than the late components. At threshold, only the late positive 'on' and 'off' components are detectable (Fig. 7.2(d)); it will be seen that these components are separated by a time (500 ms) corresponding to the stimulus duration. Waves of such long latencies could be artifacts not related to the visual stimuli at all and several controls were carried out to eliminate such possibilities. All subjects were in a Faraday cage, away from switching circuits. To avoid the possibility of expectancy potentials (Walter 1964) the stimulus repetition rate was semi-randomized. Finally, to test if the electroretinogram (ERG) or electrooculogram (EOG) were contributing to the evoked potential, additional recordings were made. Contamination from the ERG was excluded since they were of much shorter latencies. Similarly there was no obvious contribution of the eye-muscle potentials to these records (see Kulikowski and Leisman 1973). These experiments (Kulikowski and Kozak 1967) demonstrated a definite correlation between the VEP and the threshold detection of patterned stimuli.

The relationship of VEP components to stimulus parameters

Only the late components of the VEP are correlated with the psychophysical contrast threshold (Fig. 7.2). Possibly the early waves are the result only of transient events whilst the late components reflect the ability of the visual system to integrate weak stimuli over a period of time. This possibility was examined by varying the presentation times of various gratings. Finer gratings are considered in order to verify the conclusions of Fig. 7.2 and spatial frequencies 7·5 cycles per degree and 15 cycles per degree were selected (it is difficult to study still finer gratings, e.g. 20 cycles per degree and 30 cycles per degree, since their contrast thresholds are high, thus reducing the range of suprathreshold contrasts over which recording can be made).

Fig. 7.3(a) shows VEPs to a 7·5 cycles per degree grating at different contrasts. A contrast threshold C_0 is given at the bottom of each column. For brief presentations of 50 ms both the early and the late components are similarly reduced as the contrast is reduced. Although the early N90 disappears at higher contrasts the early positive wave P150 can be distinguished even just above threshold. It seems likely that this is the same as that labelled P120 at higher contrasts. Other experiments (Kulikowski 1972) have also shown that for presentation times of up to 50 ms the appearance of both early and late components of the VEP is correlated with threshold detection. At presentation times from 0 ms to 50 ms the contrast threshold decreases in proportion to the duration of presentation (Bloch's law) and contrast and duration are almost interchangeable (Kulikowski 1972).

For presentation times of 100 ms and 200 ms the contrast threshold is reduced (Figs. 7.3 and 7.5). Despite this the contrast level at which the early positive wave P150 is just detectable remains at the same level, so that at just suprathreshold contrast, e.g. 0·016, only the late P300–400 are detectable. Evidently the presence of early waves at threshold with short presentation times simply reflects the higher contrast threshold for the transient presentation.

This point is further illustrated when the peak-to-trough magnitudes of the early waves N90 and N120 and the late waves P200–N360 are plotted against the log of

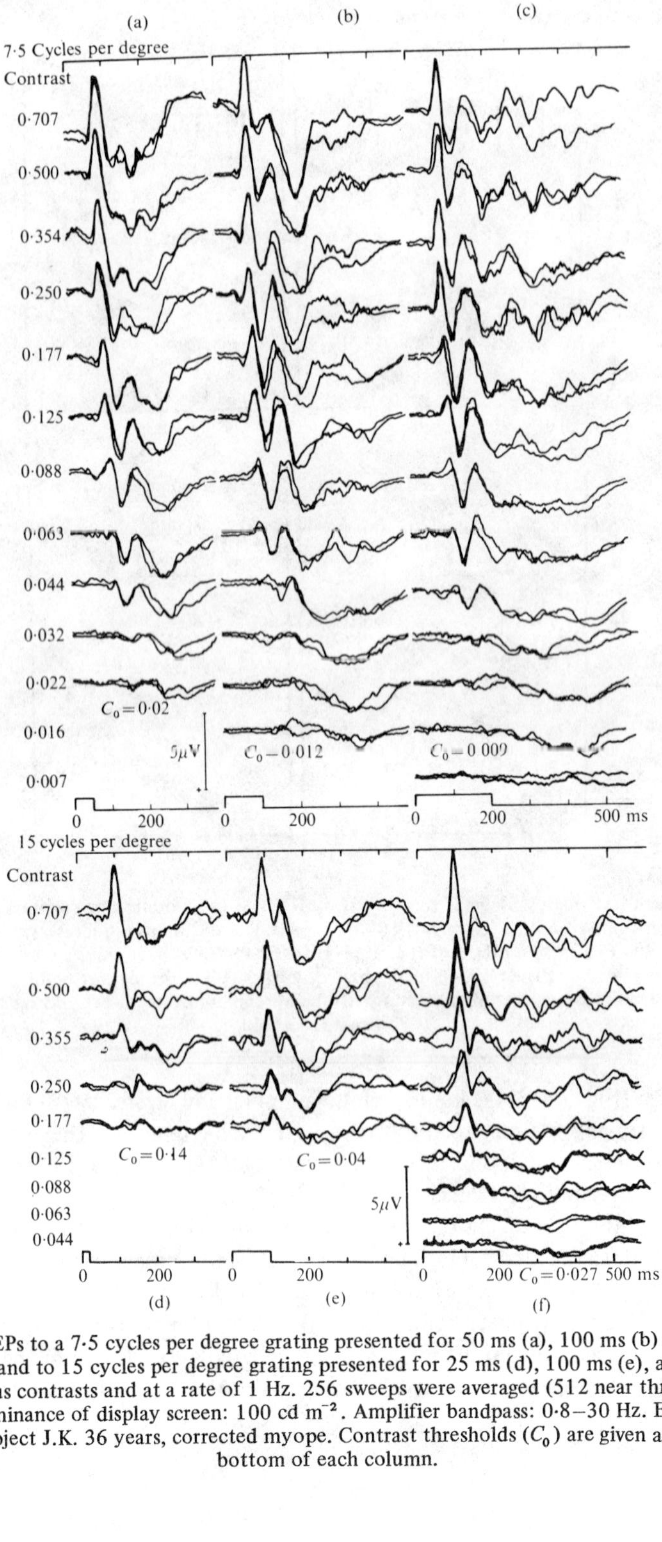

Fig. 7.3. VEPs to a 7·5 cycles per degree grating presented for 50 ms (a), 100 ms (b) and 200 ms (c) and to 15 cycles per degree grating presented for 25 ms (d), 100 ms (e), and 200 ms (f) at various contrasts and at a rate of 1 Hz. 256 sweeps were averaged (512 near threshold). Average luminance of display screen: 100 cd m^{-2}. Amplifier bandpass: 0·8–30 Hz. Electrodes, 0_Z–T_4. Subject J.K. 36 years, corrected myope. Contrast thresholds (C_0) are given at the bottom of each column.

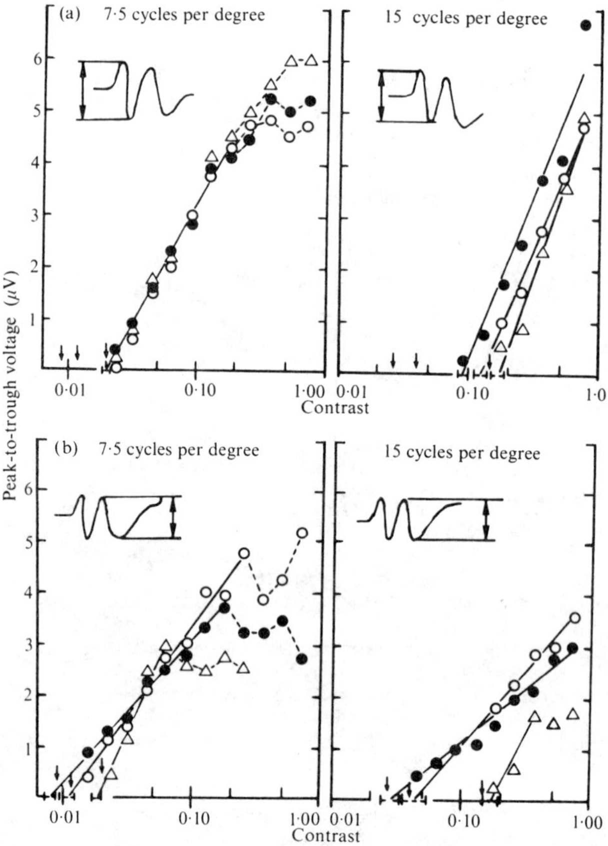

Fig. 7.4. Peak-to-trough voltage of the VEP from Fig. 7.3 as a function of contrast at presentation times of 50 ms (triangles) 100 ms (circles), and 200 ms (squares). (a) Voltage of the early N90–P130. (b) Voltage of the late N160–P200. Regression lines were fitted by the least-squares method (Fisher 1934) to the part of curves below the saturation of the system. Horizontal bars at the points intersection with the abscissa indicate ±1 S.E. Arrows indicate contrast threshold.

the contrast (Fig. 7.4). This kind of plot (Campbell and Maffei 1970) shows that the VEP is roughly proportional to the suprathreshold contrast. The early components are similar functions of contrast at 50, 100, and 200 ms (Fig. 7.4(a)) and cannot be correlated with the contrast thresholds (arrows) which are different at these presentation times. On the other hand, the late waves also decrease but they correlate with the contrast thresholds for the different presentation times (Fig. 7.4(b)). Thus the late VEP components are well correlated with subjective threshold. This has also been found for presentation times up to 500 ms.

The records at low contrast indicate that the late P400 is longer at the longer presentation times for both the spatial frequencies of 7·5 cycles per degree

(Fig. 7.3(a), (b), (c)) and 15 cycles per degree (Fig. 7.3(d), (e), (f)). As the contrast is reduced P400 tends to merge with the late off-wave to produce a complex wave. This late complex has a duration similar to the stimulus duration even though it occurs over 300 ms after the stimulus has ceased. This amplifies the results shown in Fig. 7.2. Since the increased duration of the late waves with increased stimulus duration occurs concomitantly with lowered contrast threshold these two phenomena might be related. The late VEP waves could be made up of a number of waves, possibly generated independently at various moments during the observation of a grating. Perhaps, then, the improved visibility at long stimulus presentations may simply be that the longer we look the greater the probability that finally we notice a stimulus. Alternatively the increased duration of the late VEP waves could be the result of an increase in the duration of individual neural phenomena and increased visibility may be the result of more sophisticated integrative processes.

Using classical psychophysical methods it is found that Bloch's law does not hold for durations greater than 50 ms (Fig. 7.5). The contrast threshold is no

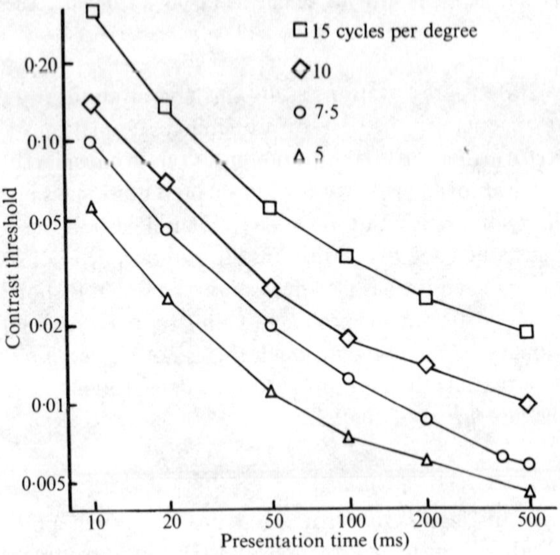

Fig. 7.5. Contrast threshold as a function of the presentation time for four spatial frequencies: 5 cycles per degree (triangles), 7·5 cycles per degree (circles), 10 cycles per degree (diamonds), and 15 cycles per degree (squares). Other conditions as in Fig. 7.3.

longer inversely proportional to the duration of the stimulus and eventually tends to level off at the longer durations. Now, as shown in Fig. 7.6, the probability of detecting the stimulus can be plotted against contrast (a) for two separate presentations of 200 ms one after the other (triangles) and (b) for single presentations of 400 ms (diamonds). The dashed line shows the probability of

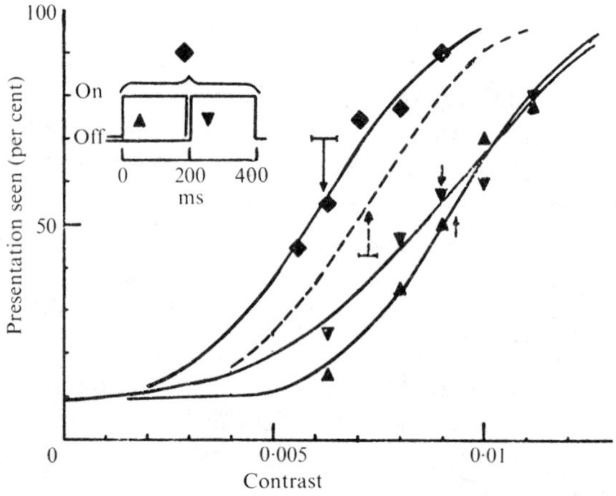

Fig. 7.6. Percentage presentations seen or probability of seeing of a grating presented either in the first or in the second half-period for 200 ms (triangles) or for 400 ms (diamonds), plotted against contrast. The continuous lines are fitted by probit analysis (Finney 1971). Arrows indicate contrast thresholds. For the 400 ms presentation, C_0 = 0·0062 ± 0·0003 (measured) as compared to predicted from the probability summation 0·0072 ± 0·0002. These values differ by more 3 S.E.

seeing the double 200-ms presentations as 400-ms presentations (by multiplying probabilities of not seeing) on the basis of probability summation. It is evident that the actual performance with 400 ms presentations is considerably better than that. Thus the improved visibility for longer presentations is not simply the result of probability summation but must have a neural basis. Some cortical neurones exhibit sustained activity in response to prolonged visual stimulation (Ikeda and Wright 1974) and it has also been observed (P. O. Bishop, personal communication) that cortical neurones may exhibit an increased excitability when exposed to a stationary stimulus even though this is not reflected by an increased number of action potentials. It is tempting to speculate that such responses might be reflected by the late waves of the VEP.

VEPs to visible gratings near threshold

VEPs become hardly distinguishable from noise near the psychophysical contrast threshold, virtually disappearing below threshold. Since the contrast threshold is determined as 50 per cent probability of seeing, the VEP might be generated only when the grating is visible. However, obtaining reliable VEPs at threshold presents considerable difficulties. Therefore in order to obtain the maximum signal-to-noise ratio both the stimulus and the recording technique must be optimized (Campbell and Kulikowski 1971).

A 3·3 cycle per degree grating stimulus was selected as having the lowest contrast threshold for a given display (screen diameter: 2°; average luminance 50 cd m^{-2}). The stimulus presentation was initiated by the observer whenever he was ready, but the precise timing was set randomly over a period of 500 ms by a PDP-8 computer to minimize any expectancy potential. The stimulus consisted of a 62·5 ms exposure to a grating followed by another exposure of the same duration but with the contrast of the grating reversed. This was followed by a blank screen of the same space-average luminance lasting until the next presentation. This rather unusual mode of presentation was found to be very satisfactory because the contrast reversal minimized possible after-images and the subject was allowed ample time to give a psychophysical response. The subject classified his response as 'seen', 'not seen', or 'uncertain', by setting a switch at one of the three corresponding positions (referred to as S, U, and N – Fig. 7.8). To prevent the subject from guessing what response should be given, the computer was programmed to vary randomly the grating contrast (Fig. 7.9) or to produce a blank (no grating) presentation (Fig. 7.8). The computer also stored the VEP to each presentation in a temporary memory before transfer into the appropriate store. At least six stores were set up: the three types of subject's responses when the grating was actually presented and another three for the false positive test when the grating was not presented. Since the amplifier bandwidth was reduced to 8–25 Hz, sampling periods of about 16 ms seemed adequate.

The accuracy of the method was first checked at eight suprathreshold contrast levels (Fig. 7.7). The points indicating mean voltages at given sampling intervals of 16 ms were compared with continuous records obtained simultaneously on an Enhancetron averager (with 1024 samples per screen). The general agreement of the discrete points and continuous lines is evident, though scatter and standard errors are quite considerable. A better agreement and smaller standard error are shown on the right in Fig. 7.7, where we averaged 327 repetitions. However a contrast of 0·01 at threshold requires more averaging since the standard error is too large to specify VEP size. The results shown in Fig. 7.7 suggest that the VEP waveform has its dominant component as P200 at latencies between 200 ms and 400 ms. Fig. 7.8 shows the VEPs to presentations reported by the subject as either 'seen', 'uncertain', or 'not seen' and were obtained in 7164 trials (Campbell and Kulikowski 1971). The whole experiment lasting over 12 hours was split into four sessions taking place on four different days and the data were pooled. The record obtained for the 'seen' presentations is a clear VEP (Fig. 7.8, S). Vertical bars indicate ±1 S.E. (standard error) over a period which was considered as containing the late wave. The VEP marked U (uncertain) is less clear and the record obtained for presentations reported as not seen (N) does not exhibit any familiar waveform at all. The correlation coefficient of the 12 relevant sampling points was calculated and found significant between records S and U: $r = +0{\cdot}727 \pm 0{\cdot}14$ ($t = 3{\cdot}35$), which indicates that the record in presentations classified as uncertain contains the VEP. On the other hand, the correlation coefficient $r = 0{\cdot}251 \pm 0{\cdot}27$ ($t = 0{\cdot}82$), between relevant points in records S and N is not significant. This means that if there was any signal in the record evoked by the not seen presentations it is too small to be detected (Campbell and Kulikowski 1971).

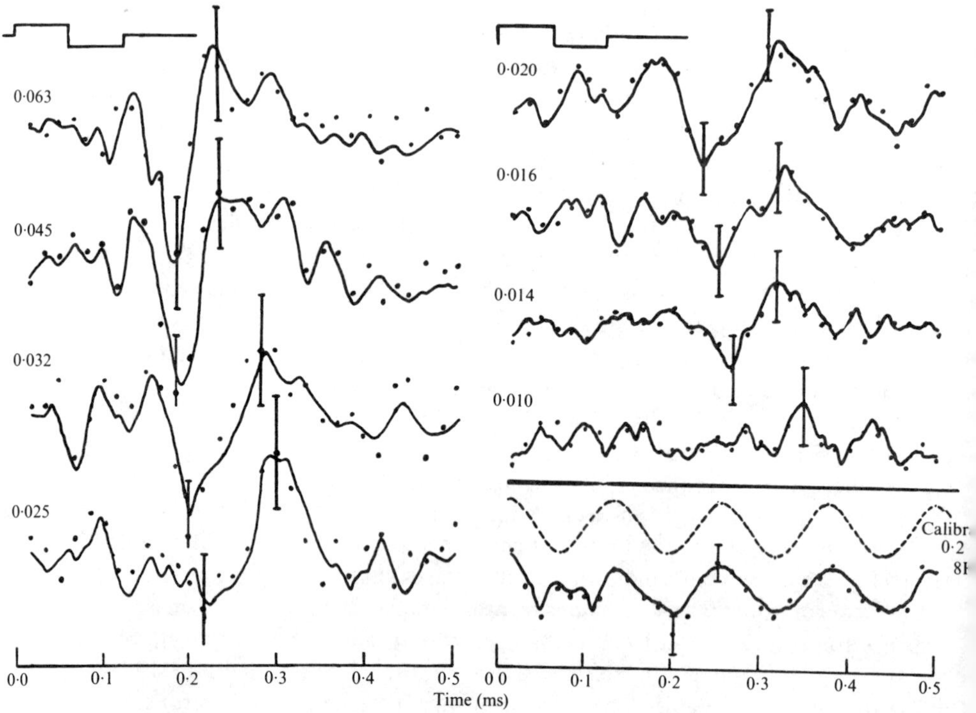

Fig. 7.7. VEPs to a 3·3 cycle per degree grating at various contrasts indicated to the left of each trace. Records on the left are averages of 100 presentations, those on the right, of 327 presentations. The continuous records come from an Enhancetron averager, the dots are PDP-8 computer averaged data points sampled every 16 ms. Vertical bars indicate ±1 S.E. in peaks and trough. Calibrating sinusoidal signal of 0·2 μV, 8 Hz. Averaged luminance of display screen: 50 cd m^{-2}. Amplifier bandpass: 8–25 Hz. Electrodes: O_Z–T_4. Subject J.K.

These results depend on the criterion of a threshold which varies with the level of confidence at which the subject chooses to operate. In record S the subject reported seeing the grating on 31·5 per cent of the presentations (1941 out of 6146) and the rate of false positive responses to the blank presentations was rather low – only 3·6 per cent (37 out of 1018). This kind of secure strategy is common in psychophysical experiments when the false-positive rate does not exceed 5–10 per cent.

The data could also be processed by taking uncertain answers for positive responses (i.e. to say: if the subject is uncertain he must have seen something) and by adding the potentials and responses corresponding to the decisions 'seen' and 'uncertain'. The resulting VEP (Fig. 7.8, S + U) is the mean of 4518 responses out of 6146 total presentations (73·5 per cent). At the same time, the rate of false positive responses rises to 31·1 per cent (316 out of 1018), since the 'uncertain' responses

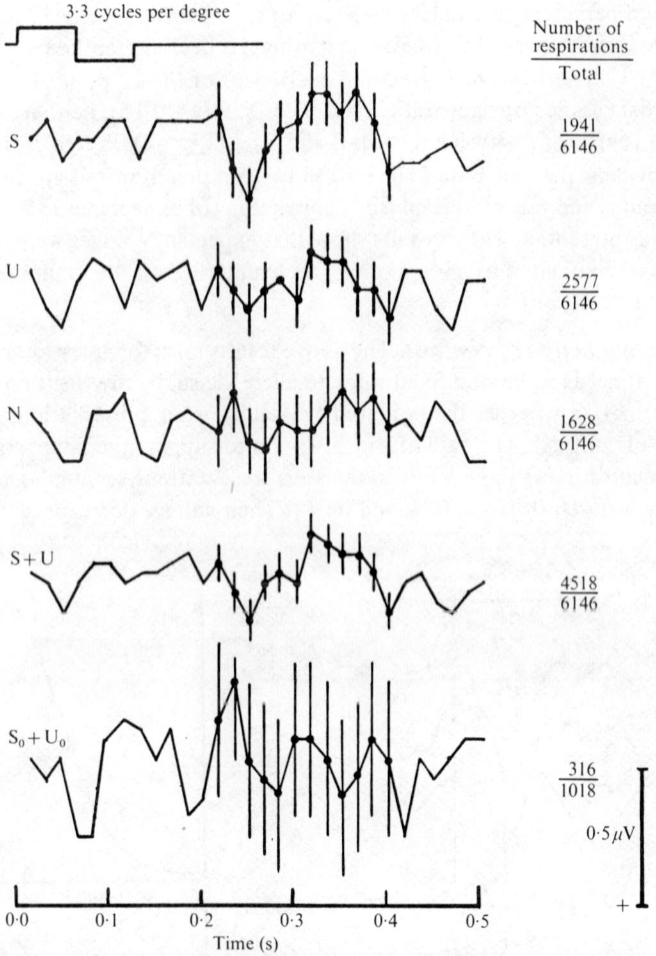

Fig. 7.8. VEPs to either a 3·3 cycles per degree grating at a contrast of 0·01 or a 'blank' false positive trial (bottom record). Records are marked as follows: S – presentation seen; U – presentation uncertain; N – presentation not seen (from Cambell and Kulikowski 1971). S + U is the weighted average of records S and U; S_0 + U_0 is the weighted average of false responses to blank presentations (seen and uncertain). Vertical bars refer to ±1 S.E. (about 0·1 μV). Figures on the right refer to the number of responses divided by the total number of presentations. Other conditions as in Fig. 7.7.

to the blank presentations (U_0)must now be added to those responses which reported 'seeing' in the absence of a grating (S_0). The potential corresponding to these false judgements is shown in Fig. 7.8 as a record S_0 + U_0. It is now relevant to enquire if there is any correlation between this record and the VEP to presentations reported as 'seen' and 'uncertain' (S + U). This control is important for testing the possible contribution of expectancy waves. In the present experimental paradigm the subject 'expects' to see a grating when he subsequently decides 'seen' and 'uncertain', whether a grating has been presented (S + U record) or not ($S_0 + U_0$ record). The correlation coefficient of the 12 points in the records S + U and $S_0 + U_0$ is not significant: $r = 0{\cdot}05 \pm 0{\cdot}29$ ($t = 0{\cdot}15$), neither is the correlation coefficient between records S and $S_0 + U_0$; $r = 0{\cdot}03 \pm 0{\cdot}29$ ($t = 0{\cdot}095$). Thus it is evident that the potentials evoked by seen presentations are generated by the stimulus and not by the subject's conviction (or expectancy) that the stimulus was presented. These results show that expectancy waves were adequately minimized or eliminated by programming the computer to time randomly the stimulus presentation.

The VEP as a function of contrast. The above results raise the question whether the potential needs to be of a fixed value to elicit the subjective decision (yes, I see the grating), or whether the potential evoked by 'seen' presentations is merely a function of contrast. The data of Fig. 7.9 seem to support the latter possibility. The first records in (a) show VEPs to the seen presentations accumulated in three stores for contrasts: 0·018, 0·014, and 0·011. Their voltage decreases with reduction

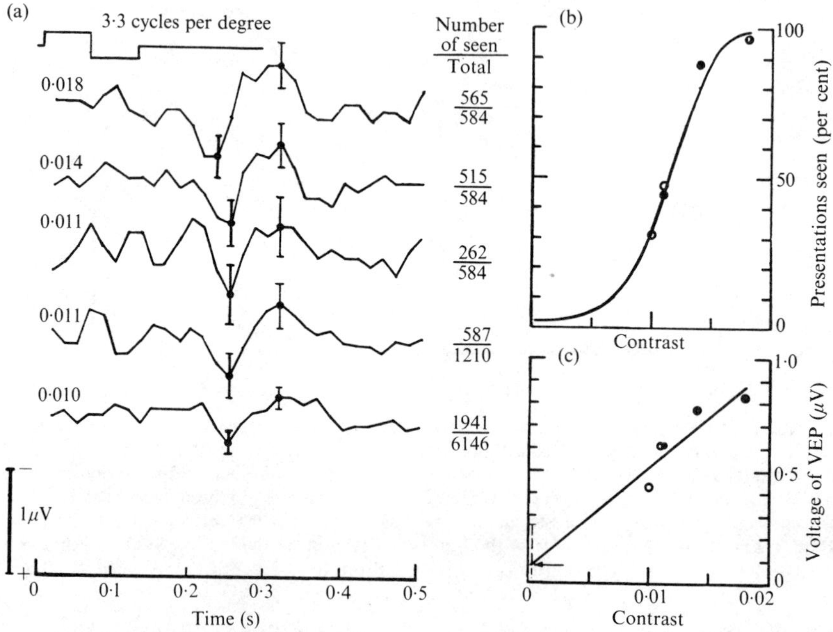

Fig. 7.9. (a) VEPs to the 'seen' presentations at various contrasts of a 3·3 cycles per degree grating. The three top records were obtained in one session. The vertical bars indicate ± S.E. in the positions of peaks and troughs of the potential. (b) Percentage of presentations seen or probability of seeing a grating as a function of contrast fitted by probit analysis. (c) Voltage of the VEP to seen presentations as a function of contrast. Filled circles correspond to the three top records in (a), the circles to the remaining records. The regression line was fitted by using the least-squares method. False-positive rate 3 per cent.

of contrast (Fig. 7.9(c)). The number of presentations seen at a contrast of 0·011 was only 262 and the standard error was rather large. Another recording obtained at the same contrast (Fig. 7.9(a)) is smoother (standard error is reduced), but its peak-to-trough magnitude remains the same, which confirms the validity of the preceding record. Recording VEPs at still lower contrasts is increasingly difficult and over 20 000 repetitions would be required at a contrast of 0·008. The percentage of presentations seen or probability of seeing is plotted in Fig. 7.10(b).

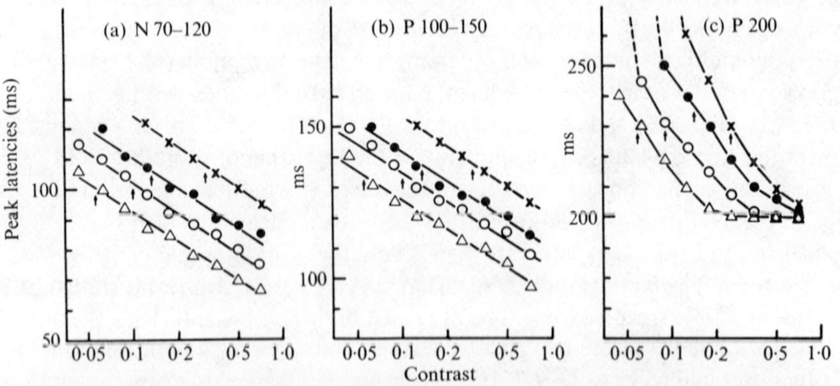

Fig. 7.10. Peak latencies in ms of three components of the VEP as a function of contrast for four spatial frequencies: 3 cycles per degree (triangles), 7·5 cycles per degree (circles), 10 cycles per degree (filled circles), and 15 cycles per degree (crosses). Other conditions are as in Fig. 7.3. (a) and (b) latencies of the early components: regression lines were fitted through the data points by the least-squares method. Arrows mark contrasts 5 times higher than the corresponding thresholds for the 50 ms presentation. The latencies at which the arrows intersect the regression lines given in the order of increasing spatial frequencies are given in ms: 101·3 ± 1·7; 102·3 ± 1·5; 106·2 ± 1·6; 108 ± 1 for the N70–120 VEP component and 133·3 ± 1·9; 135·8 ± 1·5; 137·2 ± 1·5; 137·3 ± 0·5 for the P100–150 VEP component. (c) Latencies of the late P200 component; arrows indicate contrasts 10 times above the corresponding thresholds for the 200 ms exposure.

Fig. 7.9(c) shows the peak-to-trough voltage of the VEPs on a linear scale, on the assumption that these two variables are proportional which is the simplest, but completely arbitrary, assumption (it should be borne in mind that at higher contrasts the VEP is approximately proportional to the log contrast). However, the data points can be fitted by a regression line which passes close to zero potential at zero contrast. (The vertical dashed bar indicates ±1 S.E.) Anyway, the VEP evoked by the 'seen' presentations increases in some degree of proportionality to contrast and consequently must be related by the visual stimulus and not by some decision-making process of the subject.

Latency of the VEP as a function of suprathreshold contrast

Since it is relatively difficult to determine the beginning of the VEP waves it is a common practice to specify the latency to a peak of a given component. An even more difficult task is to estimate the latency when approaching a threshold. Latencies to peaks of three VEP components, namely, early negative (N70–120), early positive (P100–150), and late positive (P200) are plotted against log contrast in Fig. 7.10. An approximate inverse proportionality over a considerable range is found for the early components ((a), (b)) and regression lines can be fitted by the least-squares method. The lower the contrast and the higher the spatial frequency of a grating, the longer is the latency. This raises the question of whether contrast and spatial frequency are in fact cross-related. To illustrate this possibility the arrows in Fig. 7.10(a) and (b) indicate the values of contrast 5 times above the corresponding thresholds for 50 ms presentation. The arrows intersect the regression lines at nearly the same latency for all spatial frequencies, i.e. at about 105 ms for N90–120 and about 135 ms for P100–150 waves. This is a convincing illustration that the latencies depend also on the logarithm of suprathreshold contrast, rather than on the absolute contrast itself (a careful examination of Fig. 7.10(a) and (b) shows, however, that there is a tendency for high spatial frequencies to have longer latencies than if only the suprathreshold contrast was the determining parameter, yet these differences are hardly significant statistically and their possible significance will be discussed in the next chapter).

The peak latency of the late positive wave P200 is a more complicated function of suprathreshold contrast (Fig. 7.10(c)) because of a marked increase in duration of the late wave at low contrasts (see dashed lines in Fig. 7.10(c)). On the other hand, at a higher contrast (near 0·7) the latencies of all the spatial frequencies examined (5, 7·5, 10, and 15 cycles per degree) seem to approach the same value, namely 200 ms. In spite of these differences the latency of the late wave (P200) also depends on the suprathreshold contrast. The arrows indicating the values of contrast 10 times higher than the corresponding contrast thresholds obtained for 200 ms presentation times intersect the latency curves at about the same latency of 230 ms.

In summary, the latencies of the various VEP components seem to be functions of the contrast above threshold as are the magnitudes of these components (i.e. latency = constant − (constant x log C/C_0, where C_0 = threshold contrast).

Functional significance of pattern VEP

It is highly probable that the occipital VEPs reflect the summed activity of cortical neurones and although perhaps also of glial cells, cf. Kelly and Van Essen (1974), since a definite correlation was found between the minimum recognizable patterned VEP and the corresponding psychophysical contrast threshold. This gross brain activity is correlated with psychophysics and can help analyse basic visual mechanisms whose significance in perception may not be apparent from single unit animal studies. The next chapter considers evidence which points to a separation of central processes concerned with (a) movement detection and (b) the detection of pattern.

Acknowledgements

The work described in this chapter was supported by the Rockefeller Foundation, Wellcome Trust, Science Research Council, and the Medical Research Council. I also with to thank Professor J. R. Cronly-Dillon, Dr. M. Tyrer, and Mr. R. Abadi for helpful comments and Dr. J. G. Robson for the loan of equipment.

8. Separation of occipital potentials related to the detection of pattern and movement

J. KULIKOWSKI

Department of Ophthalmic Optics, University of Manchester Institute of Science and Technology

The preceding chapter on VEPs to grating stimuli exceeding psychophysical contrast threshold made no attempt to analyse either the VEP itself or the detection process underlying the threshold judgment made by the subject. Yet both are complex. Criteria used to determine the threshold are often ambiguous, particularly when the stimulus is repetitive (Rashbass 1968). In fact, it is possible for the subject to set two kinds of contrast threshold: one for seeing a grating itself, the other for detecting its movement (real or apparent). The threshold for the recognition of a grating occurs at the same contrast no matter whether the grating is alternately turned 'on' and 'off' (without changing the space-average luminance) or whether its bars are shifted across, as in the case of contrast reversal. Conversely, the movement threshold depends on a transient *change* in contrast, and not on its initial or terminal value (Kulikowski and Tolhurst 1973).

This chapter analyses VEPs to gratings presented either with the on–off mode or with the contrast-reversal mode. Such VEPs under certain conditions are dominated respectively by a 'pattern' component and a 'movement' (or 'transient') component (Kulikowski 1974).

Most recent papers on VEP currently recognize this dichotomy by mentioning the contrast VEP and luminance VEP elicited by checkerboards (rather than sinusoidal gratings) (see Chapter 1). Perhaps the latter potentials could best be called 'contrast-transient' components, since they depend on a change in contrast which can also be expressed as a local change in luminance. The identification of this transient component has not always been clear in practice.

However, the method introduced for the classification of the psychophysical detection of movement (Kulikowski and Tolhurst 1973) could provide also a clear-cut criterion for the transient component of the VEP. Once identified this component could be subtracted from the total VEP, leaving predominantly pattern-evoked components.

The results will be presented in five stages:

1. A purely 'transient' VEP, or, in our specific case for grating stimuli, the

Visual evoked potentials in man: new developments (ed. J. E. Desmedt), pp. 184–96. Clarendon Press, Oxford 1977.

'movement' VEP, is defined as depending only on a transient change in contrast (or as a change in local luminance); such potentials are obtained only with very coarse gratings.

2. For less coarse gratings, the 'transient' component is subtracted from the corresponding VEP to the presentation of a grating and the resulting trace will be defined as the pattern component.
3. Since this 'pattern' component decreases after a pre-adaptation to a stationary grating (see Blakemore and Campbell 1969), the 'transient' component is shown to decrease accordingly after pre-adaptation to the contrast reversal (Kulikowski and Tolhurst 1973).
4. An increase reversal rate up to 6 Hz is shown to affect differently the pattern and the movement detectors.
5. Lastly, the superposition of various VEPs will be considered.

Methods

Vertical gratings of sinusoidal luminance profile were generated as test stimuli on the face of an oscilloscope. An additional display was provided to generate a pre-adapting stimulus, which was always similar in its spatial frequency to the test grating, but its contrast was high (0·8) and its orientation could be changed by 30° from the vertical. The contrast was defined as $C = (L_{max} - L_{min})/(L_{max} + L_{min})$ and the space-average luminance (kept constant at 15 cd m^{-2}) $L_0 = \frac{1}{2}(L_{max} + L_{min})$, where L_{max}, L_{min} are luminances of bright and dark stripes (Fig. 8.1). The spatial frequency was expressed in cycles per degree of arc. In the on–off presentation (Fig. 8.1(a)) of a grating: the grating onset (half-cycle 1) alternated with the blank screen of the same space-average luminance (half-cycle 2). In the contrast reversal (Fig. 8.1(b) of a grating: the phase of the grating is alternated by 180° (bright bars become dark and vice versa). The change in contrast for the latter mode is twice that for the on–off presentation. The same change in contrast is obtained for on–off presentation of contrast C and for contrast reversal of contrast $\frac{1}{2}C$.

The presentation rate was 1·67 Hz (full cycle 600 ms; mark-space ratio of one), since this rate activates both the pattern and movement detectors equally well.

Recording equipment

Electrodes were placed 2·5 cm above the inion (O_Z) and referred to the temporal bone (T4), according to the International 10–20 electrode convention. All experiments presented in this paper were performed on the author, J.J.K. (38 years, corrected myope). The criterion for a pure luminance-transient response was checked on another subject. Other details in the recording technique were the same as in the preceding chapter except for the amplifier bandpass chosen as 3–30 Hz.

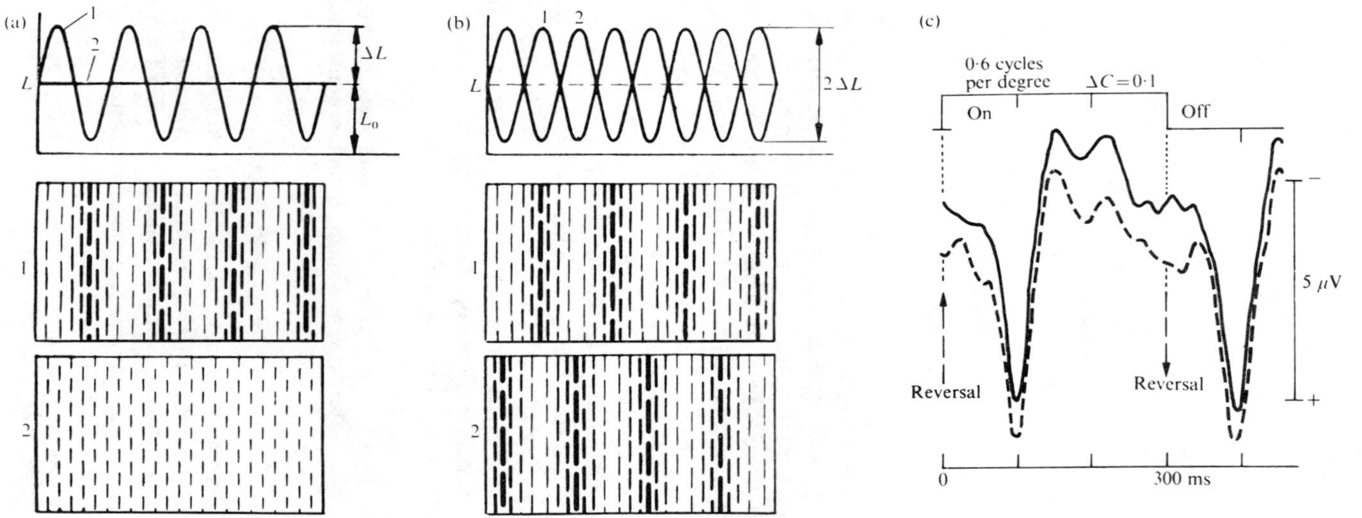

Fig. 8.1. (a) and (b) Schematic diagrams of grating stimuli and their luminance profiles. (a) Grating turned 'on' (half-cycle 1) and 'off' (half-cycle 2); L_0 = space-average luminance = $\frac{1}{2}$ ($L_{max} + L_{min}$) and is always constant (15 cd m^{-2}). (b) Grating reversed in contrast. Note that a change in local luminance (ΔL) when the grating is reversed in contrast is twice the change for the on–off presentation. (c) VEP to a 0·6 cycle per degree grating either presented 'on' and 'off' (upper record) or reversed in contrast (with interrupted line record) at the same rate (1·67 Hz). In each case the contrast changed by 0·1. The display screen subtended 15° x 15° of visual angle. In all the traces negativity is up. The contrast threshold for seeing movement was 0·003.

Results and discussion

Criterion for a purely transient response

Any VEP to a patterned visual stimulus may be defined as purely transient if it depends only on a change in the stimulus contrast and not on an initial or terminal value of contrast. Referring to an analogous example in electronics: an a.c. amplifier responds to a change in the input voltage, irrespective of any d.c. component, provided the d.c. voltage does not produce a saturation within the system. In this relation two kinds of stimuli can be studied: (a) the grating is turned 'on' and 'off' from zero to a certain contrast value, called C, and then back again to zero; and (b) contrast reversal of the same grating at half the contrast by changing the grating contrast from $-\frac{1}{2}C$ to $+\frac{1}{2}C$ and back to $-\frac{1}{2}C$. In both these cases the change in contrast is the same, that is $\Delta C = C$ (Fig. 8.1). The VEPs to either modes of presentation of a coarse sinusoidal grating (0·6 cycles per degree) whose contrast changes by 0·1 in both cases look very similar (Fig. 8.1(c)). In addition these presentations (the 'on–off' and reversal) subjectively look much the same and produce an overwhelming illusion that the bars of the grating have moved across the screen (Kulikowski and Tolhurst 1973). We may conclude that this coarse grating of a rather low contrast, when presented at a rate of 1·67 Hz, activates a transient detection mechanism which signals the presence of movement.

A pure transient response should remain similar even if the grating contrast was increased by increments, from the positive initial value (say + 0·01) and by the same amount (by $\Delta C = 0{\cdot}1$) up to a contrast of 0·11. This is usually the case, provided only the initial steady contrast is not too high to produce a 'saturation' of the VEP (analogous to the saturation of an a.c. amplifier). In fact, this method of modulating contrast about a steady level has already been used in the complementary case to show there that for a relatively fine grating (6 cycles per degree) the VEP was *not* dominated by transient components, since its size *did depend* on the mean contrast even though the contrast change is the same (Bodis-Wollner *et al.* 1973).

In practice, however, it is much easier to recognize the transient-dominated VEP by checking that the on–off and reversal potentials are similar. This method is also applicable for testing VEPs to coarse checkerboard stimuli.

Separation of pattern and movement VEPs

The similarity just described between the 'on–off' and reversal VEPs disappears when any element of a finer pattern is introduced. This may be either a square-wave grating with sharp edges, or a higher spatial frequency.

Fig. 8.2 shows VEPs to gratings with spatial frequencies 1, 2, or 4 cycles per degree and either on–off presentation, or contrast reversal. The reversal VEPs always consist of two very similar waves corresponding to the two identical reversals within one cycle. The on–off VEP consists of two different components: on- and off-waves. The asymmetry of the on- and off-waves appears in the bottom

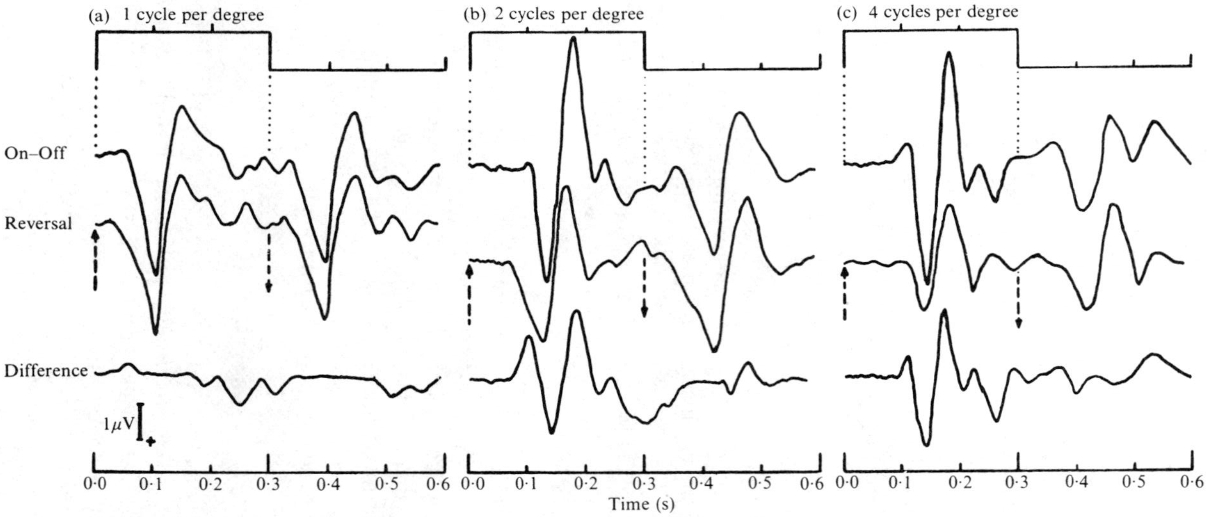

Fig. 8.2. VEP to gratings with spatial frequencies 1 cycle per degree (a), 2 cycles per degree (b), or 4 cycles per degree (c). Top records 'on' and 'off' presentation. Middle records: contrast reversal. The rate was 1·67 Hz in each case. The lowest records result from the subtraction of the middle from the upper record and they are assumed to be pattern-evoked potentials (see text). Contrast change is 0·1 for all stimuli. Screen subtended 9° x 9° for 1 cycle per degree and 2 cycles per degree gratings and 6°45′ x 6°45′ for 4 cycles per degree grating.

Constant thresholds for 1, 2, and 4 cycles per degree were respectively: pattern recognition 0·008; 0·005; 0·005 and for seeing movement: 0·0032; 0·004; 0·005.

traces obtained by subtraction of the on–off and reversal VEPs: it is hardly noticeable at 1 cycle per degree, but at 2 cycles per degree it is about the size of the reversal potential, and at 4 cycles per degree it exceeds it (Fig. 8.2). This would suggest that the transient potential component becomes less and less important for gratings of increasing spatial frequencies. It is tempting to describe the 'difference' records in Fig. 8.2 as a 'pattern VEP', since we know from psychophysics (Kulikowski and Tolhurst 1973) that the pattern detectors become more prominent than movement detectors above a spatial frequency of 3 cycles per degree. (See an independent test of this point below.)

The above hypothesis assumes (a) that the reversal VEP is dominated by transient components, and (b) that there is a linear summation between potentials evoked by the pattern- and movement-detecting systems. The first assumption is tenable for relatively low spatial frequencies for which the reversal potential cannot contain much of the pattern component (as compared with the 'on–off' potential) since it is elicited by a grating of a half-contrast (change from $-\frac{1}{2}C$ to $+\frac{1}{2}C$; see the section on methods) and we know from the psychophysical experiments that the pattern component depends on the contrast level (not on the change in contrast). Besides, the continuous presence of a grating during the contrast reversal might continuously stimulate the pattern detectors, so that little potential would be evoked (see below). For spatial frequencies above 6 cycles per degree there might be some pattern component in the reversal VEP, yet the 'difference' potential may still be a good measure of the pattern potential since such 'contamination' of the reversal potential implies that we would subtract too much, rather than too little, from the 'on–off' VEP.

The other assumption about a linear summation seems reasonable provided that the pattern and movement systems are separate. Recent experiments strongly suggest this possibility (Tolhurst 1973; Kulikowski and Tolhurst 1973).

A similar analysis has been attempted for checkerboard stimuli by Spekreijse, *et al.* (1973) and Estevez and Spekreijse (1974), who suggested that the early positive off-wave in the 'on–off' VEP is dominated by the luminance-transient component. This suggestion was based, among others, on a similarity of the shape and latency (about 120 ms) of the off-wave and the reversal VEP.

The present results also indicate that the early positive off-wave P120 contains mainly the transient component which is nearly identical with the corresponding reversal VEP for gratings 2 cycles per degree, 4 cycles per degree, and 6 cycles per degree. However, this is only part of the story, since for a 1 cycle per degree grating (and coarser gratings) both the early on- and off-waves are practically identical with the corresponding reversal waves.

Analysis of the VEPs to checkerboard onset (Estevez and Spekreijse 1974) suggests that these are not dominated by luminance transients when the checks subtend 20′. On the other hand, the VEPs to contrast reversal of a checkerboard with checks subtending 50′ (Michael and Halliday 1971) are most likely due to luminance transients, as expected.

Separation of occipital potentials related to the detection of pattern and movement

As for the late wave, P250, this is usually the first component detected when the difference between the on–off and reversal VEPs begins to be noticeable. Fig. 8.2 shows that P250 is most prominent in the difference VEP to a 1 cycle per degree grating, which is not surprising since this wave was found to be correlated with the psycho-physical contrast threshold for patterned stimuli (see Chapter 7).

Finally, the reversal VEPs tend to have slightly shorter latencies in Fig. 8.2 than the 'difference' potentials assumed to be pattern potentials. This means that the total 'on–off' VEPs to coarse gratings have relatively shorter latencies than the VEPs to finer gratings for which the influence of the reversal component becomes less and less important. This might be one of the reasons for the latencies of potentials evoked by finer gratings being longer than estimated for a given suprathreshold contrast (see Fig. 7.10, p. 181).

A test for a pattern-related component in the VEP

Blakemore and Campbell (1969) have introduced a technique of pattern adaptation to evaluate the pattern component in a given VEP. The observer is asked first to look alternately at two fixation points on the screen, where an adapting grating of a high contrast (0·8) is continuously present. The fixation points are positioned on one bright and one dark stripe to prevent a build-up of an after-image. The initial pre-adaptation lasts for 2–3 min and is followed by a 10–15 s period of averaging the VEP to a similar grating of much lower contrast (in our case change in contrast of 0·1). After this the pre-adaptation is repeated for about 30 s and followed by 10 s recording. Alternating cycles of pre-adaptation + recording are repeated many times until a stable VEP is obtained which is compared to the control VEP without the pattern pre-adaptation. Control runs should check that pre-adaptation to a blank screen will not affect the VEP.

Fig. 8.3 shows VEPs to on–off or reversal presentations following pre-adaptation to high-contrast gratings of the same spatial frequency and orientation, and compares them with VEPs (dotted lines) obtained without pre-adaptation.

The reversal VEPs for spatial frequencies of 2–6 cycles per degree were not significantly affected by the pre-adaptation to a steady grating. However, a marked reduction in voltage of the 'on–off' VEPs appears at all spatial frequencies from 2 cycles per degree and higher. As a corollary the size of the 'difference' potential is much affected by the pre-adaptation, which is indeed evidence that the difference potential is dominated by the pattern-related component.

The pattern-adaptation effect is orientation-specific: it is strongest when the pre-adapting grating has the same orientation as the test grating and it practically disappears when they differ in orientation by more than 20° (Campbell and Maffei 1970). In our next experiment pre-adaptation to a grating tilted by 30° does not affect the VEP to a 6 cycle per degree grating (Fig. 8.4).

It may be asked whether pre-adaptation to contrast reversal may be used to adapt selectively the transient system. It must be pointed out, however, that the

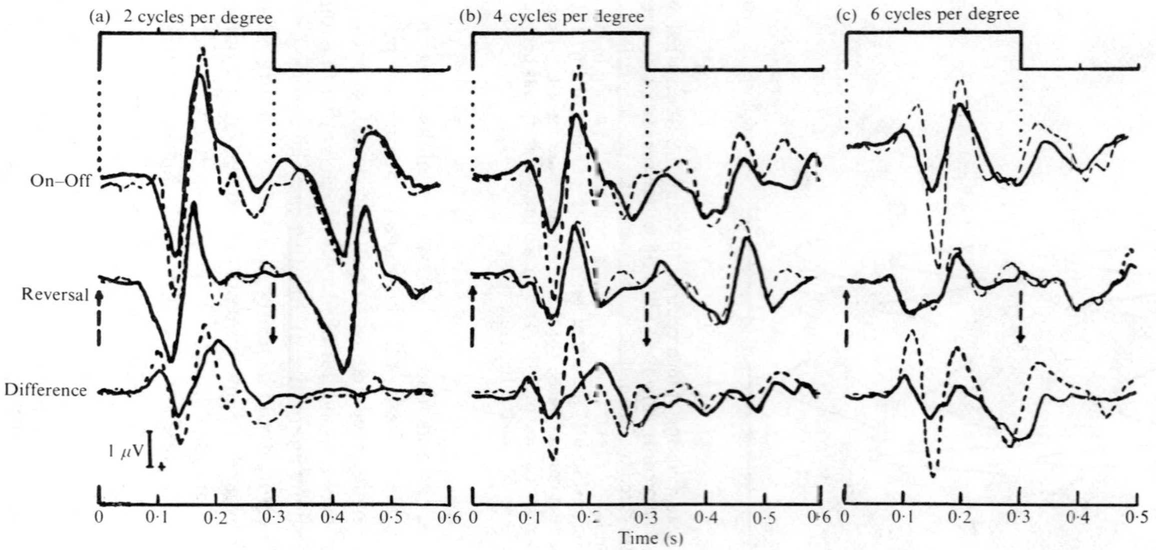

Fig. 8.3. Effect of pre-adapting to a steady grating of the same spatial frequency and orientation as the test gratings. Continuous lines show the VEP after pre-adaptation; the dashed lines the VEP before adaptation. Change in contrast was 0·1 in all cases. The test gratings of spatial frequencies 2 cycles per degree (a), 4 cycles per degree (b) or 6 cycles per degree (c) were either presented on and off (top records) or reversed in contrast (middle records) at a rate of 1·67 Hz. The lowest records are results of the subtraction of the middle from the upper record. Note that these 'difference' waveforms are drastically suppressed by pre-adaptation, whereas the reversal VEPs are virtually unaffected (only the 6 cycles per degree reversal potential shows some effect). Contrast thresholds before adaptation for 2 cycles per degree, 4 cycles per degree, and 6 cycles per degree were, respectively: pattern recognition 0·005, 0·005, 0·006, and for seeing movement 0·004, 0·005, 0·01.

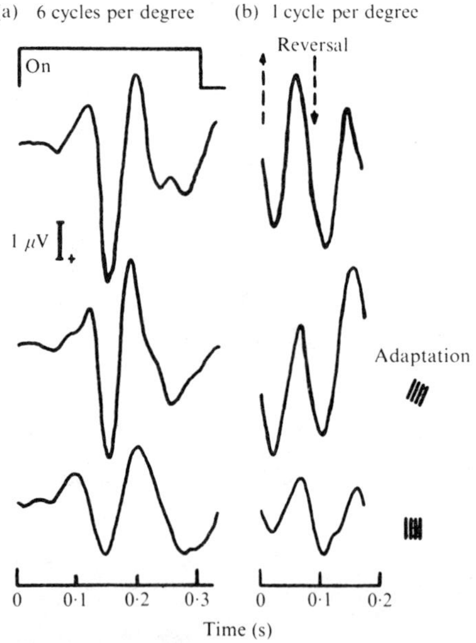

Fig. 8.4. Effect of pre-adapting to a grating of high contrast (0·8) and the same spatial frequency as the test grating. The records show the VEPs without pre-adaptation (top records), after pre-adaptation to gratings tilted by 30° (middle records) and after pre-adaptation to vertical gratings (bottom records). See text for details. (a) the potential is evoked by a 6 cycles per degree grating (having a contrast of 0·1) presented 'on' and 'off' at a rate of 1·67 Hz. The pre-adapting grating was presented continuously. (b) the potential evoked by a 1 cycle per degree grating reversed in contrast at a rate of 6 Hz. The pre-adapting grating was here reversed in contrast at the same rate.

pattern system may also respond and adapt to the reversal stimulus, even though it would contribute little to the reversal VEP. This could be because the pattern detectors may respond in a maintained manner to contrast reversal, or because different pattern detectors may respond out of phase with each other (e.g. on- and off-centre cells may respond alternatively). In either case the average level of activation of pattern detectors would be nearly constant, so that little pattern-related potential would be evoked. To minimize possible pattern adaptation due to the constant presence of a grating during the reversal, a relatively coarse grating (1 cycle per degree) was presented at a fairly high temporal frequency such as 6 Hz, at which the adaptation to temporal changes is most effective (see Fig. 8.5).

The reversal-evoked potentials in Fig. 8.4(b) show that pre-adaptation is effective only when both the test and pre-adaptive gratings do not differ much in orientation. Thus, both adaptation effects in Fig. 8.5 show their dependence upon the orientation of the adapting gratings, which suggests that both the pattern and movement VEPs may be related, directly or indirectly, to the activity of cortical

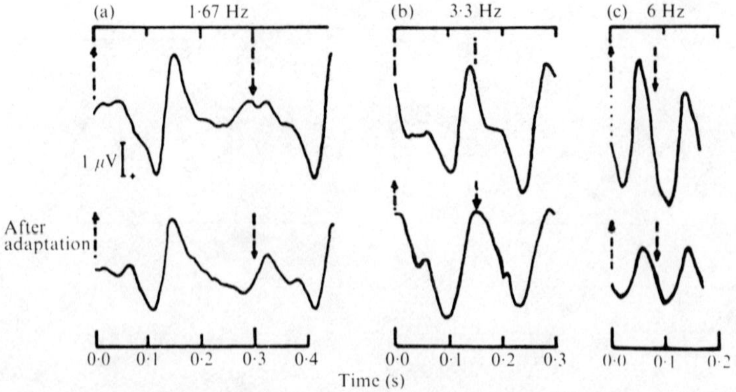

Fig. 8.5. VEPs to contrast reversal of a 1 cycle per degree grating (screen size 9°) at a variable rate: 1·67 Hz, 3·3 Hz, and 6 Hz. Top records: without pre-adaptation. Bottom records: VEPs to the same stimuli (contrast 0·025) but after pre-adapting to the contrast reversal of the corresponding grating of high contrast (0·8). The maximum contrast thresholds for seeing movement (prior to adaptation) for the 6 Hz reversal was 0·003.

cells responding to bars of specific orientation (Hubel and Wiesel 1959, 1968; Kelly and Van Essen 1974).

Effect of temporal frequency of presentations

The detection of movement is easiest when a grating is reversed in contrast at a relatively high rate, usually 6 Hz (Kulikowski and Tolhurst 1973) and the same is true for the reversal VEP (Fig. 8.5, top records). The bottom records in Fig. 8.6 show the reversal VEP recorded after pre-adaptation to a similar grating which differed from the test stimulus only in terms of contrast (0·8). The adaptation was greatest at the 6 Hz adapting stimulus. I mentioned earlier that the reversal VEP for medium gratings (e.g. 6 cycles per degree) contains a small pattern-related component. (This component would disappear with ideal fixation.) Unfortunately medium temporal and spatial frequencies produce an illusion of movement which stimulates the pursuit system, so that the eyes attempt to follow the apparently drifting grating. When this happens the reversal becomes similar to the on–off presentation in that the pattern component becomes larger.

Superposition of the VEP

The separation of pattern and movement components in the VEP was carried out with the (arbitrary) assumption that these components were linearly additive (Fig. 8.3). The television technique (see Chapter 1 of this book) was used for generating more than one pattern at a time. The superposition principle can be tested by simultaneously generating two gratings of different spatial frequencies, which were both reversed in contrast at 8 Hz (Campbell and Maffei 1970). The VEPs to the two gratings increased with an increase in the spatial frequency ratio

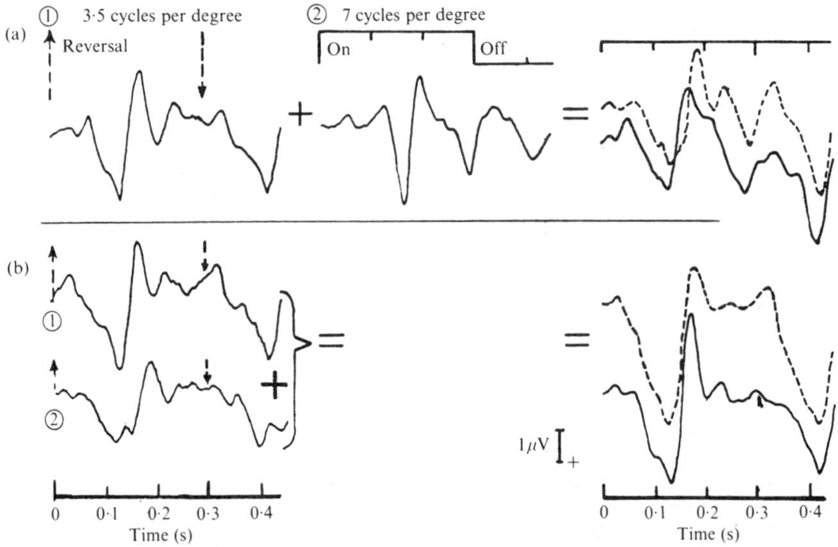

Fig. 8.6. VEPs elicited by two different grating stimuli presented at a rate of 1·67 Hz on a screen subtending 7° x 7° are shown on the left. The waveforms resulting from linear additions of 2 VEPs are shown on the right by dashed lines. Below each added waveform, the continuous record shows the VEPs to the two stimuli presented simultaneously. Notice the good agreement of the latter with the added waveforms. (a) Stimulus (1), a 3·5 cycles per degree grating, contrast 0·1, is reversed in contrast and stimulates predominantly movement detection. Stimulus (2), a 7 cycles per degree grating, contrast 0·2, is presented on and off and stimulating mainly pattern detection. (b) Both grating stimuli are reversed in contrast, so that they both evoked mostly movement potentials.

up to a factor of 2. When one grating was twice as fine as the other the maximum VEP summation was obtained, but it was always less than arithmetical. However, Campbell and Maffei did not compare the case where the potentials are evoked by each grating separately and summed.

The two main VEP components were separated in our experiments and three alternative cases of possible superposition of VEPs could thus be examined, each involving gratings of spatial frequencies differing by a factor of 2: (a) where one VEP includes the pattern component, whereas the movement component predominates in the other; (b) where the movement component predominates in both VEPs; (c) where the pattern component is considerable in both VEPs.

Fig. 8.6 shows VEPs corresponding to the first two cases. The combined VEP to the contrast reversal of a 3·5 cycle per degree grating simultaneous with the on–off presentation of a 7 cycle per degree grating is very similar to the sum of the VEPs to these stimuli presented separately (Fig. 8.6(a), dashed line). This means that the movement- and pattern-detection mechanisms for spatial frequencies of 3·5 cycles per degree and 7 cycles per degree are separate, and do not interact noticeably. A similar conclusion is reached for the summation of VEPs to the reversal of the two gratings 3·5 cycles per degree and 7 cycles per degree (Fig. 8.6(b)). However, different results are obtained when the 3·5 cycles per degree and 7 cycles per degree gratings are both presented on and off simultaneously (Fig. 8.7) which evokes a VEP smaller than the sum of the VEPs evoked

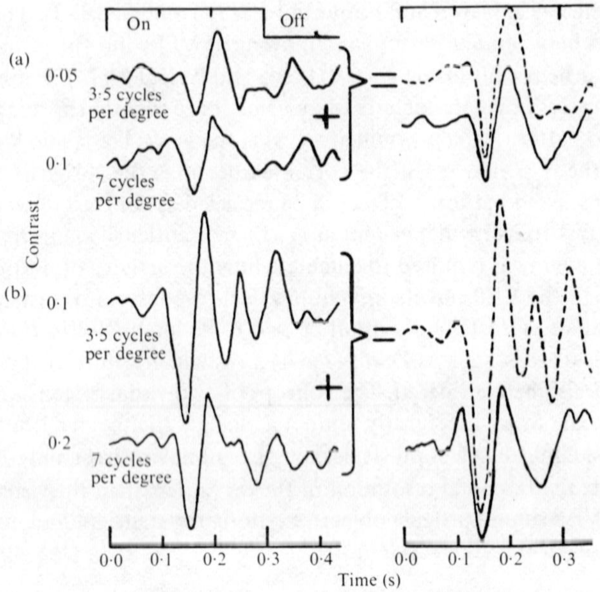

Fig. 8.7. (a) Averaged potentials evoked by presenting gratings of spatial frequencies 3·5 cycles per degree and 7 cycles per degree (contrasts 0·05 and 0·10 respectively), shown on the left, are added and the resulting waveform is shown by a dashed line on the right. Below these added waveforms the continuous record shows the average potential evoked by presenting these two gratings simultaneously. (b) As above except that the contrasts are doubled (0·10 and 0·20 respectively). Notice that VEPs to the two gratings are smaller than the added waveforms.

separately (dashed curves). Thus two pattern-detection mechanisms tuned to these spatial frequencies seem to exhibit some negative (perhaps inhibitory) interaction. This conclusion is in agreement with the subject's psychophysical report that there is a significant masking effect for gratings that differ in their spatial frequencies by a factor of two (Kulikowski 1969).

Significance of separate VEPs related to the detection of pattern and movement

The results described suggest separate mechanisms for the analysis of pattern and movement. For medium spatial frequencies, above 3 cycles per degree and below 10 cycles per degree the reversal VEP is dominated by movement components, whereas the on–off VEP is dominated by pattern-related components. It is tempting to draw a parallel between these results and those obtained in animals.

Separation of occipital potentials related to the detection of pattern and movement

Enroth-Cugell and Robson (1966) discovered two separate classes of retinal ganglion cells, the X-cells, with a rather sustained response, and the Y-cells, with nonlinear and transient responses.

Subsequently it has been suggested that the two X- and Y-systems might be involved in separate perceptual tasks such as analysis of pattern and movement (Ikeda and Wright 1972; Maffei and Fiorentini 1973; Tolhurst 1973). There are many similarities between our pattern and movement VEPs and the responses of sustained and transient cells in the cortex (Ikeda and Wright 1974). For example, latencies of the early VEP components to movement are slightly shorter than those for VEP to pattern, which would agree with the view (Ikeda and Wright, 1972 *a*, *b*) that the Y-signals reach the cortex earlier than the X-signals. Also both the X-cell responses and pattern VEP could be regarded as contrast dependent rather than contrast-transient dependent as are their 'transient' counterparts.

However, more work is required to elucidate how the activity of cortical neurones relates to the VEP and the psychophysical responses. For instance, some of the cells classified as 'sustained' cannot be said to be insensitive to transients. Specialized cortical areas, such as Zeki's (1974) area, which seems to analyse movement, must also be considered. The concept of two visual systems, one for analysis of form, the other for signally temporal changes (Schneider 1969) is also important from a clinical viewpoint. It has long been known that amblyopia ex anopsia affects the temporal resolution of flicker far less than the visual resolution. The VEP should provide objective criteria for transient and non-transient responses of the visual system.

Acknowledgements

I wish to thank the Science Research Council for a research grant (No. BI RG/1511). I also thank Professor J. R. Cronly-Dillon, Dr. P. E. King-Smith, and Mr. R. Abadi for their helpful comments and Mr. D. Carden for his expert assistance.

9. Relation of evoked potentials to pattern and local luminance detectors in the human visual system

I. BODIS-WOLLNER and C. D. HENDLEY
Departments of Neurology and Physiology, Mount Sinai School of Medicine, New York

Kuffler (1953) and Hubel and Wiesel (1959) established that single cells may be classified by the parameters of their optimal stimuli. For the majority of the cells in the retino calcarine pathway, diffuse light is not a sufficient stimulus and specific stimuli are needed to obtain optimal responses. Many cells in the visual cortex are orientation selective and their optimal stimuli are single bars or repetitive bar patterns (gratings). By employing similar stimuli in human vision research as in single-cell investigations, it has been possible to interpret human visual functions with physiological principles established through investigations on subhuman primates and carnivores (Campbell and Robson 1968; Blakemore and Campbell 1969).

There is increasing physiological evidence that cells with similar specificity are grouped together and that different groups are in parallel organization. This suggests that VEPs to non-specific stimuli express the response of more than one 'channel' in the visual system. Interpretation of such multi-component responses is difficult unless there is an adequate basis for analytically separating the components. For this reason, an understanding of physiological principles is of crucial importance to current VEP research and to the application of VEPs to the diagnosis of disorders of vision (Bodis-Wollner *et al.*, Chapter 35 of this book).

We are interested in whether the human visual cortex has a predominantly parallel or a serial organization of pattern and local luminance detectors, and in the relevance of such cortical organizations to human VEPs. What is meant by serial and parallel processing? Cells with different properties may be connected sequentially (serial processing), or may be organized into separate channels (parallel processing) from retina to cortex. The present investigations use contrast-modulated grating patterns as stimuli (Bodis-Wollner *et al.* 1972; Bodis-Wollner, Hendley, and Tajfel 1973), which makes it possible to analyse the functional relationship of psychophysical responses and VEPs to changes in local luminance and in spatial contrast of the pattern.

Visual evoked potentials in man: new developments (ed. J. E. Desmedt), pp. 197–207.
Clarendon Press, Oxford 1977.

Background

Grating patterns are easily generated on the oscilloscope screen. Only a few parameters are needed to define this type of stimulus. The sinusoidal grating has a mean or average luminance which is half of the sum of the luminance of one dark and one bright band of the pattern. The contrast of the pattern is expressed as the difference of luminance of a bright and a dark band over their sum. The *spatial frequency* is expressed as the number of cycles (a dark and bright band) in 1° subtended at the eye of the observer. *Threshold* contrast is expressed as the minimum contrast necessary to detect the grating. The inverse of threshold contrast is called *contrast sensitivity*. When this is charted as a function of the spatial frequency, a contrast-sensitivity curve can be plotted. The contrast-sensitivity curve of a single cell is a measure of the receptive field organization of the antagonistic centre-surround type (Enroth-Cugell and Robson 1966) and it can also be used to characterize orientation-selective cells in the visual cortex (Campbell, Cooper, and Enroth-Cugell 1969).

The normal human contrast-sensitivity curve has an inverted-U shape: there is an optimal range of spatial frequencies, and both lower and higher frequency gratings need more contrast to be detected. To establish the human contrast-sensitivity curve, it is customary to present the grating for 0·5 s and alternate it with a blank field of the same average luminance (on–off method). If the alternation is faster than 2–3 Hz, the contrast sensitivity falls appreciably but not uniformly. At 8 Hz, the curve becomes monotonic with a relative increase in sensitivity at low spatial frequencies: the coarser the grating, the easier it is to detect (Robson 1968). If the human contrast-sensitivity curve is the transfer function of a single channel with antagonistic centre-surround organization, then the decline in sensitivity for low spatial frequencies at slow rates may result from inhibition and, conversely, the larger response for low spatial frequencies at higher rates may be due to the temporal characteristics of the inhibitory component (Fiorentini and Maffei 1970*a*; Kelly 1971). However, the spatial contrast-sensitivity curve may also be considered as the envelope function of more than one spatial frequency channel (Campbell and Robson 1968; Blakemore and Campbell 1969). One can ask whether the low-frequency behaviour is due to a single inhibitory component and whether a single mechanism is involved in VEPs to a steadily presented grating and to abrupt changes of its contrast.

Parallel channels

Let us consider the possibility of two response mechanisms, one preferring steady stimuli, the other abrupt changes. VEPs are usually elicited by rapid changes in some stimulus parameter, e.g. onset or offset of the stimulus. There is no direct method to measure VEP to a steadily presented stimulus. Contrast-modulated gratings allow us to infer the simultaneous effects of a continuously present and an abruptly changing grating on both VEPs and psychophysical responses. This is a steady grating pattern superimposed on counterphase flicker, and both of these components have the same spatial frequency. The mean contrast of the grating defines the steady spatial contrast level, and the depth of contrast modulation defines the temporal modulation of the luminance of individual bars. These two parameters can be independently varied, which enables us to investigate the organization of local luminance and pattern detectors in the human visual system. As discussed below, these detectors may be related to two classes of cells present in the retina (Enroth-Cugell and Robson 1966) and the lateral geniculate nucleus of the cat (Cleland *et al.* 1971). It is of special interest that a similar dual organization has been demonstrated for cells in the cortex as well (Hoffman and Stone 1971; Stone 1972; Toyama, Maekawa, and Takeda 1973), although this division may be less straightforward than originally thought (Ikeda and Wright 1974).

Methods

Subjects were emmetropes or well-corrected myopes. Their age ranged from 17 years to 57 years. In a period of 4 years, we studied over 20 subjects. In this chapter a sampling of data is shown for five of them.

Vertical gratings with sinusoidal luminance profile were generated on a Tektronix 561 oscilloscope with P4 phosphor. A short horizontal black line served as a fixation point. The test screen subtended 5° at a distance of 114 cm from the observer. It was surrounded with a transparent screen of 10° diameter, back-illuminated so as to appear about the same hue and brightness as the oscilloscope screen. The space-time average luminance of the oscilloscope screen was 70 ft-L in most experiments. The subject wears a trial frame which holds lenses for refractive correction.

Contrast modulation was achieved by the successive presentation of the same grating at higher and lower contrast (Fig. 9.1) (see Chapter 1 of this book). The z-axis d.c. and a.c. response of the stimulus-display oscilloscope was calibrated with an RCA 5583 phototube. The contrast of the grating could be modulated through small steps from 1 (full modulation of the contrast) downward. The modulating signal was a square wave at the rate of 8 Hz which in these experiments switched the gratings-contrast switches between two values every 125 ms. The two values depend on both the mean contrast of the grating and the depth of modulation. The contrast C of a grating may be defined as

$$C = \frac{L_{max} - L_{min}}{L_{max} + L_{min}}, \tag{9.1}$$

where L_{max} is the maximum and L_{min} is the minimum luminance (of the bright and of the dark bands, respectively).

$$L_{mean} = \frac{L_{max} + L_{min}}{2}. \tag{9.2}$$

The depth of contrast modulation can be defined analogously as

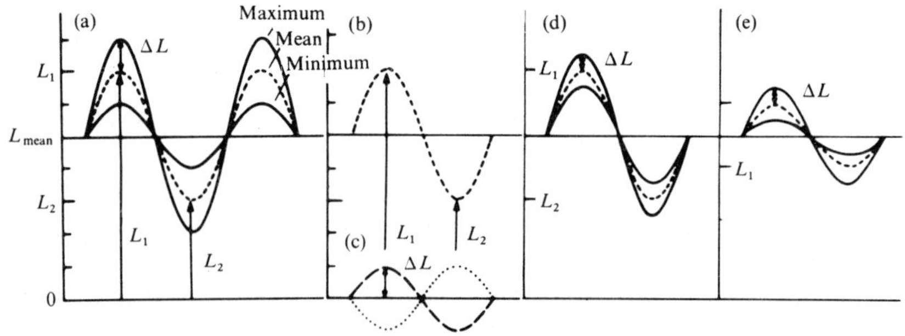

Fig. 9.1. (a) Luminance of a contrast-modulated grating. 'Max'. indicates profile of the higher-contrast state, which alternates with the lower-contrast state labelled 'Min.' The mean-contrast profile is labelled 'Mean'. The highest and lowest luminance levels of the individual bars which establish the mean-contrast profile are labelled L_1 and L_2, respectively. Peak luminance values of the grating during modulation differ from these mean levels by ΔL, which is therefore half the brightness change at the centre of each bar between the two contrast levels. Mean contrast is 0·4. Modulation depth is 0·5. This means that the maximum contrast is 50 per cent higher and the minimum contrast is 50 per cent lower than the mean contrast. Notice that ΔC is 0·2. The contrast-modulated grating may alternately be viewed as the sum of a steady grating (b) which with mean luminance $L_{mean} = \frac{1}{2}(L_1 + L_2)$ and contrast $C_{mean} = (L_1 - L_2/(L_1 + L_2)$ and a 'counterphase-flicker' grating (c) which alternates between two symmetrical states that are spatially 180° out of phase, and consequently has no standing contrast. (d) The same mean contrast (0·4) as in (a) is modulated with a modulation depth of 0·25; then $\Delta C = 0{\cdot}1$. (e) Mean contrast of 0·2 is modulated with a modulation-depth of 0·5 as in (a). Notice that $\Delta C = 0{\cdot}1$ as in (d).

$$M = \frac{C_{max} - C_{min}}{C_{max} + C_{min}} = \frac{2\Delta C}{2C_{mean}} \tag{9.3}$$

where C_{max} is the maximum and C_{min} is the minimum contrast of the grating during the modulation period.

$$\Delta C = \frac{C_{max} - C_{min}}{2} \tag{9.4}$$

and

$$C_{mean} = \frac{C_{max} + C_{min}}{2}. \tag{9.5}$$

We call ΔL the luminance difference of any bar of the grating pattern between C_{max} and C_{mean}, and similarly between C_{mean} and C_{min} conditions. Then the luminance difference of a bar can be simply related to the values of M and ΔC by expressing C_{max} and C_{min} in terms of L_{max}, L_{min}, and ΔL,

$$C_{max} = \frac{L_{max} - L_{min} + 2\Delta L}{L_{max} + L_{min}}$$

$$C_{min} = \frac{L_{max} - L_{min} - 2\Delta L}{L_{max} + L_{min}},$$

and expressing ΔC with these equations. This leads to

$$\Delta C = \frac{2\Delta L}{L_{max} + L_{min}} = \frac{\Delta L}{L_{mean}} \tag{9.6}$$

Thus ΔC is proportional to ΔL and this proportion remains constant at constant mean luminance of the pattern.

VEPs elicited by different modulation depth at a given mean contrast level were recorded consecutively. Silver-disc electrodes were placed on the scalp 2·5 cm above the inion and over the temporal bone just behind and above the ear, corresponding to the posterior temporal electrode according to the International 10–20 nomenclature. A third electrode placed in the middle of the forehead was ground. Scalp potentials were fed to a differential amplifier and filtered. Corner frequencies were usually 10 Hz and 35 Hz but were sometimes extended to a bandpass from 1·5 Hz to 60 Hz. The potentials were averaged with a Fabri-Tek 1062 computer, negativity at the active scalp electrode producing an upward deflection. The EEG was recorded using this electrode montage.

VEPs were measured as the average peak-to-peak amplitude of two humps apparent in the VEP of Fig. 9.3(a). The beginning of the sweep of the averager was synchronized with the decrease in contrast. In some subjects the VEP had only a single hump. Stimulus-locked artifacts were checked by recording potentials while the observer closed his eyes or looked away. There was a less than 1 per cent flicker (mean brightness change) at high modulation depths of the cathode ray tube screen. To estimate its influence, we recorded VEPs to a homogeneous field flickering at the same rate and amplitude by placing a diffuser in front of the cathode ray tube and found no potentials distinguishable from noise.

A contrast-modulated grating (Fig. 9.1(a)) may be regarded as a steady grating (Fig. 9.1(b)) superimposed on counterphase flicker (Fig. 9.1(c)). The spatial contrast and the modulation depth were independently varied. We asked the question: how does the level of the mean spatial contrast affect the detectability of modulation? In order to minimize pattern adaptation (Pantle and Sekuler 1968; Blakemore and Campbell 1969; Blakemore, Muncey, and Ridley 1973) the subject was asked to make his judgement in less than 30 seconds. He was allowed three binocular looks before he had to answer yes or no to the presence of modulation. Between looks he was asked to keep his eye on the evenly illuminated surround screen. Cycloplegics were not used either for psychophysical or VEP measurements. Thresholds were first roughly estimated by a method of limits. Then at least 4 modulation depths were chosen and at least 5 random presentations were given at each level. The subject was asked to decide whether he could detect any change in the contrast of the pattern. In this manner frequency of detection curves were obtained and threshold was estimated as the 50 per cent intercept value of the curve. False positive responses were checked. We call the inverse of modulation threshold the modulation sensitivity, and this was plotted as a function of mean contrast. The lowest mean contrast was well above the subject's detection threshold for the given spatial frequency. Mean contrast levels were selected 6 or 10 dB apart within the range of 30 dB above the lowest contrast. Modulation threshold curves were obtained at various spatial frequencies in the range 1·5–12 cycles per degree.

Results

Fig. 9.2(a) shows modulation sensitivity data for a 6 cycles per degree sinusoidal grating. The two sets of symbols refer to data obtained 3 years apart in the same

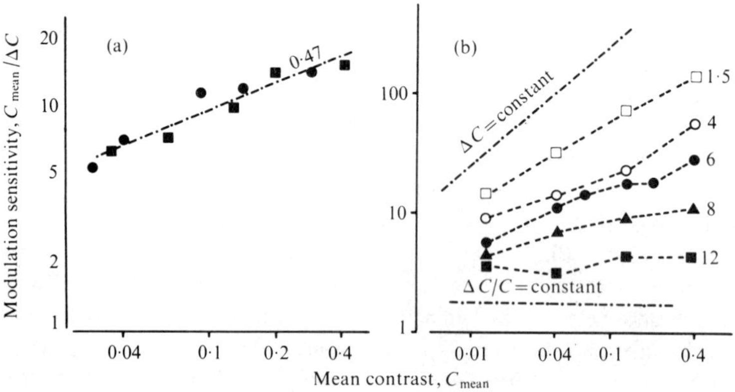

Fig. 9.2. Modulation threshold was established as a function of mean contrast of a 6 cycles per degree grating pattern. (a) Filled circles and squares refer to data obtained from the same subject 3 years apart. (b) Contrast-modulation functions plotted for different spatial frequencies. The numbers at the right represent the spatial frequency of the pattern. The two dot-dashed lines indicate the limiting slopes of these functions. (From Bodis-Wollner 1974.)

subject. In the explored mean contrast range, data points can be fitted with a straight line by the least-squares method. Absolute values are less relevant than the slope of this regression line. Let us assume that the modulation threshold is constant with ΔC proportional to the mean contrast level: this would result in a zero slope of the regression line, which is not the case in Fig. 9.2(a). If, on the other hand, ΔC was constant, the modulation threshold curve should be a line with a 45° slope. In fact the calculated regression line has an intermediate slope. An explanation for this finding is suggested in Fig. 9.2(b), where the slope of the modulation-sensitivity curves range from 45° to 0° when different spatial frequencies are tested.

Assume that there is a row of cells, each cell looking at an individual bar (half cycle) of the pattern. No cell alone could signal the luminance difference of neighbouring bars which, at a given mean luminance, is simply the spatial contrast of the pattern. If contrast modulation were detected by such cells (since $\Delta L = L_{mean}\Delta C$), then the just noticeable difference in contrast (ΔC) would be independent of C_{mean}. In other words, the slope of a modulation function should be 45°. Another possibility is that cells look at at least two bars of the pattern. These cells would be capable of signalling the spatial contrast of the pattern, and the just noticeable difference would be proportional to the mean contrast. This would result in a slope of zero of a modulation function. From Fig. 9.2(b) it is apparent that from 1·5 cycles per degree to 12 cycles per degree, with increasing spatial frequency, the slopes change between 45° and 0°. As spatial frequency increases from 1·5 cycles per degree, modulation detection seems to become more and more dependent on the mean spatial contrast of the pattern. We interpret the intermediate slope of a modulation sensitivity function as expressing a balance of detectors responding to local luminance changes and those responding to spatial contrast. Six cycles per degree appears to be near the watershed of these two types of detectors. It is interesting to note that the peak region of the human contrast sensitivity curve is about 6 cycles per degree.

VEPs to contrast modulation

At different mean contrast levels of 6 cycles per degree sinusoidal gratings VEPs were recorded at different modulation depths. The typical VEP has two humps with prominent negative and positive components (Fig. 9.3(a)). We measured VEP

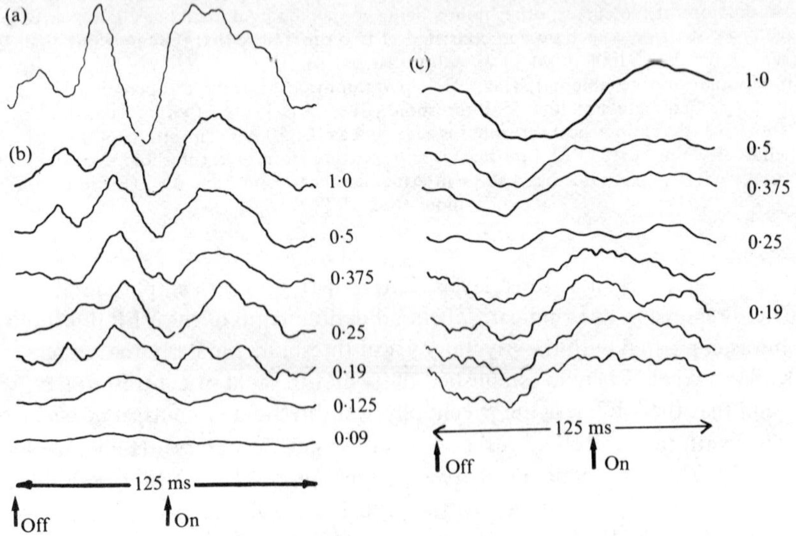

Fig. 9.3. (a) VEP to full modulation of a 6 cycles per degree grating of 0·4 mean contrast. Average of 512 responses. (b) and (c) VEPs at 0·2 mean contrast. In (b) gain is reduced for the top three records. The numbers to the right of each trace indicate the modulation depth. Note the apparent lack of response at modulation depth of 0·09. (From Bodis-Wollner, *et al.* 1972). (c) VEPs for another subject in whom the wave form presents only a single hump. The gain is doubled for the four consecutive traces at 0·19 modulation depth. Contrast decrease is synchronized with the beginning of the sweep. Negativity is recorded upwards in all traces.

amplitude following the methods of Campbell and Maffei (1971). VEP amplitude diminishes with decreasing modulation depth (Fig. 9.3(b)). Not infrequently, apparently normal subjects produced single-hump VEPs with a much reduced or even absent negative component (Fig. 9.3(c)). We have no explanation of these wave forms which were consistently present at different modulation depths in these subjects. Fig. 9.4 presents the VEP amplitude as a function of modulation

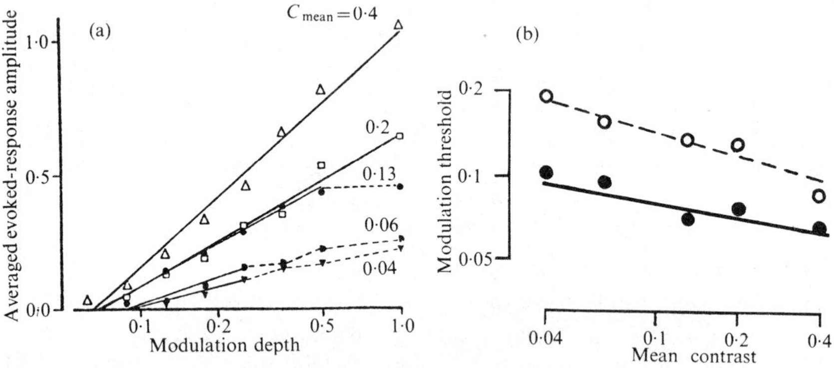

Fig. 9.4. (a) VEP amplitude as a function of contrast modulation depth at various mean contrasts (specified above each curve). Regression lines (continuous) are computed for fairly straight portions of the curves, other points being connected by dashed lines. Each curve is the average of two sessions. Each session consisted of two runs. Note that the regression lines have different slopes depending on the mean contrast level.

(b) Modulation threshold data (log scale): psychophysical threshold (open circles) are fitted by a dashed regression line; VEP threshold (filled circles) are fitted by a continuous regression line. Psychophysical threshold is accepted as the 50 per cent intercept on the frequency-of-seeing curve; VEP threshold is extrapolated from suprathreshold response curves. Note that each regression line has a slope intermediate between 0° and 45°. (From Bodis-Wollner *et al.* 1972.)

depth at different mean contrast levels. Extrapolation to zero amplitude of the calculated regression lines indicates the modulation depth of the VEP threshold, which was compared with the psychophysical threshold. Similarly to Campbell and Kulikowski (1971) who established the VEP threshold of contrast *detection*, we found that the VEP near the psychophysical threshold of contrast *modulation* correlates with the subjective 'yes' or 'no' answers of the observer (Bodis-Wollner *et al.* 1972). The correspondence between psychophysical and VEP thresholds is evident in Fig. 9.4(b). The slopes for the psychophysical modulation sensitivity function and for the VEP modulation-sensitivity function are not significantly different. As discussed above the slope of the sensitivity function indicates that the contrast-modulation psychophysical threshold is determined by the balance of pattern and local luminance detectors. This can now be extended to the VEP threshold.

When considering VEP to suprathreshold modulation, since $\Delta L = L_0 C_{mean} M$

(from $\Delta L = L_0 \Delta C$ and $\Delta C = C_{mean}M$) and if only local luminance changes determined the VEP amplitude, we should expect two features in the regression lines: at each mean contrast they should be (a) parallel and (b) superimposable by a horizontal shift proportional to the mean contrast. Inspection of Fig. 9.4 indicates that this is not the case. In fact, local luminance detectors alone do not determine the amplitude of VEPs to contrast modulation of a 6 cycles per degree grating and the mean contrast level must be taken into account as well (cf. Bodis-Wollner *et al.*, Chapter 35 of this book).

Discussion

We regard contrast-modulated grating patterns as consisting of two components: a constantly visible, steady suprathreshold grating; and counterphase flicker, both components having the same spatial frequency. What sort of cells could mediate responses to these two components? As we have shown, VEP amplitudes depend not only on the modulation depth (the transient component) but also on the mean contrast (the steady component) of the grating. Similarly, the VEP and psychophysical thresholds of modulation depend on the mean contrast of the grating. Thus there must be mechanisms in the human visual system which are capable of responding to the *steady* spatial contrast of the grating.

Detectors which respond to luminance changes of single bars are called local luminance detectors and they appear to be related to the transient cells demonstrated in the cat's visual system. This analogy is suggested by the slope of the modulation-sensitivity curve at low spatial frequencies, where ΔC is almost constant, and alone determines the modulation threshold, regardless of the mean contrast of the grating. Thus cells involved in the detection of the modulation are almost independent of the steady luminance of the pattern. Enroth-Cugell and Robson (1966) found that Y-ganglion cells of the retina signal 'almost any change in illumination of their receptive field', and Y-cells are sensitive to a lower range of spatial frequencies than X-(sustained) cells are. Our data on contrast modulation are consistent with these properties of these two types of cells. Of course, we cannot claim that the stimulus used in our experiments is as well stabilized on the retina as are the stimuli used in single-cell work. Maintained fixation does not prevent small eye movements. However, the latter could not account for the generation of 'transient' or local luminance responses. Local luminance detection dominates at low rather than at high spatial frequencies (Fig. 9.2(b)), but it is precisely at high spatial frequencies that eye movements introduce more *frequent* local luminance changes on the retina.

Tolhurst (1973), Kulikowski and Tolhurst (1973) and Kulikowski, Chapter 8 of this book (see also Rashbass 1968; Keesey 1972) established that pattern and flicker are detected at threshold by separate mechanisms, which may be analogous to sustained and transient cells of the cat. Our experiments exploring the suprathreshold range of contrasts led to the conclusion that VEPs and also psychophysical detection are determined by the balance of two mechanisms responding to the steady and transient component of a single grating (Bodis-Wollner *et al.* 1972; Bodis-Wollner, Hendley, and Tajfel 1973). The VEP data suggest that there are cortical structures which respond to both local luminance changes and to spatial contrast. There could be parallel cortical structures, but we cannot exclude the possibility that VEPs are generated in structures proximal to an interaction of the two types of detectors. There does not seem to be any major precortical interaction, since sustained and transient cells can be found in the cat's visual cortex and appear to be parts of separate information channels even at this level. This is an attractive analogy but single-cell functions are not yet completely explored. We should like to know contrast-modulation functions of single ganglion cells and also know more about the cortical organization of sustained and transient detectors in the visual cortex of the cat. It was thought that simple cells were sustained pattern detectors and complex cells were transient-luminance detectors. This has been challenged by the findings of Pollen and Ronner (1975) of narrow-band grating-detector complex cells and by Ikeda and Wright (1974), who demonstrated that both simple and complex cells can be either sustained or transient. At the moment, the analogy with the cat's cortical cells is far from clear and does not help decide whether parallel or serial organization of human cortical structures exist. Clinical VEP studies by Bodis-Wollner *et al.* (Chapter 35 of this book) suggest but do not prove that parallel processsing is maintained at the cortex. The contribution of the two types of detectors to the recorded VEP waveform at slow and fast rates of presentation has still to be analysed.

Meaningful VEP studies require the stimulus conditions to be well suited for a particular question. This is especially important for clinical research. If our conclusions about parallel pathways in the human visual system are accepted, one must also consider that parallel brain structures may be selectively vulnerable to pathology (Bodis-Wollner 1973). This is also suggested by Bodis-Wollner *et al.* in Chapter 35 and by Cook and Arden in Chapter 26 of this book). Flash stimuli appear inadequate for the demonstration of lesions which may cause selective deficits in the visual system.

Summary

Contrast modulation of grating patterns is regarded as a stimulus composed of a steady grating pattern and of counterphase flicker, both having the same spatial frequency. Detectability functions are different at different spatial frequencies and it is suggested that the balance of two mechanisms, each responding to one of the components of the stimulus, determines both the psychophysical responses and the VEP functions. These two mechanisms may be related to sustained and transient-type cells in the human visual system. It is not established whether a parallel organization exists in the visual cortex or only in precortical structures of the human visual system. The existence of stimulus specific pathways is of special importance when using VEPs in clinical diagnosis.

Acknowledgement

I. Bodis-Wollner is a recipient of an NINDS Individual Research Fellowship IF 22NS 02803-01. This work was supported by Grant NS-11631-03 from the National Institutes of Health.

Fig. 9.2 is reproduced by courtesy of the *Mount Sinai Journal of Medicine*. Figs. 9.3 and 9.4 by courtesy of *Perception*.

10. Binocular interaction: evoked potentials to dichoptic stimulation

M. R. HARTER

Department of Psychology, University of North Carolina at Greensboro

Introduction

This chapter investigates VEPs with various examples of binocular stimulation, in order (a) to ascertain how pattern information arriving from the two eyes is coded in the central nervous system to achieve binocular vision, and (b) to investigate the specificity of central neural channels in terms of the coding of pattern information. Although the studies reported here are primarily related to sensory coding, their results may readily be applied to disorders of binocularity. VEPs provide a unique, readily accessible measure of such processes in man.

A single binocular percept of the images falling on the two retinae may be obtained (a) by neural summation combining the inputs from both retinae, the binocular percept being a superposition of the two retinal images, and/or (b) by neural suppression of all or part of the inputs from one retina, the binocular percept being then based on the image falling on one eye or on a composite of elements of the images falling on one eye or the other. The extent to which summation and suppression mechanisms are brought into play depends on the nature of patterns presented to each eye. Under normal viewing conditions, virtually identical images fall on corresponding retinal areas (*dioptic* viewing conditions). Under atypical binocular viewing conditions, which may be associated with disorders of binocular vision, the images falling on the two retinae may differ in terms of sharpness of focus, size, orientation, intensity, correspondence, etc. (*dichoptic* viewing conditions). This chapter is concerned primarily with the effects of various types of dichoptic pattern stimulation on VEP indicants of binocular interaction. Data related to the corresponding psychophysical measures of binocular interaction (Blake and Fox 1973) will not be considered in detail.

White and Bonelli (1970) and Harter, Seiple, and Salmon (1973) have shown that binocularly elicited VEPs are greater in amplitude than monocularly elicited VEPs under conditions where identical patterns are presented to corresponding retinal points (dioptic viewing conditions). They also reported greater binocular summation to patterned stimuli than to diffused light, particularly for sharply focused pattern elements (White and Bonelli 1970) subtending 10–20 minutes of

Visual evoked potentials in man: new developments (ed. J. E. Desmedt), pp. 208–33. Clarendon Press, Oxford 1977.

arc of visual angle (Harter *et al.* 1973).

The effects of binocularly presenting patterned light to non-corresponding retinal points (dichoptic stimulation) on VEPs depend on the nature of non-correspondence. It has been reported that when the retinal disparity results in changes in perceived depth, VEP amplitude increases as a function of the degree of retinal disparity (Fiorentini and Maffei 1970; Regan and Spekreijse 1970). However, inducing non-correspondence under conditions which do not result in variations in perceived depth reduced the amplitude of some VEP components with latencies of 150 ms or more (Harter, Seiple, and Salmon 1972, 1973; Kawasaki, Hirose, Jacobson, and Cordella 1970), the amplitude and waveform of these components in binocular VEPs being similar to those of monocular VEPs. These data suggest the input from one eye was suppressed and support the suggestion that this form of dichoptic stimulation results in one eye contributing more to the binocular VEP than the other (MacKay 1968; Martin 1970; Ciganek 1971).

Suppression has been demonstrated more directly in studies where monocular VEPs to transient stimulation of one eye were reduced in amplitude by continuous stimulation of the other eye. Such interocular suppression has been demonstrated when the two eyes have respectively viewed diffuse and patterned light (Lansing 1964; Lehmann and Fender 1967, 1968), a small spot of light and diffuse light (Shipley 1969; Franceschetti and Burian 1971), patterns of identical spatial frequencies (Spekreijse *et al.* 1972), and striped grid patterns of opposite orientation (Riggs and Whittle 1967). Suppression of monocular VEPs has also been obtained as a function of 'spontaneous' changes in perceptual suppression in binocular rivalry experiments (Van Balen 1964; Lansing 1964; Cobb *et al.* 1967; Lawwill and Biersdorf 1968).

Although visual suppression thus occurs under a wide variety of conditions, it is not clear whether it is due to (a) differences in the effectiveness of the stimuli presented to the two eyes (e.g. patterned being more effective than diffuse stimuli), (b) the relationship between the stimuli presented to the two eyes (e.g. in terms of similarity of stimulus configuration and correspondence of points of retinal stimulation), and/or (c) attentional shifts between the two eyes. The studies described in this chapter investigate the contribution of these factors to binocular interaction. The first study is concerned with the effects of presenting different spatial frequencies dichoptically to the two eyes on both *monocular* and *binocular* VEP measures of binocular interaction. The remaining three studies are concerned with the time-course and channel specificity (in terms of spatial frequency and retinal eccentricity) of interocular suppression as measured by *monocular* VEPs.

The nature of binocular interactions indicated by VEPs were defined as follows: *binocular summation* is assumed to have occurred when binocular stimulation results in greater amplitude VEPs than when either eye is stimulated alone; *binocular suppression* is considered to have occurred when monocular stimulation of either eye results in VEPs equal to or greater in amplitude than that obtained when both eyes are stimulated. Suppression of one eye would be indicated (a) when monocular VEPs, elicited by a given stimulus presented to one eye, decrease in amplitude due to stimulation of the other eye, and (b) when binocular VEPs primarily reflect the contribution of just one eye, as indicated by similarity in amplitude and waveform of one of the monocular VEPs to that of the binocular VEP and/or by binocular VEPs being uninfluenced by the nature of pattern presented to one eye.

Methods

Subjects

Nine normal adults, consisting of graduate students and faculty staff ranging in age from 22 years to 34 years, participated in the studies. Each subject was presented all experimental conditions for 2–4 replications of each condition. The subjects had prior experience in VEP studies and had better than 20/20 visual acuities (monocular and binocular).

Visual stimulation

The patterned stimuli consisted of checkerboards or obliquely oriented, crossed-line grids which were reproduced on transparency film. Each stimulus display subtended visual angles of about 10° in length and 8° in height and was mounted in a 8·03 x 10·2 cm ($3\frac{1}{4}$ x 4 in) slide mount. The different sizes of pattern elements or 'spatial frequencies' were achieved by photographic reduction. A 'blank pattern' consisted of a diffuse transparency (neutral density filter) with luminance transmittance equal to that of the average luminance transmittance of the other patterns.

A haploscope (Harter *et al.* 1973) enabled the two eyes to be stimulated independently. The stimulus transparencies were inserted into each side of the haploscope in front of translucent diffusing screens which could be back-illuminated by two different light sources. Continuous back-illumination of the patterns viewed by both eyes was provided by two standard 40 W light bulbs connected respectively to two Variacs. This continuous back-illumination, when present, provided cues for dominance or rivalry phenomenon and for visual fixation (subjects were instructed to fixate the centre of the display). (A momentary (10 μs) increment in pattern brightness was obtained by back-illuminating the displays viewed by either the left, the right, or both eyes with light flashes produced by two Grass PS-2 photo-stimulators.) VEPs were elicited by this second light source. The order of presentation of stimulus conditions was counter-balanced across replications and subjects in order to control for the effects of time and order of conditions on VEPs.

It should be noted that the evoking flashes generated a change in average luminance in addition to making the patterned stimuli momentarily of greater contrast. The luminance and contrast effects associated with flashed-pattern stimulation could readily be dissociated, since (a) VEPs to only the luminance change (the diffuse flash) were obtained, and (b) the change in luminance was constant for all patterns used in a given experiment. The differences in VEPs elicited by the different flashes, therefore, were due to the presence and nature of the pattern and not to changes in luminance associated with presentation of pattern. The flash-stimulation technique, in contrast to constant average-luminance methods (e.g. pattern reversal and pattern onset and offset), also enabled the investigation of luminance effects *per se.* Although evidence has been offered that constance average-luminance methods may also contain luminance effects (Van der Tweel and Estevez-Uscanga 1972), such effects are always confounded with changes in contrast. Consequently, the latter technique is inappropriate for studying the effects of luminance when pattern is also varied, as in the experiments described here.

Recording procedure

VEPs were recorded monopolarly by means of gold-cup scalp electrodes placed 2·5 cm above the inion on the midline (O_Z) and/or 5 cm lateral to each side of the midline electrode (O_1 and O_2). Reference electrodes were attached to the right earlobe or to linked earlobes (when recording from O_1 or O_2). Redux electrode jelly was rubbed into the skin and applied between the electrodes and scalp in order to reduce skin resistance to less than 10 000 Ω. Cortical activity was amplified by a Grass Model 7 WC polygraph with $\frac{1}{2}$ amplitude high- and low-frequency filters set at 35 Hz and 1 Hz respectively. The amplified potentials were fed into an Alpha 16 (Computer Automation) mini-computer system or a Fabri-Tek 1062 averaging computer. The data were quantified, in terms of VEP amplitude, at particular latencies in reference to a baseline (average voltage level within 50 ms after stimulation) and statistically analysed using repeated-measures analyses of variance.

Results

Experiment 1. Dichoptic presentation of grids of different spatial frequencies

On the basis of previous work, it was predicted that the dichoptical presentation of identical patterns should result in the greatest degree of binocular summation, while the presentation of different patterns should result in binocular suppression, increasing with their degree of dissimilarity. Suppression could be evidenced either in terms of a reduction in sensitivity of both eyes or in terms of a reduction in sensitivity of one eye only (e.g. one eye being suppressed and the other dominating). Pattern-element size was selected as the stimulus parameter to be varied in this study (Harter, Seiple and Musso 1974) because (a) sustained differences in the perceived size of images falling on the two retinae (a condition termed aniseikonia when due to optical or neural differences in the two eyes), are known to result in visual suppression and amblyopia in man (Duke-Elder 1969, p. 113), and

(b) because each spatial frequency elicits a VEP of characteristic amplitude. Spatial frequencies of 1·5–3 cycles per degree (elements of 10–20′ subtense) elicit greater amplitude VEPs than more extreme frequencies or diffuse light (Rietveld *et al.* 1967; Campbell and Maffei 1970; Harter and White 1970; Harter 1970, 1971*b*) making it possible to assess the contribution of each eye to the dichoptically elicited VEP.

Rectangular-wave grid patterns with luminance transmittance of 0·40 mL were continuously presented to both eyes in order to increase the degree of binocular interaction. The grids were transparencies and consisted of white lines on a black background, the ratio of width of white and black elements being 1 to 7. The subtended distance between line centres was 0 (diffuse), 15, 30, and 60 minutes of arc. VEPs were elicited by a momentary (3·3 log units) increase in the brightness of the grid viewed by one eye (monocular VEPs) or both eyes (binocular VEPs).

Each of the 5 subjects participated in 4 experimental sessions. They were right-handed and all were found to be right-eye dominant as indicated by a visual sighting test. Each experimental session provided one complete replication of all experimental conditions wherein all combinations of the 4 pattern sizes were presented to the two eyes. Monocular and binocular VEPs to a given binocular viewing condition were obtained by sequentially presenting the increment in pattern brightness or flash to both eyes, the right eye, both eyes, the left eye, etc. at a rate of 1·96 Hz. The order of presentation of the four patterns to the left and right eye during the four replications (sessions) was determined by four 4 x 4 counter-balanced Latin squares. To ensure that subjects attended to transient stimulation of both eyes throughout the experiment, they were required to perform a synchronous tapping task in anticipation of the increment in pattern brightness to be presented to one or both eyes. Control data were obtained to ensure that muscle artifacts or motor potentials did not contaminate the data.

The results were quantified by measuring the amplitude of VEPs at two points in time after stimulation (Fig. 10.1): the most surface-negative portion of the VEP within a 20 ms epoch at approximately 110 ms after stimulation (N110); and the most surface-positive portion of the VEP within a 20–30 ms epoch (depending on the subject) at approximately 175 ms after stimulation (P175). These measures were respectively most negative and positive in response respectively to the 15′ and 30′ patterns. Amplitude was measured in reference to a baseline determined by the average voltage level of the VEPs elicited by the 4 replications at trace onset. Repeated analyses of variance were performed on each amplitude measure.

Monocular VEPs and interocular suppression. The monocular VEPs were influenced not only by variations in pattern size presented to the eye receiving the increment in brightness but also by the pattern size presented to the other eye which was not flashed. These effects are illustrated by the monocular VEPs in Fig. 10.1 and 10.2. Varying the size of pattern viewed by the eye receiving the evoking stimulus (left eye in Fig. 10.1 and eye I in Fig. 10.2) significantly affected both N110 and P175

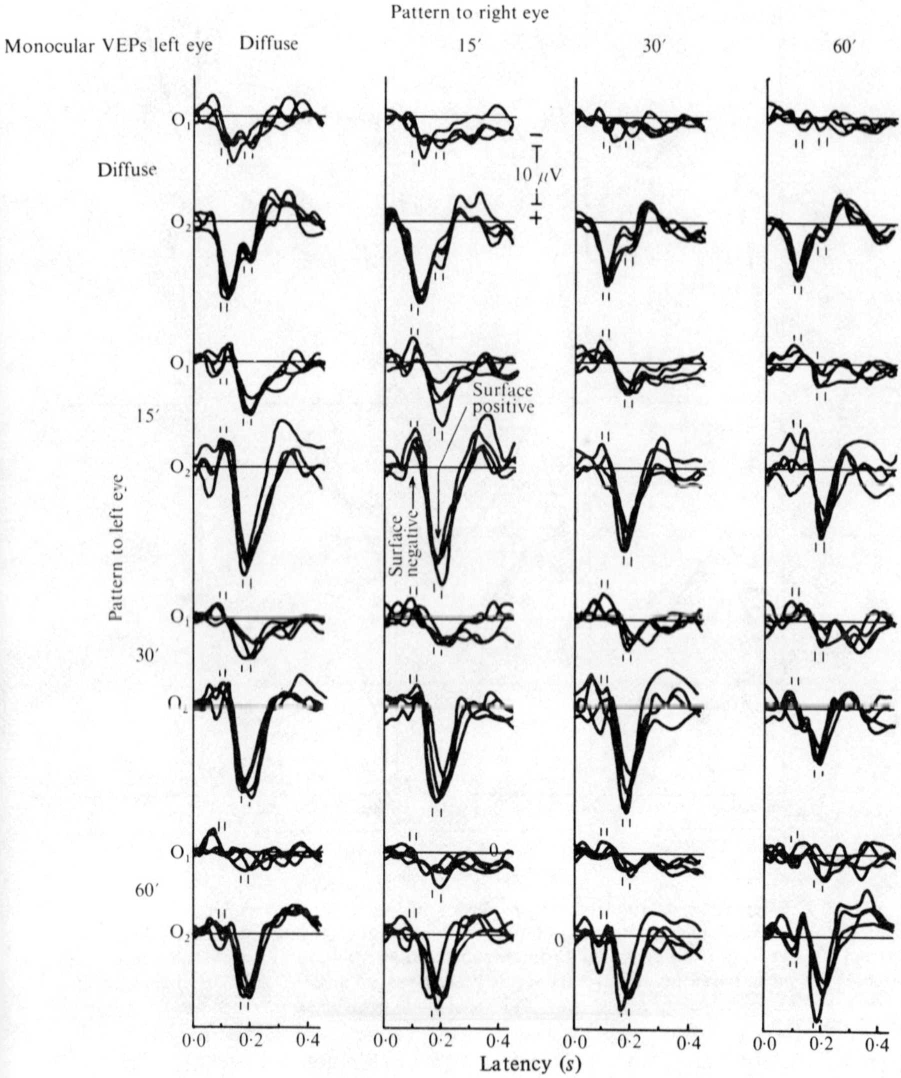

Fig. 10.1. Effects of the size of pattern elements presented to the left and right eye on monocular VEPs to momentary increments in brightness of pattern presented to the left. For example, the top row (O_1) indicates suppression of VEPs to diffuse flashes to the left eye as the pattern continuously viewed by the right eye varied from diffuse to the 60′ pattern. The first column indicates VEPs to the different patterns flashed to the left eye when the right eye continuously viewed diffuse light. The vertical marks indicate time windows in which the N110 and P175 amplitude measures were obtained. Each superimposed tracing is a replication and is an average of 64 responses. Subject B.S. Negativity up O_1 and O_2 : electrode position (see 'methods' in text).

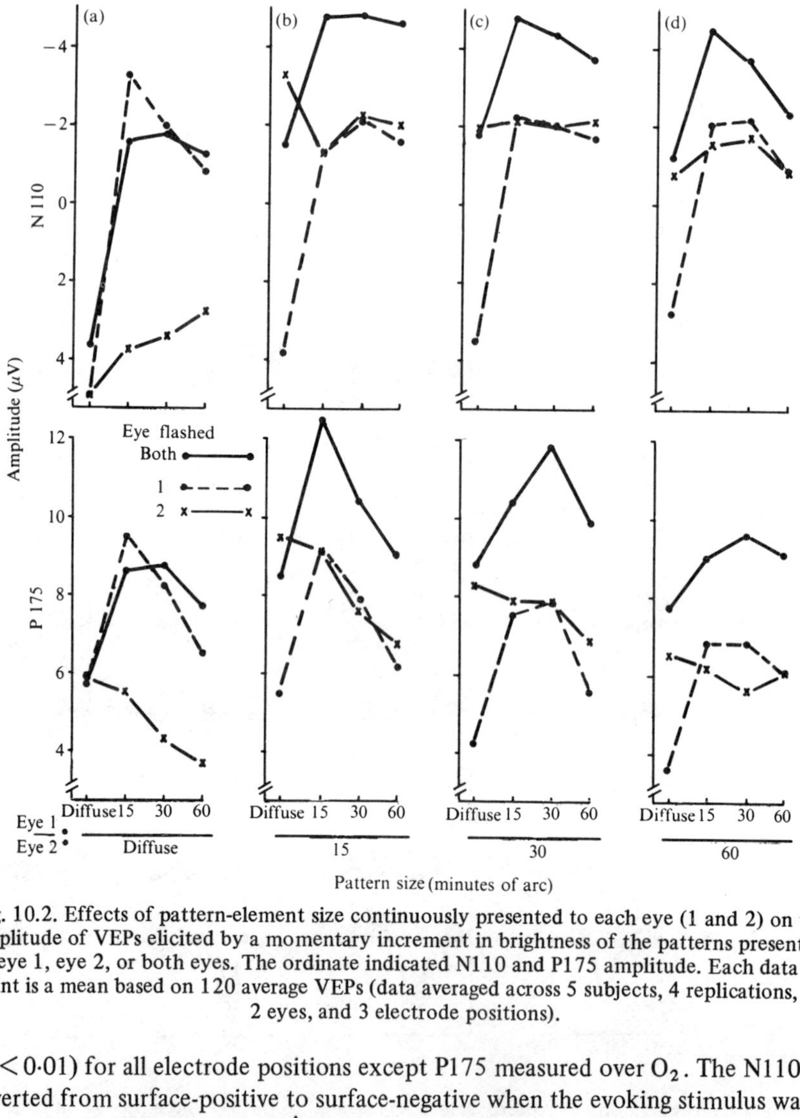

Fig. 10.2. Effects of pattern-element size continuously presented to each eye (1 and 2) on the amplitude of VEPs elicited by a momentary increment in brightness of the patterns presented to eye 1, eye 2, or both eyes. The ordinate indicated N110 and P175 amplitude. Each data point is a mean based on 120 average VEPs (data averaged across 5 subjects, 4 replications, 2 eyes, and 3 electrode positions).

($p < 0{\cdot}01$) for all electrode positions except P175 measured over O_2. The N110 inverted from surface-positive to surface-negative when the evoking stimulus was changed from diffuse to the 15′ pattern and then progressively decreased in amplitude as the pattern size was increased from 15′ to 60′. The amplitude of P175 varied similarly except that an inversion of polarity was not evidenced in this component. It has been proposed that such effects reflect the modal size of receptive field centres of cells in the visual system: VEP amplitude increases as element size is increased until it reaches the assumed modal size of receptive field centres (presumably 10–20′ subtense in the human visual system) and then it decreases as element size is increased beyond the modal field centre size (Harter and White 1970; Harter 1970, 1971; Armington, Corwin and Marsetta 1971).

The rows of Fig. 10.1 and eye 2 of Fig. 10.2 illustrate how the monocular VEPs were influenced by the size of the pattern continuously presented to the other eye. The amplitude of P175 generally decreased as the elements in the pattern presented to the other eye were varied in size from diffuse, 15′, 30′, to 60′ subtense ($p < 0{\cdot}05$ and $p < 0{\cdot}025$ for O_z and O_2 respectively). The amplitude of N110 reflected this effect only when the monocular VEP was elicited by diffuse light.

In addition to this main effect, the N110 measure indicated that the effects of varying pattern-element size in one eye depended on the size of pattern elements presented to the other eye (interaction significant $p < 0{\cdot}05$ for the O_z and O_2 electrode positions). The effects of pattern size presented to one eye (eye 1), as indicated by changes in the amplitude of monocular VEPs to increments in stimulation of the other eye (eye 2), were greater when the latter eye viewed diffuse light. This interaction between the size of elements presented to the flashed and non-flashed eye had a similar effect on the P175 measure of monocular VEP amplitude which was statistically significant ($p < 0{\cdot}05$) only for the O_1 electrode position.

This interocular suppression of monocular VEPs in part corroborates data of Lehmann and Fender (1967, 1968) indicating that VEPs elicited from the flashed eye may be reduced depending on the nature of pattern presented to the opposite non-flashed eye. The effects of contour density, however, differed in the two studies. They reported progressive suppression of monocular VEPs to diffuse light flashes as the patterns continuously presented to the opposite non-flashed eye were varied from blank, dot, cross, to grid – i.e. as pattern density was increased. In the present study, an increase in contour density resulted in increased VEP amplitude (less suppression). Lehmann and Fender (1968) proposed that the central elements activated from both eyes have limited processing capability and that one eye can load the central elements so that they would not be able to process additional information from the other eye. If this proposal is correct, an inverted-U shaped function between information load and pattern density must be assumed in order to account for the results of both studies. Such an assumption is warranted in view of the inverted-U shaped function between contour density and VEP amplitude reported in many studies.

Blakemore and Campbell (1969) reported that presentation of a high-contrast pattern of a given spatial frequency to one eye selectively suppressed visual threshold to that frequency in the opposite eye. This would suggest that the degree of interocular suppression or adaptation depends on the relative spatial frequency of the patterns presented to either eye, rather than on the absolute spatial frequency as suggested in the present study. It is difficult to know whether the interocular adaptation effects they reported were, in fact, specific to the adapting spatial frequency, since only one spatial frequency of 10 cycles per degree was used. The apparent discrepancy in the interocular transfer of pattern effects could be due to differences in the stimulus paradigms employed in the two studies, in terms of the time-course, intensity, and nature of spatial frequency of the adapting and test stimuli (see below).

Binocular VEPs. The amplitude of binocular VEPs to transient increments of the steady stimulation in both eyes (solid lines, Fig. 10.2) also varied as an inverted-U shaped function of the pattern size presented to eye 1 and eye 2 ($p < 0{\cdot}01$ for O_Z electrode position). The binocular VEPs reflected the contribution of both eyes, particularly when both eyes were presented with pattern stimuli.

The effects of varying pattern-element size presented to one eye (e.g. eye 1) on the binocular VEP depended on the size of pattern elements presented to the other eye (e.g. eye 2). This interaction was statistically significant for both N110 and P175 when activity was measured from the O_Z electrode position ($p < 0{\cdot}05$ and $p < 0{\cdot}01$ respectively). The nature of this interaction differed for the two components. The N110 measure indicated that when the 15′ pattern was presented to one eye, the stimulus presented to the other eye had little influence as long as it contained pattern; whereas, when the 60′ pattern was presented to one eye, the pattern presented to the other eye had considerable influence on the binocular N110. In contrast, the P175 measure reflected the unique effect of presenting identical-sized patterns to both eyes. Relatively large binocular P175 were elicited when both eyes were presented with patterns of the same-sized elements 15′/15′ and 30′/30′ as illustrated in Fig. 10.2(b) and (c). This enhancement was obscured when 60′ patterns were presented to both eyes, apparently because of the pattern-size effect *per se.*

Comparison of monocular and binocular VEPs. Binocular VEP amplitude was significantly greater than the mean amplitude of the two monocular VEPs elicited under comparable conditions ($p < 0{\cdot}025$ and $p < 0{\cdot}05$ respectively for N110 and P175 when data were averaged across the O_1, O_2, and O_Z electrode positions). The degree of binocular summation depended on the nature of stimuli presented to the two eyes. When one eye (eye 1) was presented patterns and the other eye (eye 2) presented diffuse light (Fig. 10.2(a)), the amplitude and waveform of the binocular VEP was always approximately equivalent to that of the monocular VEP elicited by the eye receiving pattern. The eye viewing diffuse light appeared to contribute little to the binocular VEP in this situation. This finding corroborates previous conclusions based on dichoptic stimulation (MacKay 1968; Ciganek 1971) and supports other data obtained from amblyopic subjects (Lawwill, Cox, Tuttle, Meur, and Burian 1973; Shipley 1969; Lombroso, Duffy, and Robb 1969; Franceschetti and Burian 1971; Dawson, Perry, and Childers 1972; Sokol, Chapter 22 of this book) indicating VEPs may be used as a measure of visual suppression.

When various combinations of pattern sizes were dichoptically presented to both eyes, however, the binocular VEP reflected the contribution of both eyes (Fig. 10.2(b), (c), and (d)). For N110, the degree of binocular summation appeared dependent primarily on pattern size, the smaller the size of pattern presented to either eye (up to 15′ subtense) the greater the amount of summation.

The hypothesis that binocular summation would be greatest when identical-sized pattern elements were presented to the two eyes (eye 1/eye 2 combinations of 15′/15′, 30′/30′, and 60′/60′) and least when different-sized pattern elements were presented to the two eyes (the degree of suppression increasing as a function of the degree of difference) was supported by only the P175 measure of binocular VEPs and binocular summation. This finding is consistent with previous data in which late components of binocular VEPs indicated greater amplitude (Harter *et al.* 1972) and greater binocular summation (Harter *et al.* 1973) when identical patterns were presented to corresponding as compared to non-corresponding retinal points.

The effect of hemisphere and eye differences. The effects of which eye was flashed, and recording electrode position were most pronounced on the P175 amplitude (Fig. 10.3). The amplitude of P175 recorded over the left and right hemisphere (O_1 and O_2 respectively) differed depending on the eye stimulated (hemisphere x eye interaction significant at $p < 0{\cdot}01$). Monocular stimulation of the right as compared to left eye elicited greater P175 over the right hemisphere. This eye difference was not evident in VEPs elicited over the left hemisphere.

The most pronounced hemispheric differences ($p < 0{\cdot}01$) were that overall VEP amplitude (monocular and binocular) and binocular summation were greater over the midline electrode position than the lateral two electrode positions as indicated by P175. The greater-amplitude of VEPs over the midline electrode position is consistent with earlier data (Perry, Childers, and McCoy 1968) and may be attributed (a) to summation of electrical activity from both hemispheres at the midline due to volume conduction, (b) to greater topological representation of the foveal retinal area near the midline (Ganong 1969) and/or (c) to the great contribution of the foveal retinal to VEPs in response to patterned stimulation (Rietveld *et al.* 1967; Harter 1970; Sokol 1972). The greater binocular summation on the midline may also be attributed to the greater binocular interaction between the central regions of the retinae (see below).

It may be noted that the effects of which eye was flashed, interocular suppression, and binocular summation tended to be greater in VEPs recorded over the right then left hemisphere. These trends suggest greater functional involvement of the right hemisphere in binocular interaction, a conclusion consistent with perceptual data obtained from clinical patients with cortical lesions in one hemisphere (Benton and Hecaen 1970).

Experiment 2. Size specificity, interocular suppression, and monocular VEP

Although several investigators have noted that stimulation of one eye suppresses VEP amplitude to stimulation of the other eye, the specificity of this interocular suppression has not been investigated. There is considerable evidence, however, that adaptation of one eye to a given spatial frequency raises contrast threshold in

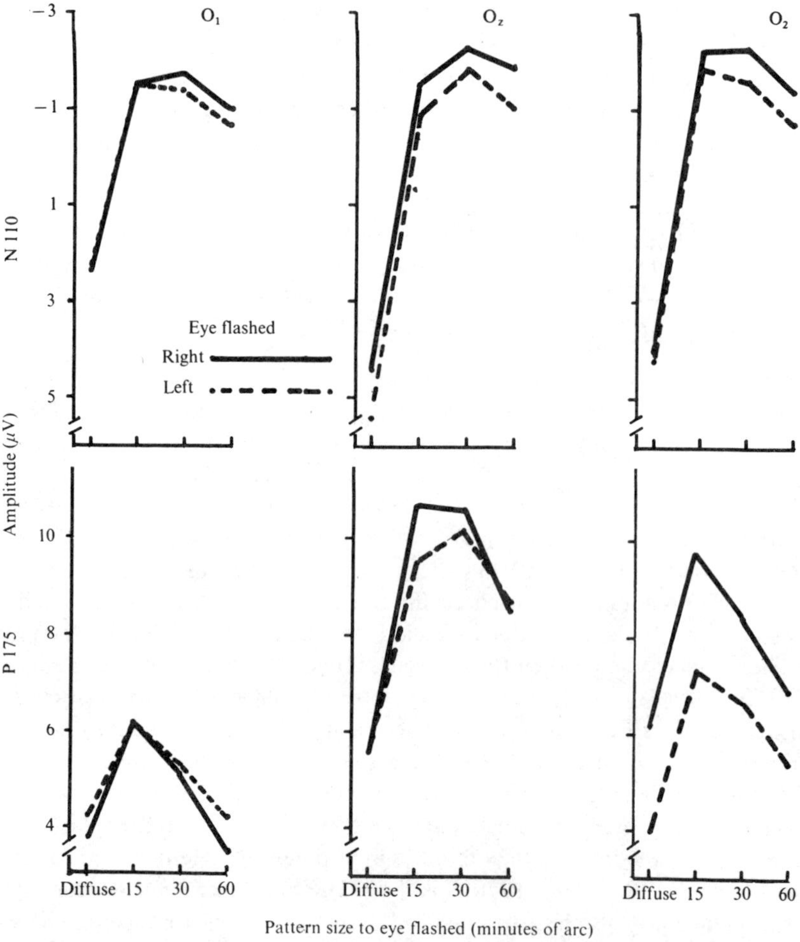

Fig. 10.3. Effects of recording electrode position (O_1, O_Z, and O_2) and eye (left/right) receiving the evoking stimulus (increment in pattern brightness) on N110 and P175 amplitude. Each data point is a mean based on 80 average VEP (data were averaged across 5 subjects, 4 replications, and the 4 patterns presented to the non-flashed eye).

that eye to subsequently presented gratings of similar spatial frequencies (Pantle and Sekuler 1968; Blakemore and Campbell 1969; Graham 1972; Sullivan, Georgeson, and Oatley 1972; Bagrash 1973). This elevation of threshold is limited to a spectrum of frequencies with a bandwidth of about $1\frac{1}{2}$ octaves centred on the adapting spatial frequency. Channels selectively sensitive to spatial frequency have also been demonstrated using VEP (Campbell and Maffei 1970).

Experiment 1 was in part concerned with the size specificity of interocular suppression. Contrary to expectations, its results did not support the notion of size-specific central channels since exposure of one eye to the 60′ pattern reduced the response of the other eye to all stimuli, not just the 60′ pattern.

The purpose of experiment 2 (Harter, Towle and Musso 1976) was to further investigate the size specificity of interocular suppression under conditions more similar to the above studies in which intraocular size-specific adaptation effects were reported. The conditions of Experiment 1 were changed as follows toward this end: the mean luminance transmittance of the continuously presented adaptation stimulus was increased from 0·40 mL to 35·00 mL; the line grid patterns were changed to checkerboard patterns; the continuous adaptation stimuli were presented monocularly to the right eye only, thus eliminating cues for binocular rivalry; the evoking test flash was decreased in intensity from 3·3 log units to 1·5 log units above contrast threshold and was always presented to the left eye (which was in darkness); subjects attended the flash presented to the left eye at all times as required by a reaction time task to the flash; and the range of 'suppressing' pattern sizes was increased from 15–60′ to 9–95′. The effects of continuously presenting this range of suppressing or conditioning checkerboards to the right eye on VEPs to two test stimuli (checks subtending 12′ and 35′) flashed to the left eye were investigated. The test flash was flashed every 1500 ms on the average (range 1350–1650 ms).

Nine subjects participated in this experiment and all but one subject had monocular visual acuities of better than 20/20. All the combinations of test and conditioning patterns were presented to each subject for 4 replications conducted on different days.

A sample of VEPs from 2 of the 9 subjects is shown in Fig. 10.4. The changes in the VEPs across the rows illustrate the effects of continuously presenting various check sizes to the right eye on VEPs elicited to either the 12′ (a) or 35′ (b) checkerboards flashed to the left eye. A variance-analyses procedure (Harter *et al.* 1972; Musso and Harter 1975, see experiment 3) was conducted by our minicomputer to determine which portion of the VEP elicited from one eye was influenced by changing the check size of the adaptation pattern presented to the other eye. The results of these analyses, indicating the variability (in microvolts equivalent to 1 standard deviation) due to interocular adaptation at successive 5 ms delays after the presentation of the test flash, are illustrated by the dotted curves in the right-hand portion of Fig. 10.4. The variance measures of all subjects indicated a peak at about 160 ms after stimulation. Inspection of the VEP data indicated this variability was due to changes in amplitude of a surface-negative component (indicated by vertical dashed lines in Fig. 10.4). Other investigators have noted that VEP amplitude between 120 ms and 180 ms after stimulation is particularly sensitive to dichoptic stimulation (Lehmann and Fender 1968; Regan and Spekreijse 1970; Harter *et al.* 1972).

The changes in amplitude of N160, in reference to the baseline, are indicated for the grouped data in Fig. 10.5. When potentials were evoked by the 12′ or 35′ test checkerboard N160 amplitude was lowest when the checkerboard presented

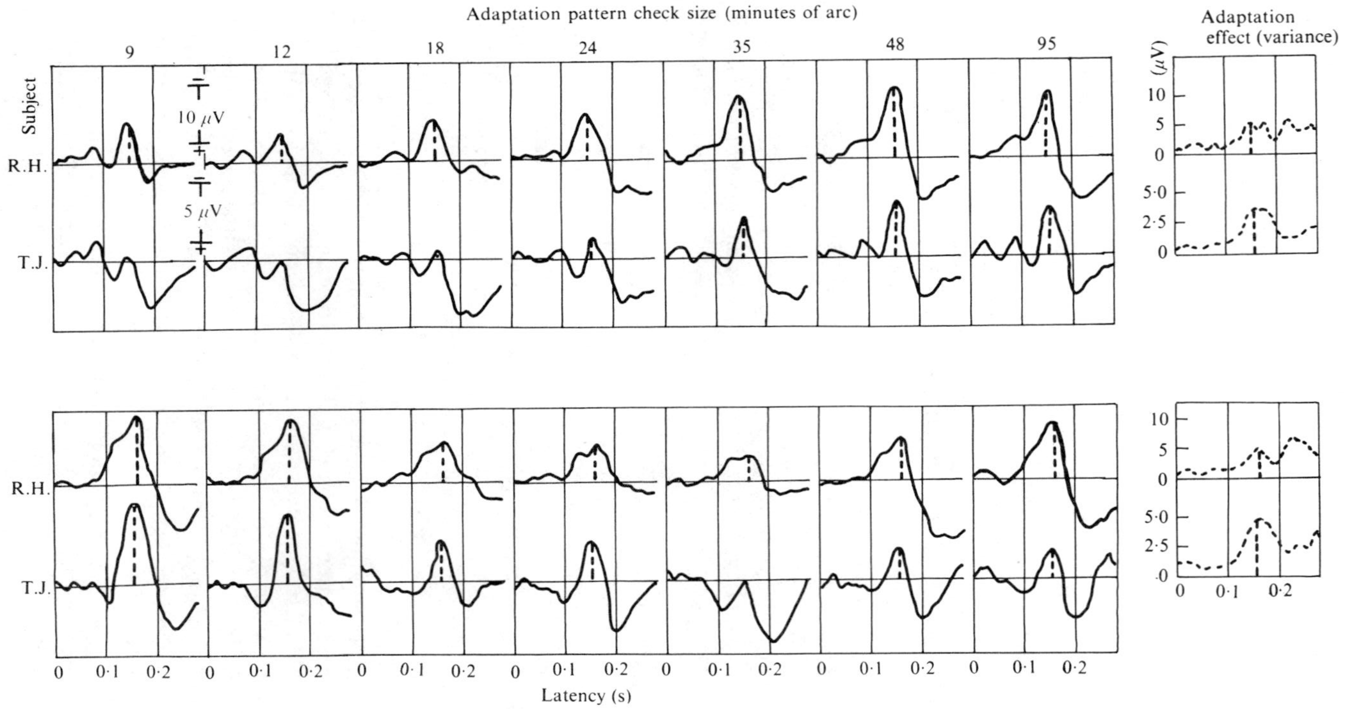

Fig. 10.4. Changes in monocular VEPs due to interocular suppression. The VEPs are elicited by a 12′ (a) or a 35′ (b) checkerboard flashed to the left eye. Data from two subjects (R.H. and T.J.) are shown. Changes in VEP from the left to right of the figure are a function of the check size of patterns continuously presented to the opposite (right) eye. Note that N160 amplitude (vertical dotted line) was smallest when the test and adaptation pattern contained the same sized checks. Each tracing is the average VEP to 256 flashes (4 replications of 64 flashes each). The dotted tracings in the right portion of the figure indicate the variability (one standard deviation) of the 7 VEPs about their mean and thus the magnitude of the interocular effect (see text).

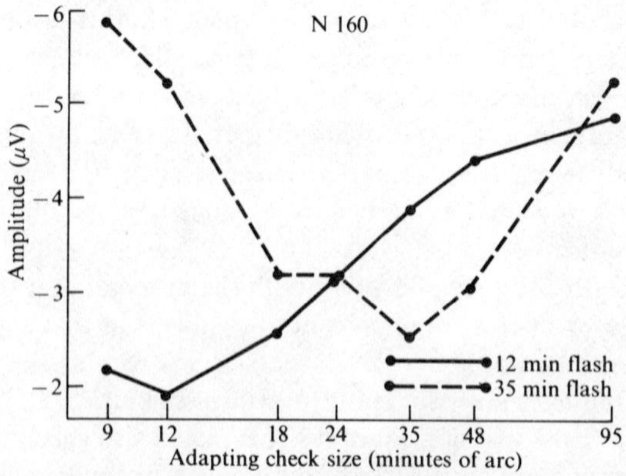

Fig. 10.5. Suppression of N160 amplitude to either the 12′ or 35′ test flash as a function of the check size continuously presented to the opposite (right) eye. Each plotted point is a mean based on 9 subjects and 4 replications. Suppression progressively increased as the check-size of the adapting stimulus approached that of the test stimulus.

to the other eye also contained respectively 12′ or 35′ checks. Suppression of N160 amplitude progressively increased as the check size of the conditioning checkerboard presented to the opposite eye approached that of the test checkerboard. Suppression was greatest when identical check sizes were presented to the two eyes. Subjects reported that the contrast or sharpness of the checks in the test flash was poorest under these conditions.

Four other measures of VEP amplitude were also made on these data: three were at other latencies (approximately 80 ms, 120 ms, and 210 ms after stimulation) and the fourth was the overall average amplitude (average absolute integral of successive 5 ms intervals for the first 300 ms of the VEP). Overall amplitude reflected the same trends observed with the N160 measure. The other latency measures, however, yielded different results which were not related to the subject's perception of the test flash. The fact that different VEP measures indicated different trends emphasizes the importance of the measure chosen to quantify VEP changes.

The tuning curves in Fig. 10.5 are quite similar to those of Blakemore and Campbell (1969) based on contrast-threshold measures obtained under dioptic viewing conditions. These investigators, however, reported little specificity of adaptation for spatial frequencies less than 3 cycles per degree and that the harmonic components of a square-wave pattern caused elevation of threshold in the region of the third harmonic frequency. The data from the present experiment indicate interocular suppression with spatial frequencies as low as 0·86 cycles per degree (the 35′ test checkerboard) and there was little evidence of the effects of the third harmonic (which would be the effect of the 12′ adapting checkerboard when the test stimulus was the 35′ checkerboard).

Binocular interaction: evoked potentials to dichoptic stimulation

Size-specific interocular transfer effects were obtained in this second experiment and not in experiment 1, perhaps because more intense adaptation stimuli were used in experiment 2. Psychophysical studies indeed indicate that the intensity of the adapting pattern influences the specificity of spatial frequency adaptation (Bagrash 1973). The different types of patterns used to elicit VEPs and the different VEP latencies measured in the two experiments also may have contributed to the different results.

The results of Experiment 2 are consistent with the proposal that size-specific signals from the two eyes share a common central channel and that activation (saturation) of the central channel by a given spatial frequency presented to one eye will selectively suppress the response of the central channel to stimulation of the other eye with the same spatial frequency. This model also accounts for the fact that *binocular summation* results when identical spatial frequencies are flashed to *both* eyes (experiment 1). In such situations the stimuli flashed to both eyes possibly were not of sufficient duration or intensity to saturate the central channel. This suggests that critical variables in interocular suppression are the duration and intensity of the adapting stimuli.

Experiment 3. Time-course of interocular suppression and monocular VEPs

Blakemore and Campbell (1969) and Blakemore *et al.* (1973) reported that the duration of an adapting grid influenced both the magnitude of suppression of contrast threshold to that grid and the duration of recovery from such suppressions. Adaptation increased to a near asymptotic level as the duration of the adapting pattern was increased up to 60 s. Further increases in duration had little additional effect. Recovery from this condition took up to 60 s. The purpose of experiment 3 (Harter, Musso, and Towle) was to investigate the time-course of the interocular suppression effect on VEPs. The stimulus conditions in this experiment were identical to those of experiment 2 except that the adaptation pattern (presented to the right eye) was turned on and off once every 7·5 s. VEPs were obtained to flashes presented to the left eye on the average 1·5, 3·0, 4·5, and 6·0 s after both the on- and offset of the adapting checkerboard (Fig. 10.6). The test and adaptation stimuli consisted of 12′ checkerboards. The 7·5 s adaptation interval was considerably shorter than the optimal interval reported by Blakemore and Campbell (1969) and Blakemore *et al.* (1973). The 7·5 s interval was selected since pilot data indicate that the interocular effects were near maximum within this period of time after the on- or offset of the adapting stimulus. Lansing (1964), who investigated the effect of interocular suppressions on unaveraged EEG responses to flickering light, presented raw data which also indicate such effects occurred within 1 s after the on- or offset of the suppressing stimulus.

Fig. 10.6 illustrates the VEPs obtained from all 6 subjects studied. The variance-analysis procedure mentioned in experiment 2 was utilized to determine (a) if turning the adaptation pattern on and off in one eye influenced the waveform of VEPs to flashing the other eye, and (b) which latencies of the VEP were most

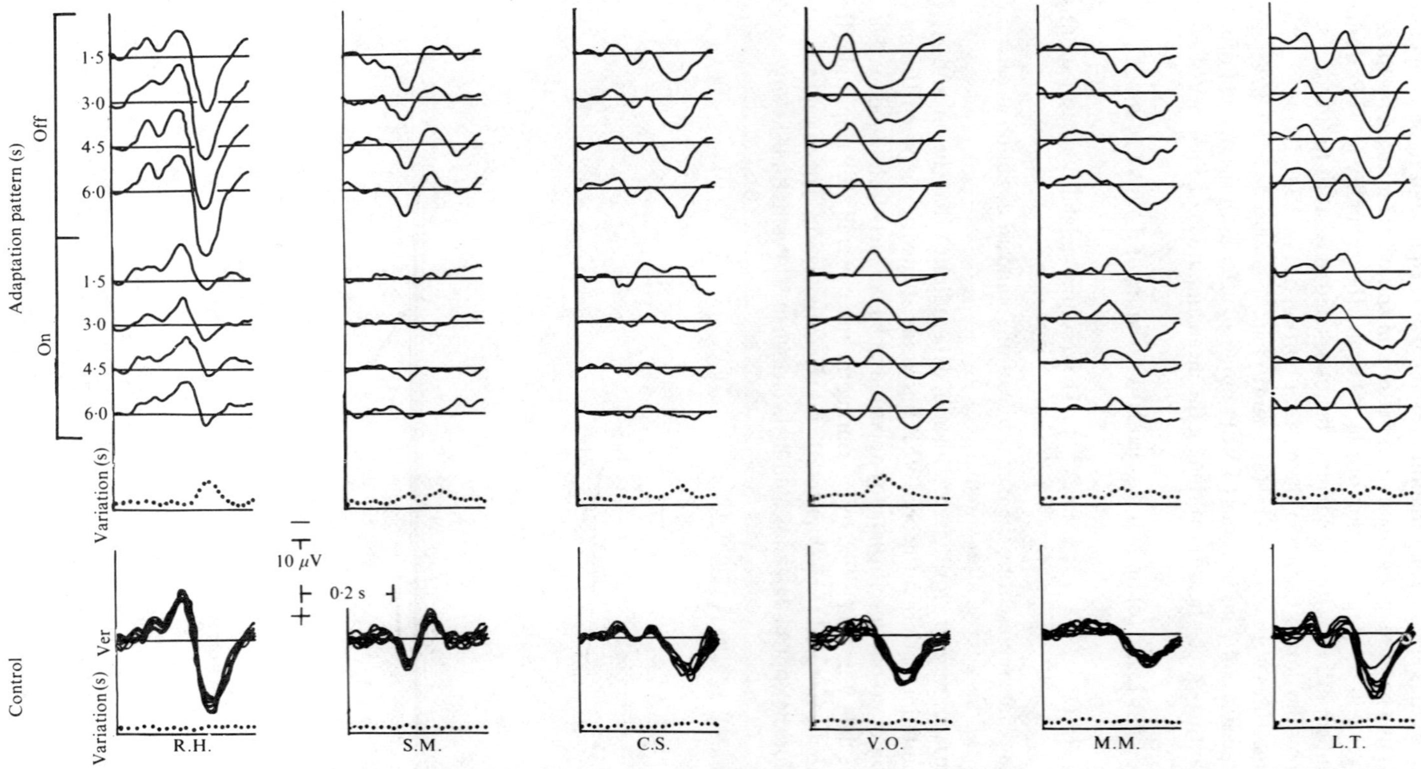

Fig. 10.6. All solid line tracings are monocular VEPs (averaged across 4 replications with a total $N = 256$) to the 12′ checkerboard flashed to the left eye. Changes in VEPs are a function of the offset and onset of a second 12′ checkerboard presented to the right eye. The dotted lines indicate the change in VEPs (1 standard deviation unit) due to the interocular effect at each latency of the VEP (see text). In the control conditions (*bottom*), the adaptation light was occluded. The six columns are data from different subjects.

influenced by this effect. The variability (in microvolts equivalent to one standard deviation) due to turning the adaptation pattern on and off is indicated by the dotted tracing in the upper portion of Fig. 10.6, and the variability in VEPs during the control conditions with the adapting light occluded in front of the eye is indicated by the dotted tracing in the bottom portion of Fig. 10.6. These variance measures were obtained by (a) quantifying the amplitude of all 8 averaged VEPs at successive 4·7 ms intervals (4 VEPs obtained after both the on- and offset of the adapting checkerboard) (b) finding the mean amplitude of these 8 VEPs $\left(\sum_{i=1}^{N} X_i/N = \bar{X}\right)$, and (c) finding the standard deviation of the 8 VEPs about their mean $\left(\text{S.D.} = \sqrt{\left\{\sum_{i=1}^{N} (X_i - \bar{X})^2/N\right\}}\right)$. The resulting variability measure consisted of 64 data points representing the magnitude of one standard deviation at each successive 4·7 ms interval after stimulation.

The variance measure for the experimental data indicated that the on- and offset of the adaptation pattern influenced VEP amplitude at latencies between 100 ms to 225 ms. Since no one specific latency appeared to be uniquely influenced by this effect, the data were quantified by measuring the mean overall VEP amplitude (the mean absolute integral) from 0 ms to 300 ms after stimulation. The variance measure for the control data indicated little change in VEP amplitude at any latency.

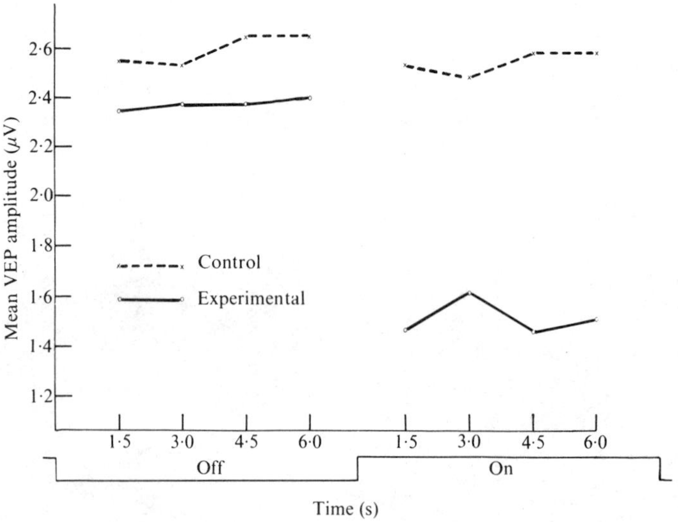

Fig. 10.7. Mean VEP amplitude (absolute integral) of data from Fig. 10.6 which have been combined across 4 replications and 6 subjects. All VEPs were elicited by 12′ checkerboard flashed to the left eye. Changes in amplitude are due to offset and onset of 12′ checkerboard presented to the right eye. The right eye was occluded (in darkness) in the control conditions.

The mean overall VEP amplitude for the grouped data are shown in Fig. 10.7. The interocular suppression (solid line) was rapid, being near complete within 1·5 s after the adapting light was turned on. Recovery also was near complete within 1·5 s after the offset of the adapting light. No significant changes in VEP amplitude were noted during the course of either the adaptation or recovery interval.

The extremely rapid time-course of this interocular suppression effect suggests that it is mediated by mechanisms different from those mediating adaptation in experiments when both the adapting and test stimuli were presented to the same eye. A more plausible explanation of interocular suppression appears to be that intense stimulation of one eye saturates the binocular central channels processing the information presented to that eye (Lehmann and Fender 1968; Ciganek 1970), so that activation of the corresponding channel of the other eye cannot further activate the central channel.

Caution should be exercised in interpreting the results of the present experiment in terms of size-specificity. Since the on- and offset of the adapting checkerboard was confounded with the on- and offset of a change in luminance, it cannot be determined from the present data whether the response to the luminance, contrast, or both aspects of the test flash was suppressed.

Experiment 4. Effects of correspondence and eccentricity of retinal areas stimulated on interocular suppression

The data above suggest that interocular suppression is specific to the nature of the suppressing stimulus. Two studies may be cited indicating interocular suppression of VEPs is also restricted to the corresponding area of the opposite eye. Lehmann and Fender (1969) mentioned this effect although supporting data were not presented. Spekreijse *et al.* (1972) reported data suggesting VEPs reflect point-to-point interocular suppression but the effects of varying the degree of non-correspondence of retinal areas stimulated were not investigated.

Experiment 4 (Shuttlesworth 1974) was an investigation of two problems. First, to find the areal extent of interocular suppression. Should corresponding retinal areas be suppressed and not the entire eye, the areal extent of the suppression could reflect the size of binocular receptive fields of central neurons innervating that retinal region. It is known that the size of retinal receptive fields generally increases from foveal to peripheral retina. The second purpose of this experiment was to investigate the effects of eccentricity of retinal stimulation on the areal extent of interocular suppression.

The VEPs to a small (2·86′) spot flashed to the foveal or peripheral region (5° temporally) of the right eye was measured as a function of the degree of correspondence of a similar spot of light continuously presented to the other (left) eye. The method was similar to that employed by Sanderson, Bishop, and Darian Smith (1971) to investigate the binocular receptive fields of lateral geniculate nucleus units in cats. The test flash was 10 μs in duration, had a luminance of

9·65 mL, and was presented aperiodically at random intervals (mean intervals 1·25 s) to a fixed location of the retina of the right eye (foveally or 5° temporally). The continuously presented suppressing light had a luminance of 2·74 mL and was presented either ipsi-ocularly or contra-ocularly (by means of a haploscope) to points 0′ to 50′ above or below the test flash. Fixation points were presented continuously to corresponding points of both retinae, which enabled the displays presented to the two eyes to be binocularly superimposed. The median latency of a reaction-time response and the average amplitude of the VEP to the test flash were measured. In one-half of the conditions, subjects were required to release a reaction-time key as fast as they could in response to the flash. In the other half, subjects were required to count the flashes. This was in order to ascertain, through this implicit response, that the results were not contaminated by the overt reaction-time task. VEPs were recorded from O_1 and O_Z electrode positions, which roughly correspond to the projection areas for the foveal and right eccentric (5°) retinal areas stimulated. The O_2 electrode also was selected since Experiment 1 and clinical data (Benton and Hecaen 1970) indicated binocular interaction in humans is greater in the right than left cerebral hemisphere.

The VEP amplitude was quantified as follows: first the algebraic average of the amplitude of each data point during the 448 ms following stimulus onset was used as a baseline; then the absolute average amplitude of each data point of the entire VEP above or below this baseline was used as a measure of overall VEP amplitude. This measure was used since visual inspection indicated that changes in amplitude were evident in all components of the VEP.

Fig. 10.8 and 10.9 indicate that when the test flash was presented to the fovea (0° eccentricity), VEP amplitude progressively decreased and reaction time progressively increased as the conditioning stimulus was moved from 30′ above or below the test flash toward the test flash ($p < 0{\cdot}05$). Little suppression was noted beyond a distance of 30′; responses to the 30′ and 50′ non-correspondence conditions were similar to those under the control condition (conditioning stimulus withheld). This trend was present when the conditioning stimulus was presented to the same (monoptic condition) or opposite (dichoptic or bioptic condition) eye as the test flash. These findings are consistent with psychophysical data which indicate that metacontrast results from both monoptic and dichoptic stimulation and decreases as a function of the distance between the test and masking stimuli (McFadden and Gummerman 1973).

Interocular interaction was not indicated by either the VEP or reaction-time data when stimuli were presented to the peripheral retina. The effects are consistent with the proposal that VEP measures of binocular interaction reflect activity originating from the foveal (cone) region of the retina.

The notion that interocular suppression is restricted to the corresponding region in the opposite eye and does not involve the entire eye is supported by the present data. The suppression was not point-to-point, however, since it was evident with up to 30′ non-correspondence. This suggests that the test flash could be

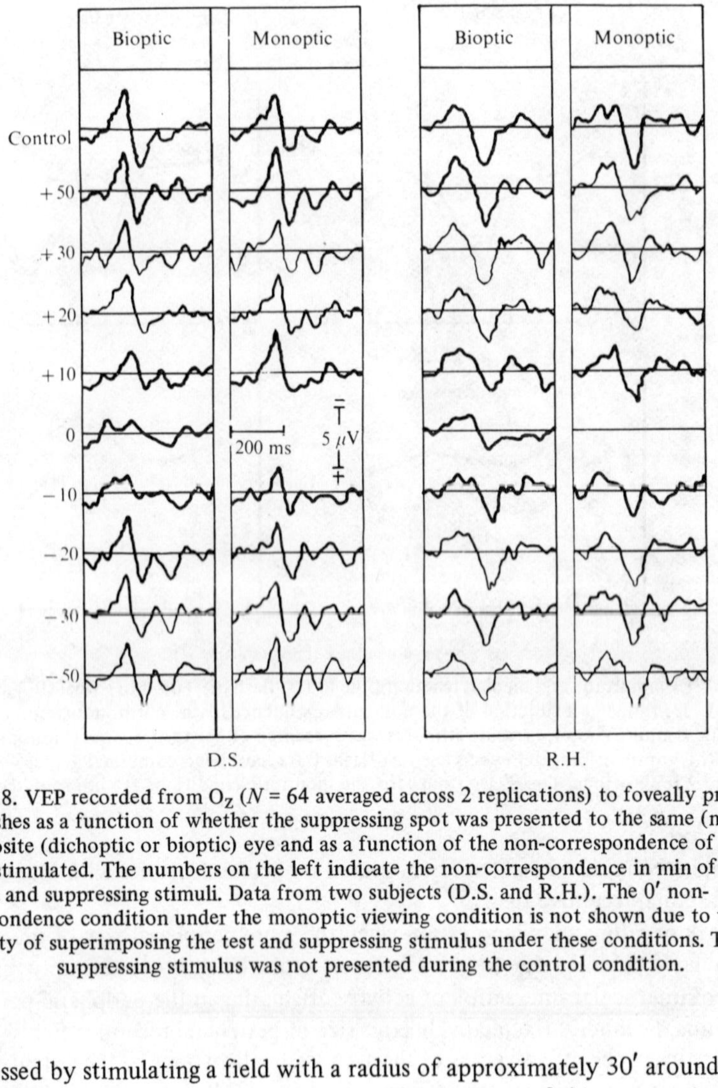

Fig. 10.8. VEP recorded from O_Z ($N = 64$ averaged across 2 replications) to foveally presented test flashes as a function of whether the suppressing spot was presented to the same (monoptic) or opposite (dichoptic or bioptic) eye and as a function of the non-correspondence of retinal points stimulated. The numbers on the left indicate the non-correspondence in min of arc for the test and suppressing stimuli. Data from two subjects (D.S. and R.H.). The 0′ non-correspondence condition under the monoptic viewing condition is not shown due to the difficulty of superimposing the test and suppressing stimulus under these conditions. The suppressing stimulus was not presented during the control condition.

suppressed by stimulating a field with a radius of approximately 30′ around the corresponding point in the opposite retina. The diameter of this suppressing field would then be 60′ of arc, which is consistent with the relatively large suppressing fields noted in Experiment 1.

The localized nature of interocular suppression found in the present study could be due to the nature of stimulation employed. Campbell and Maffei (1970) have shown that adaptation of one portion of the retina to a given spatial frequency will reduce the sensitivity of other portions of the retina to that spatial frequency and they speculated that this was due to the non-localized nature of the cortical neurone activated by such stimulation. Possibly the diffuse light

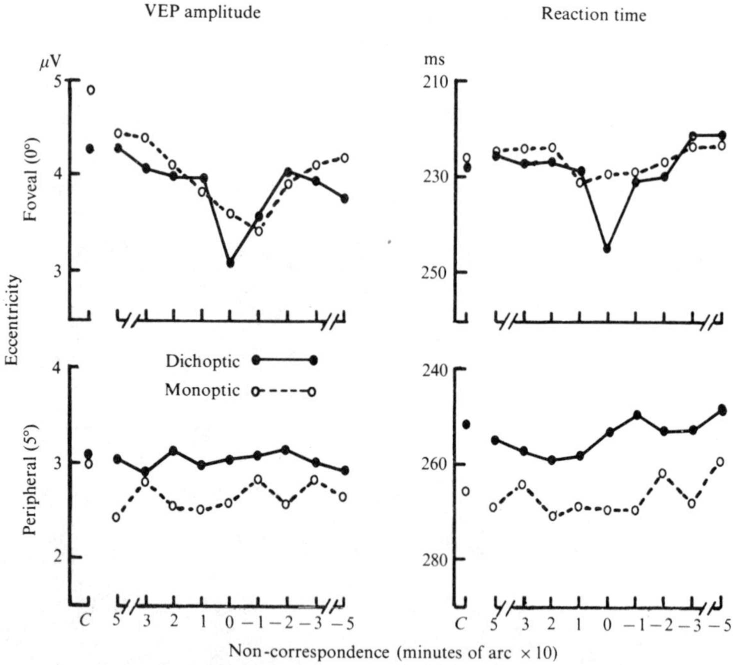

Fig. 10.9. VEP amplitude and median reaction time to test flash presented to foveal (0°) and peripheral (5°) retina as a function of the non-correspondence of the continuously presented suppressing stimuli. The suppressing stimulus was presented either to the same (monoptic) or opposite (dichoptic or bioptic) eye as the test flash. Data have been combined across 4 subjects and 2 replications. The 0′ arc values for the monoptic conditions are interpolated.

spots employed in the present study activated binocular neurones with more localized retinal receptive fields.

The lack of interocular suppression when the more peripheral area of the retina was stimulated could be due to at least three factors. First, it could simply reflect the lack of interocular interaction of activity originating in the peripheral portions of the retina. Secondly, the relatively large size of peripheral receptive fields possibly reduced the effectiveness of the suppressing light spot to the extent that its effects were not evidenced by VEPs. A third but less likely possibility was that the two recordings electrodes used (O_Z and O_2) were not appropriately placed to record activity projecting from the more peripheral part of the retina. It may be noted that the O_Z and O_2 data did not differ significantly.

Discussion and conclusions

(a) Greater binocular summation of VEPs results when pattern, as compared to diffuse light, is dioptically presented to both eyes (White and Bonelli 1970; Harter *et al.* 1973; experiment 1).

(b) Under conditions of *dioptic stimulation* with pattern light, binocular summation was greatest when pattern elements subtended 10–20′ (Harter *et al.* 1973) and were in sharpest focus (White and Bonelli 1970).

(c) The effects of dichoptic stimulation with different patterns depend on the nature of dichoptic stimulation.

(i) When patterned light is presented to one eye and diffuse light to the other, both binocular and monocular VEPs indicate the response to diffuse light is suppressed. The amplitude and waveform of the binocular VEP was approximately the same as that of the monocular VEP to the patterned light alone (MacKay 1968; Ciganek 1971; experiment 1); and the amplitude of monocular VEPs to diffuse light flashed to one eye was progressively reduced as stimulation of the other eye was changed from diffuse to the 60′ patterned light (Experiment 1).

(ii) When patterned light is *dichoptically* presented to both eyes under conditions which result in changes in perceived depth (e.g. conditions of retinal disparity), VEP amplitude increased as a function of the degree of retinal disparity (Fiorentini and Maffei 1970; Regan and Spekreijse 1970).

(iii) When patterned light is *dichoptically* presented to the eyes under conditions in which the images falling on the retinae are not perceptually fused, the amplitude of *binocular VEPs* (primarily at latencies of about 200 ms) is *reduced.* Such suppression has been demonstrated with dichoptic stimulation with patterns of different sizes (Ciganek 1971; experiment 1), with patterns of different orientations (Kawasaki *et al.* 1970; Harter *et al.* 1972, 1973), and with patterns presented to non-corresponding retinal points (Harter *et al.* 1972).

Monocular VEP amplitude (primarily at latencies of about 160 ms) was *greater* in response to *dichoptic* stimulation with patterns of different spatial frequencies or sizes (Regan and Spekreijse 1970; Fiorentini and Maffei 1970; experiment 2), and when non-corresponding retinal points are stimulated (Lehmann and Fender 1969; Spekreijse *et al.* 1972; experiment 4). Monocular VEPs are smallest in amplitude with dioptic stimulation.

The size specificity of interocular suppression of monocular VEPs varied as a function of the absolute size of pattern elements presented to the suppressing eye and increased as the size was increased from 15′ to 60′ (experiment 1). In apparent disagreement, suppression was also found to vary as a function of the relative size of pattern elements presented to the two eyes and was greatest when identical patterns were presented to the two eyes (experiment 2). The difference in results in these two experiments is attributed to the different stimuli (cross-line grids versus checkerboards), measures of VEP amplitude (P210 versus N160) and/or intensity levels of the test and suppressing stimuli (bright–dim versus dim–bright) in experiments 1 and 2 respectively.

(d) The time-course of interocular suppression was found to be relatively fast in comparison to that indicated by psychophysical data on intraocular adaptation effects. Interocular suppression and recovery from such suppression was nearly complete within 500 ms after the on- and offset of the suppressing stimulus respectively.

In comparing the results of different studies it should be noted first that different investigators select different components of VEPs to quantify in terms of amplitude changes, and secondly, that once a component is identified, a given change in amplitude may be interpreted as indicating either facilitation or suppression. Thus, it is possible for an investigator to search for and sample that change in the VEP which best supports the hypothesis he is testing. This possibility emphasizes the importance of using multiple measures of amplitude and of quantitative perceptual or behavioural measures of the phenomenon being investigated. The latter then can be used to validate interpretations of changes in VEPs.

These problems raise some concern about the apparent enhancement of binocular and suppression of monocular VEPs in response to dioptic stimulation since these two trends, in part, were based on different measures of amplitude, e.g. P210 and N160 respectively. In each situation, however, it was reported that the measure used reflected the subject's perception, as indicated by introspective reports by the subjects. These two trends, therefore, will be assumed to be valid indications of perceptual processes and not to be the result of different quantitative procedures.

A number of models have been offered as explanations of suppression and facilitation which may be relevant to the binocular interactions reported here. Binocular summation in response to transient stimulation of both eyes may adequately be explained by excitatory effects originating from each eye in the convergence and summation of central neural mechanisms (spatial summation model).

Four models have been offered which may be relevant to the type of interocular suppression reported in the above studies.

(a) *Selective attention model.* Selective attention to information presented to one eye could account for reduction in VEP amplitude in response to information presented to the other, unattended eye. Such selective suppression could be mediated by efferent inhibition of inputs from one eye. Attention, however, was controlled for in all our studies, which makes this an unlikely explanation of the effects of dichoptic stimulation on binocular interaction. Also, it does not explain why interocular suppression is greatest when identical stimuli are presented to the two eyes – a condition in which it would be most difficult to discriminate which eye was being stimulated and to selectively attend to that eye.

(b) *Adaptation model.* The input from one eye could adapt the binocular central channel so that it would be less responsive to inputs from the other eye. Implicit in this model is that adaptation increases as a function of the duration of stimulation. Although adaptation may be a likely explanation of intraocular effects with a relatively long time-course, it appears less likely to account for interocular effects, which have a relatively short time-course and involve central mechanisms. Neither does adaptation account for binocular summation of VEPs to an increment in brightness of dioptic pattern stimulation as reported in Experiment 1 – a condition which should result in greatest adaptation of the binocular channel.

(c) *Inhibition model.* The responsiveness of the central channel to the excitatory influence of inputs from one eye could be actively inhibited by inputs from the other eye. Although such a mechanism might explain interocular suppression and has been reported at the lateral geniculate nucleus and cortical levels in animals (see below), its main limitation is that it does not explain binocular summation when both eyes are stimulated simultaneously.

(d) *Occlusion model.* The binocular occlusion model appears to be most consistent with the types of binocular interaction reported in the above studies. In this model, input from one eye activates elements in the central channel, so that fewer elements in the central channel are free to respond to inputs from the other eye. Ciganek (1970) and Lehmann and Fender (1968) have proposed this type of model as an explanation of interocular suppression. In contrast to the inhibition model, occlusion provides an explanation of binocular summation when both eyes are stimulated simultaneously. In this situation, occlusion would not be operating since it requires prior activation of the central binocular channel.

An adequate explanation of binocular interaction must account for the specificity of the interaction, and suggest physiological mechanisms which might underlie it. Lehmann and Fender (1969) provided evidence based on human data that interocular suppression was dependent on the convergence of projecting afferents from corresponding areas of each eye. Interocular suppression was not evidenced by a subject with a split optic chiasma.

The lateral geniculate nucleus is the first known structure in the visual projection system which is involved in binocular interaction. Sanderson *et al.* (1971) reported that many dorsal lateral geniculate nucleus cells in the cat had binocular receptive fields in approximately corresponding retinal areas of the two eyes. In the majority of these cells (72 per cent), the receptive field of the dominant eye was concentric with an excitatory centre (subtending up to 60′) and an inhibitory surround. The receptive field of the non-dominant eye did not contain a centre-surround organization and was inhibitory in influence. Inhibition due to stimulation of the non-dominant eye was fairly weak, had a latency of 50 ms and lasted about 400 ms, and presumably was mediated by interneurones in the lateral geniculate nucleus whose axons crossed the borders from one cell layer to another.

The features of interocular inhibition in the cat appear consistent with some of the characteristics of interocular suppression in human VEPs: inhibitory receptive fields were relatively large in size which is consistent with the greater effectiveness of relatively low spatial frequencies in suppressing VEPs as reported in experiment 1; and stimulating the dominant eye reduced the effectiveness of interocular suppression in the single unit data just as a more effective evoking stimulus (pattern versus diffuse flashes) reduced the amount of interocular suppression of the VEP data.

A number of the characteristics of the interocular inhibition at the dorsal lateral geniculate nucleus level, however, are not consistent with the VEP data: (a) the lack of centre–surround organization in the non-dominant eye indicates that this inhibition cannot account for the size specificity of interocular suppression of VEPs noted in experiment 2; (b) the inhibition was transient and subsided within about 400 ms after the onset of the inhibitory stimulus, which is not consistent with the sustained nature of interocular suppression noted in experiment 3; and (c) such inhibition is not consistent with the binocular summation of VEPs when both eyes are flashed simultaneously with appropriate stimuli. Neither were the receptive fields of the binocular lateral geniculate nucleus units orientation specific; they therefore cannot account for the effects of dichoptic stimulation with patterns of different orientation on VEPs (Kawasaki *et al.* 1970; Harter *et al.* 1972).

Binocular interactions related to the orientation and size of patterns presented to the two eyes and to binocular summation are probably mediated by cortical mechanisms. The binocular receptive fields of some cortical units in animals are organized so that they are maximally stimulated when patterns of appropriate size and orientation are presented to corresponding retinal points (Hubel and Wiesel 1962; Barlow, Blakemore, and Pettigrew 1967; Pettigrew, Nikara, and Bishop 1968; Bishop, Henry, and Smith 1971; Minke and Auerbach 1972). If such organization may be assumed to exist in the human visual system it could account for the binocular summation of VEPs obtained when patterns of the same size (experiment 1) and orientation (Harter *et al.* 1972, 1973) are flashed to both eyes. Typically, studies of single cortical units in animals have not investigated interocular suppression.

Other cortical units have binocular receptive fields organized so that stimulation of slightly disparate or non-corresponding retinal points optimally activates the units (Barlow *et al.* 1967; Hubel and Wiesel 1970; Pettigrew *et al.* 1968). If such receptive field organization exists in the human visual system it would provide an explanation of the enhanced amplitude in response to retinal disparity in human studies (Fiorentini and Maffei 1970; Regan and Spekreijse 1970).

In marked dichoptic situations, when the stimuli to either eye activate different cortical units (or channels) there would be little, if any, binocular interaction, but such a situation may result in binocular rivalry. Evidence has been offered that during conditions of rivalry VEPs are greater from an eye when perceptually dominant than when it is suppressed (Lansing 1964; Cobb *et al.* 1967; Lawwill and Biersdorf 1968). Suppression during rivalry appears to be mediated by different mechanisms than those used to explain the above results. Rivalry involves interaction between different information channels – e.g. channels processing vertical as opposed to horizontal contour information. The more discrepant the information presented to the two eyes the greater the rivalry. The nature of binocular interaction discussed in the above studies involves interaction within the same information channel – the more similar the two patterns presented to the two eyes the greater the amount of interaction.

11. Evoked potential indications of the processing of pattern, colour, and depth information

D. REGAN

Department of Communication, University of Keele

Pattern and colour

Summary of conclusions

Colour coding of pattern VEPs. The model illustrated in Fig. 11.1 is a simplified illustration of the model that has been proposed for the colour coding of pattern VEPs (Regan 1972*a*, 1975*a*).

Light striking the eye is eventually absorbed by three photo-pigments that are preferentially sensitive to red, green, or blue light respectively. At this peripheral stage the effect of a visual stimulus upon the eye is no more than a simple response to local light intensity. It is at a more central level in the visual pathway that signals from nearby retinal areas converge and are compared at a stage sensitive to spatial contrast or edges. The main point illustrated in Fig. 11.1 is that signals from red and green photoreceptors are still segregated when they arrive at these first contrast detectors. The segregation may be total or almost so.

One function of this peripheral colour segregation might be to minimize the degradation of visual acuity caused by the eye's chromatic aberration. Red and green lights from a pattern are never simultaneously in sharp focus on the retina, so that a pattern detector sensitive to a wide range of colours would always be fed from a blurred retinal image. If, however, the most peripheral stage were segregated into two colour channels, then at any moment either the red or the green channel would receive a sharper image and preferentially feed the next stage. The function of the gate in Fig. 11.1 is preferentially to transmit the stronger pattern signal, possibly by means of mutual inhibition between red and green pattern channels. This notion would explain why visual acuity has been reported to be little worse in white than in monochromatic light, why acuity for one colour can be unaffected by superposing light of a different colour, why the eye's depth of focus is greater in white than in monochromatic light, and would also be in accord with the McCollough effect (see May, Chapter 13 of this book).

Visual evoked potentials in man: new developments (ed. J.E. Desmedt), pp. 234–49. Clarendon Press, Oxford 1977.

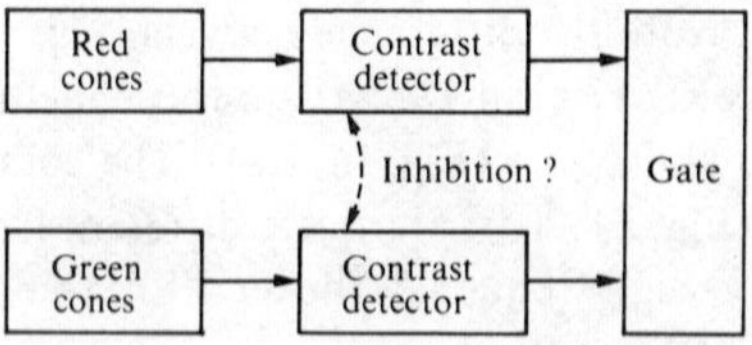

Fig. 11.1. Pattern VEP: simplified model of colour organization.

Colour coding of flicker VEPs. Flickering the intensity of an unpatterned patch of light gives VEPs whose colour properties are quite different from the colour properties of pattern VEPs. One explanation for this difference is that colour signals from spatially unpatterned and spatially patterned light stimuli are handled differently by the eye and brain.

Flicker produces large VEPs in three frequency regions (Fig. 11.2(a)). 'High-frequency' flicker VEPs (Van der Tweel and Lunel 1965; Regan 1968*c*) are those falling in the resonant-like peak between 35 Hz and 60 Hz shown in Fig. 11.2(a). The colour properties of high-frequency VEPs are illustrated in Fig. 11.2(b). Signals from red-sensitive, green-sensitive, and blue-sensitive photoreceptors are pooled

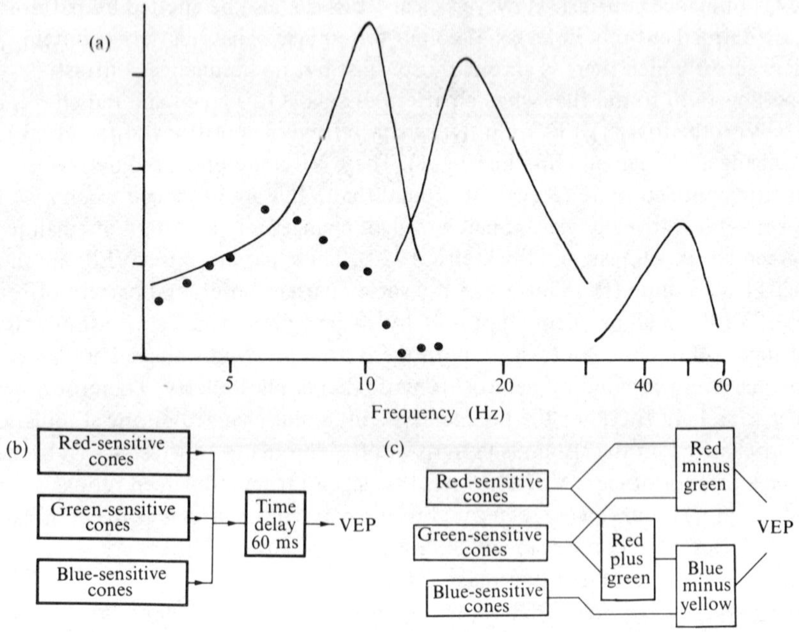

Fig. 11.2. (a) Amplitude (ordinate, arbitrary units) versus frequency plots for steady-state VEPs. Dots are pattern-reversal VEPs. Continuous lines are flicker VEPs showing low-frequency (8–12 Hz) region, medium-frequency (13–25 Hz) region, and high-frequency (35–60 Hz) region. (b) High-frequency flicker VEPs: simplified model of colour organization. (c) Medium-frequency flicker VEPs: simplified model of colour organization based on opponent colours theory (cf. Graham 1965).

very early in the system. Note the difference between Figs. 11.1 and 11.2(b).

'Medium-frequency' VEPs (Regan 1968*a*) are those included in the resonant-like peak between 13 Hz and 25 Hz (Fig. 11.2(a)). The colour properties of medium-frequency flicker VEPs (Fig. 11.2(c)) are quite different from the colour properties of both pattern VEPs and high-frequency flicker VEPs (see Regan 1972*b*; Spekreijse, Estevez, and Reits, Chapter 2 of this book).

Colour properties of pattern VEPs

Chromatic-contrast VEPs. It is well known that clear transient VEPs can be recorded from the scalp overlying the occipital cortex when a uniform patch of light changes into a pattern of bright and dim checks or bars, even when there is no change of total light flux. These are variously called pattern-appearance VEPs, or VEPs to an increase of spatial contrast. Disappearance of pattern also elicits VEPs, though with different properties. It is also well known that exchanging the positions of adjacent elements in a pattern of bright and dim bars or checks can give a clear VEP at each pattern reversal. All these VEPs are elicited by patterns composed of bright areas bordered by dimmer areas, in other words, patterns containing borders across which there is luminance contrast. However, clear VEPs can also be elicited by patterns that are defined entirely in terms of colour differences. These patterns contain borders across which there is chromatic contrast but no luminance contrast.

Sperling and I found that when a pattern of small (12′) green and red checks or bars falls on the fovea, VEPs are produced each time the positions of the checks are exchanged (Regan and Sperling 1971). These VEPs are produced by reversing chromatic contrast. More recently we found that VEPs are produced when a uniform yellow, foveally viewed patch of light changes into a pattern of small red and green checks (Regan and Spekreijse 1974). These pattern-onset VEPs are shown in Fig. 11.3 (column (f)). Thus pattern-reversal, pattern-onset, and pattern-offset types of VEP can all be elicited not only by changing luminance contrast but also by changing chromatic contrast. In both these stimulus conditions red and green luminances were equated by heterochromatic flicker photometry. Therefore neither total light flux, nor the luminance at any point changed during stimulation. All that changed on the stimulus pattern was the chromatic contrast across borders and the existence of clear VEPs suggests that signals from red–green retinal photoreceptors (cones) were segregated to some extent on arrival at the contrast detectors (Regan 1972*a*; Regan and Sperling 1971). However, there are several objections to this argument that must first be considered.

Are chromatic-contrast VEPs caused by inappropriately matching the red and green lights? Although heterochromatic flicker photometry is a standard method for equating the luminances of differently coloured lights, it might not be appropriate here. Pattern VEPs were therefore recorded while the luminances of the red and green lights were progressively unbalanced. The results illustrated in Fig. 11.4 show that chromatic-contrast VEPs were not luminance-contrast VEPs

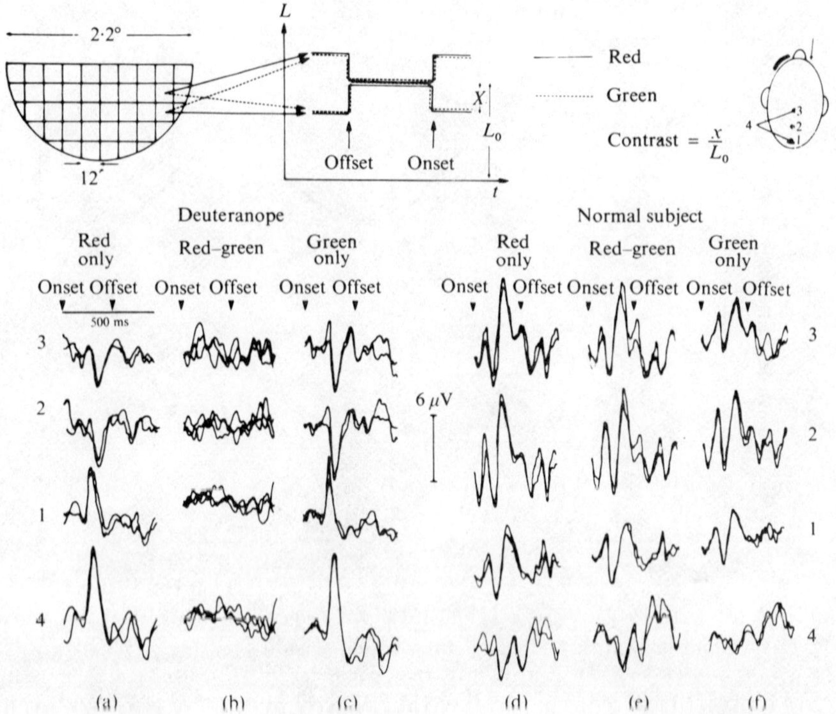

Fig. 11.3. Transient VEP to chromatic contrast elicited by onset and offset of a pattern of red and green checks ('red–green' column). These are clear in the normal subject, but absent in the colour-blind subject (deuteranope). Different electrodes marked 1–4. In both normal and colour-blind subjects the monochromatic red and green parts of the stimulus by themselves give clear VEPs, marked 'red only' and 'green only'. (From Regan and Spekreijse 1974.)

due to mismatched luminances (Regan 1972*a*, *b*, 1973*a*).

A further point is that the familiar white light stimulus patterns give VEPs whose properties begin to resemble those of flicker VEPs rather than pattern VEPs when check size is too large (larger than roughly 25–40′) (Spekreijse 1966; Regan and Richards 1973). Smaller checks were used in the present study for this reason. A further distinction between pattern and flicker VEPs is that the largest pattern-reversal VEPs were obtained at about 5–8 Hz, whereas flicker VEPs were largest at much higher frequencies (Fig. 11.2(a)). Thus chromatic-contrast VEPs were different from frequency-doubled flicker VEPs.

Are chromatic-contrast VEPs due to the eye's chromatic aberration? Because of ocular chromatic aberration, the differently coloured parts of a stimulus pattern would normally not simultaneously be in sharp focus on the retina. Thus the patterned stimulus could act as though one colour were absent and normal luminance-contrast VEPs would masquerade as chromatic-contrast VEPs. Fig. 11.5 (a) shows that ocular chromatic aberration does indeed have a large effect upon

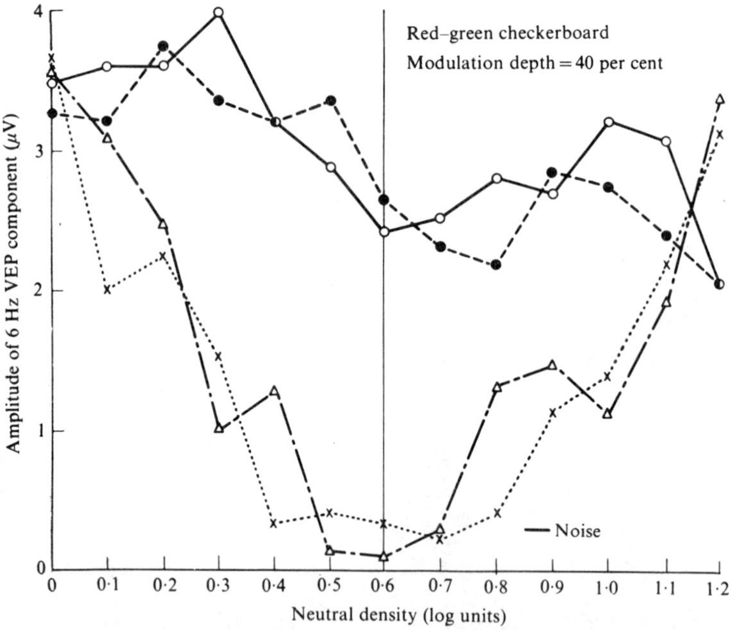

Fig. 11.4. Chromatic contrast VEPs are not due to a luminance mismatch. At 0·6 on the abscissa the subjects viewed a 3° foveal pattern of equiluminant 11′ red and green checks that exchanged places 6 times per s. Clear 6 Hz VEPs were elicited (open and filled circles). VEP amplitude did not fall to a minimum when the luminance of the green light was varied by up to ± 0·6 log units about the equiluminant point.

pattern VEPs (Regan 1973*a*). It is clear from Fig. 11.5(a) how, for example, a pattern of equiluminant red and blue checks could give large VEPs that were due almost entirely to the red part of the pattern. In that case the blue light might just as well not be present.

Fig. 11.5(b), however, shows that when the ocular chromatic aberration was cancelled, a pattern of red and green checks still gave clear VEPs. Thus chromatic-contrast VEPs are not due to ocular chromatic aberration, though this can be an important artifact.

Are red and green signals completely segregated at the first contrast-sensitive stage? From the above it seems that coloured patterns can elicit VEPs which are pattern specific and which are not artifacts of intensity changes, chromatic aberration or luminance contrast. This means that some proportion of the signals from red-sensitive and green-sensitive photoreceptors are still segregated when they arrive at the first contrast-sensitive stage. The following evidence suggests this segregation holds for all, or at least the great majority, of such signals (Regan and Spekreijse 1974). Fig. 11.6 shows VEPs elicited by a pattern of adjacent, equiluminant red and green checks. But this time red checks stayed red at all times, and green checks stayed green. However, when the luminance of the red checks

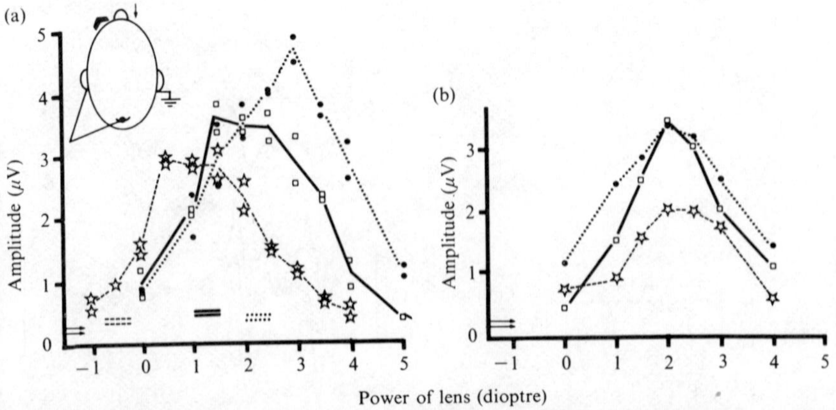

Fig. 11.5. Effect of the eye's chromatic aberration upon pattern VEP. The subject whose accommodation was paralysed viewed a semicircular pattern of 12′ checks restricted to the lower half of the fovea. The pattern-reversal frequency was 7 Hz. In (a) the amplitude of the 7 Hz VEP component is plotted versus the power in dioptres of a trial lens placed before the eye for red (dots), green (squares), and blue (stars) checks. Ocular chromatic aberration clearly has a large effect on VEP amplitude. In (b), although the eye's chromatic aberration has been cancelled optically, a pattern of red and green checks gives clear VEPs.

increased, the luminance of the green checks decreased by an equal amount and vice versa. To a colour-blind subject this stimulus looked like conventional monochromatic pattern-reversal and he gave normal pattern-reversal VEPs (Fig. 11.6(a)). For the normal subject the situation was quite different. This stimulus gave no VEPs at all (Fig. 11.6(b)). This meant that the normal subject's contrast-sensitive mechanism did not accept equiluminant red and green checks as being equally effective stimuli.

This finding implies that the percentage of red and green signals still segregated at the first contrast-sensitive stage must be high, possibly even 100 per cent. For if an appreciable proportion of red and green signals were pooled prior to the contrast-sensitive stage, then the equiluminant red and green checks of Fig. 11.6 should have given measurable VEPs in normally sighted subjects. The absence of VEPs under such conditions in normal subjects could be predicted by the model of Fig. 11.1. Equiluminant red and green checks 'seen' through, say, the red channel would appear monochromatic with one set of checks (green checks) much dimmer than the other. Therefore the contrast between adjacent checks would never reverse. However, if the luminance of the green checks were sufficiently increased, contrast reversal would occur and VEPs should then be recorded. In practice VEPs can indeed be recorded when the green checks are some 0·6 log units brighter than the red checks (Regan and Spekreijse 1974). The figure of 0·6 log units is approximately the one estimated from two independent measures of the relative sensitivities of the red and green channels of Fig. 11.1 (Regan 1974*a*, 1975*b*).

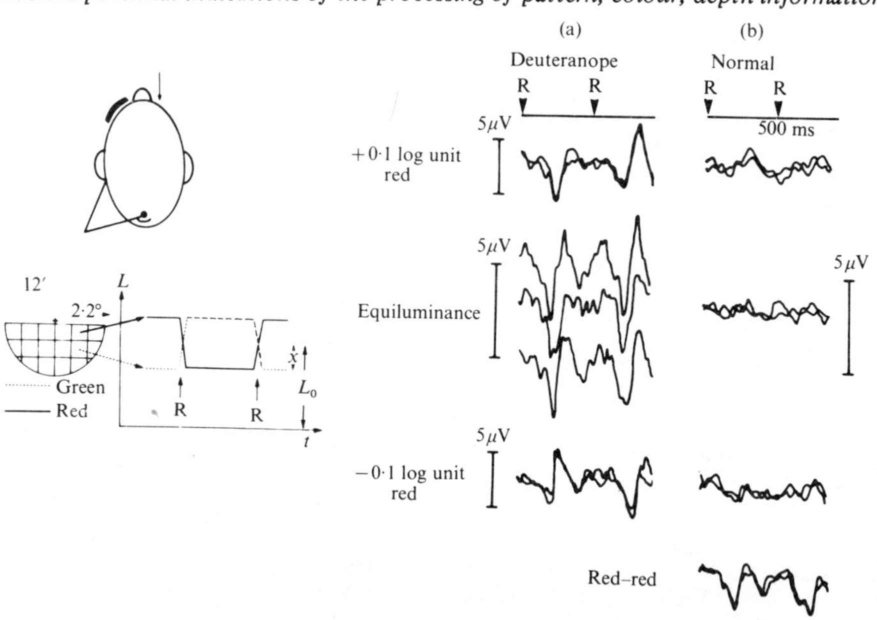

Fig. 11.6. VEP elicited by a pattern of adjacent, equiluminant red and green checks. Red checks remained red and green checks remained green at all times. When the intensities of the red checks increased (arrow marked R) the intensities of the green checks decreased correspondingly and vice versa. To the colour-blind (deuteranopic) subject this stimulus was equivalent to normal pattern-reversal of a white pattern ('equal luminance' traces). However, this stimulus gave no VEPs in the normally sighted subject. Hence for the normal subject, all or nearly all red and green signals are segregated when they reach the contrast-detector stage. (From Regan and Spekreijse 1974.)

Action spectra of red and green channels for pattern VEPs. The action spectrum for the red channel of Fig. 11.1 was measured by using as a probe VEPs elicited by a deep red (676 nm) foveal (2°) stimulus of small (9′) checks. Steady-state VEPs elicited by a pattern-reversal frequency of 7 Hz were continuously recorded. A 6° desensitizing patch of light was superposed on the pattern. Since the required measurements would be very prolonged if conventional techniques were used, a speedy method was developed for this experiment (Regan 1975*b*). The Fourier-analysis method (Regan 1966*a*, *b*) was used to give a continuous running average of the amplitude of the steady-state VEP elicited by the red pattern. This VEP then controlled the intensity of the stimulus desensitizing light patch so as to maintain the instantaneous value of VEP amplitude at some criterion level. In other words the subject was inside a feed-back loop. If VEP amplitude momentarily fell, then the intensity of the desensitizing light was reduced; if VEP amplitude increased, then the intensity of the desensitizing light was increased (see Regan, Chapter 4 of this book).

Fig. 11.7 shows how, for yellow desensitizing light (580 nm), VEP amplitude

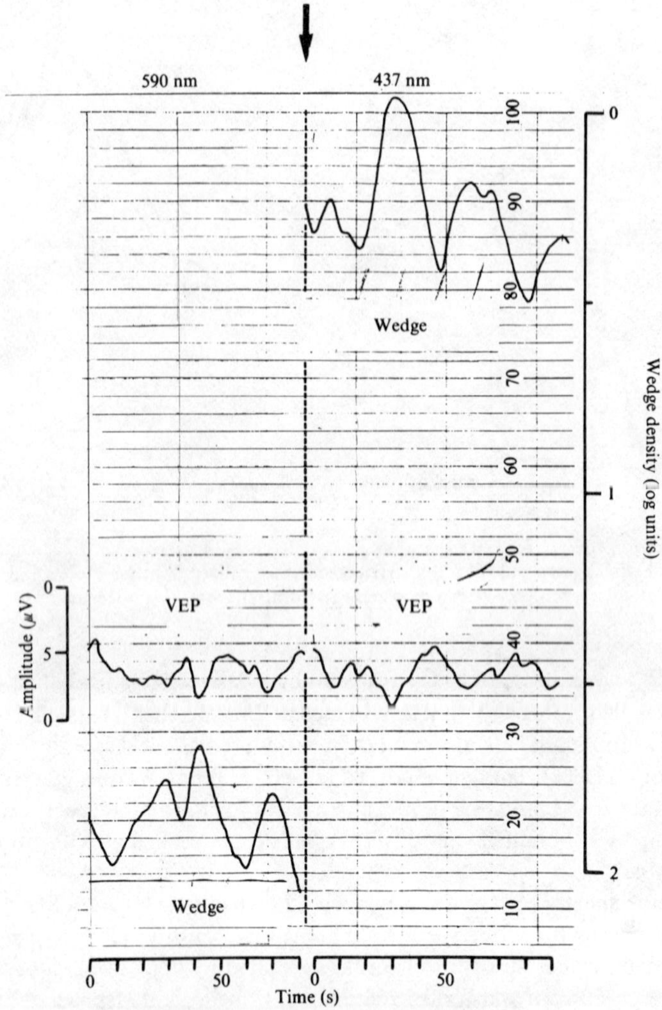

Fig. 11.7. VEP feed-back whereby the voltage of the brain responses controls the stimulus intensity. The VEP amplitude was held constant at roughly 6 μV. Right ordinate, density of the variable compensating wedge in log units. Traces marked 'wedge' show how the actual stimulus intensity was automatically adjusted by VEP so as to maintain VEP amplitude constant when the actual colour of light was changed from yellow (590 nm) to blue (437 nm). The intensity was roughly 50 times greater for the blue light than for the yellow light.

was held constant in this way, wandering about a mean level, while the intensity of the desensitizing light hunted some ± 0·2 log units about a steady value. When the colour of the desensitizing light was changed from yellow to blue (437 nm), VEP feed-back caused its intensity to be increased by some 1·7 log units (50 times) before VEP amplitude stabilized at its former value. This meant that the red

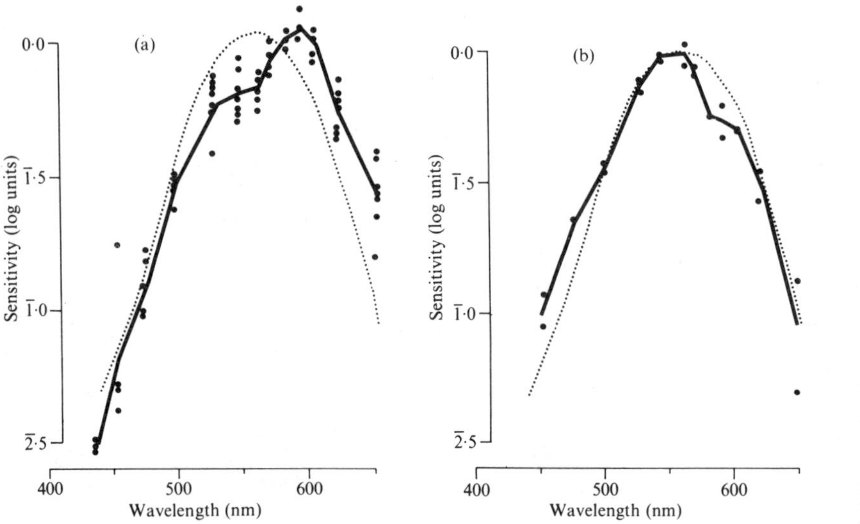

Fig. 11.8. Action spectra for red (a) and green (b) channels of pattern VEPs. The curve in (a) was obtained with a deep red (676 nm) pattern of 9′ foveally presented checks and the curve (b) with a similar pattern of green (544 nm) checks. (From Regan 1974.)

pattern VEPs were 50 times less sensitive to blue desensitizing light than to yellow desensitizing light. This experiment was repeated for desensitizing lights of different colours so as to obtain an action spectrum for the red channel similar to that shown in Fig. 11.8(a). This curve peaked at 580–600 nm. When a green (544 nm) stimulus pattern was used as a probe, an estimate for the action spectrum of the green channel was obtained (Fig. 11.8(b)). This curve peaked at 530–560 nm (Regan 1974*a*).

The action spectra for the red and green VEP channels shown in Fig. 11.8 are in fair agreement with action spectra for human red-sensitive and green-sensitive photo-pigments or colour (π) mechanisms estimated by objective and psychophysical means (Brown and Wald 1964; Marks, Dobelle, and MacNichol 1964; Baker and Rushton 1965).

It is a trivial point that separate colour channels would be observed if strong monochromatic adapting lights were used that depressed the sensitivity of either red or green cones. Such a finding would merely demonstrate the fact that red- and green-sensitive photoreceptors exist. It is important to note that Fig. 11.8 implies more. These curves are valid, not only for near-threshold patterns, but also for patterns whose visibilities far exceed the contrast threshold. The supra-threshold measurements were made by utilizing the nonlinear 'knee' in the VEP saturation curve as a marker that could be recognized even when very little adapting light had been added (Regan 1974). This showed that fine pattern is processed in parallel colour channels whether the pattern's contrast is high or near-threshold. Furthermore, the spectral sensitivities of the colour channels are to a first approximation independent of the pattern's contrast (Regan 1974*a*).

The blue channel of pattern vision was not evident when the eye was stimulated with a blue pattern, even when coarse (40′) checks were used to match the blue channel's poor spatial resolution. Presumably this was because the blue channel is insensitive. A somewhat imprecise spectral-sensitivity curve could be measured for the blue channel by using intense yellow chromatic adaptation, and this peaked at roughly 460 nm.

Colour-blindness. Chromatic-contrast VEPs provide a sensitive objective test for colour-blindness. The red–green traces of Fig. 11.3 show how the abrupt appearance of a pattern of equiluminant red and green checks gave clear averaged transient VEPs in normally sighted subjects, but produced no response at all in a colour-blind (deuteranopic) subject (Regan and Spekreijse 1974). An even more sensitive test for colour-blindness was to elicit steady-state VEPs by repetitively exchanging the positions of red and green checks six times per s (Regan 1973*a*; Regan and Spekreijse 1974).

The colour-blind subject's VEPs were abolished only when the luminances of the red and green checks were exactly balanced. This gave a measure of the eye's relative sensitivity to red–green that could be read off to better than 0·1 log unit. Such a measure of red–green sensitivity can provide an objective equivalent of the conventional psychophysical match (red + green – yellow) obtained with a Nagel anomaloscope. In this way the method of recording VEPs to chromatic contrast stimulation can not only detect defective colour vision, but can also provide objective data to diagnose the type of colour defect. The technique might well prove useful with children, uncooperative patients, and malingerers.

VEP recording can also provide clues as to the nature of colour-blindness. For example, the observation that a pattern of equiluminant red and green checks does not elicit VEPs in a colour-blind subject means that the physiological signals produced by the red and the green lights are pooled before they reach the first contrast-sensitive neurones. This pooling could be due, for example, to fusion of signals from red and green cones. Alternatively there might be only one sensitive photo-pigment in the red–green part of the spectrum. If red and green cones were present, ocular chromatic aberration would be expected to prevent complete abolition of the VEP, even when red and green luminances were carefully balanced (see Fig. 11.5(a)). Experimentally however, VEP amplitude can be reduced completely to noise level, i.e. to at least 7 times smaller than signal level (Regan 1973*c*; Regan and Spekreijse 1974). This finding favours the view that the colour-blind subject studied had only one photo-pigment at the long-wavelength end of the spectrum. This has subsequently been confirmed (Estevez *et al.* 1975) by measuring the deuteranope's spectral-sensitivity curve using a technique similar to that described here and elsewhere (Regan 1974*a*, 1975*b*).

Colour properties of flicker VEPs: experimental evidence

The colour of a patch of light was alternated 24 times per s between white and blue (460 nm). The resulting flicker VEP consisted almost entirely of two frequency components, one of 24 Hz (fundamental component) and one of 48 Hz (second harmonic component).

High-frequency (35–60 Hz) VEP components

By varying the intensity of the blue light a point could be found at which flicker could not be seen at all. At this point the luminances of the white and coloured lights are conventionally defined as equal. Fig. 11.9 shows that near this point

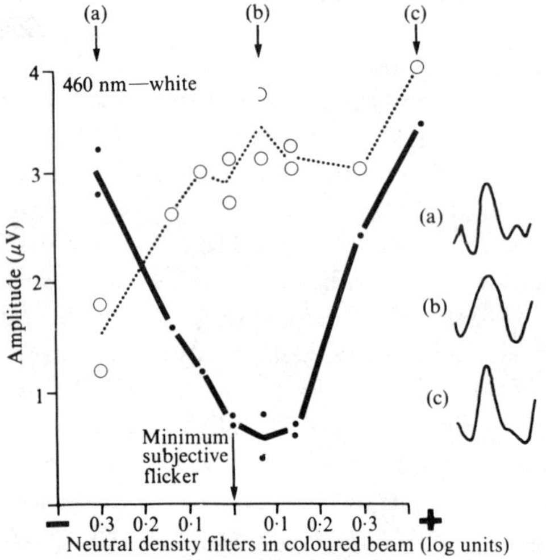

Fig. 11.9. Comparison of psychophysical and VEP heterochromatic flicker photometry data. A standard white light was alternated at 24 Hz with a blue light (460 nm) whose luminance was adjusted by the subject until he saw minimum flicker (zero on abscissa). VEP amplitudes for 24 Hz and 48 Hz components are plotted versus intensities of blue light (abscissa). The second harmonic (48 Hz) VEP component (continuous line) fell to a minimum that coincided with the point of zero subjective flicker. On the other hand, the amplitude of the fundamental (24 Hz) VEP component (dotted line) did not have a minimum at all. The two components were recorded simultaneously at the same electrode. It can be seen that the averaged VEP waveform ((a), (b), and (c)) is difficult to interpret without Fourier analysis.

(0 on abscissa) the amplitude of the second harmonic (48 Hz) component of the flicker VEP fell to a clear minimum (continuous line). In other words the amplitude of the 48 Hz VEP component indicated the point of luminance equality. This held for all colours. Thus the spectral sensitivity curve for the objectively measured 48 Hz VEP component agreed with the spectral-sensitivity curve for brightness (luminosity) perception (Fig. 11.10). This was true for any VEP component throughout the 'high-frequency' range (see Fig. 11.2(a)), whether generated as a

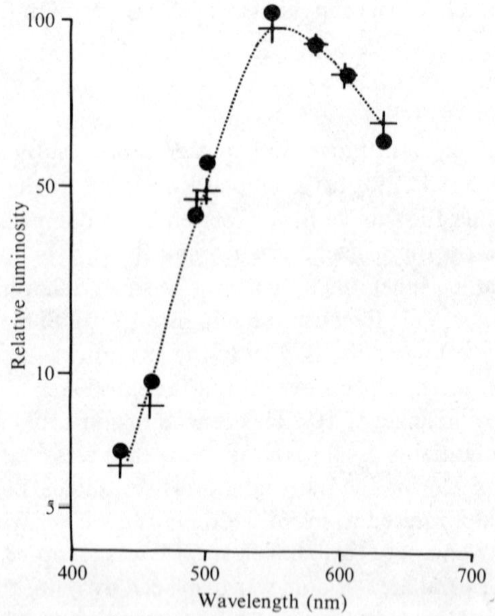

Fig. 11.10. The crosses are relative luminosities (photometric brightness) measured by psychophysical heterochromatic flicker photometry. The dotted line is drawn through these points. The filled circles are visual sensitivities measured by the VEP method illustrated in Fig. 11.9. The VEP data applies for any VEP flicker components in the 35–60 Hz range. (From Regan 1970.)

fundamental or frequency-doubled component (Regan 1970*a*). The agreement was very close (better than 0·07 log units), so that VEP recording offers a means of measuring the spectral luminosity curve that is of similar precision to heterochromatic flicker photometry, but can be much faster. Fig. 11.10 suggests that, for high-frequency flicker VEPs, colour signals are pooled as shown in Fig. 11.2(b). The latency of VEPs elicited by flickering lights of different colours did not differ by more than 2 ms (Regan 1970*a*) (mean latency was about 60 ms) (Van der Tweel and Verduyn Lunel 1965; Regan 1968*c*). This suggests that colour signals are pooled before the main latency stage, as shown in Fig. 11.2(b).

Medium frequency (13–25 Hz) VEP components

Fig. 11.9 shows that the 24 Hz component did not fall to a minimum at the point of zero flicker; its amplitude was large when no flicker could be seen. No unique spectral sensitivity could be defined for this component (Regan 1970*b*). This component showed large, frequency-independent phase shifts that could be interpreted as reflecting opponent-colour processing (Regan 1973*c*). Since the latencies for different colours differ by no more than 2 ms (in about 120 ms), the main latency stage is tentatively placed after the opponent colour stage in Fig. 11.2(c). These characteristics were not restricted to 24 Hz VEP components, but applied generally to all VEP components within the medium-frequency range shown in Fig. 11.2(a).

Illusory sideways movement

This familiar illusion of apparent movement is often produced by switching on a lamp at location A while switching off a lamp at location B. If the two lamps are sufficiently close together the subject may experience the compelling illusion that a single lamp moved across the space between A and B.

A related illusion can be generated by patterns of small, randomly arranged dots (Anstis 1970; Julesz 1971; Regan and Spekreijse 1970). Subjects viewed such a pattern with the left eye only. Suddenly the pattern was replaced by another pattern, similar in all respects except that a central area of dots had been displaced to one side by an angle of 10′. This central region could not be seen by static inspection of the initial or final patterns, since each was composed of randomly arranged dots. During the transition, however, subjects clearly saw a central area of dots that appeared to move sideways *as a whole.* When this illusion of apparent movement occurred, a clear VEP was recorded (Fig. 11.11(d)). In contrast, when the central area of dots was displaced by more than about 10 minutes of arc the central area did not appear to move as a whole. Instead there was an impression that individual dots moved in different directions so that the patterning changed. Note that in this situation, where there was no illusion of global apparent movement, neither was there a VEP (Fig. 11.11(e), (f).* Thus the VEP of Fig. 11.11(d) mainly reflects apparent movement.

Stereoscopic depth movement

VEPs may be affected by the properties of both peripheral and central sites in the visual pathway. Peripheral levels in the visual pathway often exert a strong influence on VEPs, even though VEPs may be generated by cortical neurones. For example, the frequency doubling (i.e. second harmonic generation) that is such a marked feature of flicker VEPs is caused by rectifier-like neural activities in the eye at a level at, or peripheral to, spike generation (Van der Tweel and Lunel 1965; Spekreijse 1966; Spekreijse *et al.* 1972). Those situations where visual perception correlates poorly with VEPs (Van der Tweel and Verduyn Lunel 1965; Regan 1968*c*; Regan and Beverley 1973*c*) might be explained, at least in part, if in such situations VEP properties were dominated by characteristics of the peripheral rather than central visual pathway. This argument suggested to us that attempts should be made to correlate stereoscopic depth perception and VEPs to depth.

* If there are movement-sensitive neurones that 'recognize' movement of an extended object by correlating signals from many different retinal locations, then this illusion suggests that the global correlation process is effective only up to distances of 10′ or so. Since only individual dots appear to move for displacements of 20′ and 40′, point-to-point correlations may be effective over somewhat greater distances. Braddick (1973) has discussed this point more fully.

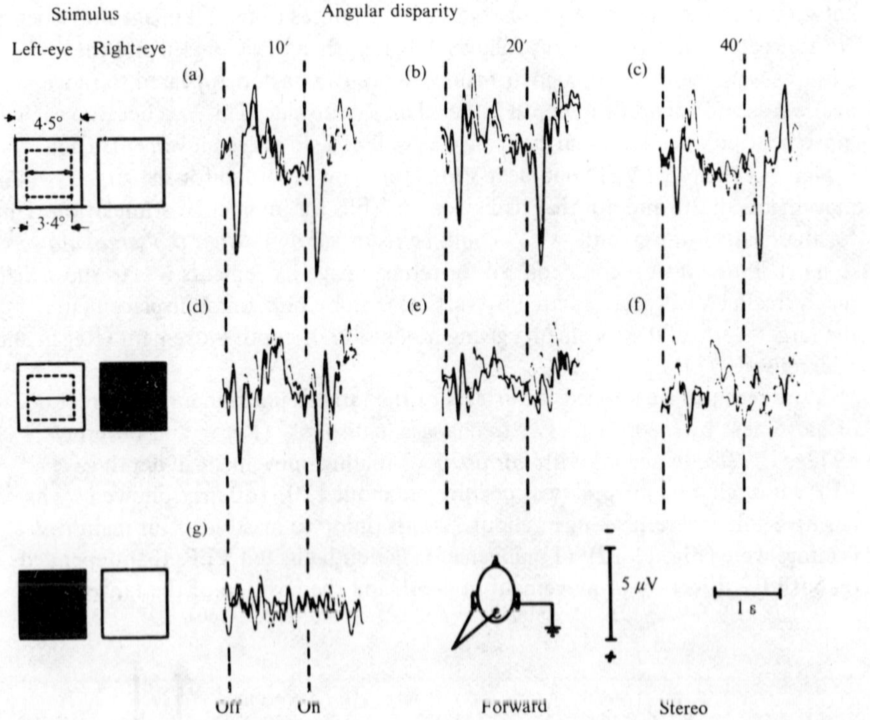

Fig. 11.11. VEP evoked by changes in stereoscopic depth and by apparent movement. (a), (b), (c) The central region of the stimulus field (dotted area) appeared to jump forward and then return at a rate of 0·45 per s. (d), (e), (f) Similar stimulus except that the eye viewing the static reference field was occluded, so that no depth changes were seen by the subject and VEP were produced by sideways movements of the Julesz pattern. For a 10′ (d) displacement there was an illusion of sideways movement and clear VEPs are seen. For 20′ (e) and 40′ (f) displacements there was no illusion of sideways movement and no VEPs were recorded. Trace (g) shows the noise level. (From Regan and Spekreijse 1970.)

When a solid object is viewed binocularly, the left and right eyes' retinal images are slightly different because of the horizontal separation of the eyes. This difference is called retinal (or binocular) disparity. It is well known that retinal disparity alone is sufficient to provide a compelling perception of depth and solidity, for example when a stereoscope is used to view two slightly dissimilar photographs in binocular fusion. If monocular cues are absent it is clear that the neural activities that give rise to this illusion of depth must occur after visual signals from the two eyes have been brought together, i.e. after the stage of binocular convergence (Julesz 1960). Thus, VEPs determined by changes in retinal disparity would be expected to reflect activities at central sites in the visual pathway and be little influenced by peripheral characteristics.

The first major problem when recording VEPs to depth was to distinguish between responses to disparity changes, and responses to retinal image movements. We approached this problem as follows. When both eyes were used and the patterns were viewed in binocular fusion, the central region appeared to move backwards and forwards in depth rather than side to side. This was because each movement produced a disparity change as well as a sideways movement. Each movement elicited a VEP, but clear VEPs were now recorded for the larger movements of 20′ and 40′ that had given no VEPs for monocular stimulation. Thus, for these larger movements, VEPs could be recorded *only when the target appeared to move in depth.* A second control for retinal image movements was to show that much smaller VEPs were elicited by vertical than by horizontal displacements of the target, vertical displacements giving no illusion of depth movement (Regan and Spekreijse 1971).

More recently we studied the effects of the target's position and its direction of movement by recording VEPs to changes in disparity (Regan and Beverley 1973*a*, 1973*b*). In accord with our previous finding, movement in depth gave a VEP whose first major peak was positive, at about 120–160 ms, followed by a negative-going wave peaking at about 220 ms (inion to mastoid). Our main new findings were (Fig. 11.12): (1) movements in depth elicited VEPs that depended on both the direction of movement in depth and the position of the target;

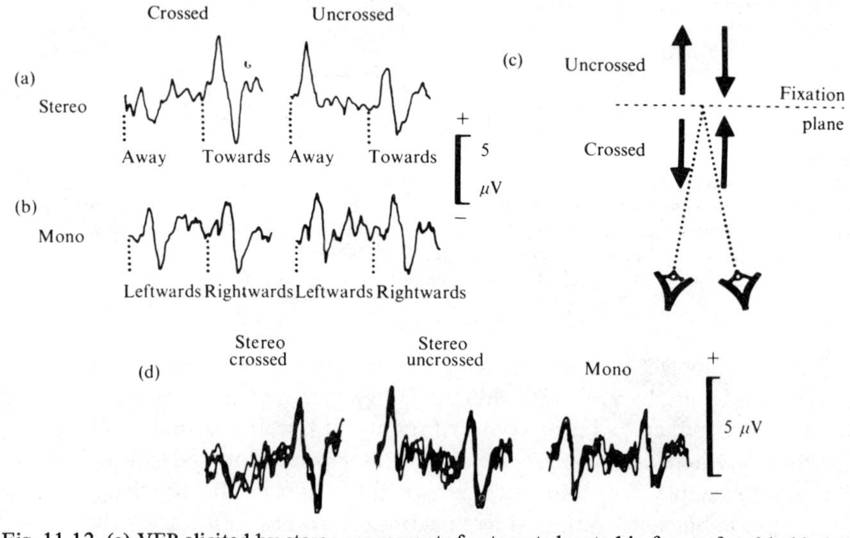

Fig. 11.12. (a) VEP elicited by stereo movements for targets located in front of and behind the plane of binocular fixation. (b) VEP elicited by monocular control stimuli similarly located in front of and behind the fixation plane. (c) Drawing to illustrate the apparent positions and directions of movement in space of the stimuli in the two stereo conditions. (d) Variability illustrated by three superposed VEP traces. Each trace is the average of 500 sweeps in (a) and 100 in (d). Stimulus frequency 0·9 Hz and sweep duration 1 s. Stimulus target was a 2° disc of random black dots surrounded by 5° annulus of dots. Stimulus displacement 10′. (From Regan and Beverley 1973.)

(2) movements in depth from either direction directed away from the plane of fixation gave VEPs whose amplitude was fully saturated for displacement of about 15 minutes of arc; (3) movements in depth from either direction towards the plane of fixation gave VEPs whose amplitude had not started to saturate for displacements as large as 20′; (4) monocular (sideways movement) stimulation gave VEPs whose amplitude had saturated for displacements less than 5′.

All these findings could be explained on the following two assumptions: (a) that the way in which the brain handles information that a target's retinal disparity has changed (i.e. that the target has moved in depth) depends on whether the target is in front of or behind the plane of fixation; (b) that information as to a change of retinal disparity is handled differently when the target is moving away from the fixation plane than when it is moving towards the fixation plane. Assumption (a) would agree with psychophysical evidence that disparity detectors are organized into two or three 'pools' (Richards 1970). Assumption (b) would accord with our psychophysical evidence suggesting that there are neurones in the human brain 'tuned' to the direction of movement in depth (Regan and Beverley 1973*a*; Beverley and Regan 1973). In particular, assumption (b) accords with the notion that there are neural mechanisms in the visual pathway that signal 'an object is moving towards the fixation plane' independently of both the actual direction of motion and (presumably) the position of the fixation plane (Beverley and Regan 1974). The function of such a neural mechanism might be to help converge the eyes accurately onto a chosen target.

It is interesting to note that cortical neurones with analogous properties have subsequently been found by Zeki (1974) in a region of monkey cortex specialized for signalling motion.

Acknowledgements

This work has been supported by the Medical Research Council. Thanks are due to Hazel Henry for assistance in preparing this chapter.

12. Colour-evoked potentials: development of a methodology for the analysis of the processes involved in colour vision

C. T. WHITE, R. W. KATAOKA, and J. I. MARTIN
Naval Electronics Laboratory Center, San Diego, California

Our group has been interested in colour effects in the VEP since we first started working in that area in about 1962, using various coloured stimuli and background conditions. The search for an adequate technique for the study of certain kinds of colour effects is very important. By the time we had completed the experiments referred to in this chapter, we felt that we were at last ready to *begin* the study of colour effects in the VEP. This chapter presents the evolution during the past 10 years of methodology for colour research as well as the findings and deductions made by our studies.

One of the aspects of the VEP considered during our early work was concerned with binocular summation under various conditions. We had already decided that if we were to deal with intensity or colour of the stimuli as such we should avoid having contamination from contour effects.* Therefore halves of table-tennis balls were put over the eyes of subjects, making it impossible for them to perceive any details of the stimulus light. This allowed us to mix stimuli on the surfaces of the translucent hemispheres in a very simple manner by having a number of small spotlight sources which could be varied in terms of intensity or spectral characteristics. Fig. 12.1 shows VEPs to flash stimuli delivered once per second from a xenon discharge tube, viewed through the obscurring hemisphere. The red and the blue stimuli had been roughly equated for apparent brightness, a rather meaningless term when dealing with coloured stimuli.

The characteristics examined were not spectral differences as such, but rather the effects of binocular versus monocular stimulation. The adding of the input from the second eye did not merely increase the amplitude of the monocular VEP

Visual evoked potentials in man; new developments (ed. J. E. Desmedt), pp. 250–72. Clarendon Press, Oxford 1977.

* Since the saturation of the coloured stimulus and of its subsequent after-image were markedly enhanced when used in a checkerboard pattern, we attempted a study of differential colour VEPs using black–red, black–green, and black–blue checkerboards (checks subtending 10–15′ visual angle). This study was rather quickly abandoned when it was found that the checkerboard VEP was practically identical regardless of the colour of the stimulus light. Minor differential effects may have been present but this was not the most effective way of obtaining such effects (see also Shipley, Jones, and Fry 1965).

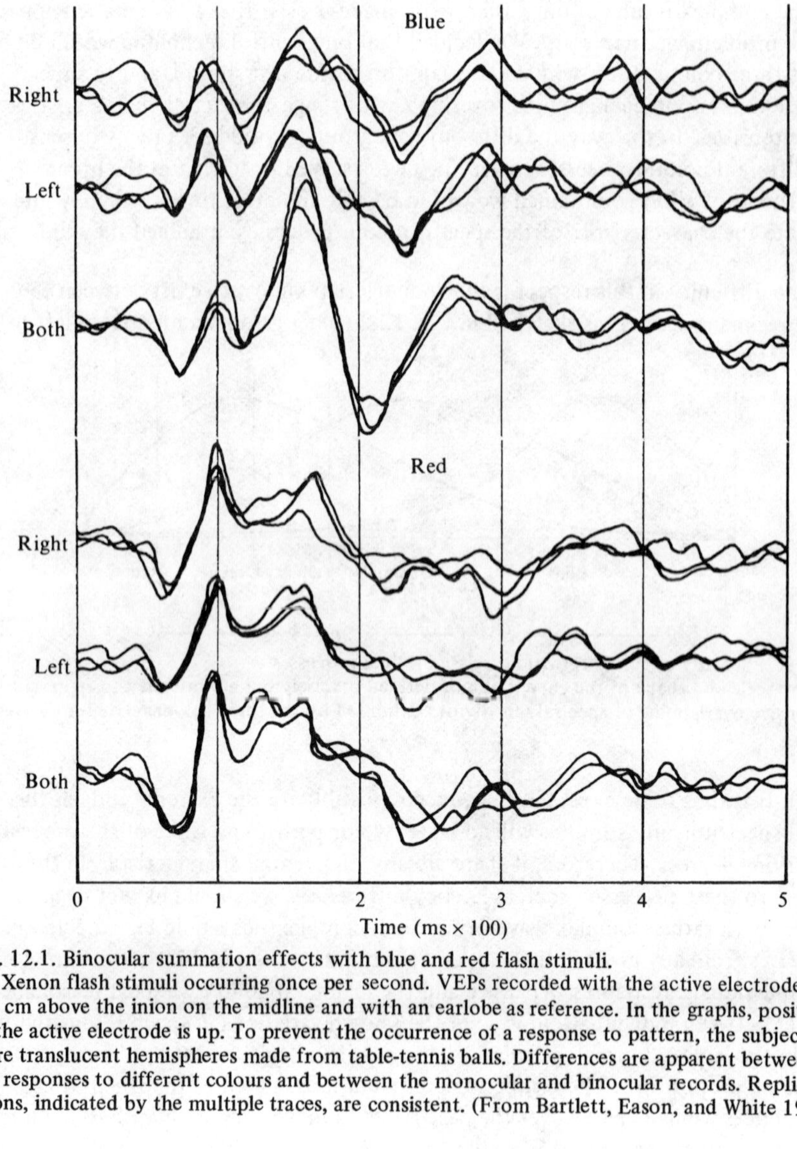

ig. 12.1. Binocular summation effects with blue and red flash stimuli.
Xenon flash stimuli occurring once per second. VEPs recorded with the active electrode 5 cm above the inion on the midline and with an earlobe as reference. In the graphs, positivity ' the active electrode is up. To prevent the occurrence of a response to pattern, the subject ore translucent hemispheres made from table-tennis balls. Differences are apparent between .e responses to different colours and between the monocular and binocular records. Replica- ions, indicated by the multiple traces, are consistent. (From Bartlett, Eason, and White 1968).

ut involved specific *components* of that waveform. Furthermore, the summation ffects appeared to occur at different times for different colours of stimulation.

A number of years later another extended series of studies was conducted in ur laboratory which confirmed that binocular colour stimulations obviously ccentuate the differences shown in monocular stimulation. This increased the nportance of finding ways to detect the specific effects of colour in the VEP.

Colour-evoked potentials

The complex results of our earlier work made it clear that a systematic approach to the problem was necessary. We decided that one fruitful technique would be to select three colour filters with no overlap, to provide test stimuli, and to superimpose them upon backgrounds covering a wide range of spectral characteristics and intensities. In this way the different backgrounds would selectively desensitize the different colour processes to varying degrees. We hoped that in the broad assortment of VEPs so obtained we would be able to detect trends which would indicate the characteristics of the specific colour processes, if indeed they did exist.

One difficulty in this respect is the wide overlap known to exist between the three retinal processes, as sketched in Fig. 12.2 (blue, green, and red from left to

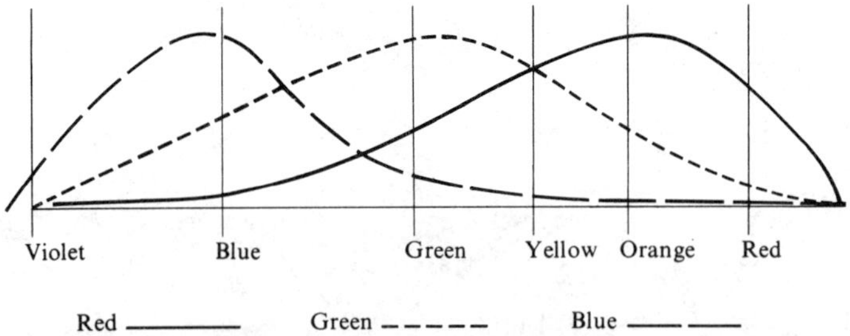

Fig. 12.2. Sensitivity curves for colour-related retinal processes.
The scale and shape of the curves are not defined precisely but are intended to represent the extensive overlapping of spectral sensitivities exhibited by the three colour-related processes.

right). It is thus to be expected that, except possibly for the extreme ends of the visual spectrum, any stimulus will activate two or perhaps all three of the processes to varying degrees. Therefore, if there are any differential characteristics in the VEP related to these processes, such as latency differences, we should expect to have to deal with rather complex waveforms. Such complexities would be expected in the VEPs from any given individual, compounded by the variability over time for that individual's responses. When we add the major variability we must reasonably expect between individuals, in view of the known variations in spectral sensitivity within the 'colour normal' population, the problem begins to take on somewhat awesome proportions. These sobering considerations, added to the frustrating experiences we had gained over the past 10 years in working with VEP to colour, helped determine new procedures for approaching the problem. Some of the things we have done will be seen by many as quite unorthodox, but we ask the concerned reader to reserve final judgment until the whole story is told.

General plan of study and methods

The general plan decided upon was as follows.

(a) A small number of colour-normal subjects, who would be available over an extended period, were tested under various specific stimulus and background conditions, with as many replications as necessary to establish that the types and trends found in the VEPs were reliable.

(b) One of these normal subjects was chosen for intensive study with various kinds of stimulus/background conditions. Such procedure is not at all unusual. A particularly good and stable 'chronic preparation' is traditional in neurophysiological research.

(c) The many background colours are useful for detecting subtle changes in a given subject's responses, but may not really be necessary for comparing individual differences. A single appropriately chosen background condition can now be used to study the VEP differences in many subjects in rather short sessions.

(d) Individuals with known colour anomalies were then tested in order to try to establish means of determining the relationships between abnormal VEP features and specific types of colour anomalies. The study of differential colour sensitivity within the colour-normal population is also relevant.

At the time of writing the stages (a)–(c) listed above have been carried out, and a good start has been made on stage (d).

Experimental procedure

The subjects were seated in a shielded room facing a window through which the stimuli were delivered. They wore goggles with frosted plastic lenses, which quite effectively removed any sharply focused patterns from the central visual field. For most of the work, a single electrode was placed about 2·5 cm above the inion on the midline of the scalp, with the two ears connected together as reference. The electrical activity was fed through an Offner DynoGraph Type R into a Nicolet 1072 averager. The frequency response of the amplifying system was 2–30 Hz. The responses were recorded with a Hewlett Packard 135C *x–y* plotter. The flashes were presented from a distance of 1·219 m (4 ft) by a Grass P-2 photo-stimulator. Fig. 12.3 shows the method of presenting the flashes and the background light. The intensity of the background light was changed by varying the voltage to a standard 60 W tungsten bulb. The resultant background intensity so obtained was measured by means of a Gamma T-500 telephotometer. The values for average luminescence (ft-L) given on the various records in this chapter refer to the brightness of the filament of the tungsten bulb measured through the background filter as viewed from the subject's regular position. The spectral characteristics of the filters chosen as stimuli and backgrounds are shown in Fig. 12.3. Wratten filters Nos. 92, 93, and 94 were selected for the red, green, and blue stimuli, respectively. The background filters were Corning glass filters, identified by the manufacturer as shown (R_2, A_2, Y_1, Y_2, etc.). All the series of backgrounds were not necessarily used with all subjects for every study, but are included in the figure to show the degree of selectivity available.

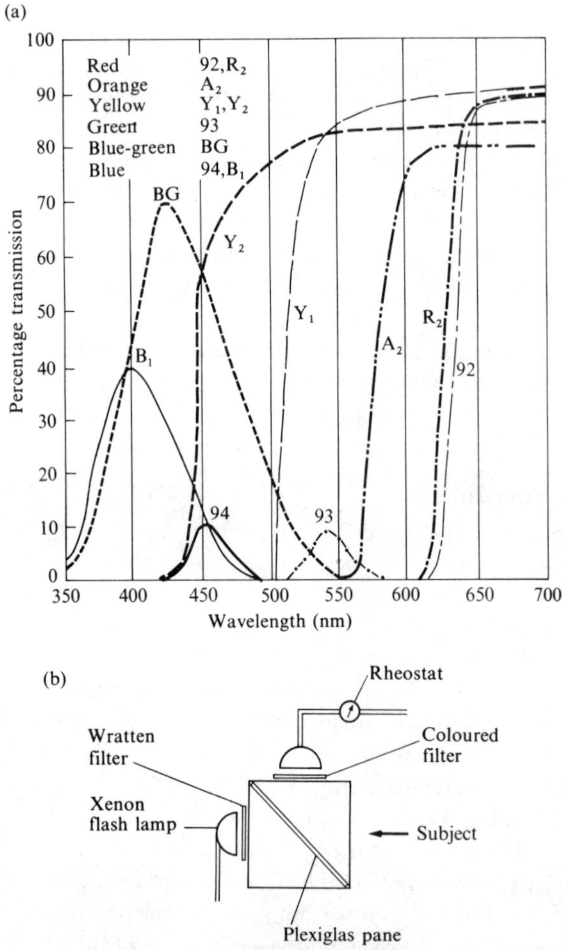

Fig. 12.3.(a) Spectral transmission characteristics of selected filters.

The Wratten filters numbered 92, 93, and 94 were used with the xenon flash lamp as the stimulus source. The remaining Corning glass filters (identified by the manufacturer as R_2, A_2, Y_1, Y_2, etc.) were used with a tungsten light to provide continuous background illumination. (b) Presentation apparatus. The subject viewed (arrow) a constant background light, the brightness of which could be adjusted by a rheostat, passed through a coloured filter and reflected off a pane of Plexiglas. Stimuli were presented by a xenon flash lamp passed through a Wratten filter and then through the Plexiglas pane. The lights from the two sources superimposed and by the subject who wore frosted lenses were viewed as a formless wash covering the entire visual field.

Results and discussion

Detailed study of subject R.K.

Examples of VEPs of this colour-normal individual to the three colour stimuli superimposed on five background colours are shown in Figs. 12.4–12.8. In each case the entire range available for the five backgrounds was used. A careful examination of the effects produced by the two backgrounds most limited in intensity range, the red and the blue (Figs. 12.4 and 12.8), will show that, even so, they provide valuable clues concerning the colour processes. The five sets of VEPs

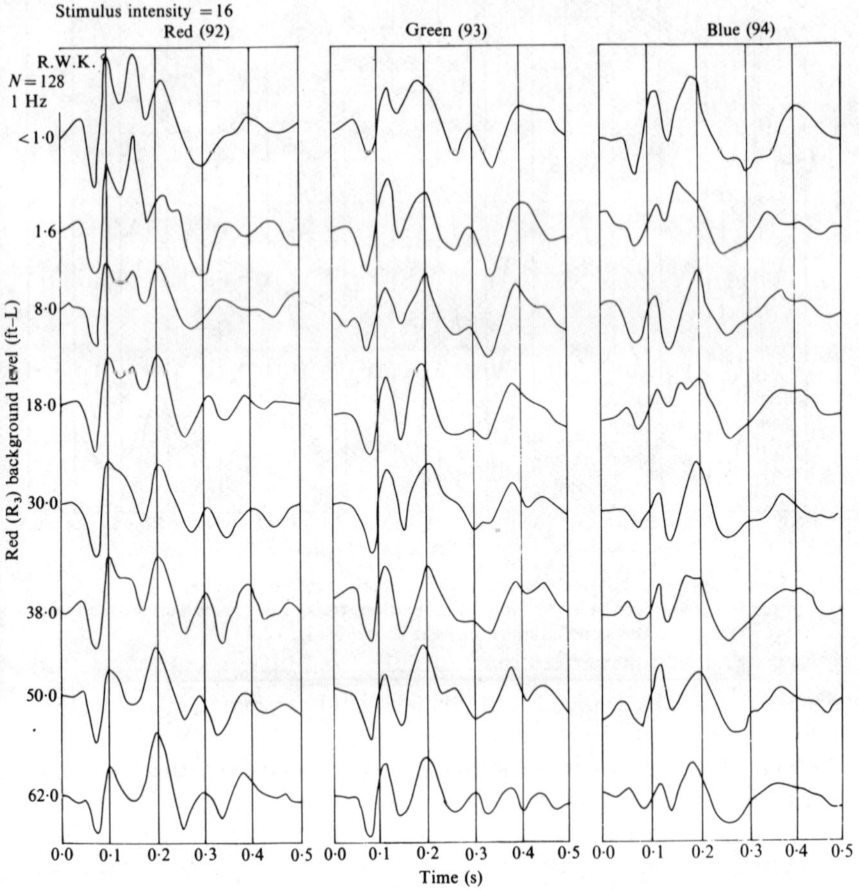

Fig. 12.4. Responses to flashes of different colours superimposed on red.

Colour-normal subject wearing frosted lenses viewed 128 presentations of flash stimuli occurring at once per second. Stimuli were passed through the Wratten filters indicated by number at the top of each column and a background light was used with the characteristics indicated at the left margin. The VEPs were recorded with the active electrode 2·5 cm above the inion on the midline and with the earlobes yoked as reference. Positive is up.

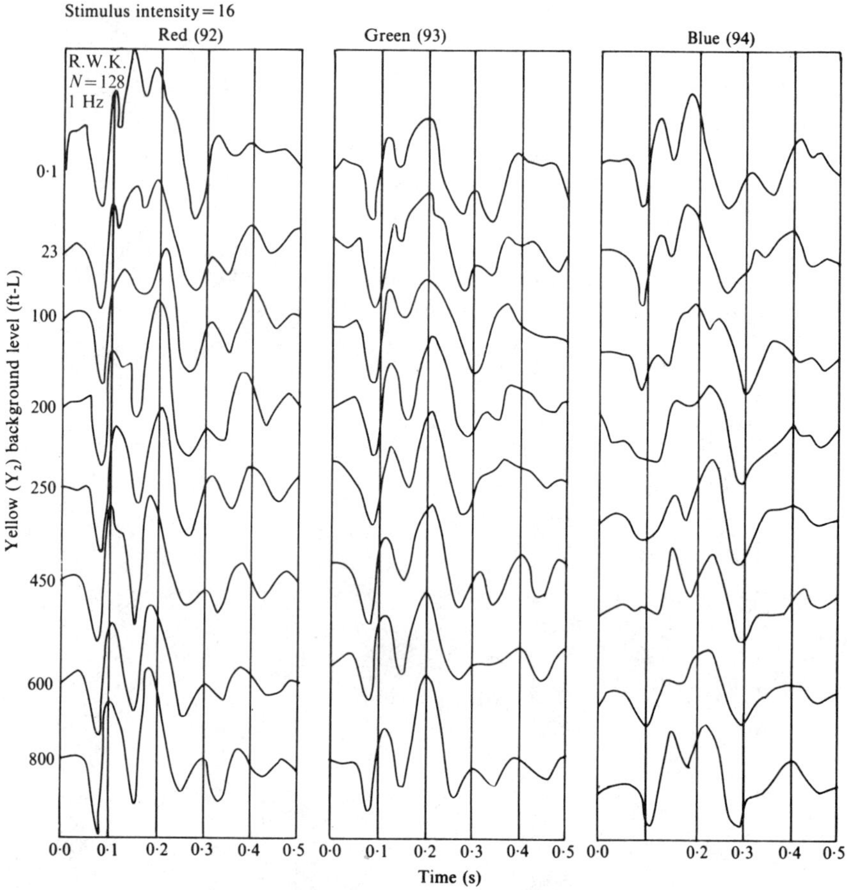

Fig. 12.5. Responses to flashes of different colours superimposed on yellow.
Except for the colour of the background illumination, these waveforms were evoked under the same circumstances as those of Fig. 12.4.

obtained in the dark background condition (< 0·1 fl-L) represent, of course, five replications.

There is a marked difference between the responses to the red stimulus and the green and blue stimuli. Considering VEP components between about 100 ms and 250 ms following stimulus onset, the responses to the red stimulus consist of three major positive components, while only two such components appear in the green and blue responses. It is also quite clear that any kind of background has a marked effect on the middle component of the red VEP, this effect being a function of the spectral and intensity characteristics of any chosen background condition. The variation in the VEP to the blue stimulus is also quite marked as a function of background conditions. The VEPs to the green stimuli appear to be least affected

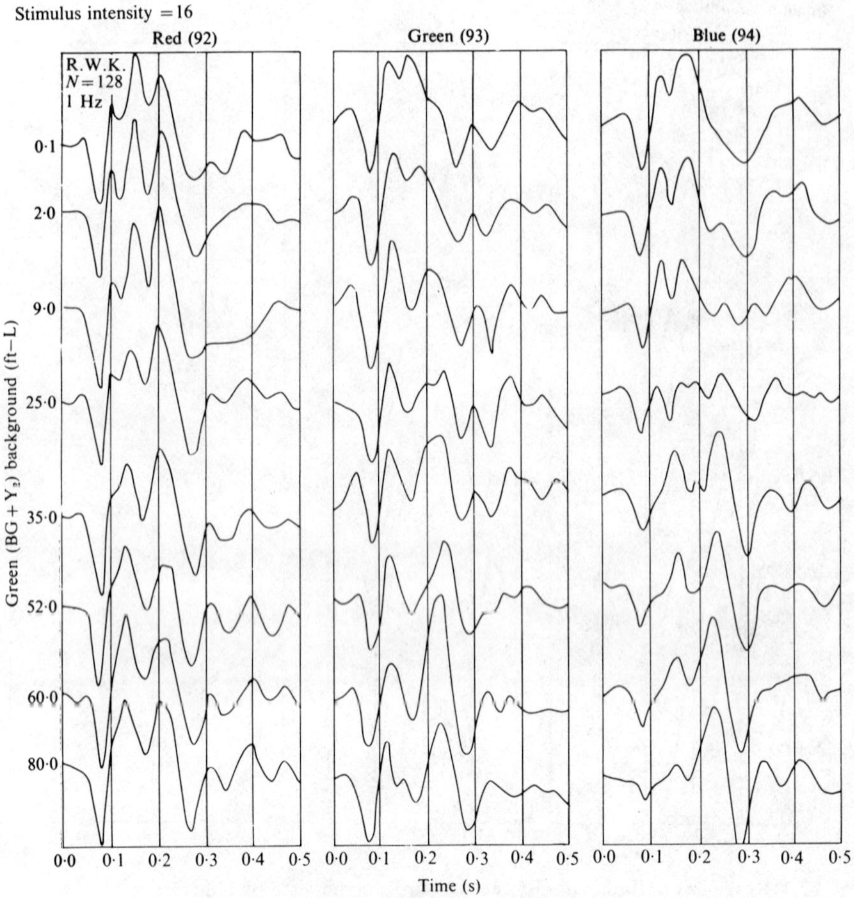

Fig. 12.6. Responses to flashes of different colours superimposed on green. Except for the colour of the background illumination, these waveforms were evoked under the same circumstances as those of Fig. 12.4.

by changes in the background conditions. It will be seen that there is a reason for this, since the green stimulus stimulates all three of the basic retinal processes.

The best approach at this point might be to examine the changes of the VEPs to a given stimulus when the backgrounds were varied systematically in order to secure information about the VEP components related to the basic colour processes.

The red response. When the blue and green processes are progressively desensitized by the various backgrounds, a rather regular VEP pattern to red begins to emerge. This consists of two positive peaks, one at about 100 ms and the next at around 190 ms after stimulus onset. These were tentatively identified as the 'red' components.

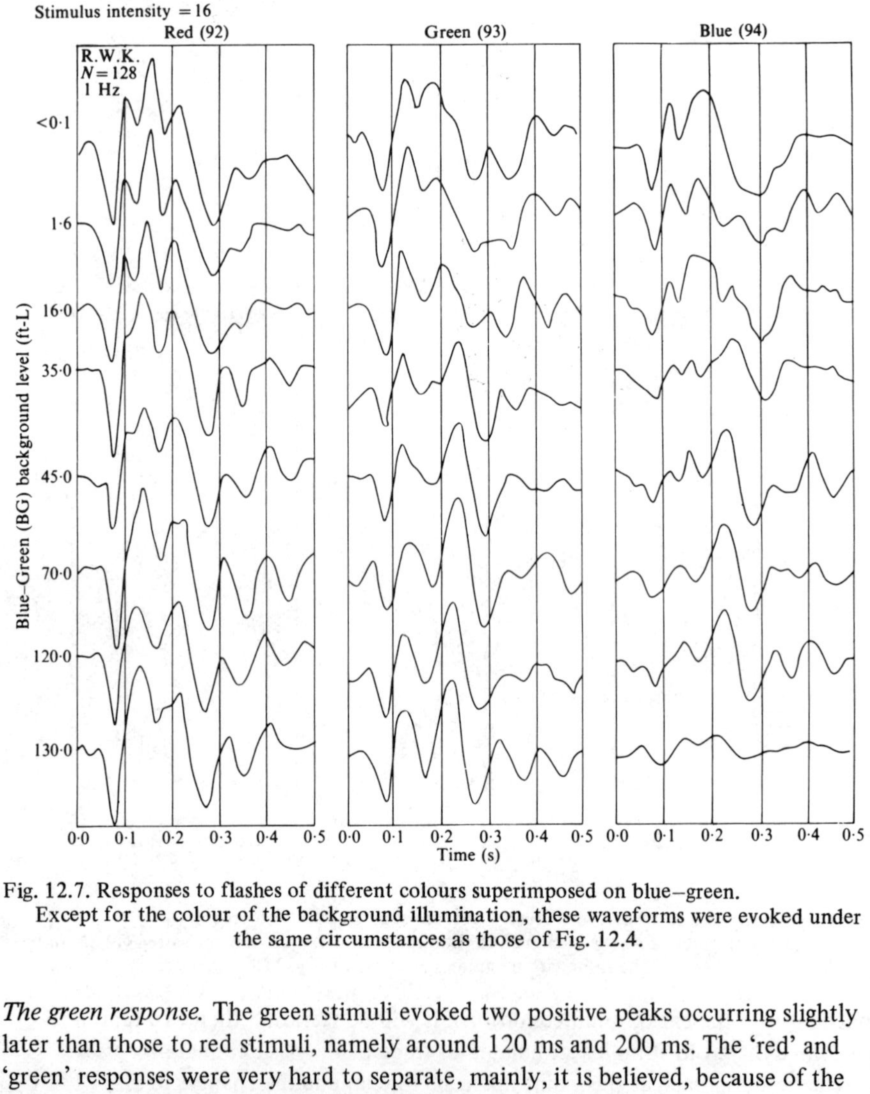

Fig. 12.7. Responses to flashes of different colours superimposed on blue–green. Except for the colour of the background illumination, these waveforms were evoked under the same circumstances as those of Fig. 12.4.

The green response. The green stimuli evoked two positive peaks occurring slightly later than those to red stimuli, namely around 120 ms and 200 ms. The 'red' and 'green' responses were very hard to separate, mainly, it is believed, because of the fact that the red and green retinal processes overlap so much.

The blue response. This may turn out to be the key to the whole situation. Since the blue process apparently has spectral characteristics quite different from the green and the red it appears possible to isolate its responses by desensitizing the red and green portion of the spectrum by a yellow background, consisting of red and green wavelengths. The other relevant factor here is that the blue stimulus, in the dark background situation, stimulates essentially only the blue and green processes. As we raise the level of the yellow background we should therefore

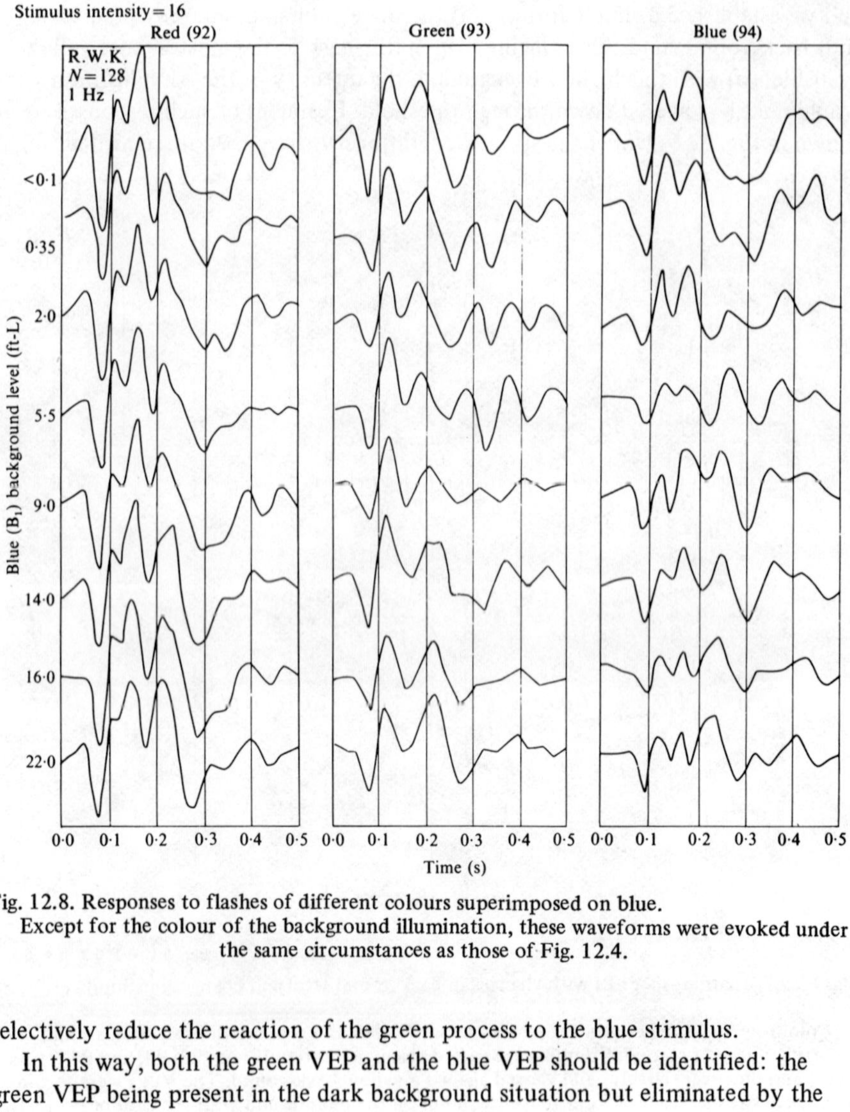

Fig. 12.8. Responses to flashes of different colours superimposed on blue. Except for the colour of the background illumination, these waveforms were evoked under the same circumstances as those of Fig. 12.4.

selectively reduce the reaction of the green process to the blue stimulus.

In this way, both the green VEP and the blue VEP should be identified: the green VEP being present in the dark background situation but eliminated by the increasing yellow background, while the blue VEP would become increasingly evident as the green VEP was removed by that increasing background.

Once identified in this way, the green VEP should be again differentiable from the red VEP, although both are strongly stimulated by wavelengths in the yellow–red portion of the spectrum.

The experiences we had with the various background colours convinced us that a yellow background was the logical one to use in any general testing programme, and we established a simple format: (a) the three colour stimuli presented upon four background conditions ranging from in the dark to the most intense yellow available; (b) with this highest background, the intensity of the stimulus flash would next be lowered down through threshold. Examples of such responses are shown in Fig. 12.9. Under the specific conditions we have used it seems that, for

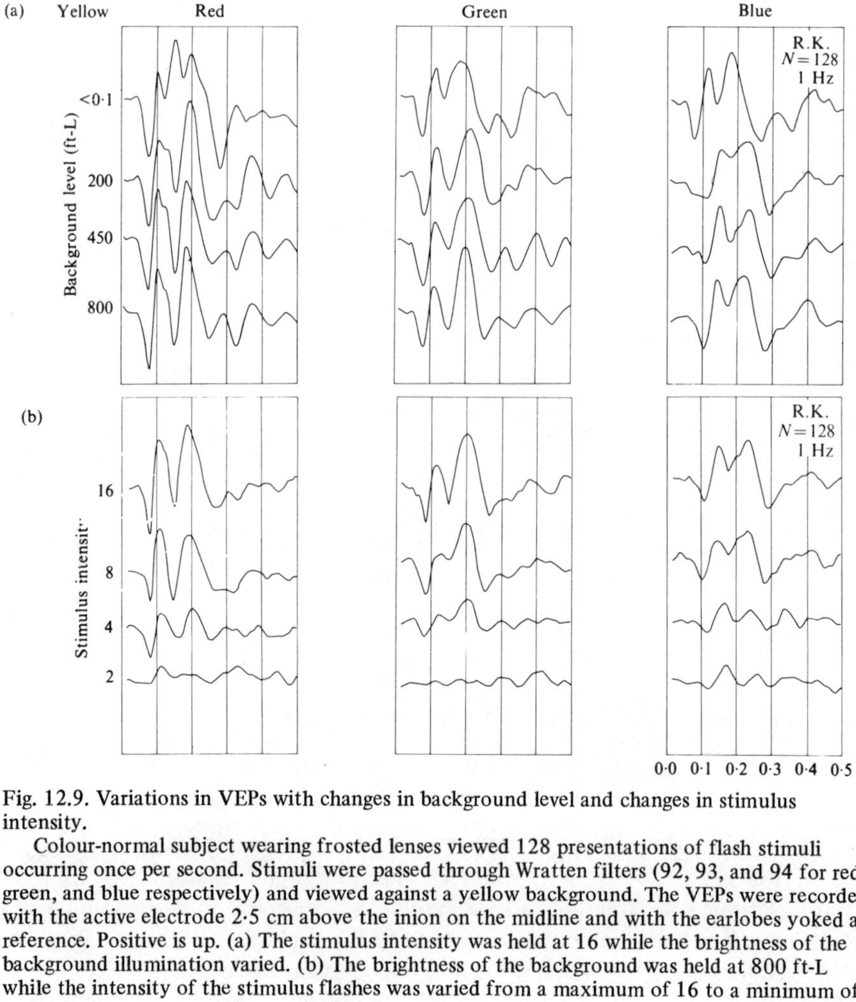

Fig. 12.9. Variations in VEPs with changes in background level and changes in stimulus intensity.

Colour-normal subject wearing frosted lenses viewed 128 presentations of flash stimuli occurring once per second. Stimuli were passed through Wratten filters (92, 93, and 94 for red, green, and blue respectively) and viewed against a yellow background. The VEPs were recorded with the active electrode 2·5 cm above the inion on the midline and with the earlobes yoked as reference. Positive is up. (a) The stimulus intensity was held at 16 while the brightness of the background illumination varied. (b) The brightness of the background was held at 800 ft-L while the intensity of the stimulus flashes was varied from a maximum of 16 to a minimum of 2.

the light-adapted situation, there are three sets of components, each consisting of two major peaks (Fig. 12.10). The red responses are the earliest, having positive peaks at around 100 ms and 190 ms, the green occurring slightly later at about 120 ms and 200 ms, and the blue with positive peaks at about 150 and 240 ms.

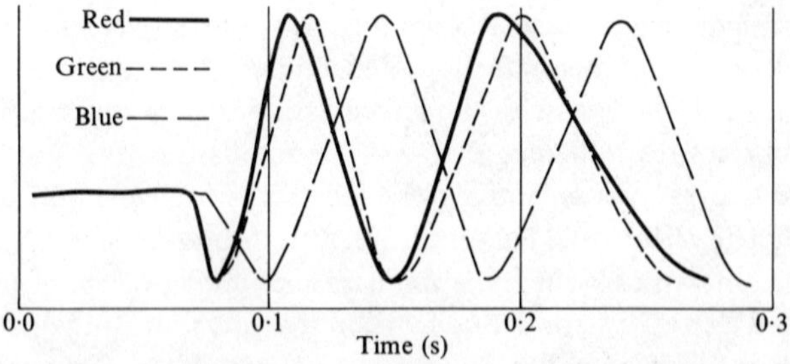

Fig. 12.10. Theoretical red, green, and blue components of the VEP to flashes of different colours.

This represents the type of recordings obtained over the occipital cortex, positive up, when the subject wears frosted lenses. With most stimuli, some contribution from each of the three components is likely to occur. By selectively adapting the eye of a subject by varying the spectral characteristics of the stimulus and of the continuous background light, one or more of the component contributions may be reduced and the more nearly pure response will be obtained. Note that the response to red precedes that to blue by 50–60 ms.

Note that we are concerned primarily with the relative (not the absolute) timing of these responses. It should be pointed out that the relative timing of the three response sets agrees with earlier determinations of the relative time-courses of the three basic colour processes (Piéron 1952).

Some of these earlier findings about time-course differentials for the different colours are discussed briefly by Mollon and Krauskopf (1973). More recent work employing techniques involving VEP (Krauskopf 1973) and responses made to paired flashes delivered simultaneously or sequentially (Krauskopf 1974, personal communication) have both indicated that a difference of 50 ms exists between the time-courses for red and blue stimuli. These data, based on rather different electrophysiological and behavioral techniques, are in close agreement with our own findings.

Possible subcortical elements in the VEP

Because of the recent evidence about brain-stem auditory responses which can be recorded from the vertex, it was necessary to enquire whether the sharp earlier peaks of VEPs to colour should be related to cortical activity. It is usually assumed when recording from the scalp over the occipital region, that only cortical reactions are being dealt with.

In our earlier work with coloured stimuli we had recorded both the VEP and the ERG (electrode taped to the lower eyelid) and noticed a sharp negative response at the lower eyelid about 100 ms after a red stimulus. Because of its temporal characteristics, we assumed that this marked reaction was not a retinal response, but its real nature was in question.

Since the negative response at the eye roughly coincided in time with a marked positive VEP component recorded at the occipital electrode, this indicated that the response might be generated at a point somewhere between the eye and the cortex. This led to the rather unorthodox technique of recording between the occipital cortex and the eye, with the linked earlobes as ground leads. It was also possible to subtract the VEP recorded with the standard cortex–ear leads from that recorded between cortex and eye. The results of such an approach are shown in Fig. 12.11. The differential colour effects were found to be much more marked than in our earlier work in which the standard monopolar occipital electrode was used, which led us to the tentative conclusion that the first components of the colour responses idealized in Fig. 12.10 represent activity at some subcortical

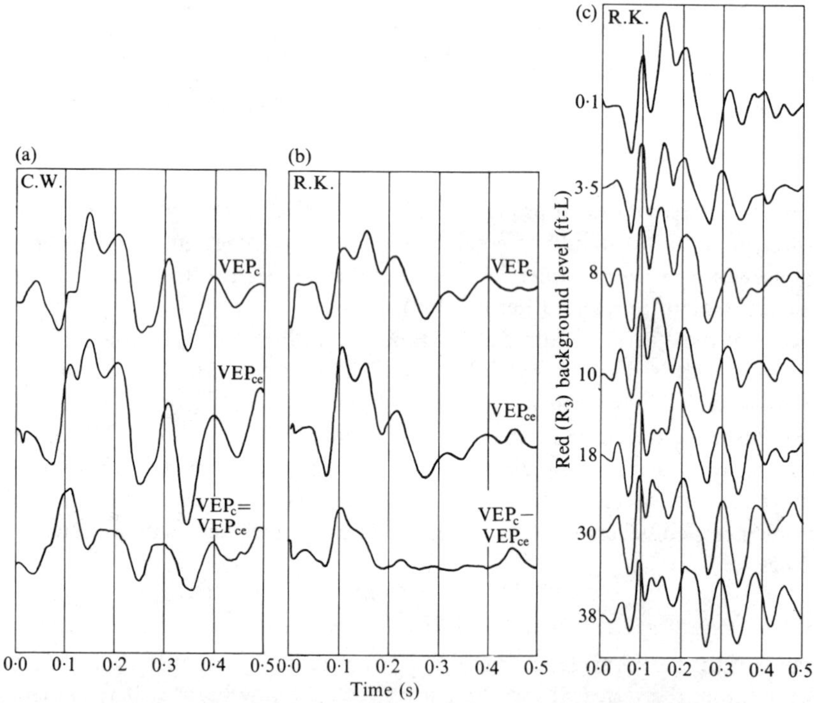

Fig. 12.11. (a) and (b) Responses to red recorded at the cortex and at the eye. Averaged responses of two colour-normal subjects wearing frosted lenses viewing 64 presentations of flash stimuli at intensity 16, occurring once per second, passed through a Wratten number 92 filter. The VEP$_c$ is defined as the category of VEP obtained with the active electrode 2·5 cm above the inion and with linked ear lobes as reference. Positive is up. The VEP$_{ce}$ was obtained with the same active electrode and with the reference at the eyelids. The third curve indicates the difference when the VEP$_c$ is subtracted from the VEP$_{ce}$. (c) Resolution of the central peak of the red response into two components. A colour-normal subject wearing frosted lenses, viewed 30 presentations of flash stimuli at intensity 4, occurring once per second, passed through a Wratten number 92 filter. Active electrode 2·5 cm above the inion on the mid-line and with the linked earlobes as reference. Positive is up. Note how, as the red background illumination is increased, the central peak of the dark condition response to red resolves itself into two distinct components.

level, possibly geniculate, while the second peaks are cortical. We have delayed publishing these results because the assumption of brain-stem components could be met with scepticism. But we have replicated the studies many times with many variations, always with the same results.

The objection usually raised to the interpretation offered here is that the latency of the processes may be too large for a subcortical mechanism. A number of observations can be made which make this objection less formidable. First, we are discussing the latency of certain positive peaks, chosen because they have been most easy to detect, but which could represent the later phases of the relevant processes. Secondly, the electrophysiological response to visual flash presentation may extend over a considerable period of time and will reach a peak considerably after the onset of the stimulus. Recording directly from the lateral geniculate nucleus, De Valois, Smith, Karoly, and Kitai (1958) found that a burst of spikes would begin 40–100 ms after stimulus onset (see also Sheppard 1968). Thirdly, a close examination of the records indicates that each positive peak considered follows a smaller negative peak occurring about 30 ms earlier. The beginning of the negativity leading to these peaks in turn occurs about 30 ms earlier than that. In other words, we are probably dealing with processes that commence about 30–70 ms following the onset of stimulation. Even earlier estimates of the beginnings of such processes will be obtained when using higher frequency cut-off. Our techniques are obviously too crude to determine where the various processes may be occurring, and direct studies of higher primates which have a colour system similar to man are called for.

Detailed description of the response to red in one normal subject

A number of workers have commented on the distinctive characteristics of the response to a red stimulus, as compared to the responses to green and blue, which are reported as being rather similar. Presumably such observations were made with the subjects in a darkened room (cf. VEP in the top rows in Fig. 12.4–12.8). All the colour normal subjects studied have produced a VEP to the red stimulus in the dark similar to those shown for subject R.K., with, of course, the expected variations in the relative amplitudes of the three major positive peaks.

At high background level, essentially the first and third positive peaks remain. We looked more closely at the marked positive peak, occurring about 150 ms after red stimulus onset, which is so much affected by variations in background conditions. Even though it was not feasible to have identical ranges of brightness levels for the various background colours, interesting features can be observed by studying all the conditions, keeping in mind the great variations in absolute background levels.

First, the middle peak does not relate to a single process but represents the interaction of two components, as shown by the red background series (Fig. 12.11(c)). Secondly, the middle peak does not just drop out as the background is increased, but instead appears to move forward in time, eventually merging with the first peak. There is reason to believe that only the first of the two components making up the middle peak actually does merge with the first major peak, however. For example, in the yellow background series the waveform has changed markedly between the 10 ft-L and 50 ft-L levels. The middle peak is now a very small bump while the first major peak has broadened noticeably, presumably because the first component of the second peak has merged with it. Further evidence for this can be seen at the two highest background levels, where a shoulder begins to appear on the trailing edge of the first major peak and the first peak itself becomes much narrower again.

In the case of the green and blue–green backgrounds, increasing the background level leads to a marked decrease in the latency of the second peak, with no noticeable decrease in amplitude. In the green background situation we did not have high enough intensity for the two peaks to merge completely. At the highest level available, 80 ft-L, the first major peak was still to be seen as a shoulder on the leading edge of the combined peak. With the highest blue–green background available, 130 ft-L, the merging was complete, with a single, much-broadened peak.

When considering the nature of the middle peak, it must be remembered that the rather broad-spectrum colour stimuli used will activate at least two, and probably all three basic colour processes to varying degrees and therefore elicit rather complex responses except under certain extreme stimulus/background situations. Assuming the red background to selectively desensitize the red process, and the stimulus light to stimulate all three processes, we might expect a point to be reached, as the red background was increased, when all three processes were activated nearly equally. With the highest level of red background used in Fig. 12.11(c) the middle peak now consists of two components occurring at the times which have, by other means, been related to green and blue components respectively.

The changes in latency noted for the middle peak under variations in backgrounds of blue–green, green, and yellow lead to the same conclusion. The first component of the middle peak reacts as if it were related to the green process since it finishes in the high background conditions, at the relative time of occurrence assigned to the green process in other experiments.

If the above analysis is correct, we have discovered some unusual attributes of this 'green process': the speed of reaction of this process, when stimulated by red light, is apparently accelerated up to a point, by increasing the amount of green light in the background and with no marked decrement in amplitude. Beyond that point, however, the amplitude begins to fall off, leaving only the responses of the red process itself at the highest background levels and when the intensity of the red stimulus is reduced. A similar phenomenon was noted for the blue response: as higher levels of backgrounds containing blue or green wavelengths were used the blue response decreased markedly in latency, until approaching threshold conditions.

Preliminary work with colour-weak subjects

As we felt fairly sure about the ways in which the VEPs of the colour-normal subjects vary under the various conditions, we studied VEP of subjects with various types of anomalies.

The results more than justified our expectation that we might find gross differences between their responses and those of our colour normals. Even more interesting, perhaps, is the fact that there are such marked individual differences between the VEPs of colour-weak subjects nominally belonging to the same class of disorder. Some general comments will be made about the VEPs of three volunteers reporting red deficiencies (Fig. 12.12). Identical results of each subject on the Ishihara pseudo-isochromatic charts indicated a profound colour disorder, possibly protanopic or red-weak condition. On the anomaloscope all three subjects accepted every combination, even the purest red and green, as matching a standard yellow light source. The variation in the setting of the intensity level indicated a deficiency to the red end of the spectrum. The VEPs revealed some rather remarkable features which would indicate that the colour deficiencies were quite different in the three cases, a finding which would have been impossible with conventional testing.

Colour-weakness or colour-blindness may involve different stages in the visual system: the retinal receptors for particular colours may be either absent or not functioning because of lack of the necessary pigments or neurones; neurones in visual pathways or in higher centres may have failed to develop, may have degenerated, or may be blocked and non-functioning. Any or all of these defects may combine in a given case of colour deficiency. Thus a red-weak individual may differ from another red-weak individual in the mechanism of the defect, even though the resultant is the same.

Response to the red stimulus. In the dark background none of the three subjects exhibited the three positive components of latencies between 100 ms and 200 ms, which typifies the normal response to red, and none of them showed much evidence of the first red peak itself.

As shown in Fig. 12.12, subject C.J.'s VEP seemed to consist almost entirely of the green response, and this continued to be the case as the yellow background was increased in intensity. Subject J.S. showed a massive green response in the dark, but the presence of the background markedly reduced its amplitude. As the green component was progressively eliminated another component became more and more prominent. Its timing and its reaction to the yellow background strongly suggest that it is the blue component (see later).

Subject R.W.'s in-dark reaction to the red stimulus showed little evidence of the first part of the red component (positive peak at 100 ms), but this component seemed to appear sporadically as the background was increased. The interesting thing about this subject, however, was that his responses to all the colours showed little if any positive peaking around 200 ms.

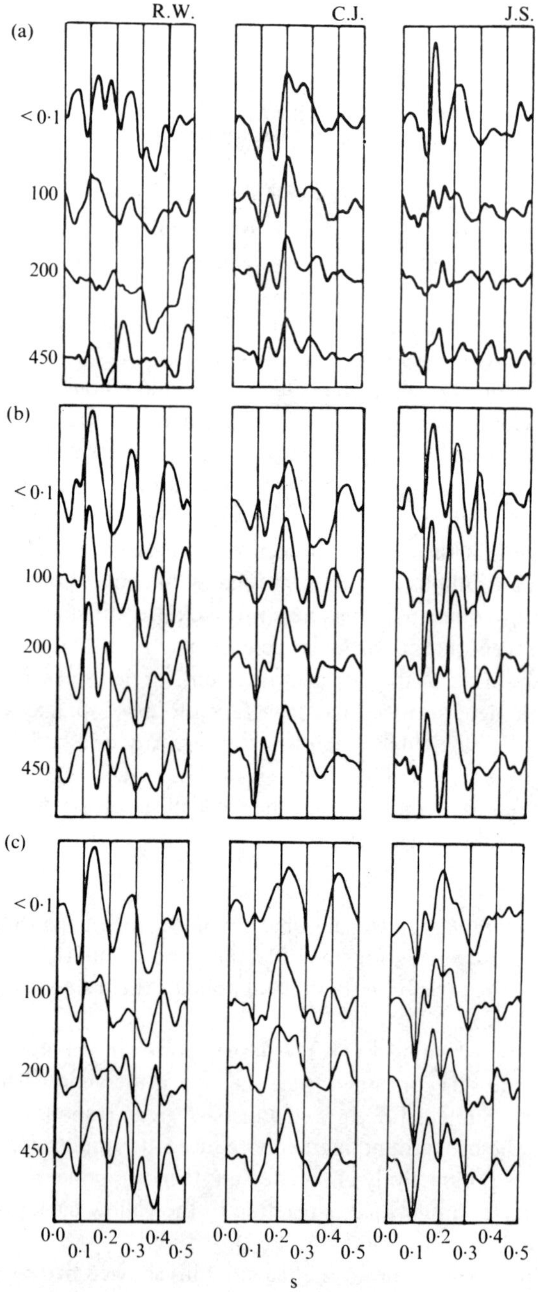

Fig. 12.12. Averaged responses of three colour-weak (protanope) subjects wearing frosted lenses, viewing 64 presentations of flash stimuli at intensity 16, occurring once per second. (a) Red stimulus (Wratten filter 92). (b) Green stimulus (93). (c) Blue stimulus (94). The yellow background level of illumination varied throughout each session as indicated on the left margin. The active electrode was 2·5 cm above the inion and linked earlobes were the reference. Positive is up.

Response to the green stimulus. The three subjects again showed different response patterns. J.S. showed strong green components which were maintained over the entire range of background intensities. What are interpreted to be elements of the blue component begin to be noticeable at the highest background levels.

Subject C.J. provided a surprise in that his in-dark VEP to green resembled the colour-normal subject's VEP to red, including the sharp positive peak at 100 ms and the three-peak pattern. If this did indicate a red response to the green stimulus the effect was not a very strong one, since it was eliminated by the lowest level of the yellow background used. What remained appeared to be a summation of strong green and blue components. The marked differences in these VEP patterns for subjects C.J. and J.S. at the higher background levels could be accounted for by assuming that J.S.'s blue process was stimulated relatively little by the green stimulus.

Subject R.W.'s in-dark response was a striking demonstration of his relative lack of positive activity at 200 ms. With the introduction of the yellow background a positive peak occurred in that time-region, but it was different from those in our colour normals, and also in the other two subjects, being narrower and peaking earlier. Our tentative conclusion is that it represents the first peak of the blue component. The great variability shown by this subject's VEPs does not allow us to say much about the positive activity around 100 ms. The relatively early beginning of the positive process, as compared with the other two subjects, could mean that there is some red activity represented. The predominant aspect however, would be the green component.

Responses to the blue stimulus. Subject J.S.'s VEPs to blue with an increasing level of yellow background followed the general course observed in our colour-normal subject (Figs. 12.4–12.8). The in-dark response consisted of strong green and blue components. The increasing yellow background selectively desensitized the green process, leading to a gradual diminution of its component in the VEP (peaks at about 120 and 200 ms) and uncovering a relatively pure blue component.

Subject C.J. presented a very interesting pattern of VEPs to blue, as if his green process was little affected by the blue light. The in-dark response hinted at a slight red response at 100 ms. As the background was introduced this small red response was eliminated and a small hint of the primary peak of the green process was seen, which soon gave way to the blue component. R.W. again showed a lack of positive peaking at 200 ms and, once the green and red processes were fairly well eliminated by desensitization with the yellow background, he began to show the normal blue response pattern.

The very marked individual differences in VEP that we have just considered are important, and may correlate with subtle differences in the perception of colour. It also shows that the seemingly gross techniques used may after all be appropriate for the study of such subtleties. Reasoning from the concepts developed in our study of colour-normal subjects, a number of interesting and testable hypotheses concerning the nature of colour processes of these 3 individuals may be advanced.

First, subject J.S. showed none of the VEP components we have designated as red-related, which suggests that he has no basic peripheral red process and that the defect must occur at the retina or at some early stage in the processing of colour vision. On the other hand, subject C.J. appeared to have a quite weak peripheral red process which failed to be detected when the red stimulus was presented, and became manifest when the green stimulus was presented in the dark background (but not in the yellow background). It might be assumed that subject J.S. has a green process which is minimally sensitive in the red portion of the spectrum. A marked green response is elicited by the red stimulus in the dark background but it is eliminated in the yellow background which contains green wavelengths. If we also assume a blue process having a rather broad spectral response for this subject, we can understand that with little if any red process and with a green process very insensitive in the red region, the introduction of the yellow background might well lead to the appearance of primarily a blue response to the red stimulus. By the same reasoning C.J. would have a nearly normal green process and thus would continue to give what we would refer to as a green response to the red stimuli even as the yellow background was increased.

More information about the green process in J.S. and C.J. may be surmised by studying blue stimuli, to which J.S. gave strong green responses, even when the yellow background was increased. On the other hand, subject C.J. showed little green response to the blue stimuli. This could mean that the spectral characteristics of the green process were different for the two subjects, being more sensitive toward the longer wavelengths in C.J. and more sensitive toward the shorter wavelengths in J.S. It was earlier noted that all 3 of our subjects appeared to have 'normal' blue responses.

Consider now our third subject, R.W., who differs from the others mainly in the lack of positive VEP component around 200 ms. In our normal subject, and also in J.S. and C.J., there was a marked positive peak at 200 ms, especially in the in-dark situation. Detailed studies of the normal subject indicated that this broad positive wave was probably made up of the secondary parts of the red and the green components and the primary part of the blue component (Figs. 12.4–12.8). Subject R.W. exhibits the primary blue component (Fig. 12.12 for the green stimulus). Therefore it is assumed that the marked difference in the response of R.W. is because *his response lacks the secondary peaks of the red and the green components.* In an earlier section it was suggested that the primary and secondary peaks of the various components could represent activities at different levels in the visual system. It is hypothesized that the absence of positive peaks at 200 ms in R.W. indicates that the activity of the red and green processes did not, for some reason, go beyond some lower level in the visual system, between the brain-stem and the cortex. If so, the techniques we are discussing might thus be able to differentiate between colour-processing activities at various levels in the visual system, a view which should be further tested by more direct methods.

Preliminary work on recording at the eye

The marked enhancement of the primary peaks of the colour components by recording with a reference electrode on the eye (see above) has led to our renewed interest in recording at the eye itself. This technique gave provocative preliminary results. Fig. 12.13(a) illustrates the effect of stimulating only one eye.

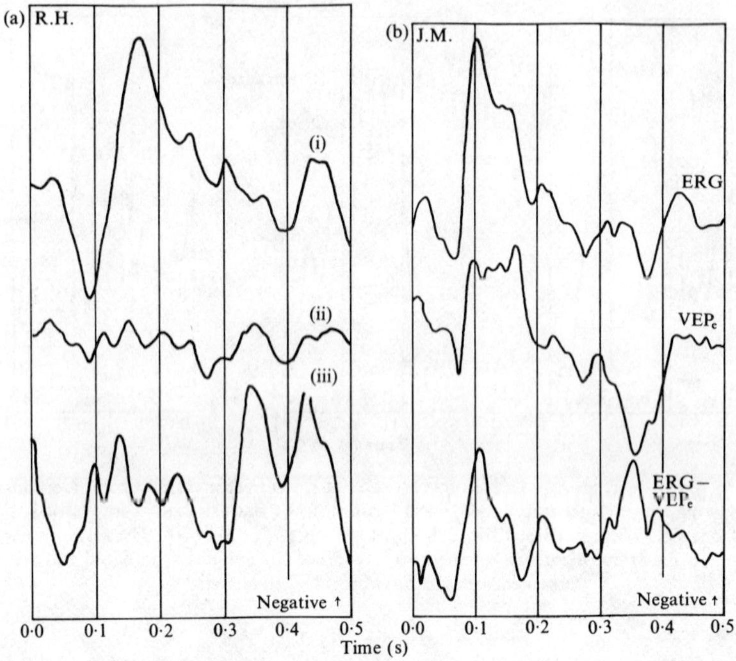

Fig. 12.13. (a) Selected responses recorded at the stimulated and non-stimulated eye. Waveforms (i) and (ii) are VEP to blue stimuli recorded at the stimulated and non-stimulated eyes respectively. Waveform (iii) is the VEP to green stimuli recorded at the non-stimulated eye. (b) Averaged responses to red recorded at the stimulated and non-stimulated eye. A colour-normal subject viewed, through frosted lenses, 64 presentations of flash stimuli at intensity 16, occurring once per second, passed through Wratten filter 92. The ERG was obtained with the active electrode on the lower eyelid of the stimulated eye. The VEP$_e$ was obtained with the active electrode on the lower eyelid of the non-stimulated (occluded) eye. The reference point for both of these recordings was the earlobes. The third waveform represents the differences when the VEP$_e$ is subtracted from the ERG. Negative is up.

The stimulated eye produces a classic ERG, with the marked positive B-wave (down in this figure) and the ensuing slow C- and D-waves. The response recorded at the non-stimulated eye is strikingly different and shows none of the characteristics of the ERG produced by green light. Instead, a number of negative peaks, from about 100 ms to a little beyond 200 ms, follow stimulus onset. The third record represents the response elicited at the non-stimulated eye by the green stimulus in the dark background. For the latter the gain was doubled to show the details more clearly.

Fig. 12.14 presents the responses recorded at subject R.H.'s non-stimulated eye for the three coloured stimuli in the dark condition. Subject R.H. suffers from a

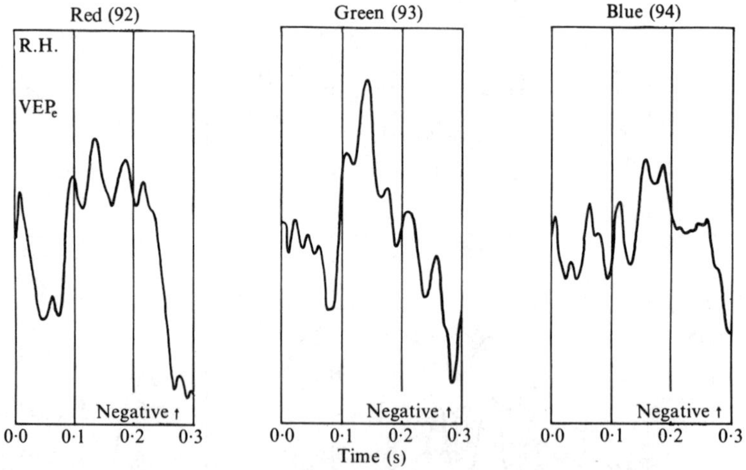

Fig. 12.14. Averaged responses to colours recorded at the non-stimulated eye of a colour-weak subject viewing, through frosted lenses, 64 presentations of flash stimuli at intensity 16, occurring once per second, passed through Wratten filters 92, 93, or 94. The responses were obtained with the active electrode on the lower eyelid of the eye not stimulated and with linked earlobes as reference. Negative is up.

marked red–green confusion. Obvious similarities are seen in the responses to red and green which differ markedly from that to blue. The last example shows the different responses to the red stimulus in the dark as recorded at the stimulated and the non-stimulated eyes. The records in Fig. 12.13(b) again show that the complexities of the response are more apparent when recording at the non-stimulated eye. The third record represents the difference between the first two response patterns. The marked difference shown in the amplitude of the peak at about 100 ms is tentatively interpreted to indicate that at least part of the activity that that peak represents is taking place in the stimulated eye itself.

Discussion

In our work we now refer to three major categories of VEP:

(a) VEP$_c$: monopolar occipital active electrode, using connected earlobes as reference.

(b) VEP$_e$: active electrode placed on the lower eyelid of non-stimulated eye, with connected earlobes as reference. This recording can be differentiated from the electroretinogram (ERG) wherein the active electrode is placed on the lower eyelid of the stimulated eye.

(c) VEP_{ce}: bipolar arrangement with one active electrode over the occipital region and the other placed on the lower eyelid of the non-stimulated eye, with connected earlobes as ground. This rather unorthodox method was developed in order to analyse certain VEP components recordable at both cortex and eye level, which may relate to processes occurring in the visual system between the retina and the cortex. The various techniques discussed should be tested with more traditional electrophysiological approaches in a primate having colour vision similar to that of man.

The working hypotheses evolved have come from the data obtained in the various studies and are not derived from any specific theoretical position on the topics in question. Any rather unusual hypotheses put forth were made necessary by the consistent appearance of corresponding trends in the VEP patterns. Sometimes these patterns indicate things that we would feel more comfortable to ignore. One such phenomenon is that under certain stimulus conditions in a subject with normal colour vision, the latencies of the green component of the VEP to red, and the blue component in the VEP to blue decrease markedly as the background intensity is increased (Figs. 12.4–12.8). These shifts in latencies do not occur in the VEP to green for this subject.

When describing this unusual behaviour of the supposed green component in the VEP to the red stimulus it was first suggested that some potentiating effect was taking place. That this is not the whole story is indicated by our subjects with colour anomalies in whom the green component stimulated by the red stimulus peaked at about 120 ms and did not change latency as the background was increased (Fig. 12.13). This suggests that *the green process is inhibited when there is a strong red process.* As the strength of the red reaction is diminished by an increasing background level of yellow light, this inhibitory effect is gradually reduced and the activity of the green component moves forward in time. In those subjects having little or no red reaction to start with the green response will occur at the earlier time, even in the dark background.

The responses of subject C.J. to the green stimulus is consistent with this hypothesis (Fig. 12.13). When a marked red VEP component is evoked in the dark background the second peak, assumed to be part of the green component, is significantly delayed. When the red response is diminished by the background, the green component occurs much earlier in time.

This 'primacy effect' appears to be quite marked in the interaction of the red and green systems. A similar kind of relationship might be functioning between the green and blue systems, thus accounting for the marked decrease in the latency of the blue component as the yellow background is increased (which would reduce the green response). If these results are verified this phenomenon could be of importance to colour vision theory. For the present we can only let the records speak for themselves.

Summary

Specific components of the VEP can be related to three basic colour processes. For each colour process, specific components may be related to different levels in the visual system. The three basic processes are not completely independent, since under certain conditions marked inhibitory effects were noted, tentatively called the 'primacy effect'. Preliminary work indicates that a meaningful objective colour-vision VEP test might be developed. One major advantage of such a test would be that it might not only describe the altered colour-world of a subject but might also suggest the possible source of the defect. Subtle individual differences, for example between the two eyes of a given subject, might be studied by the approaches described.

13. Evoked potential correlates of contingent after-effects and the problem of the McCollough effect

J. G. MAY
Department of Psychology, University of New Orleans

Since the seventeenth century, the relationship between parametric manipulations of physical stimuli and subjective experience has been studied in psychophysics. Much of today's theorizing is based on sensory physiology which focuses on the relationship between systematic variations in physical stimuli and physiological responses of the sensory systems in animal preparations. Modern experimental approaches to human experience represent an exciting merger of psychophysics and sensory physiology. Most of the chapters in this book can be considered to be the offspring of that marriage. Like most progeny, they often exhibit more of a resemblance to one or the other parent. This chapter deals with some of the conceptual and methodological problems involved in obtaining VEP correlates of a class of perceptual phenomena which are of central interest in current vision research.

Contour and colour contingent after-effects

Various forms of phenomenological report and recent experiments employing adaptation have been aimed at understanding how two dimensions, e.g. contour and colour are integrated or combined within the sensory system. McCollough (1965) first described what is generally termed a contingent after-effect, which was produced by observers adapting to alternating presentation of chromatic gratings in orthogonal orientations for 5–10 min. After viewing, say, red vertical gratings and green horizontal ones, the observers were shown a compound inspection figure which contained achromatic gratings oriented horizontally and vertically. Most of the subjects reported perceiving the lighted horizontal bars to be of a pinkish hue, while they reported that the lighted vertical bars were greenish. The McCollough effect is thus an orientation-specific complementary-coloured after-effect.

This phenomenon differs from the traditional Hering after-image which is viewed against a homogeneous background of light and in which the negative after-

Visual evoked potentials in man: new developments (ed. J. E. Desmedt), pp. 273–85. Clarendon Press, Oxford 1977.

image requires fixation of the adapting stimulus or very intense stimulation. The McCollough effect, however, can be obtained without fixation of a specific point in the pattern and with low-contrast stimuli. It also requires test gratings as opposed to homogeneous inspection fields. Harris and Gibson (1968) showed that the McCollough effect could be obtained by randomly presenting the adapting gratings in orthogonal orientations to different points on the retina. This procedure precluded the formation of the traditional negative after-images. Murch (1969) also demonstrated that, while Hering after-images generated by adaptation to orthogonally oriented chromatic gratings obey Emmert's law,* McCollough after-effects do not. From such considerations most investigators attempted to explain the McCollough effect in terms of brain mechanisms rather than early retinal processes, although they have been reticent to speculate as to the precise locus of the mechanisms. The evidence regarding the processing of achromatic grating orientation (Campbell, Kulikowski, and Levinson 1966; Sekuler, Rubin, and Cushman 1968; Blakemore and Campbell 1969) and spatial frequency (Pantle and Sekuler 1968; Blakemore and Campbell 1969) argues quite convincingly for a cortical processing site. Single-unit findings (Campbell *et al.* 1969; Campbell, Cooper, Robsen, and Sachs 1969) tend to support this hypothesis. Following this lead, some investigators have hypothesized that contour-contingent after-effects can be explained in terms of specific chromatic input channels to this same class of neurones.

In a recent study (May 1972), using a cross-adaptation psychophysical design, observers were asked to adapt (for 15 s) to square-wave gratings which varied in terms of orientation (horizontal, vertical, or oblique) or wavelength (620 nm or 530 nm). After adaptation, they were asked to adjust a vertical test grating of red or green to threshold. The results indicated that threshold elevations were present only under conditions involving adaptation gratings which were the same as the test grating in both wavelength and orientation (Fig. 13.1). In another experiment, spatial frequency was varied instead of orientation, and the results were similar. Only when the adapting grating and the test grating were alike in wavelength and spatial frequency was a threshold elevation observed. Thus it appeared that the orientation- and size-specific mechanisms delineated using achromatic stimuli could be selectively adapted to light of different wavelengths. Coltheart (1973) has recently argued that colour-selective cortical neurones are monocularly driven and cites data reported by Hubel and Wiesel (1968) as suggestive of this fact. He further nominates 'higher-order hypercomplex cells' located in cortical areas beyond area 17 as likely candidates. To date, there has been no definitive micro-electrode work aimed at answering this question and very little previous single-unit data bear directly upon it.

Since McCollough's initial report, numerous replications and new versions of the orientation-specific effects have been reported (Harris and Gibson 1968; Murch

* Emmert's law states that an increase in the distance of the background results in an increase in the size of the after-image in direct proportion to the square of the distance.

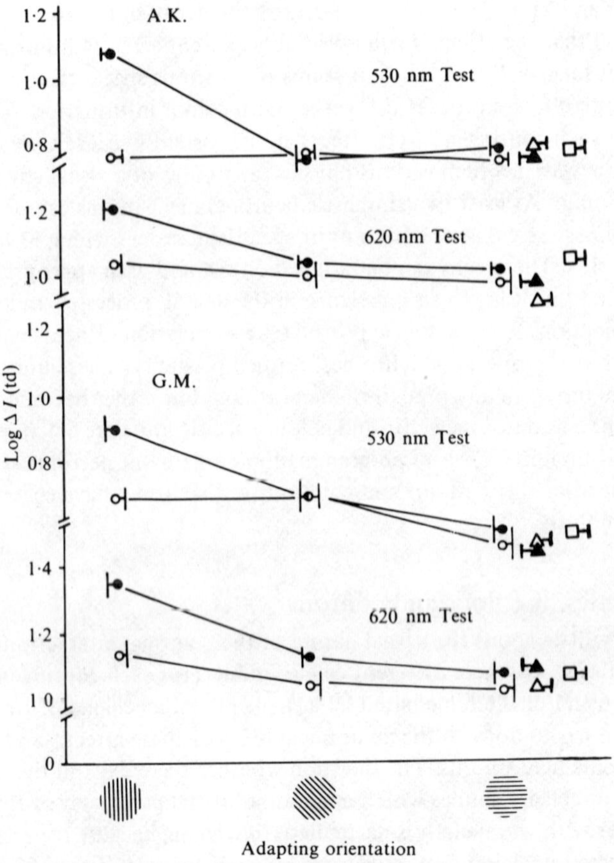

Fig. 13.1. Log ΔI at threshold for vertical green and red test gratings following adaptation to gratings of the same (closed circles) and different (open circles) wavelength as a function of the orientation of the adapting grating. Thresholds for red and green vertical gratings prior to adaptation (squares) and after adaptation to homogeneous fields of the same (closed triangles) and different (open triangles) wavelengths are also shown. Vertical bars adjacent to each data point denote ±1 S.E. (From May 1972.)

1968; Harris and Barkow 1969; Stromeyer 1969; Harris 1969; Murch 1969; Fidell 1970; Murch 1972; Stromeyer 1972; Murch and Hirsch 1972; MacKay and MacKay 1973). In addition, Held and Shattuck (1971) have reported a colour-contingent tilt after-effect; Riggs (1973) has demonstrated curvature-specific colour after-effects; numerous investigators have found colour to be linked to spatial frequency (Teft and Clark 1968; Harris 1970; Breitmeyer and Cooper 1972; Lovegrove and Over 1973; Stromeyer 1972) and others have shown that there exist colour-contingent motion after-effects (Helper 1968; Stromeyer and Mansfield 1970; Favreau Emerson and Corballis 1972; Mayhew and Anstis 1972).

Evoked potential correlates of contingent after-effects

Riggs, White, and Eimis (1973) have measured the decay of the McCollough effect. They reported that the effect is still noticeably present after 24 hours and in some cases lasted as long as 7 days. Thus, it seems that various spatio-temporal aspects of visual stimulation are processed together with colour information.

Studies of such contingent after-effects are important because they can help understand the way in which various physical attributes of a visual stimulus are coded in the brain. At least two simplistic neuronal mechanisms can be envisaged. The first assumes the existence of contour-specific neurones which have specific chromatic inputs. These cells can be fatigued or adapted with appropriate stimulation and this leads to an imbalance in the neural processes underlying veridical perception. A second view postulates a population of neuronal units characterized by a property which is best termed plasticity. These units do not react to visual inputs in any predetermined fashion, but rather become recruited and fire whenever contour-specific and colour-specific units are activated conjointly. These association units, once so programmed, modulate our perceptual experience for some time after the contour- and colour-driven neurones have ceased to be activated conjointly.

VEP correlates of colour and contour

We know very little about the actual nature of the neuronal interactions underlying these perceptions. Are there different cell assemblies for each contingent after-effect or are many of them mediated by a single neural mechanism? An even more basic question has to do with the anatomical locus of these effects, and VEP results might shed some light on this. The question whether there exist in the brain specific cells or cell assemblies which code some spatial parameter of the visual input together with wavelength is particularly intriguing because it parallels to a significant degree single-unit investigations in lower animals. If the VEP did prove to be a meaningful covariant of both single-unit activity in animals and psychophysical measures in humans, reliable VEP correlates of contour-specific chromatic adaptation would constitute an important step forward.

There have been many reports relating VEP characteristics to colour vision using spatially unstructured fields (e.g. Siegfried, Tepas, Sperling, and Hess 1965; Armington 1964, 1966; Cavonius 1965; White, Kataoka, and Martin, Chapter 12 of this book). Relatively few studies have dealt with VEPs elicited by contoured stimuli differing in wavelength. Riggs and Sternheim (1969) made observers match the luminance of adjacent heterochromatic bars in a grating stimulus. When this pattern was then reversed (i.e. abruptly moved in a direction perpendicular to grating orientation over a distance of one bar width), a steady-state VEP was recorded from electrodes above the occiput, and an ERG was evoked at the cornea. Riggs and Sternheim reported that very small differences in wavelength between heterochromatic bars were needed to obtain an observable VEP, whereas rather large wavelength differences were needed to produce criteria ERGs.

May and Siegfried (1970) recorded VEPs using similar pattern-reversal techniques. Chromatic gratings were superimposed upon an achromatic photopic background and amplitude–radiance and latency–radiance functions were obtained using wavelengths selected from across the spectrum. Photopic spectral-sensitivity curves, which agreed quite well with psychophysical results, were computed from criterion amplitude measures.

Contour-specific VEPs evoked by heterochromatic checkerboards equated for luminance have been obtained (Regan and Sperling 1971; Regan 1973*a*, Chapter 11 of this book), and VEPs can also be produced by an increase in chromatic contrast *per se* (Regan and Spekreijse 1974; Spekreijse, Chapter 2). The psychophysical contrast threshold is well correlated with the amplitude of VEPs obtained by these methods (Regan 1973*a*). Regan concluded that the visual system processes colour information differently if colour is associated with contour rather than unstructured fields.

While there have been many investigations of VEPs resulting from various contoured visual stimuli (e.g. Spekreijse 1966, and Chapter 2 of this book; Halliday and Michael 1970; Rietveld, Tordoir, Hagenouw, Lubbers, and Spoor 1967), very few experiments have been aimed at assessing the effects of chromatic after-effects on the VEP. Blakemore and Campbell (1969) reported that prolonged viewing of a high-contrast grating reduced the amplitude of the steady-state VEP elicited by a low-contrast grating of the same spatial frequency and orientation. This technique was employed in the study described below.

VEP correlates of adaptation to wavelength and orientation

May, Leftwich, and Aptaker (1974) used a design derived from previous psychophysical work (May 1972), by having observers adapt to stationary square-wave gratings (1·0 cycles per degree) presented by means of a two-channel Maxwellian view optical system. The gratings were composed of red (620 nm) or green (530 nm) bars superimposed upon a 300 td white background. Adapted orientations were either horizontal or vertical and, in some control conditions, blank homogeneous chromatic fields were presented during adaptation. The luminance of the grating was set at 1·8 log units above the pre-adaptation luminance threshold for a grating image. Following adaptation, there occurred a 4 s blank period during which the observer viewed only the 300 td background, then a 9 s period during which a test pattern of red or green vertical stripes was presented. This test grating was reversed at a rate of 7 Hz by means of an oscillating mirror (see Chapter 1 of this book). There were eight adaptation and test combinations per session. In each session, the observers were tested under either a red or green vertical test grating following adaptation to red vertical, green vertical, red horizontal, green horizontal, red unstructured, green unstructured, or white unstructured adaptation stimuli. Eight trials were run under each adaptation condition for each test stimulus.

The recording techniques were similar to those of May, Forbes, and Piantanida

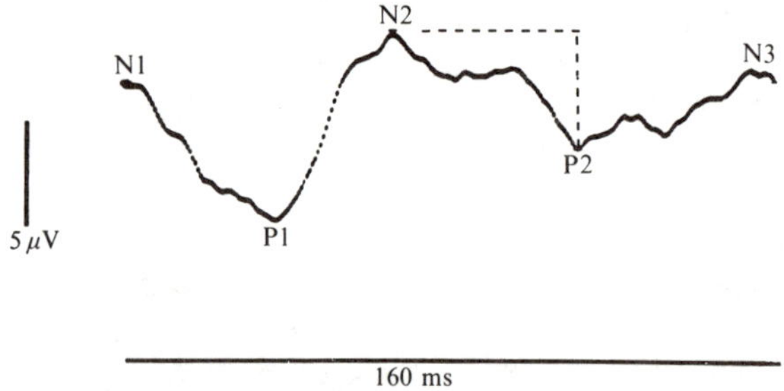

Fig. 13.2. An example of the VEP waveform recorded in the study by May *et al.* (1974). Peaks and troughs were labelled N_1, P_1, N_2, P_2, and N_3 to indicate their polarity.

(1971). The active electrode was located 2·5 cm above the inion and a mastoid reference was used. The subjects were grounded by a plate affixed to the left leg. The data were stored on a Hewlett-Packard, Model 3960 FM tape recorder. Responses were then summed with a Nicolet Model 1072 averager. Signals were played off the tape into quarters of the averager memory at 4 times the recording speed (recorded speed = 23·81 mm s^{-1} (15/16 in s^{-1}), playback speed = 44·45 mm s^{-1} ($3\frac{3}{4}$ in s^{-1})). The response epoch was 160 ms. Each average included 64 sweeps. The VEPs presented two positive peaks and two negative peaks which were labelled N_1, P_1, N_2, P_2, N_3 (Fig. 13.2).

The amplitude of N_2–P_2 was selected for measurement because the N_2 peak was always apparent which was sometimes not the case for N_1 or N_3. To counteract inter-session variability, the amplitude of each VEP under the conditions involving adaptation to chromatic stimuli (gratings on blank fields) was normalized to the average amplitude of VEPs obtained after adaptation to only a blank white field. The averaged normalized amplitude under all red test conditions was compared to that obtained under all green test conditions for each subject. These measures were not significantly different. The data for each condition were, therefore, grouped on the basis of whether or not they were obtained under heterochromatic or homochromatic conditions for each subject. It is readily apparent from the data in Fig. 13.3 that the normalized amplitude of the VEP is reliably suppressed in both subjects under only one condition – on homochromatic trials with vertically oriented gratings during both adaptation and test periods.

Data were also collected using the same adaptation and test stimuli in an interocular transfer paradigm. Observers adapted with the right eye and were tested in the left eye. Homochromatic conditions were not significantly different from heterochromatic conditions, which is consistent with the failure to find interocular transfer of wavelength-specific orientation effects psychophysically.

The VEP results agreed quite well with previously reported psychophysical results from our laboratory. VEP amplitudes were diminished under the same conditions that resulted in a significant elevation in luminance thresholds. Since the

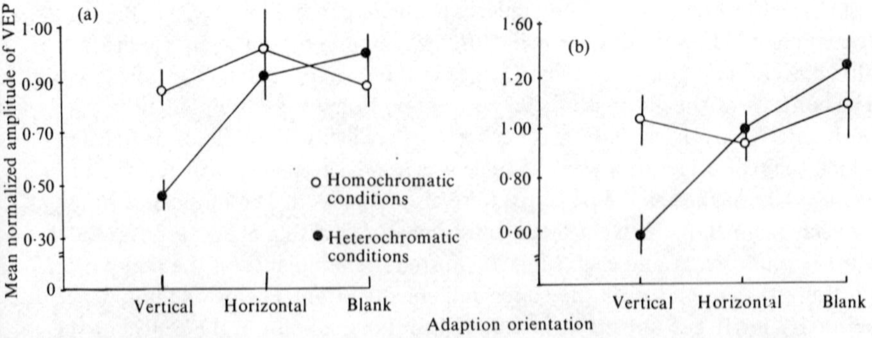

Fig. 13.3. Mean normalized amplitude of the VEP as a function of adaptation orientation (vertical, horizontal, and blank chromatic field) and chromatic condition for two subjects. Vertical bars represent ±1·0 S.E. (From May *et al.* 1974.)

procedures in both the psychophysical and VEP experiments involved adaptation to chromatic gratings oriented orthogonally, it was quite tempting to conclude that VEP correlates of the McCollough effect had been obtained. The cross-adaptational design, however, required observers to adapt for relatively brief durations to all wavelength-orientation conditions and this would not be expected to yield the McCollough effect.

Other investigators at Brandeis University have shown that the McCollough effect can be demonstrated in the absence of any threshold elevations (Timney, Gentry, Skowbo, and Morant 1974). Apparently, then, the mechanisms mediating the McCollough effect and those responsible for the threshold elevations are different. The threshold elevations could be accounted for with a traditional after-image explanation. A vertical grating would be easier to detect, if a horizontal, rather than a vertical after-image was present. Bleaching red receptors would reduce sensitivity for vertical red gratings and so on. If this is the case then the VEP changes observed might best be viewed as correlates of adaptational changes occurring at early stages in the visual system.

A new experimental approach

An experimental design allowing concomitant study of the McCollough effect and of VEPs to similar stimuli seemed indicated. The Jeffreys approach to component analyses for pattern-specific VEPs (Jeffreys, Chapter 6 of this book) appeared quite promising for searching for VEP concomitants of the McCollough effect, since it was reported during discussions at the Brussels Symposium on Cerebral Evoked Potentials (April 1974) that prolonged pattern presentation raises the thresholds of certain components (C2 and C3) whose attenuation varied according to the alignment and orientation of the pre-exposed and test patterns.

An initial experiment was carried out to confirm that the VEPs recorded were pattern specific. Achromatic square-wave grating stimuli (2 cycles per degree of visual angle) were presented binocularly to the upper and lower visual fields of five subjects. The stimuli were tachistoscopically presented (Scientific Prototype Model 800-F two-channel tachistoscope) in the form of rectangular fields (4° x 8°). The contrast of the gratings was 96 per cent and they were oriented either horizontally or vertically. Control conditions involving blank fields or fields in which the half upper or lower rectangle was non-patterned, but of the same space-averaged luminance as the patterns, were also employed. The luminance supplied by each channel of the tachistoscope was measured with a Spectra-spot (Model UB 1½) photometer and each subject adjusted the luminance of the non-pattern portions of the fields until they appeared equally bright.The overall luminance was about 1·3 log ft-L. Subjects were required to fixate a point in the centre of the field.

The stimuli were presented for 25 ms (with onset and offset times of less than 0·1 ms) at a rate of once every 650 ms. The VEPs were recorded from a single electrode 5 cm above the inion on the midline referenced to the right mastoid. The left mastoid was grounded. The signals were fed to two model 122 Tektronix low-level pre-amplifiers in series. The upper and lower bandpass were set at 50 Hz and 0·8 Hz and the nominal gain was 100 000. Four averaged VEPs (each based on 64 stimulus presentations) were recorded under each condition. The data stored on FM tape were analysed off-line using a 200 ms epoch. As was the case with Jeffreys' results, VEPs to patterned stimuli exhibited reversals in polarity for C1 (65–80 ms) and C2 (88–100 ms) for upper and lower field stimulation while VEPs to non-patterned stimuli resulted in VEPs which did not vary significantly in waveform for these retinal positions. Four superimposed VEPs obtained with (a) vertical gratings presented to the upper field, (b) vertical gratings presented to the lower field, and (c) non-patterned blank field presentations are presented in Fig. 13.4 for two representative subjects. No significant differences in waveform, amplitude, or latency were noted for horizontal as opposed to vertically oriented gratings (cf. Jeffreys and Axford 1972*a*, *b*; Jeffreys, Chapter 6 of this book).

The central experiment involving adaptation to wavelength and orientation was then carried out. Wratten filters (55 for green or 26 for red) were inserted into both fields to provide a situation which allowed for grating stimuli to be alternated with a blank field of the same wavelength. The overall luminance for the red and green stimulus conditions was 0·5 log ft-L and 0·9 log ft-L, respectively. Four averaged VEPs were recorded from 5 subjects with normal colour vision (4 of whom participated in the initial experiment) under each of the following conditions (a) red-vertical lower-field stimulation, (b) green-vertical lower-field stimulation, (c) red-horizontal lower-field stimulation, and (d) green-horizontal lower-field stimulation. The subjects were then shown a compound stimulus composed of vertical and horizontal gratings in white light and asked to make judgments regarding the hue of each type grating. All subjects reported that the two gratings did not differ in hue at this point.

Thereafter, the subjects adapted to vertical stripes in the lower half of a red

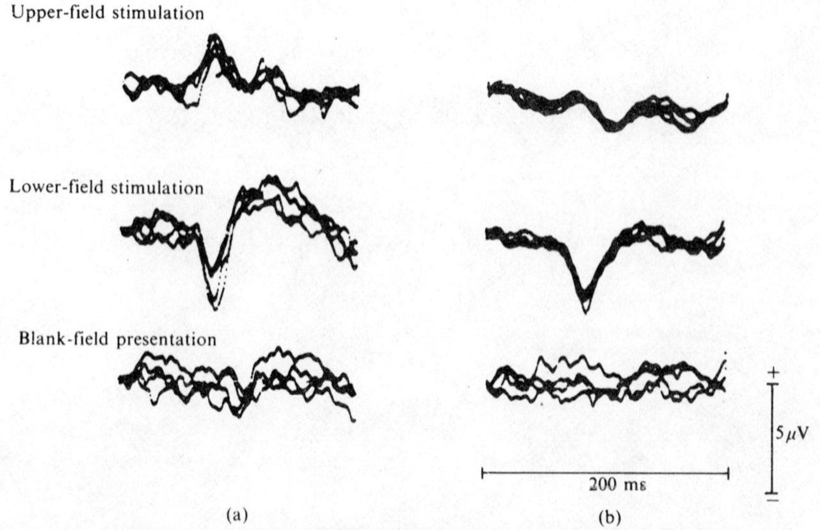

Fig. 13.4. Four superimposed averaged VEPs elicited with (a) achromatic vertical gratings presented to the upper and lower visual fields, and (b) flashes of unpatterned light. Data are presented for two observers.

field followed by horizontal stripes in the lower half of a green field cycled at a rate of 0·2 Hz for 10 min. They were instructed to allow their gaze to wander back and forth along the top of the patterned portion of the field to avoid the formation of after-images. After such adaptation, 4 of the subjects reported strong McCollough effects when once again asked to view the compound inspection figure. Each of these 4 subjects said that the vertical stripes appeared green and the horizontal stripes appeared pink when asked to describe what they saw. The fifth subject said that there was only a faint pink hue in the horizontal grating, no hue was apparent in the vertical grating. The subjects were invited to rotate their heads 90° and once again report what they saw. All 4 subjects viewing the entire effect reported that the induced hues 'exchanged positions' when the head was rotated. Five to 10 min after adaptation the VEPs were again recorded in exactly the same manner as they were prior to adaptation. At the end of the session, the subjects were again asked to view the compound inspection figure and all reported that the effect was still clearly present.

Each averaged VEP was inspected visually and baseline measurements were made within the first 40 ms of each trace. The first component (C1) appeared as a positive peak between 65 ms and 80 ms; C2 was always negative and occurred between 88 ms and 100 ms; C3 was usually positive but somewhat more variable. It was found between 135 ms and 155 ms. Representative data for two subjects are presented in Fig. 13.5. The amplitude and latency data for all conditions and all subjects were grouped for statistical analyses. Three analyses of variance

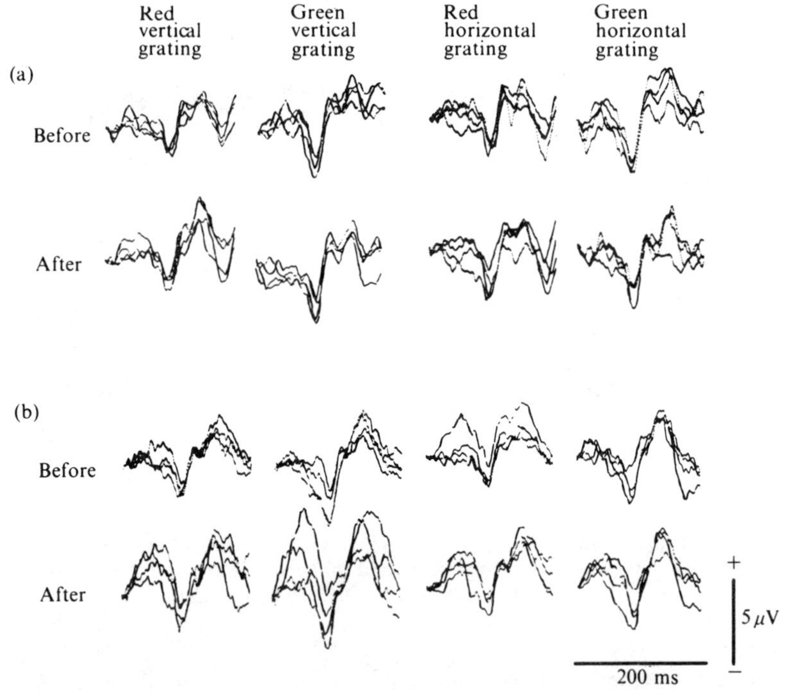

Fig. 13.5. Four superimposed average VEPs elicited under each of four stimulus conditions before and after the induction of the McCollough effect. The data for two observers are presented.

(conditions x replications x trials) were performed on the amplitude and latency data for each component. The data are summarized in Fig. 13.6. The amplitude and latency of VEPs were unaffected by adaptation conditions and did not vary significantly over repeated measures within a condition. The main effect for conditions was significant in the C1 ($F = 3{\cdot}55$, $df = 3{,}12$, $p < 0{\cdot}05$) and C2 ($F = 4{\cdot}86$,

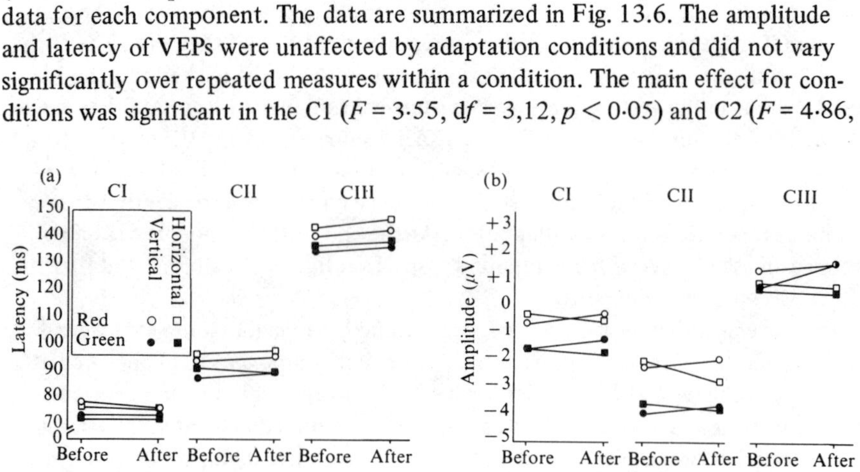

Fig. 13.6. Mean amplitude and latency data for three components of the VEP elicited with different chromatic gratings before and after the induction of the McCollough effect.

$df = 3, 12, p < 0{\cdot}025$) amplitude analyses and also in the C2 ($F = 9{\cdot}29$, $df = 3, 12$, $p < 0{\cdot}005$) and C3 ($F = 4{\cdot}53$, $df = 3, 12, p < 0{\cdot}05$) latency analyses. These significant differences were probably the result of the differences in overall luminance between red and green conditions. None of the two- or three-way interactions in any of the analyses was statistically significant (i.e. $p > 0{\cdot}05$).

All subjects reported the chromatic after-effects in association with the orientations predicted for the McCollough effect and these after-effects lasted at least 1 hour. The lack of difference in amplitude or latency between the adapted (red vertical grating and green vertical grating) and unadapted (red horizontal grating and green vertical grating) stimuli constituted a failure to uncover VEP concomitants of this contingent after-effect. Apparently, the pattern-specific VEP obtained in this study recovers quite rapidly from adaptation and in that regard resembles the steady-state VEP used in the previous study (May *et al.* 1974).

Discussion

Upon obtaining negative results regarding what originally appeared to be a feasible hypothesis, an investigator usually questions the validity of the methods used or the theory held. In this case, it may prove fruitful to do both. Given, for the moment, that it is possible to obtain VEP correlates of the McCollough effect, what methodological flaws could have obscured the fact? The overall luminance in the study reported above was lower than that used by Jeffreys and Axford (1972*a*, *b*), but the contrast was quite high. Many VEP studies have shown that the relationship between intensity and amplitude is not linear over the entire range of intensities used. A saturation level occurs at some point, such that further increments in stimulus intensity no longer lead to increases in VEP amplitude. While overall luminance seems to exert some influence on pattern-specific VEP characteristics, it is the contrast which has the greatest influence on amplitude. It could be that adaptation effects as subtle as the McCollough effect can only be observed if VEPs are recorded below the saturation point. Most researchers would prefer to work with large, reliable VEPs, but this is perhaps contra-indicated when looking for correlates of phenomena as elusive as the McCollough effect.

Most observers report that the McCollough effect is rather weak (pale or low in saturation), but clearly perceptible. Psychophysical measurement is quite crude in this regard. The effects are usually reported to be either present or not in some stated percentage of the subjects. Riggs *et al.* (1973) have reported a procedure whereby observers may cancel out chromatic after-effects by adding complementary hues to compound inspection gratings. This technique may eventually provide information about the degree of saturation or loss of sensitivity involved in contingent after-effects. Perhaps similar procedures might be employed in VEP work.

The VEP to pattern stimuli is quite sensitive to spatial frequency or check size and also the retinal locus of the stimulus. For example, May *et al.* (1971) found that gratings containing bars which subtended 11–22′ of arc were most effective in eliciting a VEP and that the area–amplitude relationship of centrally fixated stimuli saturated at about 5°. Harter (1971) found that the optimal check size depended to some extent on retinal eccentricity. As the stimulus was applied more extrafoveally, the optimal check size increased. The McCollough effect does not seem to be dependent upon a restricted retinal area around the fovea and seems to be perceived over retinal areas somewhat larger (about 20°) than that needed to saturate the pattern-related VEP. It is possible, therefore, that the perceptual phenomena reported as the McCollough effect and the VEPs recorded with pattern stimuli originate from different retinal areas and cortical projections.

The recording site employed here was chosen in the belief that the mechanisms underlying the McCollough effect were likely located in the striate or extrastriate areas of the cortex. At least two studies have speculated about the source locations of the various components in the pattern-specific VEP (see Chapters 5 and 6). If the McCollough effect derives from 'association' neurones, perhaps more lateral and anterior leads would provide VEPs which would be more sensitive to wavelength and contour adaptation. Zeki (1971) reported that there are visual projections from primate striate cortex to the superior temporal sulcus, and Pribram (1971) made some suggestions concerning the role of inferior temporal cortex in modulating visual processes. The relative dearth of information about cortico-fugal mechanisms in the visual system precludes more than speculation.

There are some reasons to think that VEP correlates of the McCollough effect are unobtainable. Coltheart (1973) has recently suggested that colour-contingent after-effects must derive from a class of cortical neurones which are exclusively monocular. This is supported by the observation that such effects do not transfer interocularly. Achromatic orientation adaptation does show interocular transfer and it is suggested that these effects must be mediated by binocularly driven cells. Unfortunately, apparently few cortical neurones are exclusively driven by monocular inputs. Current estimates are on the order of 20–30 per cent. If so, the neural pool available to respond selectively to colour and contour adaptation must be small relative to the other elicited activity unrelated to the conjunctive processing of these features.

All cerebral VEPs must be time-locked to an objectively observed stimulus event. This is not the case with phenomenological demonstrations of contingent after-effects. The important thing here seems to be one of the dimensions to which the subject has adapted. This suggests the possibility that such effects derive from the steady-state activity of central neurones or, perhaps, are triggered by the activity of internal events for which we have no objective indicator. Thus, the advantage which is associated with careful temporal control of synchronous events may not be present in this situation.

The attempt to obtain VEP changes which reflect subtle perceptual experiences such as the contingent after-effects may well push evoked potential technology to its limit. We do not know, at this point, how many cerebral neurones act in consort to give rise to an illusion of this sort. Given the redundancy and plasticity evident in some investigations of the nervous system (e.g. Galambos, Norton, and Frommer 1967; Chow 1970; Morrell 1967), it is difficult to believe that the activity of a single cell can mediate a fairly universal sensation of colour, tilt, size, or motion. It is even more difficult to think that a single unit is responsible for coding integration of that kind of information. The EP technology assumes the existence of a rather large number of neural units acting synchronously and on command. Future investigations can tell us whether such assumptions are valid.

14. Visual cortical potentials and electroretinograms triggered by saccadic eye movements

J. C. ARMINGTON
Department of Psychology, Northeastern University, Boston

Bright, intense flashes of light have often been used to study the visual system. Such stimuli are not suitable for investigating certain visual problems for several reasons. When the eyes are used in the normal fashion, they scan a structured visual field which fills much of the retina and which produces a pattern of more-or-less constant overall illumination. Stimulation is produced by displacements of the retinal image, even though the total light flux entering the eye does not change appreciably. Stimulus flashes, on the other hand, produce an increment in the total light entering the eye and their effect is considerably different from the stimuli encountered in the everyday world. Furthermore the flashing stimuli introduce problems of stray light and of arousal. As is well known, light which is imaged on one area of the retina spreads widely as a result of scattering and reflection within the eye. The intense flickering stray light associated with typical flashing stimuli produces increments of illumination of sufficient magnitude to activate a large population of receptors lying beyond the primary stimulus area (Fry and Bartley 1935; Bartley 1941; Armington 1966). The VEP is extremely sensitive to stimuli applied to the central retina, but stimulation of peripheral receptors will aslo produce potentials which contribute to its waveform. Stray light is an even more serious concern for the electroretinogram and must always be taken into account in studies concerned with pattern vision and with regional differences in sensitivity.

Stimuli which flash or change abruptly may also startle or arouse the subject. Long before computers were used to isolate VEPs, the K complex was recognized as a startle-related component of the electroencephalogram (EEG) (Whitteridge and Walsh 1963). In fact, many aspects of the EEG are responsive to the general level of activity and arousal of the subject. The VEP may be subject to a variety of effects related to startle, arousal, task relevancy, and attention (Regan 1972*a*). Thus, it is important to compare VEPs to stimuli which have a greater or lesser potential for arousing the subject with VEPs produced when there is no external event to startle the subject.

Visual evoked potentials in man; new developments (ed. J. E. Desmedt), pp. 286–300. Clarendon Press, Oxford, 1977.

This chapter will consider recording methods which avoid certain of the difficulties encountered with conventional recording, particularly those of stray light and, to some degree, those of startle. Emphasis is placed on the eye-movement method which is an outgrowth of the method of stimulus alternation (sometimes called pattern alternation or phase reversal). Results obtained by both methods will be interpreted in terms of response additivity. Most of the work features simultaneous recording of the VEP and the electroretinogram (ERG).

Methods

Alternation

The method of stimulus alternation employs a striped stimulus pattern which appears as shown in Fig. 14.1. A checkered pattern (Armington, Corwin, and Marsetta 1971) or one composed of zig-zag stripes (Moskowitz, Armington, and Timberlake 1974) may be used in place of stripes. Stimulation is produced by interchanging the dark and bright stripes abruptly and periodically. This stimulates the receptors upon which the stripes are imaged by changing the amount of light falling upon them. The averaging computer system is synchronized to the mechanism which interchanges the stripes. The Maxwellian view apparatus used to produce alternating stimuli involves a pivoted mirror (Fig. 14.1(a); see also Chapter 1 of this book) which moves the stripes back and forth within the field-stop with a square motion. The excursion is exactly one stripe-width. When the equipment is properly adjusted the subject does not perceive the movement but sees an interchange of stripe luminance. Optical filters are used to vary the luminance and spectral composition of the stimulus. The light arises from a ribbon filament lamp and is directed to the eye through a series of lenses. The subject holds his eye in proper position by viewing a steady point of red light arising from a small filament introduced into the main optical path by an unsilvered mirror.

Alternating stimuli have been adopted because they have several advantages over ordinary flashing stimuli (Spekreijse 1966; Johnson, Riggs, and Schick 1966). For instance, they may be used to control stray light. When the retinal areas occupied by the bright and dark stripes are equal, there is no change in the total light flux entering the eye as the stripes are interchanged. Light that is deflected before it reaches the retina as well as light that is reflected from the stimulus area is constant and non-fluctuating. Alternation is particularly suited for isolating photopic potentials, although under certain conditions it may be used to obtain scotopic ones (Wooten 1972). Because of its freedom from scotopic and stray light interference, it lends itself to the investigation of stimulus pattern, spatial frequency, and acuity. It also has value for the investigation of colour vision, since responses may be elicited by stimuli which differ in hue but not luminance (Riggs, Johnson, and Schick 1966). There is one disadvantage to the method of alternation. Since some of the receptors within the stimulus field receive an increment in stimulation and others a decrement, it is difficult to separate on- and off-effects.

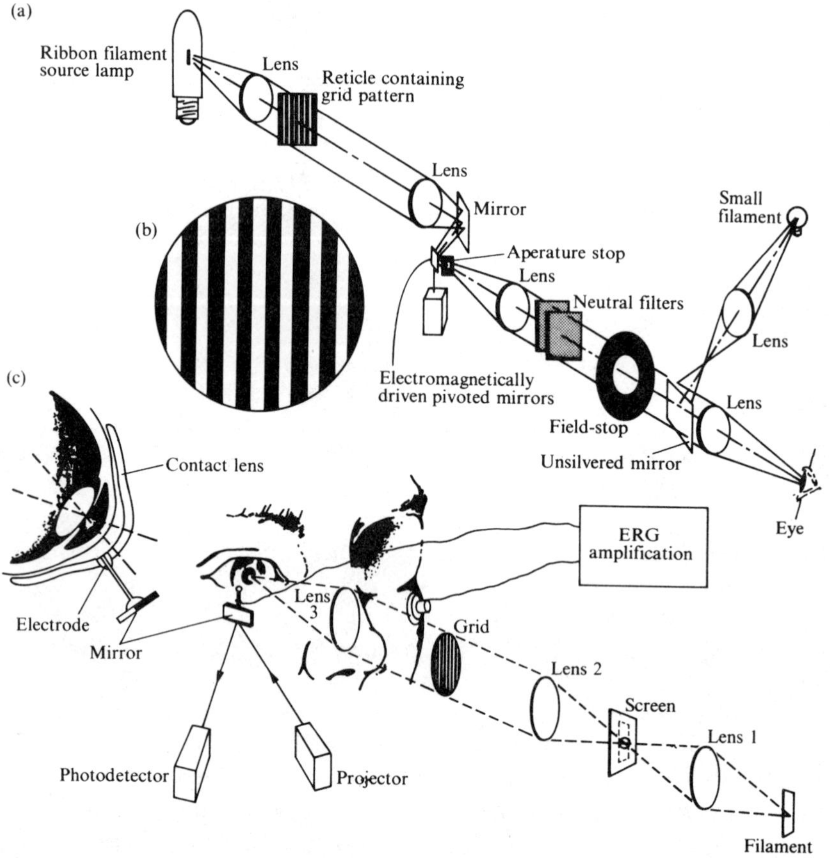

Fig. 14.1. (a) Maxwellian-view stimulator. Exploded view of the main optical components for producing alternating stimuli. (b) Shows how stimulus appeared to subject. (c) Apparatus for recording saccade-contingent responses. The subject views a steady stimulus grid through Maxwellian-view optics. Eye movements are recorded photoelectrically with the aid of a mirror attached to a tightly fitting contact lens.

Eye-movement method

Both ERGs and VEPs can be elicited by saccadic eye movements. The procedure resembles the method of alternation, but the pattern is kept steady and its image is displaced on the retina whenever the subject makes a voluntary or involuntary saccadic eye movement. An averaging computer triggered by the saccades displays the responses elicited by this stimulus alternation (Fig. 14.1(c)).

The system in current use has been described in detail (Armington 1972) and can be broken down into four parts: an assembly for recording eye movement, a stimulator for presenting the eye with a steady pattern of vertical stripes, an amplifier system for recording VEP and ERG, and an on-line computer for analysis.

The stimulator is of conventional Maxwellian-view design. It presents the subject with a pattern of vertical stripes produced by a square-wave grating placed in the plane of the field-stop. Components not shown in Fig. 14.1 permit control of the field luminance, field diameter, the spatial frequency and contrast of the stripes, the position of the stimulus on the retina, and other stimulus parameters. A contact lens which supports a light-weight mirror is tightly fitted to the eye of the subject. A pencil of infrared light, projected to the mirror and reflected back across a straight edged opening to a photocell, acts as an optical lever. The arrangement is such that the photocell produces an electrical signal proportional to the horizontal position of the eye. Upon differentiation, this signal forms trigger pulses at the onsets of successive saccades. The saccade trigger produces one pulse whenever a saccadic eye movement exceeds some pre-set lower level and a second pulse on a separate line whenever a saccade exceeds some pre-set upper limit. Because of this dual feature, the computer may be programmed to respond to all eye movements or only to those falling within defined amplitude limits. Responses to right and left saccades may be processed together or separately.

VEPs are picked up with standard EEG silver-cup electrodes, usually one on the inion and the other also on the midline, about 6 cm anterior. The ERG is recorded with an electrode mounted in the same contact lens. An EEG electrode attached to the cheek serves as reference. The potentials are amplified with standard differential amplifiers (bandpass from 0·8 Hz to 250 Hz; time-constant 0·2 s) and sent to a general-purpose computer having an external disc memory and digital interface units. A telephone connection makes it possible to deposit data in the central computer of the University. The system has evolved from earlier simpler versions. An important feature of the general-purpose computer used here is that the records are sampled continuously, thus making it possible to obtain the average response in front of, as well as following the saccadic eye movements. Since the pulses from the saccadic trigger cannot occur at the very onset of the movement, early response components could not be seen without this feature. In addition, search can be made of the brain potentials which precede eye movements.

Results

Alternating stimuli

Results from experiments with alternating stimulus fields of different size and with patterns of differing spatial frequency have a particular pertinence for explaining the eye movement VEPs. Alternating stimuli elicit purely photopic responses which are released by the activity of the cone systems of the retina, except under narrowly prescribed conditions (Armington, Marsetta, and Schick 1970). Analysis is consequently simplified because results are not confounded by an admixture of photopic and scotopic effects.

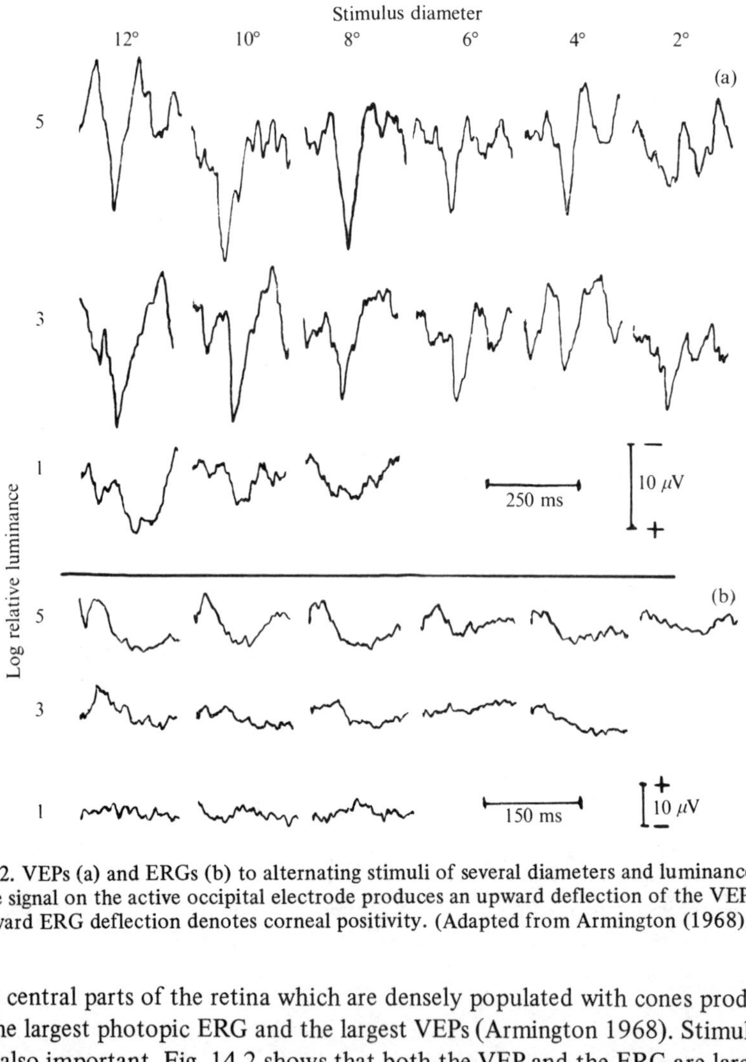

Fig. 14.2. VEPs (a) and ERGs (b) to alternating stimuli of several diameters and luminances. A negative signal on the active occipital electrode produces an upward deflection of the VEP. An upward ERG deflection denotes corneal positivity. (Adapted from Armington (1968).)

The central parts of the retina which are densely populated with cones produce both the largest photopic ERG and the largest VEPs (Armington 1968). Stimulus area is also important. Fig. 14.2 shows that both the VEP and the ERG are largest when the stimulus field is large and when the stripes are bright. Despite this similarity, responses from the two recording sites do not behave in exactly parallel fashion. The ERG more than doubles in size as the field diameter is increased from 2° to 12° for a fixed luminance condition. The VEP also grows but the change is less than 50 per cent (Fig. 14.3). The insert in Fig. 14.3 shows a replot of B-wave amplitude data with the scale on the abscissa changed to the number of cone receptors lying within the image area. The linearity of this plot indicates that the ERG amplitude is roughly proportional to the number of cones within the stimulus field for stimulus fields up to 60° in diameter. Consider the

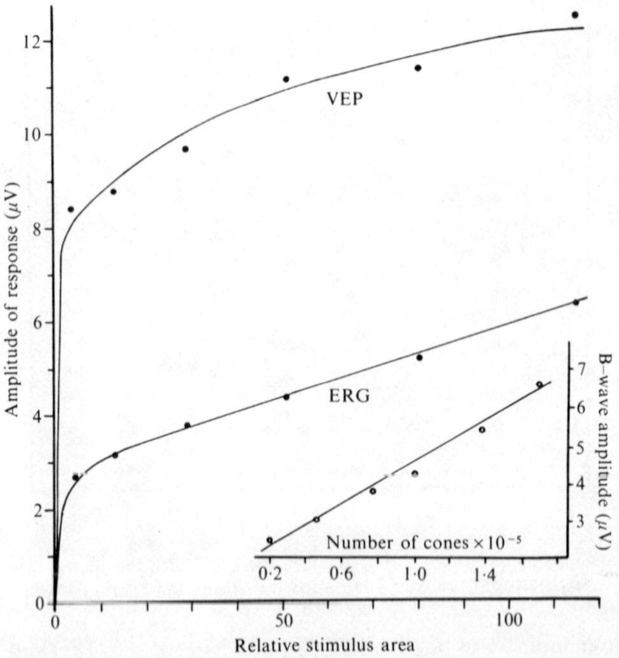

Fig. 14.3. Dependence of the VEP and the ERG amplitude on the relative area of the retinal stimulus. The data for the ERG have been replotted in the insert to show how response amplitude relates to the number of receptors stimulated. (Adapted from Armington (1966).)

ERG to be a summation of elemental waveforms. Then, it can be calculated that the responses to stimulation of each cone add together, each making a contribution of approximately 50–75 pV to the ERG (Armington and Bloom 1974). Such a simple calculation cannot be made for the VEP because stimulation of the central parts of the retina contributes more to VEP than stimulation of peripheral areas (the occipital projections from the fovea being more extensive) and because central processes may intervene. The VEP amplitude is positively associated with, but not simply proportional to, the number of receptors stimulated in this experimental situation.

Experiments with flashing stimulus displays have shown that some patterns are more effective than others in producing large VEPs (Van Hof, Van der Mark, and Rietveld 1962; Harter and White 1968). The same result obtains with alternating stimuli (Armington *et al.* 1971). Specifically, it has been found that recurrent spatial patterns are stronger stimuli than unstructured fields, that the spatial frequency of such patterns is an important parameter, and that checks are more effective than stripes having the same spacing (Fig. 14.4). This spatial tuning of the VEP may be partially explained in terms of a matching between the sizes of the stimulus elements and of the receptive fields which underlie vision, but

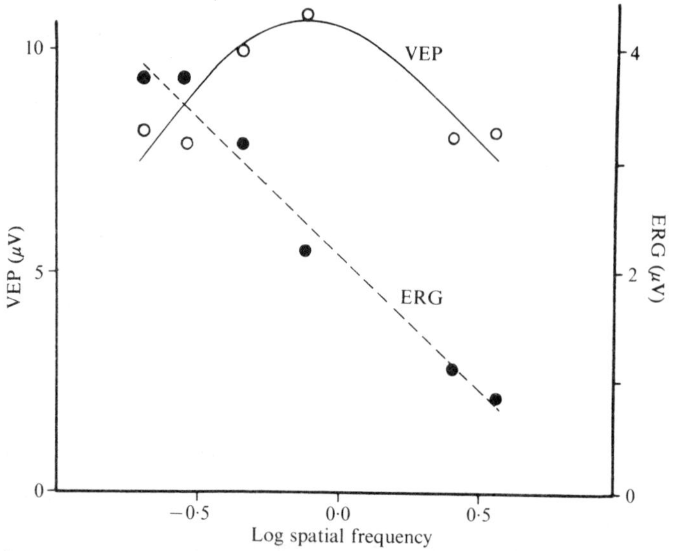

Fig. 14.4. Change in the amplitude of the VEP and the ERG with the spatial frequency of an alternating stimulus. (Adapted from Armington *et al.* (1971).)

additional factors must also be involved (Moskowitz *et al.* 1974). The ERG responds best to coarse stimulus patterns; it is not tuned to a narrow band of spatial frequencies and does not distinguish between striped patterns and checked patterns of the same spatial frequency (Armington *et al.* 1971).

Saccade-contingent responses

Saccade-contingent responses (Gaarder, Krauskopf, Graf, Kropfl, and Armington, 1964) were found to vary in a systematic way with stimulus parameters. Fig. 14.5 shows typical responses obtained with up-to-date equipment. The ERG (top line) has a prominent B-wave followed by a late negative component. The averaged saccades in the second line have the characteristic waveform of single saccades. The VEPs shown on the bottom have a waveform that is quite like that seen with alternating stimuli when using the same scalp electrode placement, and the waveforms are substantially independent of the direction of the saccadic movements. This provides evidence that genuine VEPs rather than eye-movement artifacts are being dealt with since the latter would invert with the direction of eye movement. The only evidence for artifact is seen in the early part of the ERG tracings which contain a small pulse (apparently due to the changed position of the eye in the orbit) at the time the saccade occurs. It does not distort the B-wave measures described below. No sign of eye movement is evident in the VEP tracings. Early recordings obtained with more primitive equipment resolved less detail, and there was a delay of several milliseconds between the onset of the saccades and the triggering of the computer (see p. 289).

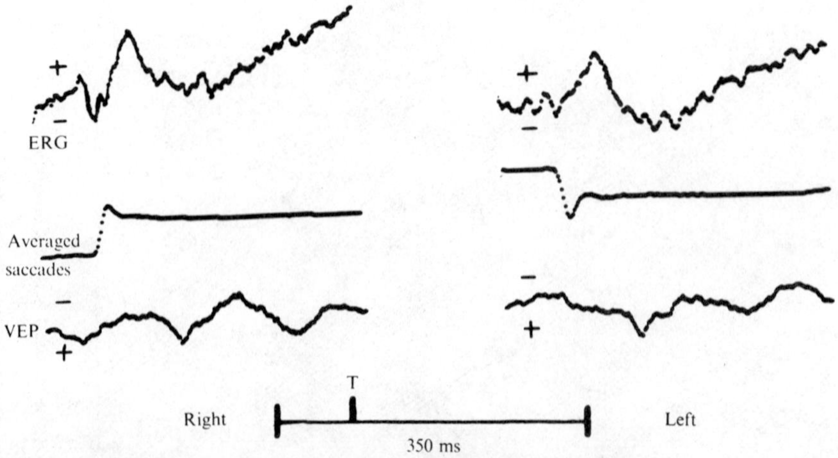

Fig. 14.5. Examples of responses accompanying right and left saccadic eye movements. T on the time-scale shows when the trigger pulse which indicated the presence of a saccade was produced. (Adapted from Armington and Bloom (1974).)

Saccade-contingent VEPs were first obtained using a stimulator that presented a single luminous dot or in some cases multiple-dotted patterns (Gaarder *et al.* 1964).When neutral filters were interposed the amplitude of the VEP decreased with luminance and its latency increased. Some subjects gave very small responses with a single-stimulus dot, but when several dots were placed in the field, the response was considerably larger. A subsequent investigation of saccade-contingent VEPs and ERGs used high-contrast vertical stripes as stimuli (Armington, Gaarder, and Schick 1967). The spatial frequency and the luminance of the patterns were experimental variables, and the computer was triggered by all fixation saccades that exceeded the noise level of the eye-movement recording. Fig. 14.6 shows the data for ERG and VEP. The columns show responses produced as the subject viewed stripes of three different widths. The rows show responses to several luminances. Both the ERG and the VEP were large when the stripes subtended about 13′ per cycle and when the patterns were of high luminance. Any departure from this optimum condition reduced the responses. The changes of spatial frequency changed primarily the amplitudes but not the latencies.

Fig. 14.7 is a plot of several response measures against the size of the stripes in the test field at a constant-luminance condition. The pattern-dependent changes in the amplitudes of ERG and VEP components parallel one another closely. To explain these data, consider the following: if the stripe width is selected so that a saccade turns the eye through an angle equal to one-half of the angle subtended by a cycle of the stimulus grid, then the positions on the retina which were occupied by bright bars before the saccade will be exactly filled by black bars after the movement and vice versa. Such a movement will produce a maximal change of retinal stimulation because all of the receptors within the stimulus field undergo

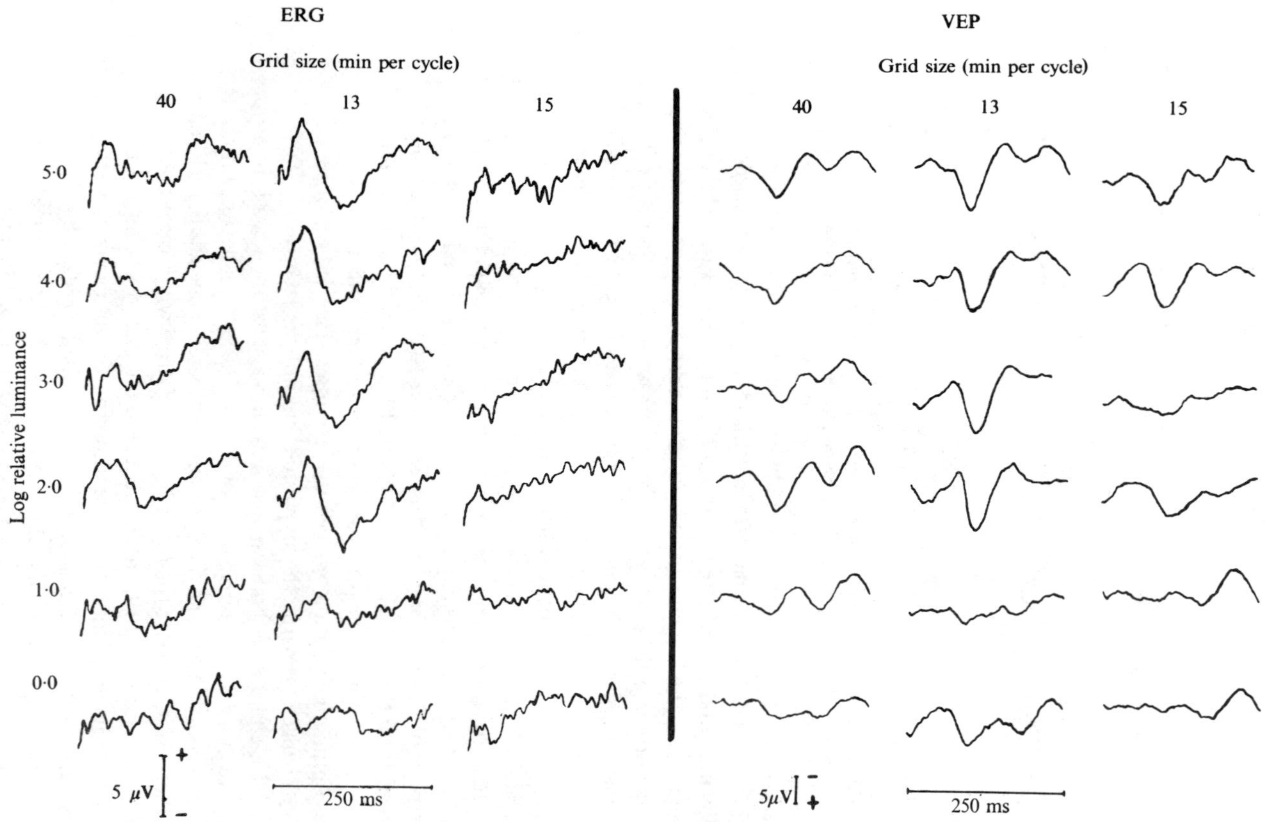

Fig. 14.6. Simultaneous recordings of saccade-contingent ERGs and VEPs for several spatial frequencies (grid size) and luminances. (Adapted from Armington *et al.* (1967).)

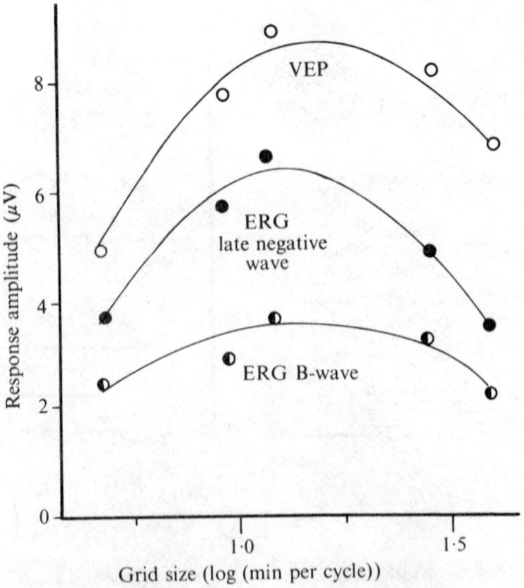

Fig. 14.7. Dependence of the amplitude of saccade contingent responses on the size of the stripes making up the stimulus pattern. (Adapted from Armington *et al.* (1967).)

a change in illumination. If the stripes subtend a much larger angle than that of eye movements, stimulation will only take place only along the stripe edges, and a smaller response will result. Very small stripes, approaching the limit of visual resolution, will also produce little change in stimulation. Thus the maximum responses would occur with the spatial frequency which matches the amplitude of typical fixation saccades. This explanation assumes that the response activities resulting from stimulation of adjacent areas add together (see above). Although consistent with the concept of additivity, the results of Fig. 14.7 do not provide a direct test. Therefore direct experiments have been conducted to determine whether the VEP and ERG amplitudes are proportional to the size of the active receptor population. Saccades are not all of the same size, and those which move the receptors over a large fraction of the stripe width should be more effective stimuli to the retina.

Fig. 14.8 shows average ERGs and VEPs sampled from the same period of fixation and which have been sorted out according to the size of the saccadic rotation. Both the ERG and the VEP grow with the size of the eye movement. The responses maintain the same latency and waveform characteristics regardless of eye-movement amplitude. Fig. 14.9 shows plots of amplitudes of the B-wave of the ERG and of the VEP, each point being the average of several measurements, and measures for left and right movements being combined. The straight lines drawn through the points have been fitted by the method of least squares. Values

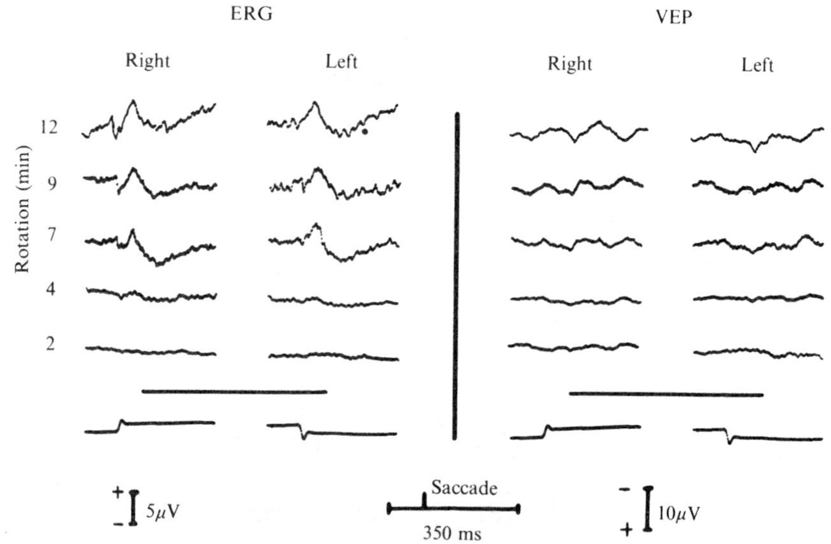

Fig. 14.8. ERGs and VEPs produced by right and left spontaneous saccades of several amplitudes. The size of the response increases with the size of the saccade. (From Armington and Bloom 1974.)

are given for the slopes M of these lines in microvolts per minute of arc of the eye's rotation.

The plots reveal three significant findings. The amplitudes of both ERG and VEP are proportional to the amplitude of the saccades which triggered them. The slope depends on the spatial frequency of the stimulus pattern. The slope relations are not the same for the ERG and the VEP when the results for different stripe size are compared. This latter finding reflects the different spatial frequency characteristics (Fig. 14.4) of the two responses. Direct comparison of the responses released by movements of fixed angular size across the three stripe sizes has been made for the B-wave and for the VEP (Fig. 14.10). The upper graph in each case is a plot of the M-values, taken from Fig. 14.9, against the spatial frequency of the stimulus. Such slopes measure the response amplitude produced by a fixed movement, since the dimensions of slope are microvolts of response per minute of rotational movement. The graphs show that the response elicited by an eye movement of fixed size increases with the spatial frequency of the stripes, but no correction has been made for the dependence of response sensitivity on spatial frequency. The importance of this correction is indicated by extrapolating the plots to the left so as to intersect the ordinate scale. They do so a considerable distance above the origin, an impossible result since there can be no response when there is no movement. When an adjustment is made by multiplying by factors taken from Fig. 14.4 which corrects for spatial frequency effects, the plots extrapolate through the origin. Hence, it may be concluded that there is a proportionality of

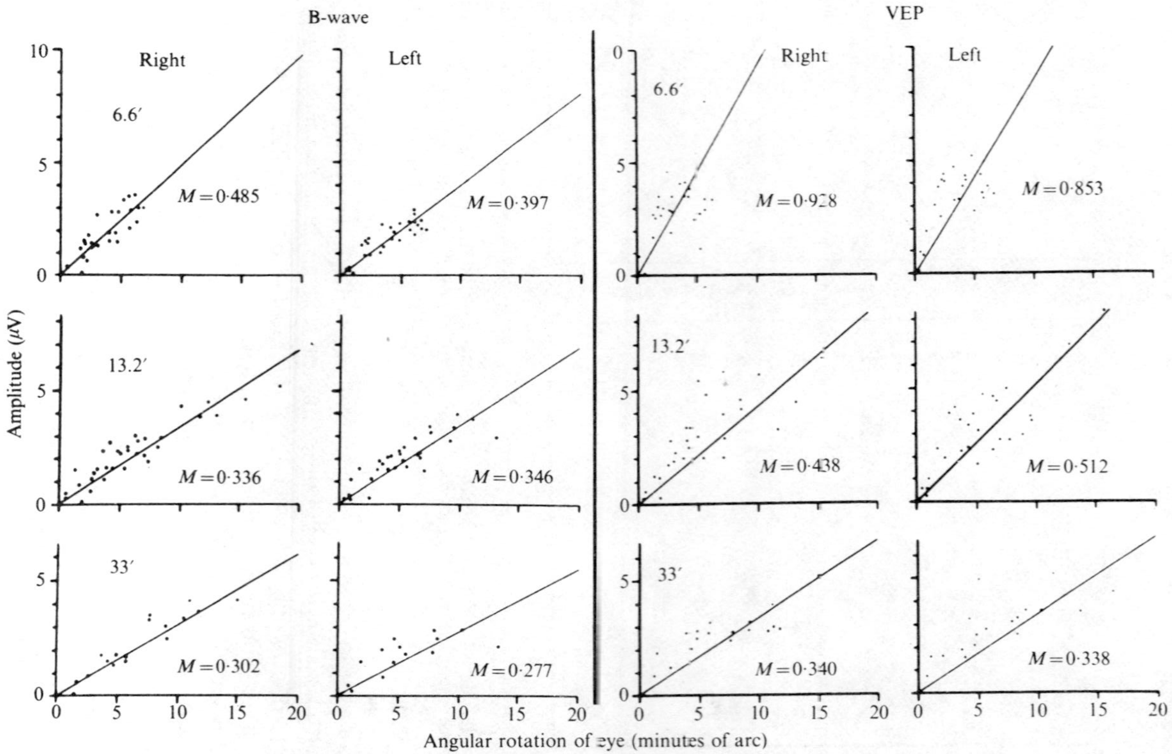

Fig. 14.9. Plots of response B-wave and VEP amplitudes comparing saccades of differing size. Straight lines have been fitted to the experimental points by the method of least squares. The slope *M* of each of the lines is given. Data are shown for three stripe sizes: 6·6 minutes of arc, 13·2 minutes of arc, and 33 minutes of arc. (Adapted from Armington and Bloom (1974).)

response amplitude to spatial frequency, and to the numbers of receptors that are stimulated by fixed image displacement. An estimate was made above of the contribution of each stimulated cone to the ERG and a new estimate can be made from data such as presented in Fig. 14.10. Armington and Bloom (1974)

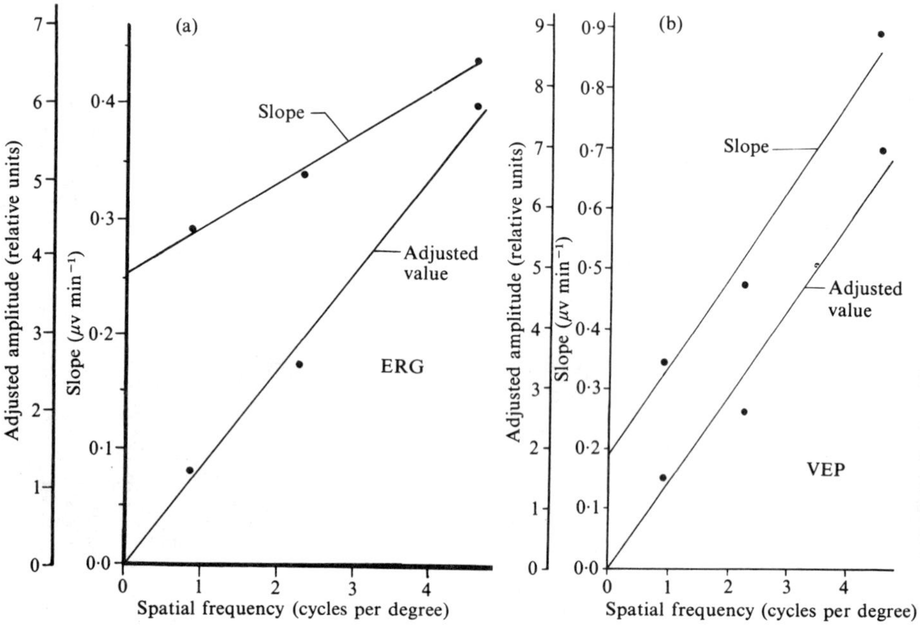

Fig. 14.10. (a) Size of the B-wave produced by a saccade of fixed amplitude as a function of the spatial frequency of the stimulus pattern. (Adapted from Armington and Bloom (1974).) (b) Amplitude of the VEP produced by a saccade of fixed size as a function of spatial frequency.

obtained a value of 22 pV per cone when the elements of the stimulus pattern subtended a visual angle of 33′. Considering the technical problems encountered in this type of recording the agreement of this value with those obtained with alternating stimuli may be regarded as satisfactory.

This type of estimate is difficult for the VEP. But in the present case, a linear plot can be obtained because there is no change in the size of the stimulus field with saccades of differing size. This again points to a type of additivity. Large saccades bring in more receptors throughout the stimulus field so that variations in receptor density and in retinal–cortical projection become unimportant. Nevertheless, it must be recognized that neural processes which depend on the orientation of the stimulus and other complex aspects of the stimulus pattern influence the VEP (Moskowitz *et al.* 1974). The present results only hold when these complex variables are held constant.

Paced and unpaced movement

The experiments described so far were conducted with the subject fixing a spot in the centre of the striped stimulus field. Thus, the eye movements may be called fixation saccades. Similar experiments may be performed by triggering the computer with the larger saccades that are produced as the subject shifts his eye back and forth between two fixation points. This has been done using saccades made periodically in step with an auditory pacing signal. The spacing between the two fixation points, and thus the movement of the stimulus stripes across the retina, was subjected to experimental variation. The VEP waveforms to paced saccades were reasonably similar to those obtained with other recording methods and the EEGs were virtually identical (Flamm 1971). As with spontaneous saccades, the ERG and the VEP both grew regularly in amplitude with increased image displacement (Fig. 14.11). Thus, the additive nature of the potentials is revealed

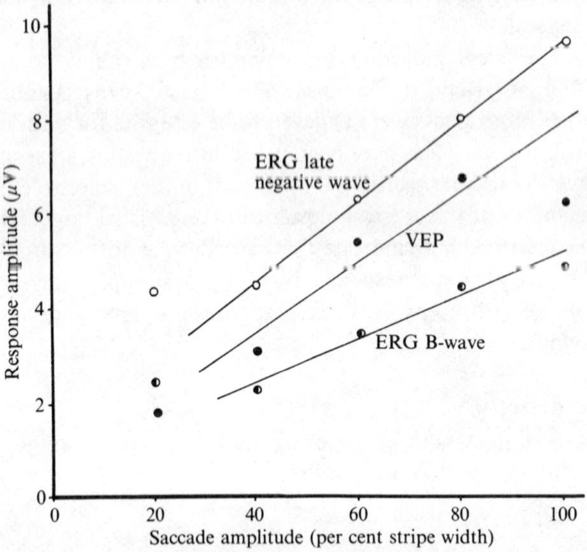

Fig. 14.11. Dependence of the amplitude of response components on the excursion produced by paced saccadic eye movements. Saccades were made between fixation points spaced at fractional intervals across the pattern's centremost stripe. The largest responses accompany the largest eye movements (measured as a percentage of the stripe width). (Adapted from Flamm (1970).)

once more. The apparently minor differences that were seen in the VEP mostly involved latency. When considering latencies, however, one must remember that stimulation is not instantaneous with the eye-movement methods but lasts for the duration of the saccade. The trigger pulse used to synchronize the computer occurs when the saccade reaches some pre-set angular magnitude. Therefore, small differences in apparent latencies are not necessarily significant. Further experiments specifically designed to compare the response waveforms produced by different recording methodologies might prove useful.

Discussion

Saccadic eye movements produce visual responses at the retina and at the visual cortex because they displace the retinal image. The responses have many properties in common with those obtained by stimulus alternation and they are related in a lawful way to stimulus parameters such as average luminance, spatial frequency, and field size. The angular extent of a saccade is of particular importance because it determines the numbers of receptors stimulated, and hence the amplitude of the response waves.

The methods reviewed here, in addition to providing information regarding evoked potentials themselves, provide a way of investigating the transmission of visual information to the cortex and the interaction between vision and eye movements in general.

The role of saccadic eye movements in vision has been subject to much recent controversy (Steinman, Haddad, Skavenski, and Wyman 1973). At one time saccades and other movements were believed to be essential for several critical visual functions, but these ideas have been called into question since a number of experiments have shown that saccades do not play an important role in visual acuity or in the ability of the eye to hold position on a visual target. Nevertheless, the experiments described here indicate that saccades cannot be discounted entirely. Saccades trigger visual responses by abruptly sweeping the retinal image over large populations of receptors. These responses probably underlie much of our visual behaviour.

Acknowledgements

Much of the research reported was supported by PHS grant EY00589. Fig. 14.2 is reproduced by permission of Pergamon Press.

15. Vision and visual evoked potentials during saccadic eye movements

B. A. BROOKS
Department of Physiology, University of Texas Health Science Center, San Antonio

Transmission in the primary visual pathway during saccades

Changes in neural activity associated with saccadic eye movement can be recorded in brain sites other than the oculomotor nuclei. While some activity changes in the primary visual pathways during saccades are due to visual input generated by retinal image motion, others cannot be so readily classified. An example of the latter are the 'PGO-waves' which occur in lateral geniculate nucleus, occipital cortex, and also the pontine reticular formation during eye movements in the dark (Berlucchi and Strata 1965; Brooks 1968*a*), following optic-tract transection, enucleation, and removal of the extra-ocular muscles (Michel, Jeannerod, Mouret, Rechtschaffen, and Jouvet 1964; Brooks 1967, 1968*a*) and which are not related to parameters of eye movement such as amplitude and direction (Brooks 1968*b*; Brooks and Gershon 1971). Anatomical pathways between the brain-stem reticular formation and lateral geniculate nucleus (Bowsher 1970) probably subserve many of these potentials, as well as those recorded in the lateral geniculate nucleus during the rapid eye movements of sleep (Mikiten, Niebyl, and Hendley 1961; Brooks and Bizzi 1963; Bizzi and Brooks 1963; Bizzi 1968).

Brain-stem input to the primary visual system is potentially a mechanism for control of visual activity during normal behaviour. Results from several recent studies provide evidence regarding the nature of the control in the alert animal. Two important points become clear from the studies of Doty's group (Bartlett, Doty, Pecci-Saavedra, and Wilson 1973; Doty, Wilson, Bartlett and Pecci-Saavedra 1973; and Wilson, Pecci-Saavedra, and Doty 1973) who have evaluated responses in the lateral geniculate nucleus produced by brief optic-tract stimulation while stimulating the mesencephalic reticular formation of monkeys. First, when mesencephalic influence is seen in the lateral geniculate nucleus it is *facilitatory* (except under anaesthesia); secondly, the effect depends on level of alterness, and fully alert animals show no further enhancement of response to optic tract stimulation, suggesting that the facilitatory effects are, in some tonic manner, already maximal. A similar facilitatory influence in the lateral geniculate nucleus of the cat follows stimulation of the mesencephalic reticular formation (Singer and

Visual evoked potentials in man: new developments (ed. J. E. Desmadt), pp. 301–13.
Clarendon Press, Oxford 1977.

Drager 1973), an effect which appears almost identical to those following saccades performed without intentional mesencephalic stimulation (Singer and Bedford 1974). Thus it would appear that comparable excitatory mechanisms may be activated both during experimental stimulation of the brain stem and during saccadic eye movement. Mohler (1975) has recently described facilitated responses in the lateral geniculate nucleus of the monkey to visual stimulation during saccades.

The role of darkness was stressed by Cohen, Feldman, and Diamond (1969) who noted that the response to optic tract stimulation in the lateral geniculate nucleus of the awake monkey was affected neither by simultaneous brain-stem stimulation nor by saccadic eye movements performed by the animals in the dark. Adey and Noda (1973) used comparable methods to come to identical conclusions (see Fig. 15.1 and below). Bartlett and Doty (1974) report that brain-stem facilitatory influences on responses to optic-tract stimulation can be seen in the striate cortex of monkey, but as in the case of the lateral geniculate nucleus they are less evident in the alert animal. Since very little effect was noted when the optic radiation was stimulated regardless of level of alertness, it was concluded that brain-stem influence on monkey visual cortex is largely mediated via the lateral geniculate nucleus (Bartlett and Doty 1974). Thus if the brain-stem is sometimes mediating *phasic* excitability changes in the primary visual path during saccades (in a way that might explain the PGO-waves) it seems clear that its influence is mainly facilitatory, and that it is inversely related to level of alertness and attentiveness.

Transmission in the lateral geniculate nucleus may be affected in a different way when saccades are made across a visual background. Further data from Adey and Noda (1973) show that postsynaptic responses elicited by optic-tract stimulation in the lateral geniculate nucleus of the alert cat are *depressed* during saccades if a visual background is present, and that a similar depression is found when the background is rapidly displaced while the eye is fixating. However, the same authors report that signs of a facilitatory influence during saccades may be seen in the cortex whether or not a visual background is present, and when the animal is alert. The findings of Adey and Noda (1973) (Fig. 15.1) would imply that the depression in visual *sensitivity* ('saccadic suppression') commonly observed in psychophysical experiments during saccades is due to visual input, since for the lateral geniculate nucleus the suppressive consequences of eye movement across a background are the same as background movement.

Lambda waves

Sharp and complex waveforms ('lambda waves') can be recorded in the occipital EEG of most alert humans when eye movements are made in an illuminated environment. Computer averaging techniques have disclosed low-amplitude lambda waves. It is generally agreed that pattern and contrast in the visual background are sufficient to produce lambda potentials (Chatrian 1975) but complex backgrounds

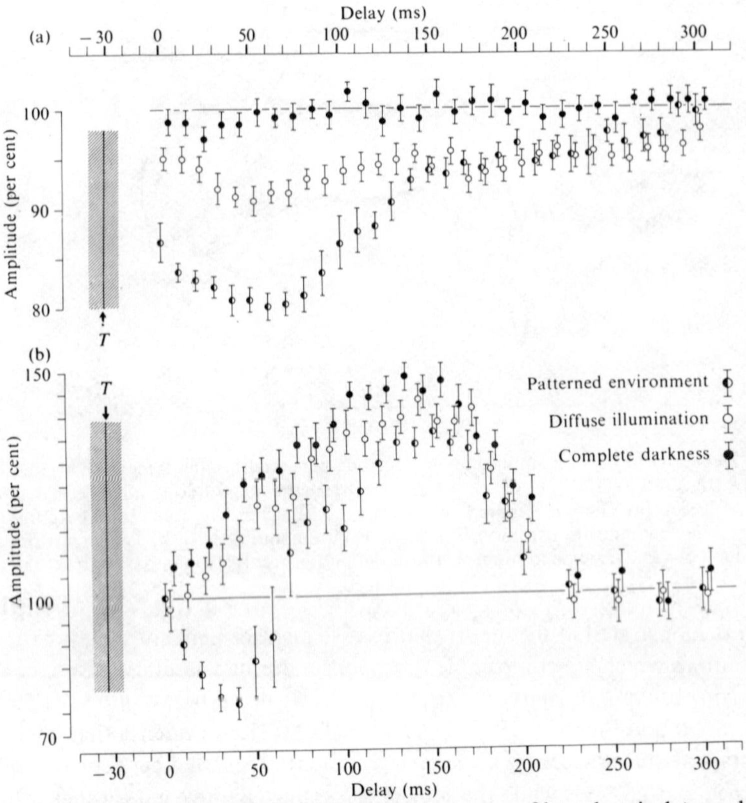

Fig. 15.1. Changes in amplitude of the post-synaptic response of lateral geniculate nucleus (a) and C_4–C_5 components of the post-synaptic response of the visual cortex (b) to electrical stimulation of the optic chiasm, during the period following saccadic eye movements. The stimulator was triggered by the potentials shifts in the horizontal EOG and a single shock was delivered to the optic chiasm with variable delays indicated by the abscissae. Each circle represents an average amplitude of 30 responses and the vertical bar represents 1 S.D. *T*, average time of saccade onset (shaded area = one s.d.) before the moment when the stimulator was triggered (delay 0). Geniculate transmission is not affected during eye movements in the dark but is reduced during saccades over either a diffuse background or patterned background of vertical stripes. Cortical responses are *facilitated* during saccades over all backgrounds but show an initial depression if the background is patterned. (From Adey and Noda 1973.)

are not necessary. Rémond, Lesèvre, and Torres (1965) and Scott and Bickford (1969), as well as myself (Fig. 15.2), have recorded lambda potentials over patternless backgrounds which may be smaller and somewhat different in configuration than those registered in the presence of pattern (Rémond *et al.* 1965). Lambda amplitude is generally reported to be attenuated when luminance is reduced and to be eliminated in darkness (Evans 1952, 1953; Cobb and Pampiglione 1952; Roth and Green 1953; Groethuysen and Bickford 1956; Rémond and Lesèvre 1956, 1971); drowsiness and fatigue have similar detrimental effects on amplitude (e.g. Scott, Groethuysen, and Bickford 1967). The role of visual input

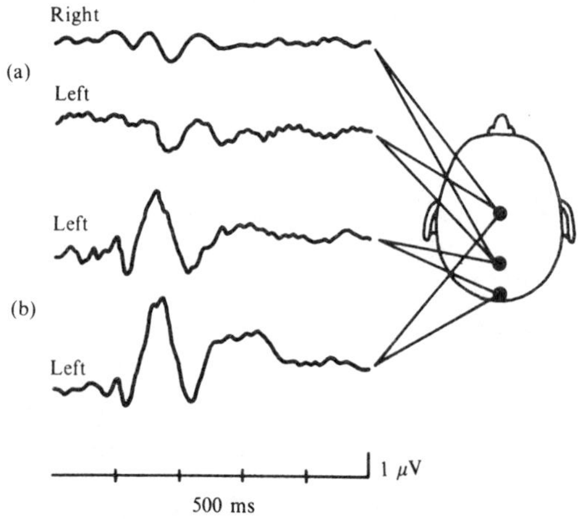

Fig. 15.2. Dependence of VEP amplitude on electrode placement. Each trace is an average of 100 sweeps triggered by a 5° saccade across an unpatterned background luminance of 1·0 log ft-L (see methods). (a) There is a similarity of cortical VEP when triggered either by a right or left saccade. Electrode positions: inion, 7·5 cm above inion and vertex. (b) The largest potential was recorded between vertex and inion. Upward deflection results from a positivity at the inion. Subject B.B.

is further demonstrated in the report that passive displacements of the eyeball elicit potentials which are comparable to responses during voluntary movement over the same backgrounds; passive displacements do not produce potentials in darkness (Scott and Bickford 1967, 1969). Finally, there is evidence that lambda waves obtained during saccades are similar to potentials elicited by displacement of patterned backgrounds while the subject is fixating (Barlow and Ciganek 1969; Rémond and Lesèvre 1971; Kurtzberg and Vaughan 1973, and Chapter 16 of this book; Morton and Cobb 1973). This kind of data does not deny subtle differences which may exist between 'displacement' potentials and responses during saccades (see Kurtzberg and Vaughan, Chapter 16 of this book, and Fig. 15.8). The point is that the evidence indicates that substantial *visual activity* accompanies a normal saccade over illuminated backgrounds and that this activity is reflected in the occipital potential.

Visual activity during eye movement and 'saccadic suppression'

Visual processing proceeds without conscious interruption and the environment remains subjectively stable during normal saccadic activity. Several investigators have proposed that a central inhibitory or compensatory mechanism could cancel or 'suppress' any visual disturbances resulting from the eye movement. Proponents of a central inhibition theory view the *increase in visual threshold* that often accompanies saccades ('saccadic suppression') as a sign that central inhibition is in action (Volkmann, Shick, and Riggs (1968) and Riggs, Merton, and Morton (1974) provide a review).

Saccadic suppression is psychophysically determined by comparing thresholds to stimuli delivered at the time of eye movement to thresholds for the same stimuli presented during fixation. There is variability in reports of the strength and time-course of suppression. Increases in luminance threshold reported during rapid eye movement over illuminated backgrounds range from about 0·1 log unit (Richards 1969) to more than 2·0 log units (Zuber, Stark and Lorber 1966). Very intense stimuli given during a saccade are not suppressed at all (Chase and Kalil 1972; Michael and Stark 1967). A near absence of suppression has also been reported during both involuntary (Krauskopf, Graf, and Gaarder 1966) and voluntary (Mitrani, Mateeff, and Yakimoff 1971; Brooks and Fuchs 1975) eye movement in dark or dim conditions. When suppression does occur, it is not only during large voluntary saccades but also during small involuntary microsaccades of fixation (Ditchburn 1955) as well as passively induced movements (Richards 1968). The duration of suppression in different studies is also variable, but there is evidence that it is inversely related to at least one *visual* parameter, the intensity of the test stimulus used to assess it (the stronger the test stimulus the shorter the suppression (Zuber *et al.* 1966). MacKay (1970) has found when the eye fixates and the background is rapidly displaced, thresholds rise in a way comparable to the elevation observed during saccades (see also Brooks and Fuchs 1975).

There is an obvious implication in these results that visual factors play a large role in the phenomenon of saccadic suppression. This point, taken in conjunction with the evidence regarding the visual contribution to the lambda wave and the facts regarding transmission in the primary paths clearly indicates a closer examination of the influence of visual background conditions during saccades. None of the transmission studies discussed earlier shows a suppression of the primary path during saccades in alert animals except when a visual background is present (Adey and Noda 1973). The lambda wave is strongly dependent upon a visual background. It would then seem reasonable that the psychophysical threshold increase associated with saccades over backgrounds is determined by the background itself. The remainder of this chapter will discuss support for this view, obtained by systematically manipulating parameters of visual background during saccadic eye movements and comparing VEPs with psychophysical measures of sensitivity.

Experimental method

The subject was seated comfortably with his head at the centre of a translucent, hemispheric dome (65 cm diameter) so that his entire visual field was covered. Two small black fixation points were located on the dome to subtend a standard 5° of horizontal visual angle. The distance from fixation points to eyeball was 27 cm, allowing good focus.

Steady backgrounds consisting of unpatterned luminance were projected on the dome from the side opposite the observer. The luminance at the fixation points (dome centre) was 0·7 log units greater than that at the periphery, providing smooth but not absolutely linear gradient. Diffuse test flashes were regulated by a Grass photo-stimulator (model PS-2) which could be triggered by an eye movement in either the right or left direction. The luminance of the test flash and background was controlled by Kodak neutral density filters.

The EEG was recorded conventionally by Beckman Ag–AgCl electrodes, amplified differentially, filtered by a bandpass filter (0·1–100 Hz, 3 db), and averaged by a Hewlett Packard Signal Analyzer 5040B. All records are the average of at least 100 sweeps.

The bi-temporal EOG was differentiated and the resultant velocity signal activated the sweep of a Tektronix oscilloscope whose trigger level was set at the earliest possible position in the EOG waveform. All saccades were 5° in amplitude and the trigger occurred approximately midway through the saccade. The oscilloscope in turn triggered the averager and stimulator.

Experimental results

Fig. 15.2 indicates the position of electrodes recording a potential which is time-locked to saccades performed against an illuminated background. Fig. 15.3 shows that the amplitude and latency of the major waves of the saccadic potential are systematically related to luminance level, so that increases in luminance are correlated with increases of potential amplitude and decreases of latency. No potential was evoked during saccades performed in darkness.

Fig. 15.4 refers to the difference between visual thresholds for a diffuse test flash during saccades and during fixation, at several background luminances. Fixation threshold was first determined, then the diffuse test flash was triggered by the saccade and the subject was asked to report on the visibility of the flash during his eye movement. Fixation threshold values were subtracted from saccadic values and the difference plotted as threshold elevation on the ordinate. If the eye movement was made in the dark with the subject completely protected from extraneous light, sensitivity during saccades and fixation was almost identical (left symbols near zero; eye movements were made without fixation points and monitored on an oscilloscope by an experimenter). However, as background luminance grew, the amount of flash luminance necessary for visibility during a saccade as compared to fixation also increased. It is the threshold elevation during saccades which some investigators would accept as evidence of saccadic suppression.

It is evident that both threshold elevation and VEP amplitude during saccades show an increase with background illumination, within the limitations of our experimental conditions. In Fig. 15.5, contrast threshold values and VEP amplitude are both plotted relative to background luminance, to emphasize the relationship. These data suggest that increases in threshold may be causally related to the saccadic potential, but require that we make considerable assumptions regarding the mechanism. Our current idea is that the potential observed during saccades

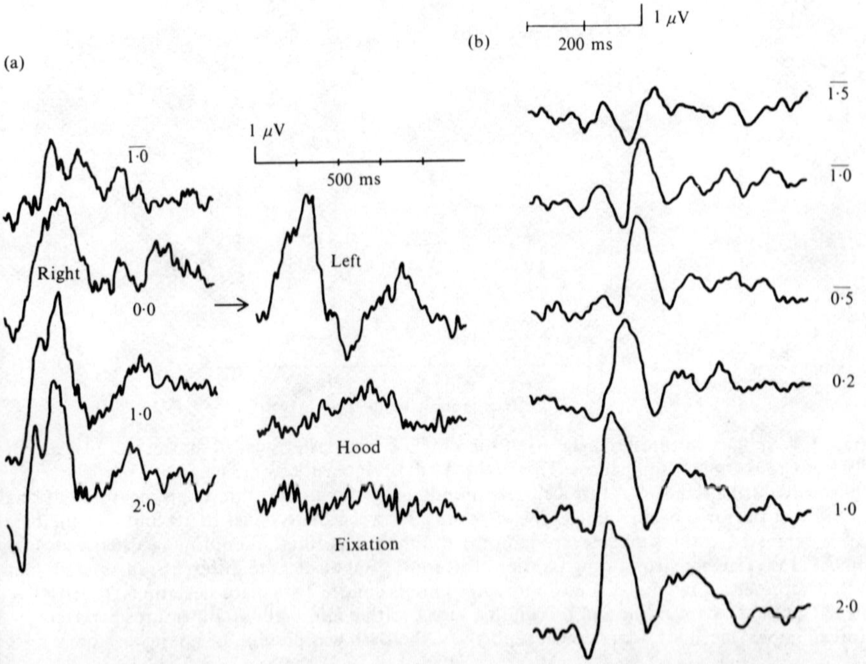

Fig. 15.3. Dependence of saccade VEP amplitude on background luminance. (a) The value of the background luminance (ft-L) appears next to individual traces in left-hand column. Records labelled 'right' and 'left' show similarity of response whether triggered by right or left eye movements. The trace labelled 'hood' was obtained when voluntary saccades without fixation points were performed in a darkened room with the head wrapped in thick black felt. The control trace, labelled 'fixation' was triggered by a stimulator while the subject steadily gazed at a point centred on the 1·0 log ft-L background. Subject J.J.K. (b) Results showing amplitude dependence on background luminance (log ft-L; right-hand column) for subject B.B.

results from the activation of visual elements sensitive to rapid, saccadically produced shifts of luminance across the retina. In the dark there is no luminance, therefore no potentials. The regular dependence of potential amplitude on background luminance is difficult to explain and probably best left open. If, however, we assume that activation in the visual system during saccades is proportional to VEP amplitude we may begin to explain the increase in threshold for diffuse test flashes. Assume that the diffuse test flash activates the same group of elements that are responsible for the potential. If the elements are already activated due to the saccade, they may be refractory to *additional* stimulation from the flash which arrives almost simultaneously. While the neurophysiological mechanisms are obscure, it is well known that closely timed visual stimuli presented to the fixating eye can show inhibitory interactions; these are referred to as 'masking phenomena' (Raab 1963; Kahneman 1968; Boynton 1973).

An essentially similar point of view was proposed by Vaughan (1973) who

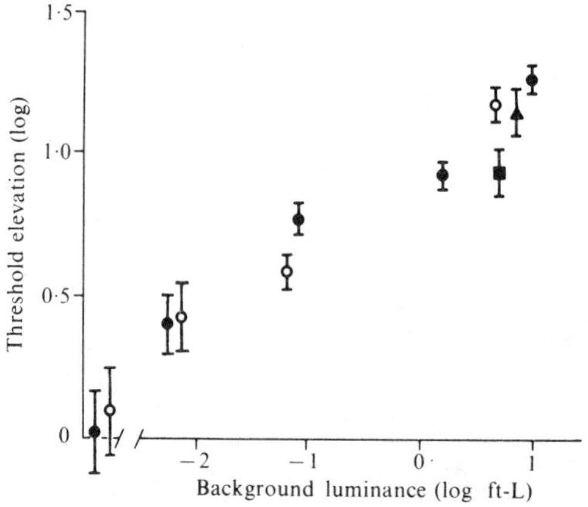

Fig. 15.4. Subjective threshold elevation for a diffuse test flash triggered during saccades at different background luminances. Threshold test flash intensities were measured psychophysically during fixation at various backgrounds and compared to thresholds measured during saccades at the same backgrounds. The *difference* between these values in log units (to the base 10) is expressed as threshold elevation on the ordinate. The threshold during saccades was almost always higher than during fixation. Different symbols denote different subjects; subject B.B. is represented by circles. Lines through symbols denote 2 standard deviations. Psychometric method of ascending and descending series, with a minimum of 7 measures per average (forced choice method; subject must report yes, the flash was present, or no, it was absent).

showed that in humans eye movements over a *striped* background pattern produced a lambda potential, which could be mimicked when the same background was 'saccadically' displaced while the eye was fixating. When a test stimulus was paired with *either* movement, its subjective intensity *and* its VEP were attenuated in comparison to a fixation control. As the time between displacement (or saccade)

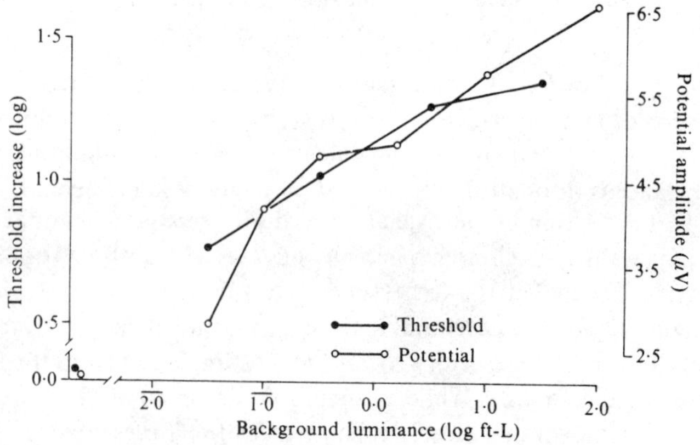

Fig. 15.5. Subjective threshold increase during saccades and saccade VEP amplitude, as a function of background luminance. Potential amplitude measured from the base to peak of the first major positive deflection. Note that neither the potential nor the threshold elevation is seen during saccades in darkness (far left abscissa). From subject S.H.

and test stimulus increased, the test VEP showed recovery. The time-course of change in test VEP was traced in both situations and found to be almost identical. Vaughan inferred from these interactions that changes in visual sensitivity measured psychophysically during saccades might be explained by physiological mechanisms independent of actual eye movement.

Fig. 15.6 compares a VEP to test flash presented during fixation and a VEP to

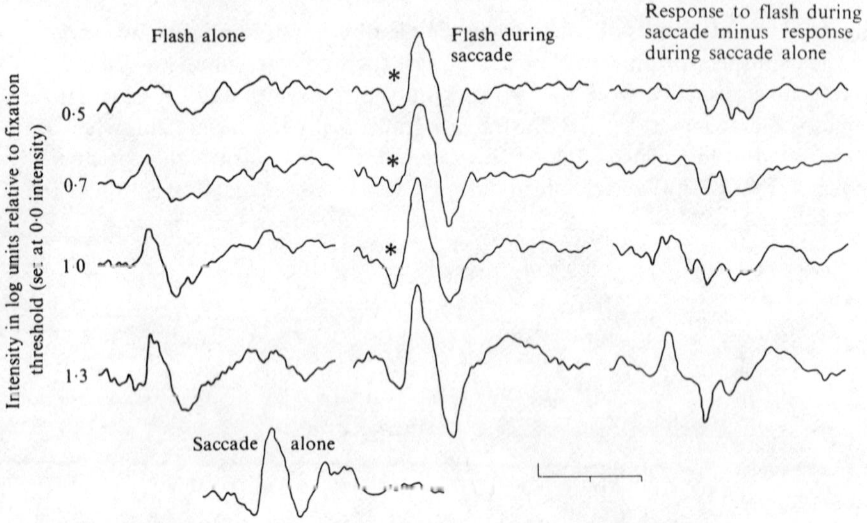

Fig. 15.6. Comparison of VEP to test flash during fixation and when test flashes were triggered by saccades. *Left column*: VEPs to increasing intensities of flash given alone during fixation. *Middle column*: VEPs recorded when the flash value shown to the left was triggered during saccades. Asterisks signify that the flash was not seen during saccades. Only the flash 1·3 log units above fixation threshold was seen during eye movement. *Right column*: difference after the computer has subtracted the saccade VEP obtained alone from the saccade plus flash VEP. *Below left*: saccade alone control. From subject B.B.

flash during saccades on the same pattern-free background of earlier figures. The record for saccade alone is seen at lower left. Responses to various intensities of test flash presented during fixation are seen at left. When the test flash was paired with the saccade an unexpected result occurred – in many instances the resultant potential was larger than the saccadic potential alone, even when the flash was not perceived during the saccade. In Fig. 15.6, this condition is marked with asterisks in the middle column. Flashes at 0·5, 0·7, and 1·0 log units above fixation threshold were not seen as separate events during the saccade. Nevertheless they appear to contribute to the combination potential amplitude.

The nature of this interaction will remain in doubt until neurophysiological evidence is obtained from single visual units. Repeated summing and subtraction by computer did *not* provide evidence of an algebraic summation between flash and saccadic VEPs obtained separately, and this may be taken as evidence that we are not dealing with two independent subsystems. For instance, in the right-hand column of Fig. 15.6, the response obtained during the saccade alone has been subtracted by computer from the response to flash and saccade as combined by the visual system. If the brain had done an algebraic summation, the resultant would equal the response to flash alone; but it does not.

The retinal area represented by the saccadic potential

Fig. 15.7 depicts results obtained when the distribution of luminance was varied on the hemispheric dome. In this case, no test flash was present and saccades were made as usual between the two fix points. Stripe width was 12° of visual angle. The drawings at the left illustrate diagramatically the visual field. When a background of luminance 1·0 log ft-L was present without stripes the potential shown in Fig. 15.7(a) was obtained during saccadic movement. Restriction of the

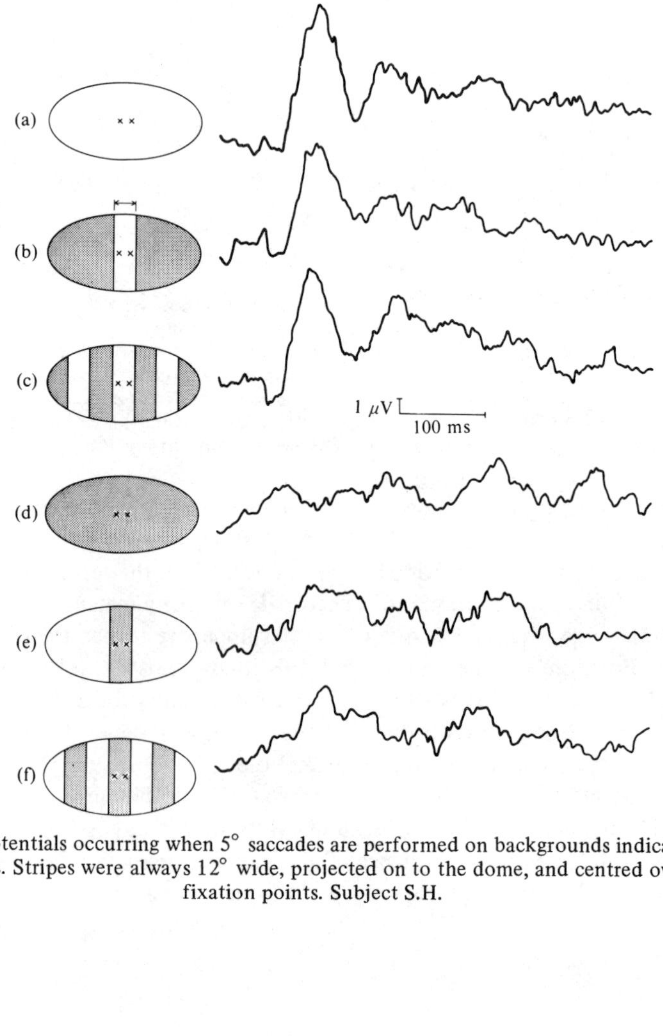

Fig. 15.7. Potentials occurring when 5° saccades are performed on backgrounds indicated in the left diagrams. Stripes were always 12° wide, projected on to the dome, and centred over the tiny fixation points. Subject S.H.

illuminated field to a single 12° light stripe overlapping the two fixation points did not greatly change the potential (b), nor did the addition of further light stripes to either side of centre (c). When the whole background was darkened, the potential disappeared as usual (d), and the record remained relatively flat even when luminance was replaced around a single dark stripe straddling the fixation points (e). Addition of dark stripes did not have much further effect (f). Finally, a single *horizontal* light stripe 20° in diameter and centred on the fixation points allowed full potential amplitude (not shown).

These results suggest that the saccadic potential is concerned with a relatively small area (not more than 12° horizontal or 20° vertical extent) of the visual field centre, and confirm that luminance is necessary for the potential to appear. We may also infer that the movement of borders close to this critical area is of little significance, since the potential failed to be affected when border movement was maximal (Fig. 15.7(c)), controls showed that the fix points could be removed without significant change of the potential.

Displacement potentials during fixation

The suggestion has been made that the interaction between the saccade VEP and the test flash is a visual one; if this is so, it should be possible to see similar interactions between test flashes and potentials evoked by rapid, 'saccadic' displacements of background.

It was possible to produce a VEP similar to that accompanying a saccade by projecting a light gradient on the dome via a mirror–galvanometer system. Rapid 5° horizontal displacement of the mirror effected a diffuse luminance change amounting to 0·5 log unit at every retinal position across the central 25° of the visual field. The potential evoked by this displacement is shown in Fig. 15.8(a). Fig. 15.8(b) shows the response following a 5° saccade made over the same background. Responses to circular test flashes of 12° diameter presented alone at 1·0 and 0·9 log units above *fixation* threshold without movement, are shown in Fig. 15.8(c) and (d); both of these test flashes were 0·1 log ft-L below psychophysical threshold during the movement, i.e. they were perceived neither during eye movement nor during background displacement. When the flash was presented during either movement the traces labelled (e) and (f) were recorded. Except for a consistent tendency for the combination displacement plus flash VEP to be *smaller* than the displacement VEP alone, there is nothing remarkably different among the two sets of records. Traces (g) and (h) show the residual of the flash VEP when the movement potentials are subtracted by computer from the combination (movement and flash together) VEP.

These data show that (a) displacements of luminance 'mask' test flashes in a comparable manner whether produced by a saccade or a rapid background displacement during fixation; and (b) there is nothing dramatically different in the VEPs to suggest that the mechanism of masking during saccades is any different

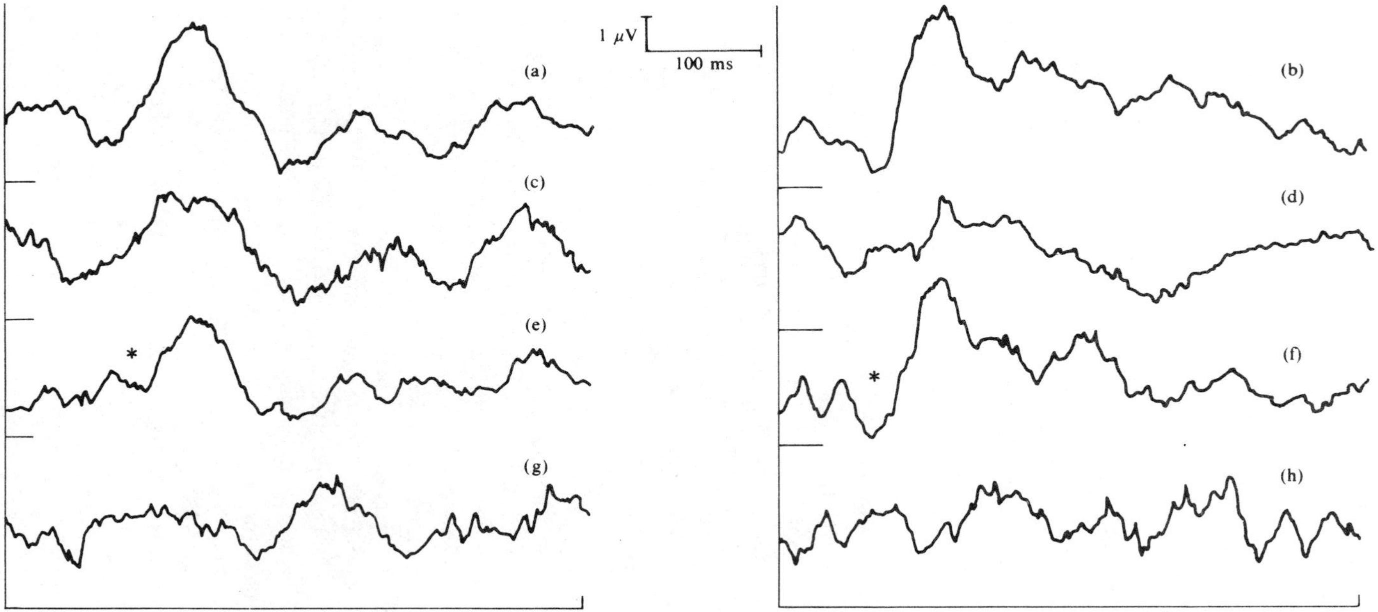

Fig. 15.8. Background displacement VEPs during fixation compared to saccade VEPs over the same background. (a) Displacement potential; (b) a saccade potential. (c) and (d) Flash potentials during fixation at 1·0 log units (c) and 0·9 log units. (d) above fixation threshold. These flash values were 0·1 log unit *below* the thresholds during displacement and saccades, respectively. (e) and (f) Potentials obtained when the same flashes were triggered by either the displacement (e) or the saccade (f). The asterisk signifies that the flash was not seen during movement. (g) and (h) The movement VEPs in (a) and (b) have been subtracted by computer from the combined (flash triggered by movement) VEPs of (e) and (f). The resultant shows little sign of the flash response alone. Subject S.H.

from that at work during background displacement during fixation. It was, however, commonly observed that the potential obtained during saccades was better defined, had a larger amplitude, and was in general crisper than that produced by a background displacement during fixation. Nevertheless, the background displacement was at least equally able to 'mask' a superimposed test flash, as determined by psychophysical measures of flash threshold during either type of movement.

Discussion

The experiments above suggest that there is substantial input to the visual system during rapid eye movements over illuminated backgrounds, even when no pattern is present in the visual field. The input is manifest in a VEP in the occipital region which is not present during saccades in the dark and the amplitude and latency of which show an orderly dependence on background luminance.

The fact that amount of threshold change for test flashes during saccades increases directly with VEP amplitude provides evidence that the two may be causally related. The similarity between psychophysical and electrophysiological events during background displacement and saccadic movement suggests that the underlying mechanisms affecting changes in visual sensitivity are the same in both situations, and is consistent with several recent studies in animals which compare saccadic activity to changes evoked in the primary visual system by rapid saccadic displacement of the background while the eye is fixating (Wurtz 1969; Jeannerod and Sakai 1971; Ebersole and Galambos 1973; Jeannerod and Chouvet 1973; Adey and Noda 1973). The contention that special inhibition accompanies eye movement to produce increases in visual threshold (e.g. Volkmann *et al.* 1968; Zuber *et al.* 1966) or reduction in the amplitude of VEP to test stimuli presented during saccades (e.g. Chase and Kalil 1972; Michael and Stark 1967) would appear questionable in the light of our results. Rather these events may be explained in terms of visual masking.

Visual activation during eye movement dependent only upon luminance in the background such as we have described has also been observed in the monkey cortex (Cohen and Feldman 1971). This discharge might well provide the 're-afference' to match an efferent command as conceived by von Holst and Mittelstaedt (1950) or to compare with the 'corollary discharge' proposed by Sperry (1950). Exact relevance to an outflow model of visual stability (as basically conceived by Helmholtz (1866)) requires future investigation.

Acknowledgement

This research was supported in part by the National Institutes of Health grant R01EY-01497 to Dr. B. Brooks. The work was initiated in the laboratory of Dr. Albert Fuchs, University of Washington, with support from Grant R01EY-00745 from the National Institutes of Health.

16. Electrophysiological observations on the visuomotor system and visual neurosensorium

D. KURTZBERG and H. G. VAUGHAN, JR.

Departments of Neuroscience and Neurology and the Rose F. Kennedy Center for Research in Mental Retardation and Human Development, Albert Einstein College of Medicine, Bronx, New York

Introduction

During the past 20 years, major strides have been made in our understanding of the neural mechanisms of vision. These have been achieved principally through microelectrode studies of the response of single neurones at various levels of the visual system to precisely controlled photic stimulation of the retina. Only recently, however, has neuronal unit activity been recorded from the cortex and subcortical structures of animals engaged in active vision. Wurtz (1968) was the first to compare the response of single cortical neurones to active saccadic displacement of the retinal image with the response to passive shifts of the visual field in monkeys trained to fixate and execute specific shifts in gaze. Bizzi (1968) and Bizzi and Schiller (1970) examined the neural activity in the frontal eye field of monkeys during spontaneous scanning. These and a number of more recent studies have begun to elucidate the complex relationship between oculomotor activity and the processing of visual information.

Despite the undeniable importance of investigations in experimental animals, there are good reasons to pursue the analysis of certain aspects of visual neurophysiology in man. From a purely technical standpoint, the recording of neuroelectric activity with the concomitant assessment of perceptual variables (e.g. Vaughan 1966; Gross, Vaughan, and Valenstein 1967; DeVoe, Ripps, and Vaughan 1968; Vaughan and Silverstein 1968) can be readily carried out in human subjects without the laborious training required for behavioural testing of vision in experimental animals. Since correlative behavioural and neurophysiological studies of vision in subhuman primates are virtually nonexistent, animal neurophysiological studies are generally interpreted in terms of human perceptual phenomena. Such *ad hoc* interpretations are often of doubtful validity. Although the electrophysiological indices available in human subjects are usually limited to scalp-recorded EEG data which must be interpreted with caution (Vaughan 1974),

Visual evoked potentials in man: new developments (ed. J. E. Desmedt), pp. 314–31. Clarendon Press, Oxford 1977.

correlative studies in man can provide guidelines for the design and interpretation of definitive neurophysiological analyses in experimental animals.

An adequate formulation of the neural mechanisms of vision must take into account the constraints upon visual processing introduced by ocular movements. In normal viewing of a stationary visual scene, the retinal image is abruptly shifted 2–5 times per s by saccadic eye movements. Thus, a new spatial pattern of excitation must be processed by the visual system every 200–500 ms. Despite this input discontinuity, there is often no awareness of any spatial or temporal interruption in the continuity or stability of the visual scene.

Although moving contours are potent stimuli for the visual system, the observer is ordinarily unaware of the shifting of the visual image during saccades. In recent years, discussions of the mechanisms underlying the maintenance of visual stability and continuity in the face of saccadic shifts in the retinal image have invoked the explanatory construct of 'corollary discharge' (Sperry 1950). Some investigators have considered saccadic suppression as well as image stabilization to be a manifestation of the corollary mechanism, whereas others (Richards 1968; MacKay 1970; Vaughan 1972, 1973) have argued that saccadic suppression does not require the operation of a central mechanism and thus constitutes a process distinct from the corollary mechanism underlying image stabilization.

A consideration of the processes underlying the control of ocular fixations and the central processing of the information derived from the ensuing retinal images led to the suggestion (Vaughan 1972) that the neural mechanisms of vision can be divided into two distinct domains. The 'visuomotor system' encompasses the afferent and efferent processes which are temporally linked to saccades, whereas the 'visual neurosensorium' comprises the central mechanisms subserving visual experience *per se.*

The visuomotor system comprises five distinct processes:

(1) saccade generation;
(2) the corollary discharge;
(3) afferent processes related to shift of the retinal image during saccades;
(4) afferent inflow during fixation;
(5) programming of the next saccadic vector.

Taken together, these processes comprise what may be called the saccadic loop, a series of neural events circumscribed by successive saccades in which information derived from the preceding fixation is utilized for the programming of the ensuing saccadic vector. Each segment of the loop must bear a close temporal relationship to specific portions of the preceding or succeeding saccade.

In contrast to the visuomotor mechanism, the visual neurosensorium must often manifest a smooth flow of neural activity relatively unperturbed by the abrupt spatial and temporal discontinuities in the sequence of retinal images which accompany saccadic scanning. When the saccades are relatively small the afferent activity generated by the new retinal image is presumed to interact with the information on saccade size and direction contained in the corollary discharge to achieve this subjective stabilization. However, with larger shifts in the retinal image where there is less overlap between the pre- and post-saccade fields, the percept begins to manifest both spatial discontinuity and a perceptible 'gap' in the temporal structure of the visual image. This circumstance also obtains in reading, where there is little or no overlap in the word-clusters processed during successive fixations. This differs markedly from the situation in which a visual target is scanned by relatively small saccades. Here, there may be no awareness of the saccades themselves, so smoothly are the pre- and post-saccade fields merged into the ongoing percept. Thus, the characteristics of neural activity within the visual neurosensorium must be affected by saccade size, with the image stabilization effects of the corollary discharge being restricted to relatively small saccades in which the pre- and post-saccadic images are substantially overlapping. It is also noteworthy that the corollary mechanism seems to be inoperative in night vision, inasmuch as apparent motion of the visual field can be readily perceived with voluntary saccades performed under scotopic conditions.

The foregoing considerations lead to specific inferences which can be put to empirical test concerning the neural processes related to the various components of the visuomotor system and visual neurosensorium. By recording brain potentials synchronized to saccades as well as to externally programmed visual stimuli, the timing and localization of some of these neural processes can be analysed. Hypotheses concerning the electrophysiological manifestations of each component of the visuomotor system and the visual neurosensorium are outlined below before presenting our experimental observations.

The visuomotor system

Saccade generation

Each saccade is generated by a brief phasic burst of neural activity in the relevant brain-stem oculomotor nuclei resulting in a specific saccadic vector (Schiller 1970; Fuchs and Luschei 1971). More proximal structures which have been implicated in saccade generation are the pontine reticular formation (Cohen and Feldman 1968; Cohen and Henn 1972) and superior colliculus (Schiller and Koerner 1971; Schiller and Stryker 1972; Wurtz and Goldberg 1972). The time-course of neural activation relative to saccades has been well defined in the latter structure by Schiller and Koerner (1971) who found that the rate of firing slowly built up over the 200 ms preceding saccades, suddenly bursting as a phasic discharge about 20–40 ms prior to the ocular movement. To date, animal studies of cortical participation in the events immediately preceding saccades have produced negative results (Bizzi 1968; Bizzi and Schiller 1970; Mohler, Goldberg, and Wurtz 1973). Consideration of the information required to encode saccadic vectors, which includes higher-order cognitive data, as well as data on the effects of cortical ablation and stimulation on oculomotor activity (Kennard and Ectors 1938; Latto and Cowey 1971*a*, *b*; Robinson and Fuchs 1969), suggests that these results may reflect technical limitations of the experiments rather than representing firm evidence for the lack of cortical implication in saccade initiation.* Indications that this is so have been found in human studies of antecedent saccade-linked potentials (Barlow and Ciganek 1969; Becker, Hoehne, Iwase, and Kornhuber 1972; Kurtzberg and Vaughan 1973).

Corollary discharge

These neural events signal the characteristics of the saccadic vector to the portions of the nervous system which will receive information derived from the succeeding fixation. The initiation of the corollary discharge will also be time-locked to saccade onset, but must persist for the time required for completion of the saccade and arrival of the afferent information at the appropriate processing stage. Saccade duration is linearly proportional to amplitude, ranging from approximately 30 ms for a 3° saccade to 150 ms for a 70° movement. The retinal–cortical delay varies as a power function of luminance over a range of approximately 50 ms under photic conditions (Vaughan 1966). Considering the magnitude of these delays, it would seem necessary for the corollary discharge to persist in its influence over a period of 150–200 ms following saccade onset. It is possible that the breakdown of image stabilization which occurs with large saccades and under scotopic conditions is due to delay in the fixational afferent volley which exceeds the effective temporal span of the corollary discharge.

Under ordinary conditions of viewing the corollary discharge will be confounded by the concurrent afferent processes. It will be disclosed in isolation only when saccades are performed in the dark.

Afferent inflow with shift of the retinal image

Moving contours are potent stimuli for discharge of neurones in retina and visual cortex (Wurtz 1969). The gross potential correlate of this discharge is the lambda wave synchronized to saccade onset. The lambda wave is enhanced by the presence of contour in the visual field and it is absent in the dark (Scott and Bickford 1969). The functional significance of this activity has been debated, but it has been most persistently and cogently related to the elevation of visual threshold during saccades. Examination of pure saccade-linked afferent activity is not possible with the relatively small eye movements which have usually been studied due to the temporal overlap of fixation-linked onflow. However, by systematically varying saccade size, those portions of the cortical response related to fixation should be distinguishable from those which are time-locked to the onset of movement.

*Since this paper was written antecedent neural activity has been found in parietal area 7 of the monkey in association with visually triggered saccades (Mountcastle, Lynch, Georgepoulos, Sakata, and Acuna 1975), and in the frontal eye field, area 8, with spontaneous non-triggered saccades (Arezzo, Dowling, Kurtzberg, and Vaughan, unpublished).

Electrophysiological observations on the visuomotor system

Visual input during fixation

On *a priori* grounds we would expect that information concerning the visual scene is derived from afferent inflow during each fixational pause. Yet there is little evidence in the literature for neural activity specifically related to fixation, i.e. to the end of the saccades. Since saccade duration can vary over a range of 100 ms or so with changes in the size of the movement, those aspects of cortical activity which are time-locked to fixation should vary in timing with respect to the saccade onset over the same range.

Programming of the ensuing saccade

This process has been included in the visuomotor system although it must in fact represent a bridge between information derived from the visual neurosensorium, i.e. the perceived visual image, and the mechanism for generating the next saccadic vector. In view of the discrete timing of the latter, it may be anticipated that some degree of time-locked antecedent brain activity will reflect the processes which encode the features of the saccade. This activity might be expected to vary depending upon the nature of the information utilized in a given situation for saccade programming. Thus, in some circumstances, such as when the subject is reading, significant cognitive determinants may operate, whereas in others, such as orienting shifts of gaze to unexpected visual or auditory stimuli, quite different neural mechanisms might be involved. Again, systematic experimental variation of the factors associated with saccade programming should disclose features of timing and localization of antecedent activity relevant to the specific neural mechanisms operative in each case.

The visual neurosensorium

One of the most exciting, if as yet unfulfilled, possibilities of human brain-potential studies is the identification and characterization of neural activity underlying conscious perceptual and cognitive processes. In this endeavour, the mechanisms related to visual perception represent an especially useful target for study due to the contrast between the discontinuous nature of the input processes and the continuity of visual experience. The former can be identified through their consistent temporal relationship to saccades, whereas the neural activity within the visual neurosensorium should, under conditions of subjective stability and continuity of the visual scene, be invisible in recordings of saccade-linked activity. Only when the visual experience itself manifests aspects of discontinuity which can be utilized for referencing the ensuing neural activity, may processes within the visual neurosensorium be disclosed for analysis.

Such circumstances occur with VEPs to brief photic stimuli. Under these conditions, a discrete visual percept is generated whose duration has been estimated by psychophysical methods to be in the order of 200 ms (Efron 1970), varying with the state of adaptation and with relationships between stimulus and the pre-

and post-stimulus fields (Haber and Standing 1970). When a visual stimulus is passively received, the corollary discharge which serves to smooth and stabilize the image received during active viewing, is absent. Thus the surge of neural activity generated by the photic stimulus should invade the entire visual neurosensorium and be recorded as a stimulus-locked VEP. By comparing the spatial extent of potentials recorded under active viewing in which the image stabilization and continuity are observed with the topography of the VEP it should be possible to identify the cortical regions comprising the visual neurosensorium (Vaughan 1972). Similarly, when saccades are large and the visual percept is no longer continuous and stable before and following a movement, fixation-locked activity should become increasingly prominent within the visual neurosensorium.

Method

The studies reported here were undertaken to provide information on the temporal sequence of cortical processes involved in the processing of visual information under conditions of normal viewing. Cortical potentials occurring in synchrony with saccadic eye movements (Kurtzberg and Vaughan 1973) were extracted from the EEG by averaging, and these 'eye-movement potentials' were topographically mapped from arrays of 23 electrodes placed over one hemisphere. In supplementary studies the potentials recorded concurrently from both hemispheres were compared and the activity observed in the peri-orbital region was mapped. The electro-oculogram (EOG) was recorded between electrodes at the outer canthus of each eye and utilized to synchronize the averaging process, which included activity preceding and following the onset of saccades. The effects of saccade size and field characteristics were investigated. Saccades of constant amplitude were obtained by voluntary shifts of gaze between two fixation points. Employing this method, saccades ranging in amplitude from 3° to 70° were studied. These movements were performed across various field configurations, the usual stimulus being a vertical grating displayed on a hemi-cylindrical field. For movements less than 10° a tachistoscopic viewer was also employed, permitting the comparison of eye-movement potentials (EMPs) with VEP elicited by shifts of the patterned field. The effects of changes in luminance and pattern on both EMP and VEP were also studied employing the tachistoscope.

Cortical responsiveness during and after 6° voluntary saccades was evaluated by presenting brief (10 ms) test stimuli at predetermined delays from the EOG onset (Gross *et al.* 1967). In contrast to other studies the test stimuli utilized pattern changes which did not alter the total luminous flux. Since cortical potentials are associated with the eye movements *per se* it was necessary to present the test stimuli on random trials and to subtract the potentials recorded on these trials from the activity associated with eye movements in the absence of the test stimulus. The magnitude of suppression effects was assessed psychophysically by varying the test stimulus duration until the test stimulus was no longer visible. The visibility of the test stimuli was also evaluated following pattern shift (Vaughan 1973) so as to compare the temporal course of saccadic suppression with the change in visibility and cortical response associated with passive movement of a pattern across the retina.

Results

Potentials synchronized with voluntary saccades are observed both preceding and following the onset of the eye movements (Fig. 16.1). We designate the activity prior to movement as 'antecedent potentials' and that which follows the saccades as the 'lambda complex'.

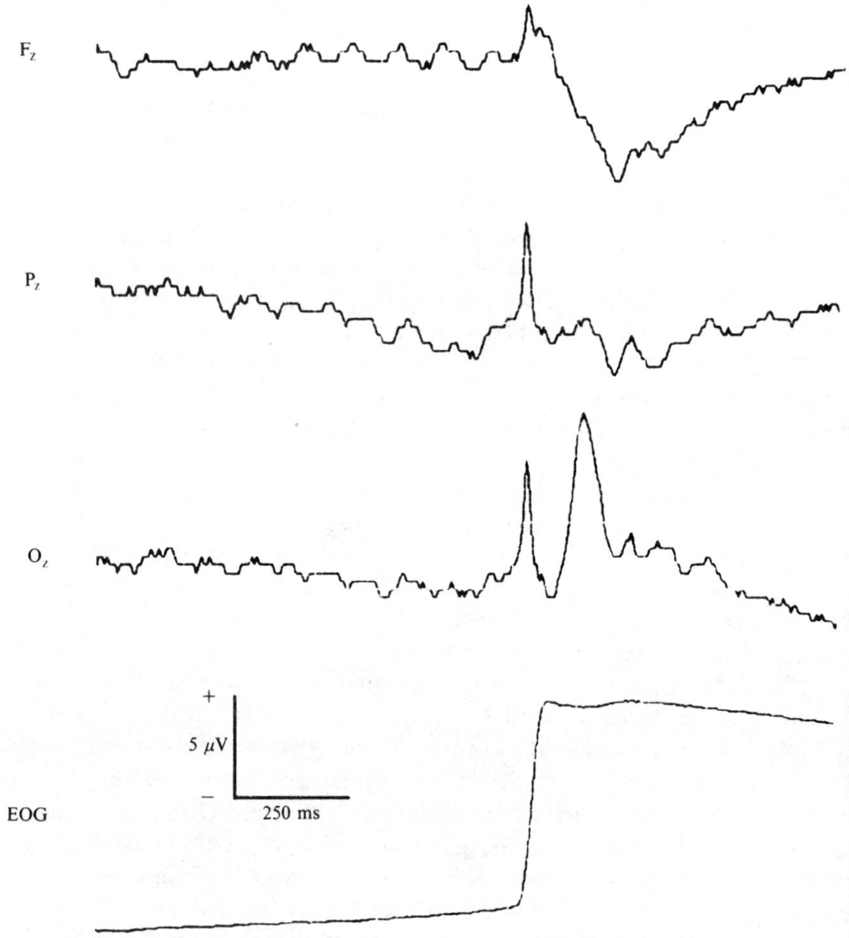

Fig. 16.1. Averaged saccade-linked potentials recorded from three cranial sites and the concurrently recorded electro-oculogram associated with 3° saccades performed across a vertical grating. Grand mean of 1500 epochs recorded from 5 subjects.

Antecedent potentials

Characteristic potentials preceding the voluntary saccades are observed with movements across either a plain or a patterned field and in the dark as well. When saccades are performed at intervals exceeding 2 s, potentials are seen which precede the saccades by a substantially greater period than could occur in normal viewing. We often observe slow potential shifts which precede the eye movements by 600–1000 ms. These are rather variable, but are usually negative in polarity and less than 5 μV in amplitude.

Following the slow shift a phasic positive complex is seen within which two distinct components can often be identified: a positive ramp-like deflection followed by a sharp positive wave. The initial positivity begins 60–190 ms before the saccade but its exact time of onset is often difficult to define precisely. The positive sharp wave begins between 10 ms and 40 ms before the EOG onset. At times, the two components are difficult to differentiate, with the sharp wave appearing as the latter portion of a smoothly accelerating positivity. The phasic positive antecedent potentials are most prominent and earliest in onset over the posterior parietal region. Frontal activity is more variable in its morphology and is often contaminated by potentials arising in the orbital region. Careful analysis of the topography and timing of these frontal potentials permits us to distinguish between activity of cerebral and orbital origin, but the antecedent potentials emanating from the frontal region are always less prominent than those observed over the posterior scalp.

The mid-sagittal distributions of the three components of the antecedent potential are presented for one subject in Fig. 16.2. Note that the maximum amplitude of each component is achieved over the parietal cortex, with a secondary maximum over the posterior frontal region. Most subjects do not show such clear differentiation of the anterior and posterior distributions of the slow negativity due to its variability and small size. On the other hand, the distribution of the phasic positive antecedent potentials is similar across subjects as shown in Fig. 16.3 which depicts isopotential maps of the phasic positivity for three subjects.

The intracranial sources of these potentials were estimated by comparing the empirical potential distributions with theoretical field configurations derived from a multi-shell volume conductor model (Vaughan 1974). The major source appears to lie within the pre-occipital and posterior parietal regions. The secondary focus includes a wide area of the posterior frontal cortex. These zones closely conform to the electrically excitable eye fields defined by electrical stimulation in man and subhuman primates (Penfield and Boldrey 1937; Crosby and Henderson 1948; Crosby, Yoss, and Henderson 1952). Although the cranial distribution of both the positive ramp and spike appears to be essentially the same and thus consistent with their cortical origin as delineated above, the identification of the sources of the antecedent spike is complicated by the fact that a potential of similar timing, but of opposite polarity is regularly recorded near the orbit. This potential diminishes

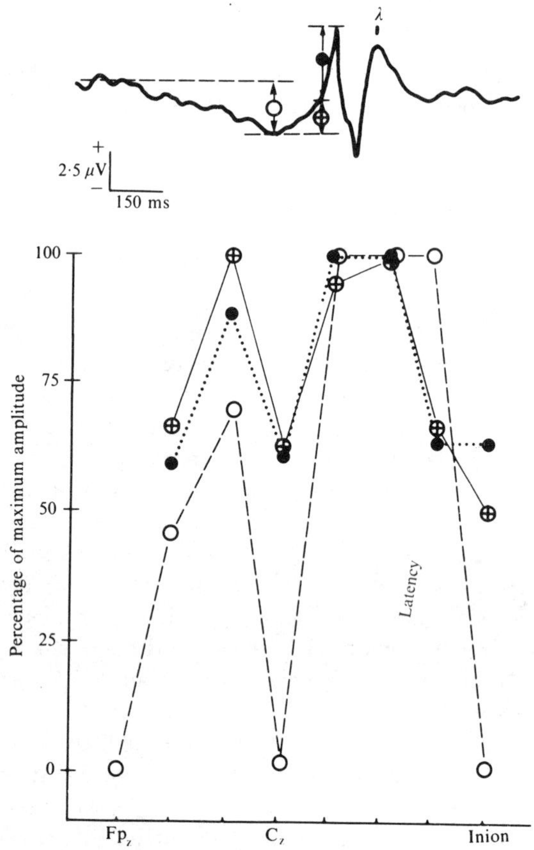

Fig. 16.2. Mid-sagittal distribution of the antecedent eye-movement potentials expressed as a percentage of the maximum amplitude of each component. 3° saccades across grating.

sharply in amplitude with distance from the immediate peri-orbital region, does not invert in polarity with eye movements in opposite directions, but does invert just behind the posterior margin of the orbit. These characteristics indicate that the peri-orbital spike represents neural rather than muscular potentials but their anatomic source remains in doubt.

The lambda complex

When saccadic movements are small, i.e. 10° or less, the potentials following their onset are fairly simple in form and distribution, comprising a positive deflection which is maximal in amplitude over the occipital pole. The amplitude and timing of this peak is dependent upon field luminance (Rémond *et al.* 1965; Gaarder *et al.* 1964) in much the same way as is the VEP. Indeed, the waveshape and distribution of this lambda wave are rather similar to that of the VEP elicited by a passive shift

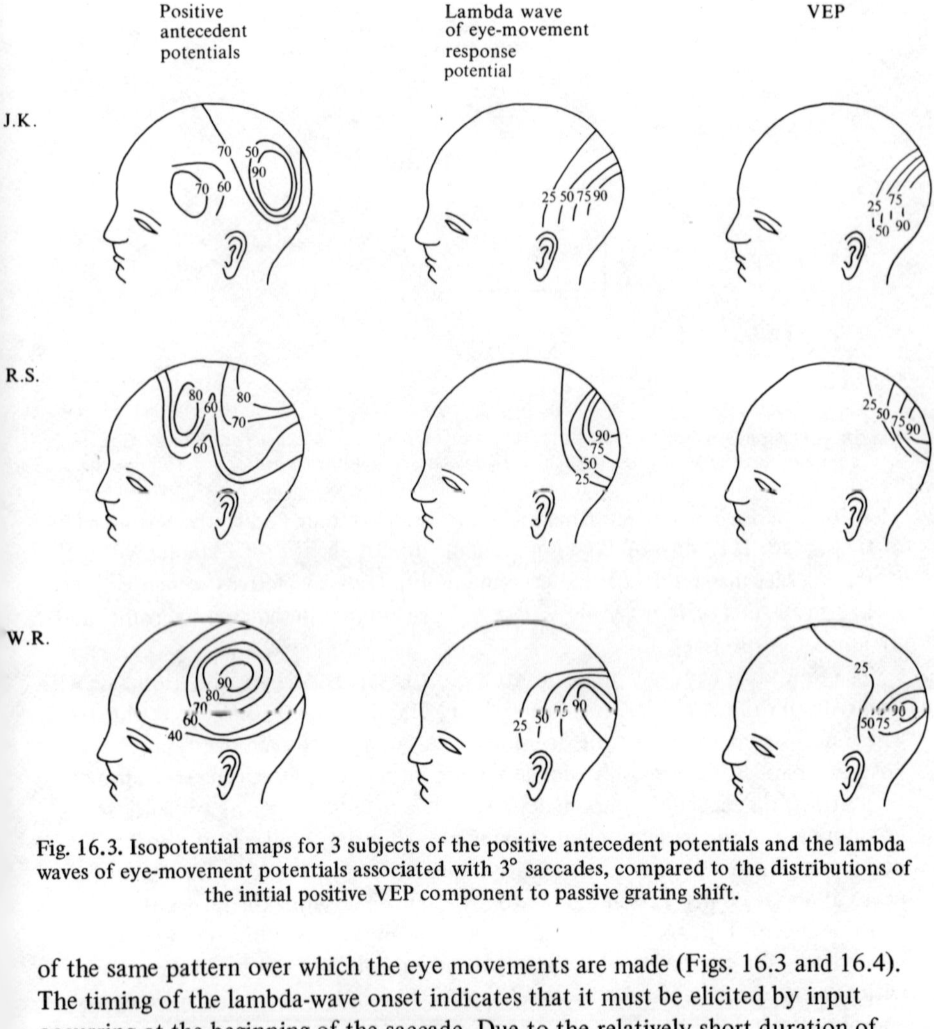

Fig. 16.3. Isopotential maps for 3 subjects of the positive antecedent potentials and the lambda waves of eye-movement potentials associated with 3° saccades, compared to the distributions of the initial positive VEP component to passive grating shift.

of the same pattern over which the eye movements are made (Figs. 16.3 and 16.4). The timing of the lambda-wave onset indicates that it must be elicited by input occurring at the beginning of the saccade. Due to the relatively short duration of the smaller eye movements it is not possible to detect activity associated with input occurring at the beginning of the fixation. As saccades are increased in size, however, the lambda wave begins to take on a complex configuration and distribution (Lesèvre and Rémond 1973). As shown in Fig. 16.5, movements which exceed 20° are associated with a complex series of potentials which differ in their relative timing with increases in saccade duration and also show somewhat different spatial distributions.

Analysis of this lambda complex requires careful examination of the form and distribution of the potentials associated with saccades over a large range of magnitude. With the largest movements studied it is possible to unequivocally

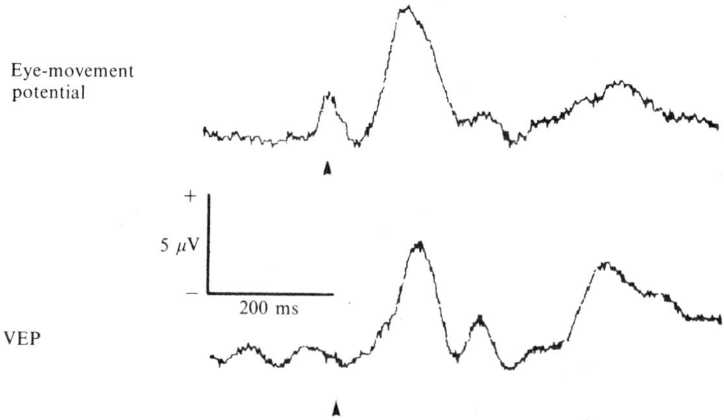

Fig. 16.4. Occipital eye-movement potential associated with 3° saccades across a grating compared to the VEP to grating shift. Each trace represents an average of 400 epochs.

identify potentials which are time-locked to the beginning and to the termination of the saccade. The onset-linked components do not change their latency with increasing saccade size, but are altered in amplitude by the activity which is time-locked to the end of the saccade. These components are designated 'saccadic' and 'fixational' respectively.

The fixational components manifest a positive–negative–positive sequence with peaks at approximately 100 ms, 150 ms, and 200 ms after the saccade termination. These peaks are largest over the occipital pole, but are also seen overlying the posterior parietal region. They increase in amplitude with increasing saccade size. In contrast, the saccadic components associated with the larger movements are predominant in the parietal region, having a distribution similar to the antecedent potentials. These also comprise a positive–negative–positive complex but with peaks at about 80 ms, 120 ms, and 150 ms after the onset of the saccades.

Reference to Fig. 16.5 shows that these saccadic and fixational complexes are most clearly differentiated with the larger movements, but can be discerned even with the 20° movements. A striking change in distribution of the early saccadic component can be seen in the 20° recording, however, in that the initial positivity appears at large amplitude over the occipital pole. This prominent saccadic component is also seen for all smaller movements and indeed appears to comprise the major portion of the relatively simple lambda wave seen with small saccades. An interpretation of the functional significance of the lambda complex will have to account for this shift in the relative size and distribution of the saccadic and fixational components as a function of saccade amplitude.

Corollary discharge

Saccades performed in total darkness are associated with antecedent potentials which are indistinguishable from those associated with movements across an illuminated

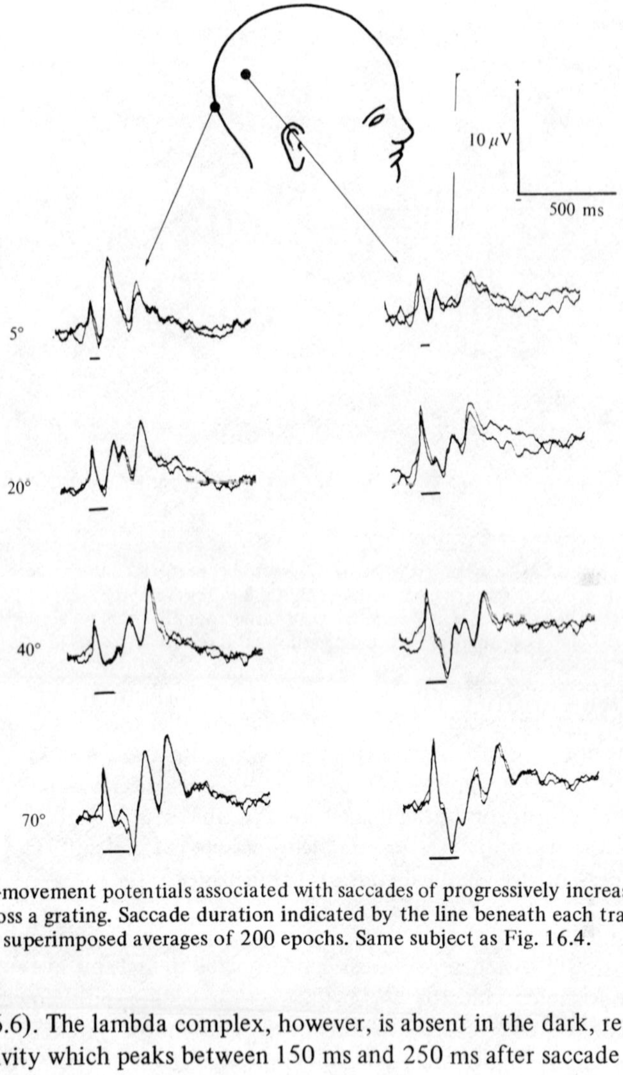

Fig. 16.5. Eye-movement potentials associated with saccades of progressively increasing size performed across a grating. Saccade duration indicated by the line beneath each trace. Two superimposed averages of 200 epochs. Same subject as Fig. 16.4.

field (Fig. 16.6). The lambda complex, however, is absent in the dark, replaced by a slow negativity which peaks between 150 ms and 250 ms after saccade onset and is maximal in amplitude over the parietal region.

This activity reflects the presence of a corollary discharge, the effects of which are presumably maximal during the period of peak amplitude, between 150 ms and 250 ms after the beginning of the eye movement.

Saccadic suppression

When eye movements are made across a patterned field a substantial elevation of threshold for pattern reversal detection is observed, as much as 2·5 log units, which is associated with a marked reduction in amplitude of the VEP to test stimuli

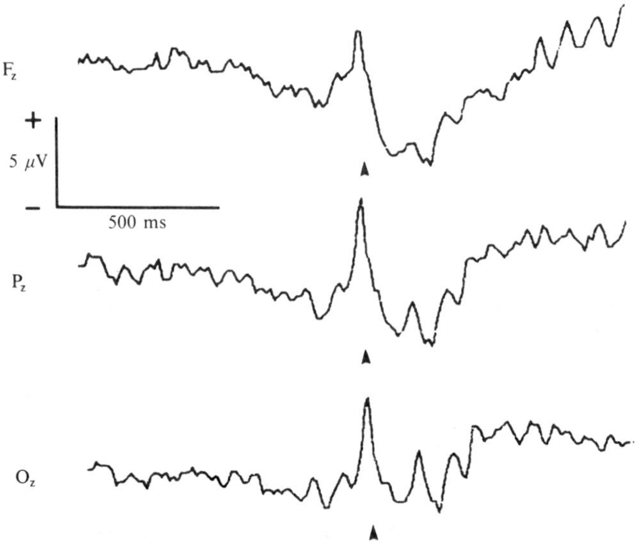

Fig. 16.6. Averaged EMP associated with 400 3° saccades performed in the dark. Same subject as Figs. 16.4 and 16.5. Note absence of the occipital lambda wave (compare with Figs. 16.1 and 16.4). A negative wave appears in P_Z and O_Z with some concurrent alpha activity. Frontal potentials are not changed in the dark (see Fig. 16.1).

presented during the saccades (Gross *et al.* 1967). Under the same conditions of field luminance and saccade size active movements are associated with minimal reductions in test VEP amplitudes and a threshold elevation which does not exceed 0·5 log units. Comparison of the magnitude and time course of the changes in measures of visual sensitivity associated with passive pattern shifts (Vaughan 1973) indicates an essentially identical effect as for saccades.

Discussion

Averaging of scalp-recorded potentials synchronized to saccadic eye movements has made it possible to identify cortical activity preceding and following saccades which may be related to specific aspects of the visuomotor system and visual neurosensorium. Although saccade-related potentials have been described by a number of investigators, there has been no consensus concerning the significance of either the antecedent potentials or the lambda complex. We will now try to interpret these phenomena within the functional framework outlined in the introductory remarks.

The principal issue posed by the observation of antecedent cortical potentials in human scalp recordings concerns the role of the cerebral cortex, and especially the classical frontal and posterior eye fields, in the programming and initiation of saccades. The failure to detect significant numbers of single frontal eye-field neurones which increase their firing prior to saccades, in contrast to the presence of such neurones in the superior colliculus of monkeys (Schiller and Koerner 1971; Wurtz and Goldberg 1972; Schiller and Stryker 1972), has been taken to exclude the frontal cortex from a role in saccade initiation. These studies have not, however, conclusively ruled out the presence of cortical saccade encoding mechanisms.

Since stimulation of either the frontal eye fields or the superior colliculus produces short-latency saccades whose amplitude and direction are specific to the locus of stimulation (Robinson and Fuchs 1969; Robinson 1972; Schiller and Stryker 1972), it is probable that a relatively small number of neurones encode a given saccadic vector. It would be necessary to identify the parameters of the saccades elicited from a particular site in order to know whether or not a neurone had, in fact, been recorded in relation to the expression of its specific functional characteristics. Since the latencies of frontally elicited saccades are even shorter than those elicited from stimulation of the superior colliculus, further examination of the role of the frontal eye fields in saccade control seems indicated.

The situation in the posterior eye fields is even muddier, since this region is complex in its functional organization with respect to eye movements, as judged from the stimulation data (Crosby 1953) and has been relatively little studied in relation to oculomotor functions in recent years. The human antecedent potential data suggest that phasic neural activity occurs in both the frontal and parietal regions prior to saccades. Some of this activity, notably the ramp-like positivity, could represent the process of saccade programming.

The sharp potential is harder to understand, both in terms of its origin and its functional significance. Since a spike of similar timing, but of opposite polarity, is recorded around the eyes, it has been suggested (Becker *et al.* 1972; Riggs, Merton, and Morton 1974) that the parietal spike represents a volume-conducted potential from the ocular region. Our data do not rule out this possibility since the timing of the peri-orbital and parietal spikes is virtually identical and a polarity inversion of the peri-orbital spike is present posterior to the orbit. However, this spike closely resembles the phasic pre-movement discharge in superior colliculus of monkeys. It could be supposed that the antecedent spike potentials represent a phasic discharge which is related to activation of the ocular musculature and is concurrently transmitted to other parts of the nervous system which are directly concerned with the programming of saccades. Thus, this spike would represent the initial portion of the corollary discharge, providing the rest of the visual system with precise information on the timing as well as on the direction and amplitude of each saccade. Although our finding of parietal and frontal maxima for the cranial distribution of the sharp positive wave is suggestive of a projection of this pre-saccadic discharge to the cortical eye fields, this speculation cannot be definitively tested in human subjects and will require study in experimental primates.

Turning to a consideration of the potentials which follow the onset of saccades, we have seen that the lambda complex comprises a series of deflections, some of which are time-locked to the initiation of the saccades and others to their termination. Both the saccadic and fixational components of the lambda complex are influenced by the size of the saccades as well as by the characteristics of the visual field over which these movements are made. In view of the fact that both the size of the lambda wave and the magnitude of threshold elevation are markedly enhanced by the presence of pattern in the visual field, it is reasonable to postulate that the saccadic lambda component may play a role in saccadic suppression. We originally showed (Gross *et al.* 1967) that the presence of a pattern field is required for an elevation of threshold sufficient to account for the absence of perceived movement of the field during saccades. Richards (1968) and MacKay (1970) demonstrated that small threshold elevations were observed following passive movement of an unpatterned field. Richards directly compared the effects of active with passive eye movements and found the magnitude of threshold elevation to be essentially the same under both conditions. Vaughan (1973), employing the same grating fields utilized in the earlier study of saccadic suppression, found that the magnitude and time-course of threshold elevation for detection of grating shifts and of reduction in VEP amplitude to the test stimulus were the same for passive grating shifts as for active saccades. Brooks (Chapter 15 of this book) has shown that field luminance affects both threshold elevation and lambda-wave amplitude, further supporting the idea that saccadic suppression is due to neural activity generated by movement of the visual field.

In cats, Adey and Noda (1973) have demonstrated the critical role of the visual field in diminishing geniculate and cortical responses to chiasmal shock during spontaneous eye movements. Their experiment evaluated excitability during eye movements in the dark and across a diffusely illuminated field as well as across a patterned field. Postsynaptic responses in the lateral geniculate body were reduced in amplitude when saccades were performed across the pattern field, unaffected in the dark, and only slightly reduced with movements across the unpatterned field. A virtually identical reduction in geniculate response was obtained by rapid passive shifts of the pattern field.

An interesting difference between geniculate and cortical excitability was observed (Adey and Noda 1973). Whereas only movements across the patterned fields were associated with reduced cortical responses to the chiasmal stimulation, all active movement conditions displayed a slowly rising facilitation which reached its peak about 150 ms following the onset of eye movements. This cortical facilitation was absent following passive pattern shifts. The authors suggest that this cortical facilitation might represent a manifestation of the corollary discharge.

Duffy and Burchfiel (1975) have reported direction-specific inhibition of spontaneous firing in a substantial proportion of neurones in striate cortex of monkeys performing spontaneous eye movements in the dark. This inhibition began about 20 ms following the phasic discharge of the oculomotor nucleus and usually lasted between 150 ms and 220 ms. Although Duffy and Burchfiel interpret these findings as evidence for a central mechanism subserving saccadic suppression, they present no evidence to show that the eye-movement related reduction in spontaneous activity is associated with a diminished responsiveness to afferent input. Indeed, reduced spontaneous firing might just as well be associated with enhanced cortical responsiveness, as found by Adey and Noda. Thus, Duffy and Burchfiel's observations may have little or nothing to do with saccadic suppression, but do reflect the effects of the corollary discharge on neurones within visual cortex. It seems likely that the parieto-occipital negative wave observed in human subjects with eye movements in the dark reflects the changes in cortical activity and responsiveness found in the cat and monkey.

The preponderance of evidence in both human and animal studies supports the conclusion that saccadic suppression reflects a reduction in responsiveness to retinal stimulation during saccades which is directly due to activity generated by movement of the retinal image. Indeed, the studies in which active and passive conditions of movement have been studied under the same experimental conditions (i.e. Richards 1968; Vaughan 1973; Adey and Noda 1973; Brooks, Chapter 15 of this book) have shown the effects to be virtually identical. Thus, one must question the functional significance of excitability changes which have been described during active eye movements in the dark (Riggs *et al.* 1974).

Despite the fact that the threshold elevation during saccades is largely mediated by a reduction in excitability of the visual system concurrent with the saccadic lambda component, it is by no means clear what happens to the visual information represented by the burst of neural activity generated at the initiation of saccades. There is no reason to suppose that this activity makes no contribution to perception. Indeed, the progressive diminution in amplitude of the early occipital saccadic lambda components with increasing saccade amplitude indicates that the saccade-linked input is itself modified with larger eye movements. Since both the saccadic and fixational lambda components change in their relative size and distribution with variation in saccade amplitude, the interaction of neural activity generated at the beginning and end of the eye movement must be a complex one which depends upon the spatial and temporal relationships of the pre- and post-saccade field.

In the case of small movements, there is a broad overlap. Therefore, little of the representation of the pre-saccade field needs to be erased from the visual neurosensorium. There is only the requirement for maintaining visual continuity by shifting the new retino-cortical input into its appropriate position within the perceived visual scene. Thus, it seems plausible that the spatially overlapping inputs from the pre- and post-saccadic retinal images might summate within striate cortex, possibly at the level of the complex cells (Hubel and Wiesel 1968). We hypothesize, therefore, that the large occipital lambda wave observed for small ocular movements represents a fusion of activity generated by the overlapping portions of the pre- and post-saccade fields.

As saccades increase in size, there is a steadily increasing temporal as well as spatial disparity between the information derived from the pre- and post-saccade fields. This is reflected in changes in the configuration and topography of the various components of the lambda complex. With very small saccades the occipital lambda wave peaking around 100 ms is prominent whereas later components, both occipital and parietal, are quite small. We have suggested (Vaughan 1972) that the parietal and posterior frontal regions, from which both the later VEP components at 200 ms and the antecedent eye-movement potential appear to be generated, represent the cortical domain of the visual neurosensorium. The small size of late lambda components over the parietal region was viewed as consistent with the smoothing effects of the corollary discharge.

It is evident, however, that larger eye movements are associated with increasingly prominent parietal waveforms, both early and late. Fixational components peaking at 100 and 200 ms are present with 10° saccades and become increasingly prominent as saccade amplitude increases. These changes reflect the circumstance that the afferent volley derived from the post-saccade field at the onset of fixation is not only quite different in spatial information content from the pre-saccade field, but also is arriving at the cortex progressively later relative to the saccade onset. There is, therefore, an increasing amount of pre-saccade information which no longer falls within the post-saccade field and must be discarded from the visual neurosensorium.

Consideration of this requirement leads us to recognize the need for a second type of visual suppression related to saccades which we will call 'saccadic erasure' to distinguish it from saccadic suppression. The latter mechanism suppresses input from the moving retinal image during saccades, whereas the former must eliminate from the visual neurosensorium those portions of the pre-saccade image which no longer fall within the visual field after completion of the saccade. It is possible that saccadic erasure is a purely passive phenomenon dependent upon the sharply delimited persistence of the visual image. Since most saccades under the usual circumstance of vision last considerably less than 100 ms however, there will often be a temporal overlap of pre- and post-saccade processes within visual cortex. Efron's (1970) estimate for visual persistence of about 200 ms corresponds closely to the duration of the fixational components of the lambda complex. If we assume that the processes generated by the pre-saccadic image last for the same amount of time, then post-saccadic activity which arrives at the cortex less than 200 ms following saccade onset could interact with the neural activity underlying the resident visual image. A reduction in the perceived duration of brief stimuli occurs when closely followed by a patterned field (Haber and Standing 1970). Thus, the phenomenon of visual masking could account for the erasure of those portions of the pre-saccadic content of the visual neurosensorium which are discordant with the input derived from the subsequent fixation.

There are obvious limitations to the inferences which can be drawn from scalp-recorded potentials on the nature of the neural mechanisms underlying the visuomotor and perceptual processes which take place during viewing of the visual world. Nevertheless, even the superficial account of saccade-related activity presented here illustrates the value of these recordings for identifying the timing and gross localization of cortical events which take place during active vision.

Most of the phenomena reported on here have yet to be observed in experimental animals, and even in man, they have been subjected to but a preliminary analysis. Future studies of vision will increasingly have to take into account the complex visuomotor mechanisms which underly the transformation of information derived from the retinal image into the perceptual representation mediated by the visual neurosensorium.

Summary

Averaged scalp-recorded potentials synchronized to saccadic eye movements reveal at least four distinct types of cortical activity:

1. Antecedent potentials, which are maximal in amplitude over the parieto-occipital and posterior frontal regions. These potentials may reflect neural processes responsible for the programming and initiation of saccades.
2. Saccadic lambda components, which are time-locked to the initiation of eye movements. These reflect activity generated by the onset of image movement across the retina and appear to be related to the suppression of input during saccades.
3. Fixational lambda components, which become increasingly prominent with increasing saccade amplitude. These components are similar to the VEP in timing and distribution and are presumed to represent the new visual information derived from the fixational pause.
4. The corollary discharge, which is unmasked with saccades performed in the dark.

Analysis of the timing and topographic distribution of these components with varying saccade size suggests that the lambda complex reflects the degree of overlap in the pre- and post-saccadic fields. Small saccades are associated with extensively overlapping fields which can be spatially and temporally integrated within the visual neurosensorium. Little saccade-linked activity is visible over the parietal region. In contrast, larger saccades are associated with progressively increasing fixational lambda components reflecting the increasing amount of new information communicated to the visual neurosensorium.

Acknowledgements

This research was supported by USPHS Grants MH 06723 and HD 01799 and a grant from the Scottish Rite Schizophrenia Foundation.

17. Pattern visual evoked potentials in infants

M. R. HARTER, F. K. DEATON, and J. V. ODOM
Department of Psychology, University of North Carolina at Greensboro

Because of the limited ability of infants to make behavioural responses to visual stimuli, pattern vision in neonates was until about 1970 investigated almost exclusively by means of behavioural techniques based on eye movements (Berlyne 1958; Fantz, Ordy, and Udelf 1962; Hershenson 1964; Brennan, Ames, and Moore 1966; Gorman, Gogen, and Gellis 1967; Karmel 1969*a*, *b*). More recently VEPs to patterned stimuli proved particularly appropriate for investigating pattern vision in infants. Harter and Suitt (1970) reported preliminary results on pattern VEPs in one infant from his 30th to 156th day of life. A recent study on infants ranging in age from 6 days to 45 days old analysed the effects of both check size and refractive error on VEP and visual fixation. This chapter presents comprehensively the data collected by Harter and Suitt (1970) – experiment 1 – and reports the data from our second study on infants from 6 to 45 days – experiment 2.

Experiment 1

Pattern VEPs were investigated longitudinally in one full-term (2·922 Kg) normal male infant (Bryan Harter). He was born 23 January 1969 and, due to problems with laboratory equipment, was 21 days old before usable VEP data were obtained from him. This report contains data collected during 23 recording sessions up to his 156th day of life. A single session consisted of 2 blocks of 50 presentations of each of 5 stimulus patterns. This resulted in 10 averaged VEPs per session. The 2 blocks of stimulus presentations were counterbalanced in an ABCDEEDCBA manner with stimulus order being varied systematically from session to session. The stimuli consisted of 4 checkerboards (individual checks subtending visual angles of 20′, 43′, 86′, and 133′) and a blank. These stimuli were reproduced on transparencies and were back-illuminated once every 1·1 s with a 10 μs light flash. Luminance transmittance was constant for all stimuli (approximately 2·5 log units above adult threshold). The stimuli were located 63 cm from the subject's eyes and their boundaries subtended visual angles of 22° x 22°. VEPs were recorded monopolarly by a gold-cup scalp electrode, located 1 cm above the inion on the midline, right earlobe reference.

Visual evoked potentials in man: new developments (ed. J. E. Desmedt), pp. 332–52. Clarendon Press, Oxford 1977.

Electrocortical activity was amplified by a Grass Model 7WC polygraph with high and low half-amplitude frequency filters set at 35 Hz and 3 Hz respectively and averaged by a Fabri-Tek 1062 computer, and recorded with an $X-Y$ plotter. The Dawson superimposition technique was used to monitor the variability within averaged VEPs. The raw data were also recorded on magnetic tape. The subject was placed in a supine position with his head turned sideways and oriented toward the stimulus. The room was electrically shielded, partially sound-proof and darkened, except for a dim light placed above and behind the subject. This light did not illuminate objects in the subject's visual field, but enabled the experimenter to monitor the orientation and movement of the subject's head. The photic stimuli were presented only when the subject was relatively still, with eyes open and oriented toward the patterns. Visual fixation was checked by means of the image reflecting from the pupil centre. White noise masked sounds associated with the flash tube and other extraneous noise.

This flash technique, as compared to constant-luminance techniques (Chapter 1 of this book) had three advantages in working with infants: first, the flash appeared to hold the infant's attention more efficiently than a continuously presented stimulus; secondly, a VEP to diffuse light could also be obtained for comparison with the pattern VEP at different ages; thirdly and most important, the stimulus could be presented contingent on the infant fixating the stimulus. This procedure exploited the rewarding properties of the flash and enabled the collection of more data.

Results

Representative VEPs to the different patterns at different ages (Fig. 17.1) indicate that two components were particularly sensitive to these variables: a surface-positive and surface-negative component with peak latencies at approximately 160 ms and 250 ms respectively at 21 days of age. The amplitude and latency of these components, designated P120 and N210, were measured as a function of stimulus pattern and age (Fig. 17.2). The latency of both components decreased nearly linearly and quite significantly as a function of age ($p < 0{\cdot}01$). This function for P120 had two negatively accelerated trends: latency decreased most rapidly between approximately the 21st and 35th and the 45th and 65th days of age. The effects of check size became more pronounced starting at about 45 days. Check size had no systematic influence on VEP latency. The amplitude of P120 and N210 varied significantly ($p < 0{\cdot}01$) and curvilinearly as a function of age: amplitude progressively increased to a maximum at approximately 65 days and then progressively decreased for the remainder of the experiment. These changes in average VEP amplitude were inversely related to the variability of the individual responses averaged. Up to about 65 days of age, variability progressively decreased, possibly due to increased attentiveness. From 65 days on, variability progressively increased, possibly due to movement artifacts and higher-amplitude background EEG activity.

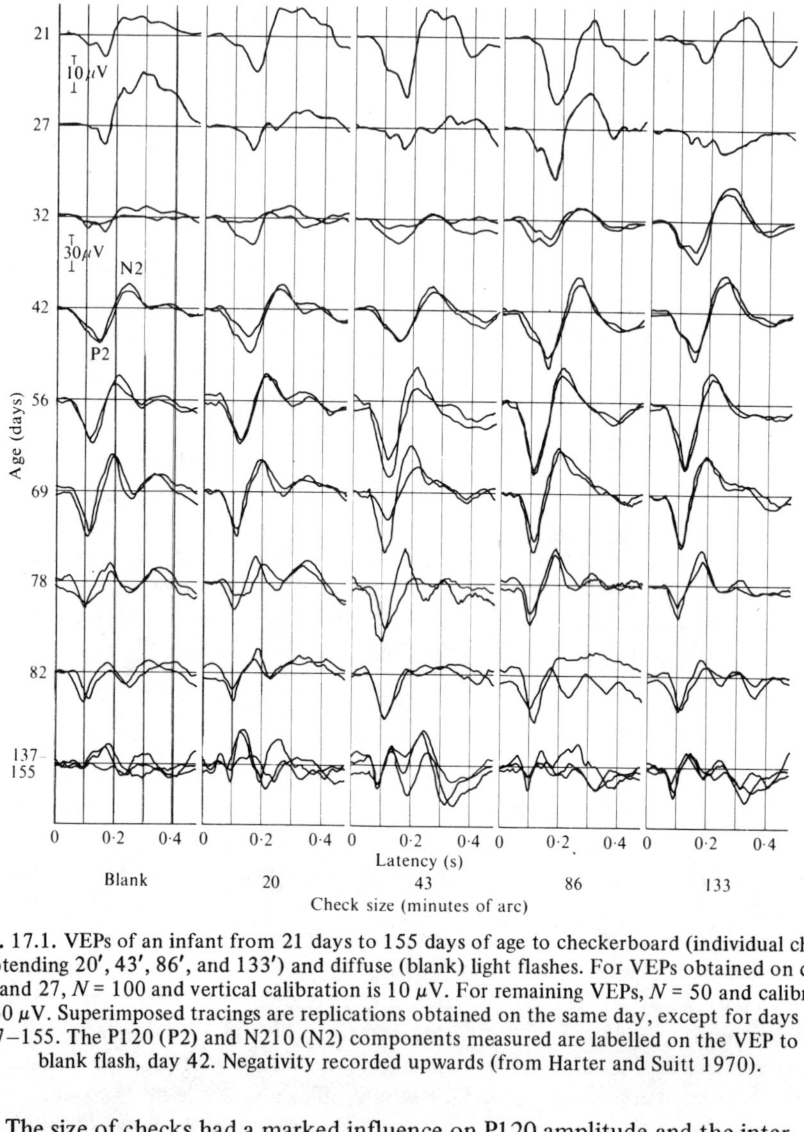

Fig. 17.1. VEPs of an infant from 21 days to 155 days of age to checkerboard (individual checks subtending 20′, 43′, 86′, and 133′) and diffuse (blank) light flashes. For VEPs obtained on days 21 and 27, $N = 100$ and vertical calibration is 10 μV. For remaining VEPs, $N = 50$ and calibration is 30 μV. Superimposed tracings are replications obtained on the same day, except for days 137–155. The P120 (P2) and N210 (N2) components measured are labelled on the VEP to the blank flash, day 42. Negativity recorded upwards (from Harter and Suitt 1970).

The size of checks had a marked influence on P120 amplitude and the interaction between check size and age was significant at $p < 0{\cdot}01$. With exception of data collected from 21 days to 40 days (see below), progressively smaller check sizes evoked the greatest amplitude VEPs as the subject matured. By the 55th day of age, the relationship between the range of check sizes employed and P120 amplitude is described as an unverted-U-shaped function. Check size had a similar effect on N210 amplitude ($p < 0{\cdot}05$) except the inverted-U-shaped function was not evident until the 75th day of life and the peak of this function occurred for

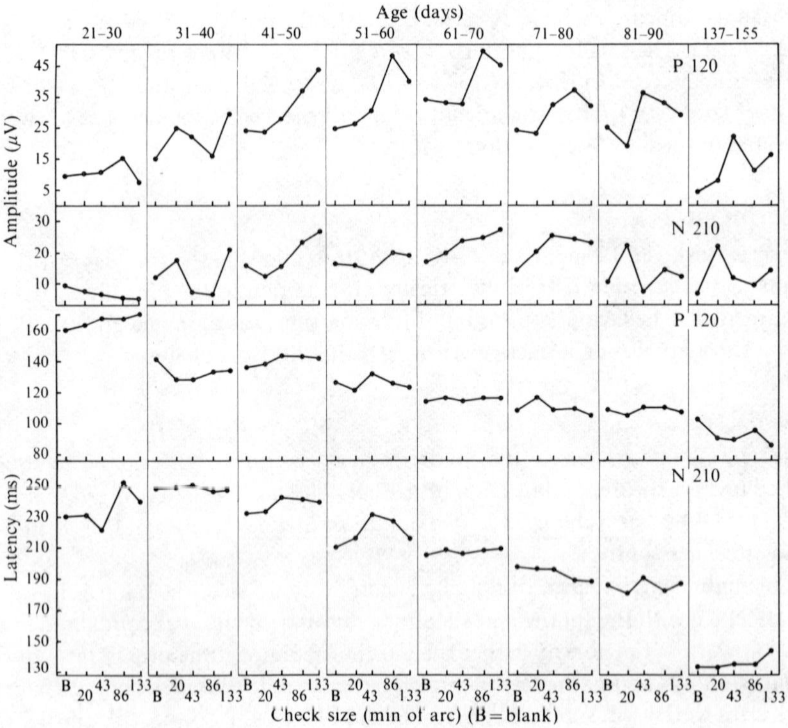

Fig. 17.2. Average amplitude and latency of P120 and N210 in an infant as a function of age and check size. Data have been grouped into 10-day blocks, except for days 137–155. The plotted points are means based on 3, 6, 5, 8, 5, 4, 2, and 3 averaged VEPs (replications) respectively for the 21–30, 31–40, 41–50, 51–60, 61–70, 71–80, 81–90, and 137–155 blocks of days.

smaller check sizes. The latter finding has been noted in adult subjects (Harter 1970; Harter and White 1970).

The effects of check size on VEP amplitude before the 40th day indicated a different trend. For the data collected from 31–40 days, both amplitude measures indicated a bimodal function – an increase, a decrease, and then an increase in amplitude as check size varied respectively from blank to 20′, from 20′ to 86′, and then from 86′ to 133′. This unexpected effect was evident in 5 of 6 replications and was statistically significant for N210 ($p < 0{\cdot}03$) and approached significance for P120 ($p < 0{\cdot}09$). Only three replications were obtained from 21–30 days and no consistent trend was evident in these data.

The following procedure was used to determine the smallest check size that elicited a response different from that elicited by diffuse light. First, the two amplitude measures were combined, resulting in a P120 to N210 peak-to-peak measure since the two measures reflect similar trends. Then a Dunnett *t*-test was used to compare each check-size VEP to the diffuse-light VEP for each 10-day block of data. The smallest check sizes were 20′ for 31–40 days ($p < 0{\cdot}01$), 133′ for 41–50 days ($p < 0{\cdot}025$), 86′ for 51–70 days ($p < 0{\cdot}001$), and 20′ for 71 to 156 days ($p < 0{\cdot}05$). These significant differences served as the bases of analyses presented in the discussion section.

Experiment 2

This series involved 10 infants of 6–45 days, thus allowing the first days of the infants' visual experience to be investigated. In addition to the procedures used in experiment 1, a behavioural measure of fixation time was obtained and the effects of contour sharpness or refractive error in the infants were analysed.

Method

Subjects were infants held in the children's nursery prior to adoption. The 10 infants studied had no apparent clinical abnormalities. The birth weights ranged from 2·4 kg to 3·4 kg (see Table 17.1). Two adults with visual acuities of 20/18 and 20/17 served as controls.

The equipment, experimental design, and procedure were the same as in experiment 1 with the following exceptions: the experiment was conducted in an isolation ward in the nursery rather than in the laboratory; the overall level of room illumination was approximately 3–5 mL (rather than in darkness); and different check sizes were used, subtending visual angles of 11·24, 22·5, 45, 90, and 180 minutes of arc. Each VEP was the average of 32 sweeps. The room was not electrically shielded nor sound-proofed. Interference at 60 Hz was minimized by maintaining skin resistance below 10 000 Ω. The electromechanical programming equipment generated an electrical artifact which was evident in the first 80 ms of the VEP.

Seven infants participated in at least four sessions with a minimum of a week's time between the first and last sessions; 3 other infants participated in two sessions. Two replications of each check-size condition were obtained during each session. If the infant was still cooperating after the check-size series was completed, VEPs were obtained to either the 45′ or 90′ checkerboard viewed through a series of spherical refractive lenses from −6 dioptre to +6 dioptre. The lenses were hand-held in front of the infants' eyes. Refraction data were obtained from 8 infants (Table 17.1). The order of presentation of the check sizes and refraction conditions was counterbalanced both within and between replications.

The handling of the infants was of critical importance in obtaining reliable noise-free data. An infant was tested at the end of a sleep period, just bejore feeding. The infant's diapers were changed and the electrodes were attached before the infant was fully awake. A 10–30 min period usually followed before feeding when the infant was awake, quiet, and orienting to the centre of the visual display. Visual fixation time was carefully monitored. The infant was held by one experimenter

TABLE 17.1 *Characteristics of the infants*

	Sex	Weight (kg)	Check-size data: Age (days) Range	Age (days) $\overline{X}$	Number of replications†	Visual acuity‡ (minutes)	Visual acuity‡ (Snellen)	Peak check size (minutes of arc)	Refractive lens data: Age (days) Range	Age (days) $\overline{X}$	Number of replications†	Best lens (dioptre)
B.R.	M	3·24	6–17	11	8	4	20/80	14	12–17	14	2–6	+ 2·00
H.A.	M	3·18	12–13	12	4	5	20/100	15		16	1	+ 1·25
T.R.	F	3·18	8–23	16	8	8·5	20/170	19	14–24	20	2–6	+ 3·00
P.E.	M	3·24	14–29	22	8	7	20/140	15	19–29	24	4–7	+ 2·00
M.I.	F	2·97	22–34	27	10	2·3	20/46	11	22–30	26	2–6	+ 1·00
A.B.	F	3·1	24–45	35	12	7	20/140	––	24–37	31	2–5	+ 1·00
J.O.	M	2·97	31–32	31	4	6·1	20/122	17	––	––		
J.I.	M	2·41	30–39	35	6	5·6	20/112	16	30–42	37	2–7	– 3·00
D.A.	M	3·41	26–41	33	10	4·7	20/94	22	26–40	35	3–5	+ 6·00
M.A.	F	3·03	37–40	39	4	8·4	20/168	22	––	––		
$\overline{X}$			6–45	26		5·8	20/117	17	12–42	25		+ 1·66 |2·41|

† Number of replication depended on the cooperation of the infant.
‡ Estimated from VEPs at a viewing distance of 63 cm.

so that its eyes were oriented toward the centre of the stimulus display. A second experimenter stopped the stimulus presentation if the subject shifted his fixation from the centre of the display, i.e. if the reflection of the checkerboard image shifted away from the centre of the pupil, or if the subject closed his eyes. As noted in experiment 1, the contingent presentation of the light flashes improved the cooperation of the infants. The amount of time the infant spent fixating (T_f) and not fixating (T_{nf}) were measured over the period of time required to obtain an averaged VEP (T_t) so that $T_f + T_{nf} = T_t$. Since each VEP was based on 32 flashes presented at 1·1 Hz, T_f was fixed at 29 s. The percentage time fixated equalled $T_f/T_t \times 100$. It is emphasized that VEPs were recorded only when the infants were fixating the centre of the display.

Equipment in the nursery was kept to a minimum: a portable Grass Model 79-2 Polygraph for amplification, an Ampex Model SP 300 seven-channel FM tape-recorder for data storage, and a variable-persistence oscilloscope for on-line monitoring of the data. The VEPs were averaged off-line in the laboratory by means of a Fabritek 1062 computer and a DataCom Minicomputer System.

Results

Representative VEPs from 2 younger and 2 older infants are illustrated in Fig. 17.3. The two superimposed tracings in each pair are VEPs to the same stimulus condition and reflect the repeatability of the data within a given session. The VEPs were more variable between sessions.

VEPs to the diffuse and 22′ checkerboard light flash for all subjects are shown in Fig. 17.4. Each tracing is an average of the four replications ($N = 128$) obtained nearest to each infant's 25th day of life. The waveform of VEPs was consistent among subjects and presented three prominent components which were respectively surface-positive, -negative, and -positive with peaks between 130 ms and 160 ms, 230 ms and 280 ms, and 320 ms and 430 ms after the flash. The amplitude of all three components varied as a function of the pattern presented. The amplitude was measured at four latencies: the most positive portion of the VEP between 130 ms and 160 ms, the most negative portion between 190 ms and 210 ms and 240 ms and 300 ms, and the most positive portion between 320 ms and 400 ms (Fig. 17.4). The baseline was the voltage level 60 ms after the flash. These four measures were then averaged resulting in a single measure of overall VEP amplitude. Repeated measures analyses of variance were performed to statistically assess the effects of check size and refractive error on VEP amplitude and on the percentage time fixated.

Effects of check size

The VEP amplitude varied as a function of check size ($p < 0{\cdot}01$) as shown for individual and grouped data in Fig. 17.5. Eight of the 10 infants gave the greatest VEP amplitude to the smaller (11′ or 22′) checkerboard flashes. A Newman–Keuls

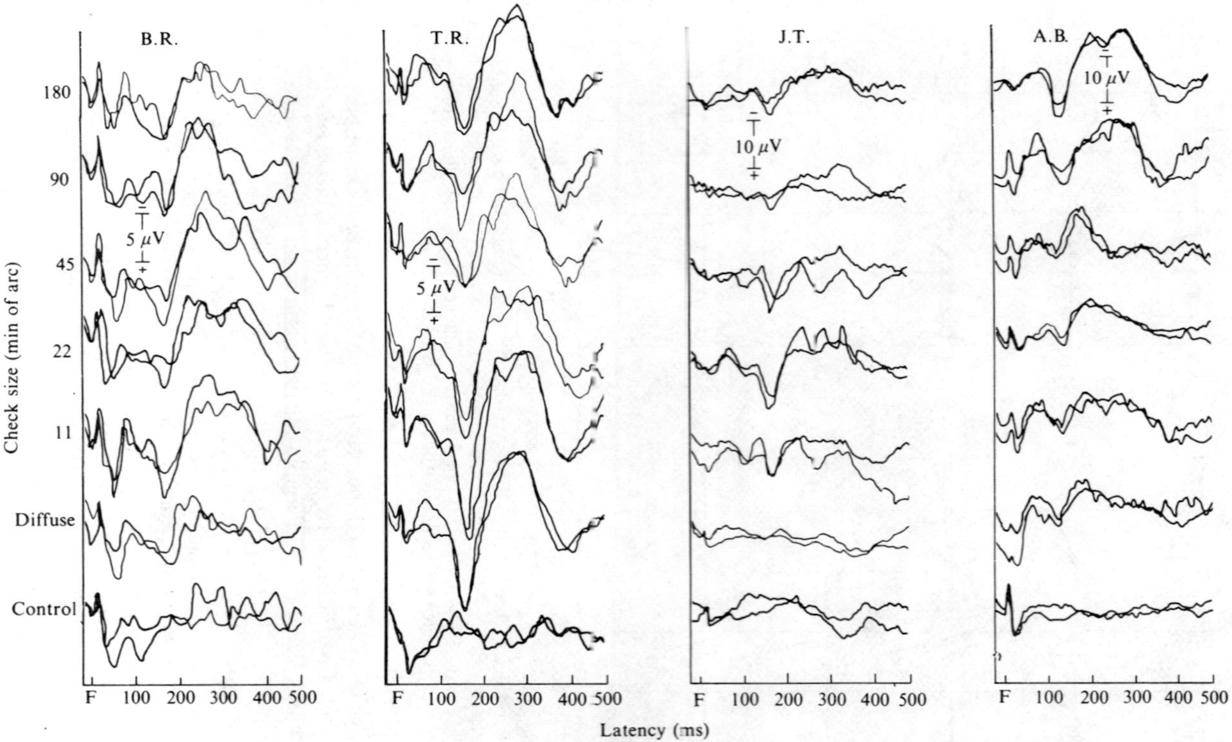

Fig. 17.3. Sample of VEPs to different check sizes from four representative subjects (B.R., T.R., J.I., and A.B.) obtained at 6, 8, 30, and 24 days respectively after birth. Each superimposed tracing in a pair is a replication with $N = 32$. The control VEPs were obtained when the flash was occluded and reflect an artifact for the first 100 ms after the light flash.

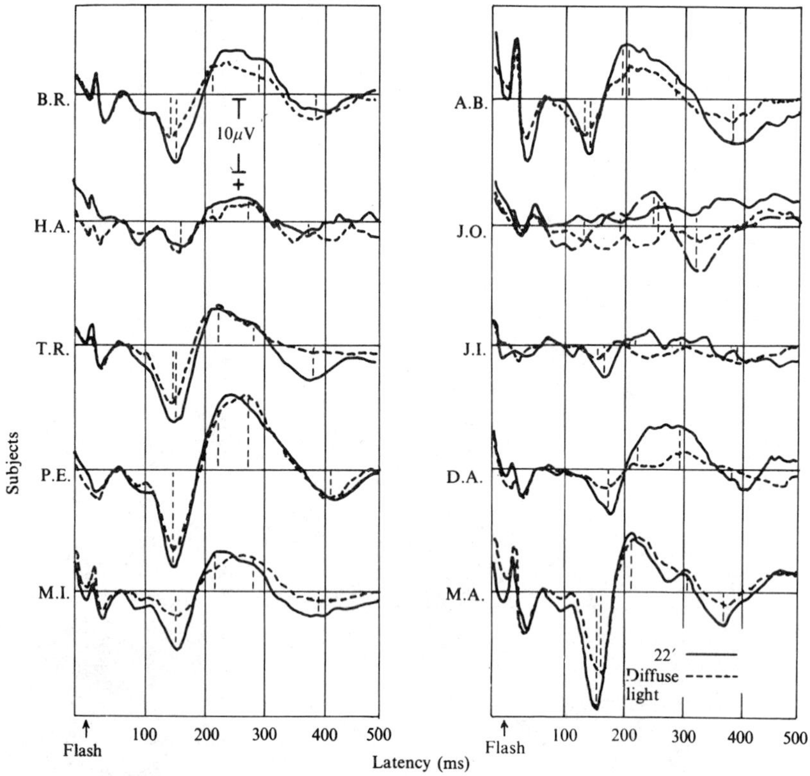

Fig. 17.4. VEP to the 22′ checks and to diffuse flash from each infant that participated in experiment 2. Each VEP ($N = 128$) was obtained nearest to 25th day of life. The extra dashed VEP for J.O. was in response to the 180′ checkerboard. The vertical dashed lines indicate latencies where amplitude measures were obtained.

Multiple Range test (Winer 1962) indicated a significant increase in amplitude when the stimulus was changed from diffuse to the 11′ checkerboard ($p < 0{\cdot}01$), the smallest check size used. VEP amplitude decreased when the check size was increased from 22′ to 45′ ($p < 0{\cdot}01$) and it then increased slightly when check size was changed from 45′ to 180′. Two of the older infants (A.B. and J.O.) gave the greatest VEPs to the larger checks. This tendency for a bimodal function between check size and VEP amplitude may explain apparent discrepancies between different studies as discussed below.

Data in Fig. 17.6 support the suggestion that greater VEPs were obtained to the 11′ check size in 6–9-day-old infants and to the 180′ check size in 42–45-day-old infants. This interaction was difficult to demonstrate statistically, however. Analyses on individual subject's data did not reflect a significant interaction between the effects of check size and age over the relatively short period of time each infant was investigated (no more than 17 days). However, a significant correlation was

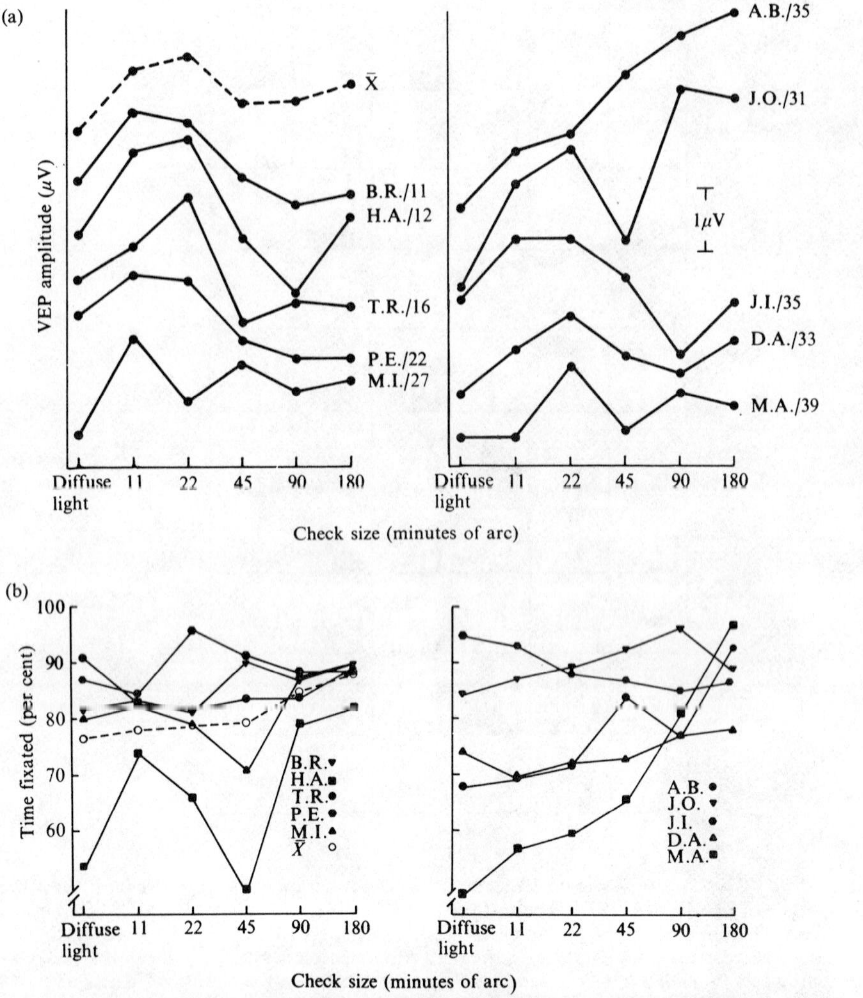

Fig. 17.5. Effects of check size on VEP amplitude (a) and on percentage time each check size was fixated (b) for each subject (solid function) and the mean of all subjects (dashed function). VEPs were obtained only when infants were fixating. Data have been averaged across replications and days, the values after each subject's initials indicating the mean age in days (see Table 17.1).

obtained between the check size eliciting the greatest VEP and the age of the infant on a given replication ($r = 0{\cdot}39$, $N = 42$, $p < 0{\cdot}01$). Age varied both within and between subjects in computing this correlation coefficient.

The percentage time fixated for both the individual and grouped data is shown in Fig. 17.5(b). It increased with check size from diffuse light to the largest check ($p < 0{\cdot}01$). This was an increase of approximately 12 per cent in the grouped data, most of which occurred from the 45′ to 180′ check. There was little difference in

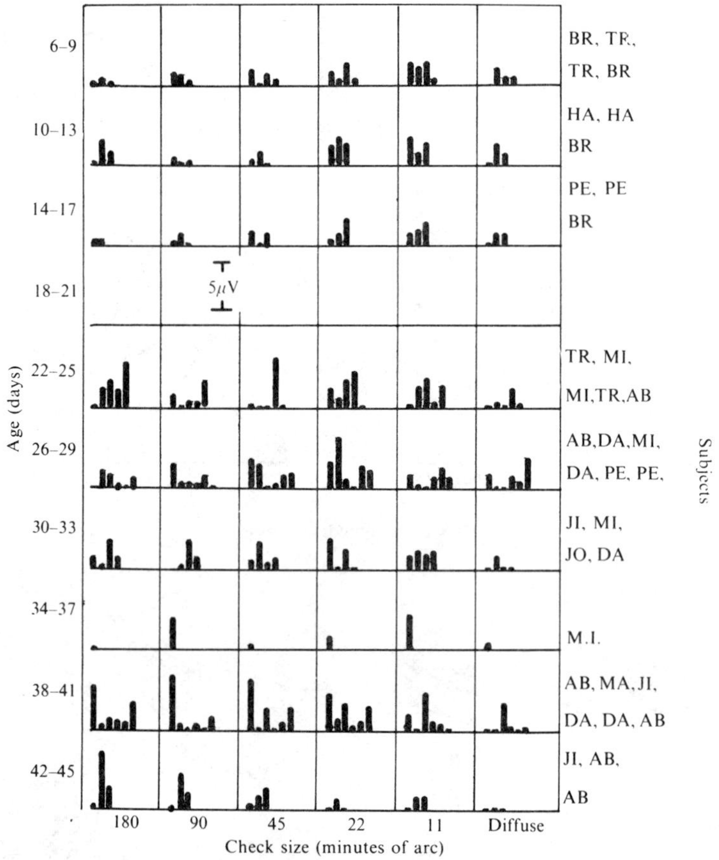

Fig. 17.6. Effects of check size on VEP amplitude as a function of age. Each vertical bar is the amplitude of one averaged VEP. The vertical bars within each square are VEPs of different infants to a given condition (age and check size). The subject from which each VEP was obtained is indicated by the initials on the right-hand portion of the figure. Note that greater-amplitude VEPs tended to be elicited by 22′ and 11′ checks from 6 days to 17 days and by 45′ to 180′ checks from 38 days to 45 days.

percentage time fixated in response to the diffuse, 11′ and 22′ patterns. Individual subjects varied considerably in how the various check sizes were fixated.

Correlation coefficients were computed for both individual subjects and the group to assess the relationship between changes in percentage time fixated and VEP amplitude as a function of check size. Only one of the 11 resulting correlation coefficients was statistically significant (A.B.: $r = 0{\cdot}85, p < 0{\cdot}05$). The correlation coefficient for the grouped data was $r = 0{\cdot}21$. It may be concluded, therefore, that the effects of check size on VEP amplitude and percentage time fixated were poorly correlated under the conditions of the experiment.

Effects of power of lens

When the infants viewed checkerboards (90′ or 45′ checks) through refractive lenses, the dioptre value of the lens significantly influenced VEP amplitude ($p < 0{\cdot}02$) (Fig. 17.7). The grouped data indicated the greatest VEPs were

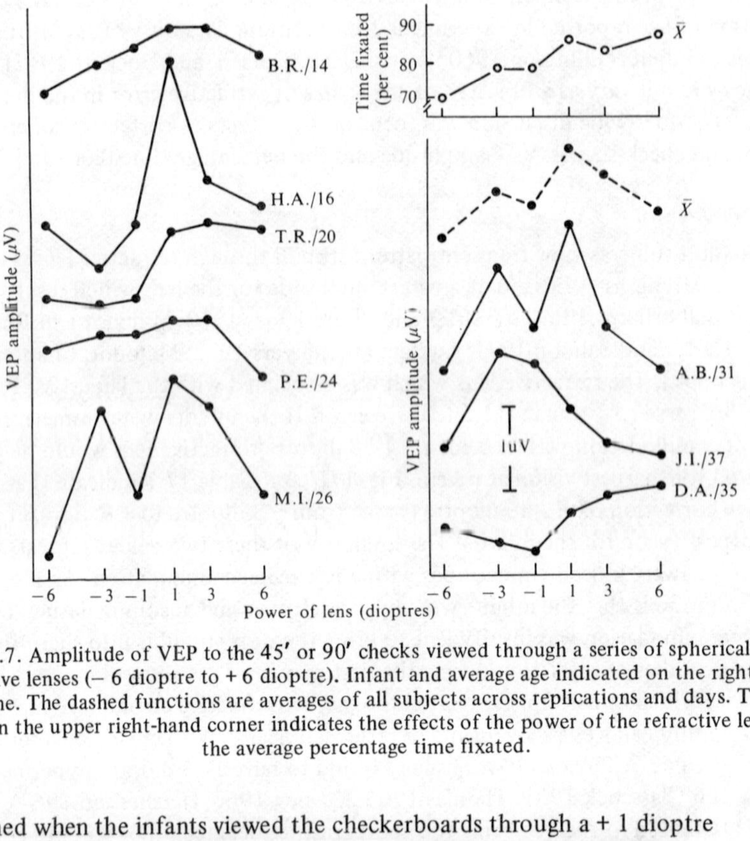

Fig. 17.7. Amplitude of VEP to the 45′ or 90′ checks viewed through a series of spherical refractive lenses (− 6 dioptre to + 6 dioptre). Infant and average age indicated on the right of each line. The dashed functions are averages of all subjects across replications and days. The insert in the upper right-hand corner indicates the effects of the power of the refractive lens on the average percentage time fixated.

obtained when the infants viewed the checkerboards through a + 1 dioptre refractive lens. Individual data indicated that all except one subject (J.I.) gave the greatest VEPs when viewing the pattern flashes through positive lenses (Table 17.1).

The changes in percentage time fixated due to the infants viewing the checkerboards through refractive lenses did not approach statistical significance. The correlation coefficient between percentage time fixated and VEP amplitude across the 6 lens values (Fig. 17.7) was 0·68. Although this value did not approach statistical significance it was larger than the one obtained across check sizes. It may be noted that these curves reflect more variability than the relationship of percentage time fixated or VEP amplitude to check size. This might be attributed to the refraction data being obtained after check-size data and involving fewer replications. Sufficient data were not obtained to assess the effects of lens diopters as a function of age on either VEP amplitude or fixation time.

Discussion

The waveform and component latencies of VEPs and the shift in VEP latency as a function of age reported in experiment 1 corroborate data on VEPs to diffuse light flashes in infants (Ellingson 1960; Ferris, Davis, Dorsen, and Hockett 1967). VEP latency did not vary as a function of check size or refractive error in the present study. The following discussion will focus on the effects of corrective spherical lenses and check size on VEP amplitude and the percentage time fixated.

Refractive error

When adult subjects view transient pattern stimuli through refractive lenses of different strengths, VEPs are of greatest amplitude for the lens which results in the perceptually sharpest image (Harter and White 1968, 1970; Millodot and Riggs 1970; Harter and Salmon 1971; Ludlam and Meyers 1972; Millodot, Chapter 22 of this book). The refractive lens which was associated with the largest VEPs may therefore serve to estimate the refractive error. If the infants were emmetropes and their accommodation was relaxed, a + 1·58 dioptre refractive lens would be required for sharpest vision at 63 cm. Fig. 17.7 and Table 17.1 indicate that an average correction of + 1·66 dioptre (range from − 3 dioptre to + 6 dioptre) resulted in sharpest vision for the infants. The similarity of these two values suggests that the infants were indeed emmetropes with a relaxed accommodation. An alternative interpretation is that the infants were hypermetropes and accommodating, but that accommodation was insufficient to bring the near stimulus into sharp focus. Previous studies of refraction during the first month of life showed inconsistencies which in part appear related to whether refractive errors were measured behaviourally using eye movements or retinoscopically. With cycloplegia retinoscopy the eye in a normal neonate was usually found to have 1–3 dioptre hypermetropia (Cook and Glasscock 1951; Thomas 1965; Keeney 1966; Hershenson 1967), this being attributed to the eye being too short for the focal length of its optical system (Duke-Elder 1963). Retinoscopic refraction without cycloplegia, however, indicated either emmetropia or myopia (Thomas 1965). Estimates of refractive error based on optokinetic nystagmus measures in newborns suggested myopia (Haynes, White, and Held 1965).

Data on accommodation in newborns are equally inconsistent. It was generally stated that infants do not accommodate during the first month of life (Scheie and Albert 1969, p. 105; Mussen, Conger, and Kagan 1969, p. 158), a conclusion supported by optokinetic nystagmus data (Haynes *et al.* 1965). Behavioural data based on visual preference techniques indirectly indicated newborns could accommodate, since infant's visual acuities did not change as a function of changes in viewing distances (Frantz *et al.* 1962).

In the present study the refraction data should be interpreted with caution. First, they were relatively variable, being obtained after the check-size data and being based on fewer replications. Secondly, relatively large checks were employed since it was anticipated that the visual acuity of newborns was rather poor and larger check sizes are required to obtain pattern VEPs when visual acuity is poor (Harter and White 1970). In fact, the visual acuity of the newborns was found to be 20/117 on the average (see below), which is better than anticipated. It would have been more appropriate to use the 11′ or 22′ checks for the VEP refraction (Regan and Richards 1973).

Effects of check size

Numerous investigators have reported an inverted-U- or V-shaped function between VEP amplitude and the size of checks in checkerboard patterns, with a peak for checks of 10–20′ in adults with normal visual acuity (Spekreijse 1966; Spekreijse, Esterez, and Reits, Chapter 2 of this book; Rietveld *et al.* 1967; Harter and White 1970; Harter 1970, 1971, Chapter 10 of this book; Armington *et al.* 1971; Harter *et al.* 1974). This same trend was obtained in infants except that checks giving the peak VEPs varied with age and that the overall change in amplitude was much smaller in newborn infants. Two aspects of the function are relevant: the check size at the peak and the check-size threshold, indicated by the extrapolated smallest check size which elicits a VEP different from that to diffuse light. The latter may be used as an estimate of visual acuity.

These measures in the present data were compared with results from other sources (Harter and White 1970; Karmel, Hoffman, and Fegy 1974; Sokol and Dobson 1976) by converting the data from each subject or each age group to standard scores ($z = x - \bar{x}$/standard deviation). The slope of the ascending and descending portions of the inverted V-shaped function was determined for the data in each study. The slopes were virtually identical except for the infants older than 160 days and adult subjects. The transformed data of experiment 2 are illustrated in Fig. 17.8 and in the bottom of Fig. 17.9. Fig. 17.9 also contains the transformed data of experiment 1 (P120 to N210 amplitude) and from other sources. The descending portion of the function extrapolated until it intersects the x axis defines the check-size threshold, and is assumed to indicate the point of transition from a pattern to diffuse response (Atkinson, Braddick, and Braddick, 1974; Regan, Chapter 11 of this book; Sokol and Dobson 1976). The numerical values next to each function indicate the check sizes associated with the x axis intersects and the peaks of the functions (see Table 17.1). These values were highly correlated (Fig. 17.10(c)) and changed systematically as a function of age (Fig. 17.10(a), (b)).

Note that in the 30–40-day-old infants (J.O., M.A., J.I., D.A., M.I.), a second peak and X-axis intersection is suggested in response to larger check sizes. The VEP amplitude by check-size functions tended to be bimodal at this age, the relative amplitude of the two modes appearing to change systematically as a function of

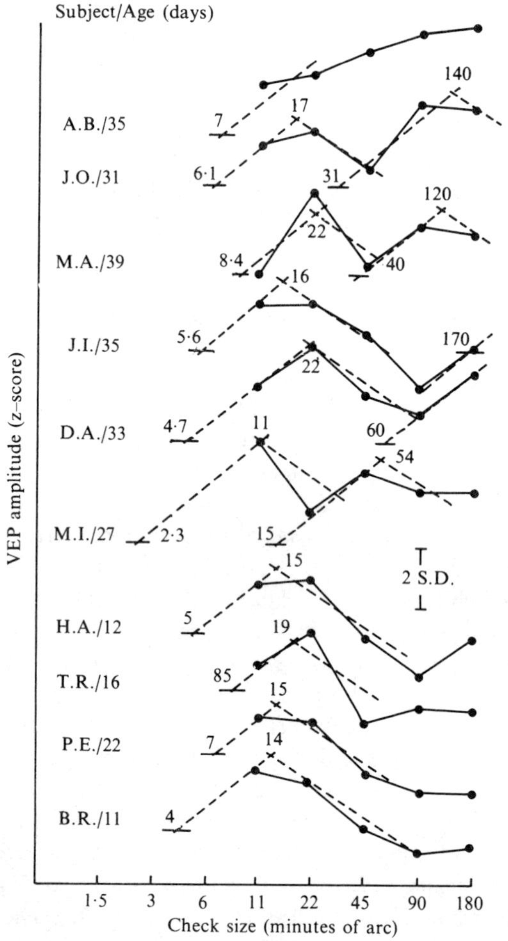

Fig. 17.8. Effects of check size on VEP amplitude and estimates of visual acuity in infants from 6 days to 45 days. Functions are *z*-score transformations of VEP data of Fig. 17.5, experiment 2. Infant and average age indicated on the left. The solid lines connect data points; the dashed lines are the inverted-V-shaped function, determined from the average slopes of all subjects (see text). The functions have been arbitrarily off-set vertically so that each may be inspected individually. The short horizontal line on the left portion of the inverted V indicates the VEP amplitude to diffuse light (baseline) for each subject. The numerical value above each baseline is the check size where the descending function intersects the baseline. This value estimates the smallest check size which elicits a VEP of greater amplitude than the VEP to diffuse light (check size threshold). The check size associated with the peak of the inverted-V-shaped function is given for each subject. Functions for the older subjects (27–39 days average age) tend to be multimodal.

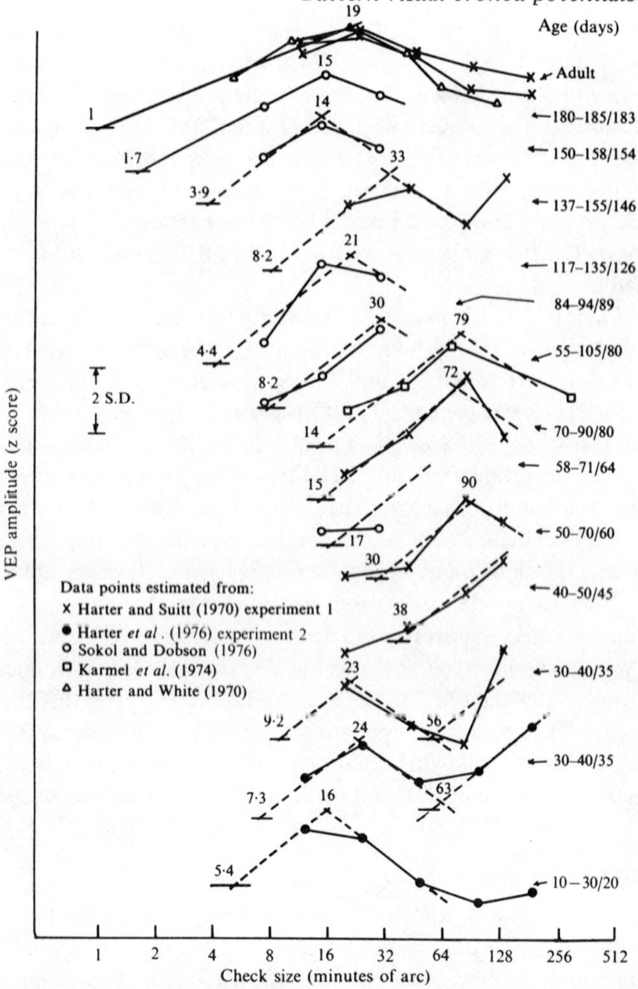

Fig. 17.9. Effects of check size on VEP amplitude and estimates of visual acuity as a function of median age (20–183 days). Functions are *z*-score transformations estimated from data presented by sources indicated on the key. The right-hand key indicates the range of ages/median age of the subject(s) from which each function was derived. The functions have been off-set vertically so that they are ordered from the bottom to top according to age (youngest to oldest). The solid lines connect data points. The dashed lines are the inverted-V-shaped function, determined from the average slopes of all subjects. The short horizontal line at the left of each inverted-V function indicates the VEP amplitude to diffuse light or zero amplitude (steady-state VEPs): the numerical value above each baseline is the check size where the descending portion of the function intersects the baseline. This value estimates the smallest check size which elicits a pattern VEP (check-size threshold) and is an estimate of visual acuity. The check size associated with the peak of each function is also given. Functions of infants from 30 days to 40 days of age tend to be multimodal. Note that the slopes used to extrapolate the check-size threshold for the adult subjects and the oldest infants (180–185 days of age) are less than with younger infants and are indicated by solid lines. The slopes indicated by the dashed lines in Figs. 17.8 and 17.9 are the same.

age (Fig. 17.9). From 10 days to 30 days, the amplitude of the first mode, peaking to the 16–24′ checks, progressively declined and the amplitude of the second mode, peaking to checks greater than 50′, progressively increased. The disappearance of the first mode to the smaller check sizes by the 40th day appears to account for the dramatic reduction of check size threshold by that day. The check-size threshold and peak-amplitude VEP based on the second mode, associated with larger check sizes, are also plotted in the left hand portion of Fig. 17.10(a) and (b) (dashed lines). The two modes apparently reflect different underlying processes (as discussed below).

Before describing the change in the inverted-U-shaped functions due to age, we should ask whether or not methodological differences in the studies represented in Figs. 17.9 and 17.10 might account for the changes – particularly the unexpected increase in the check size giving the peak response and the check-size threshold from 10 days to 45 days of age. This increase primarily was based on a comparison of data between experiments 1 and 2. The two experiments were conducted under virtually identical conditions except that experiment 2 was not conducted in darkness and the ambient illumination could have resulted in pupillary constriction, hence in greater depth of focus and less refractive error. However, this is unlikely since data from day 35 of experiment 1, obtained when the infant was in darkness, also indicates relatively good acuity (better than 20/200). The relatively good acuity in the youngest infants was not due to an artifact introduced by the transformation of raw data to z scores and method of extrapolating the check-size threshold, since VEPs to diffuse light and the 11′ checks differed in the raw data. It will be assumed for the following discussion that the changes in pattern VEPs reflect genuine changes in optical and neural factors as a function of age.

Estimates of visual acuity in infants

The Snellen equivalents for the VEP check-size thresholds for the 6–45 day-old infants in experiment 2 varied from 20/45 to 20/170 (Table 17.1) and indicated better visual acuity for newborns than that estimated from eye-movement data (discussed below). It should be noted that the infants had an average refractive error, estimated from VEPs, of 1·66 dioptre. If their less than normal acuity was the result of such optical factors only, it could have been corrected to better than 20/117. Visual acuity is reduced from 20/20 to about 20/76 by a 1·66 dioptre induced refractive error (Duke-Elder 1949, p. 4403). Three of the infants (T.R., J. I., and D.A.) had estimated visual acuities better than would be expected (20/170 or better) given their estimated refractive errors (3 dioptre or more). This suggests that one or both of the estimates was incorrect. The refractive-error estimates are less reliable since they were based on few replications and were obtained when the infants were less cooperative. Caution is recommended in accepting the estimates of refractive error for individual subjects although statistical confidence may be placed in the grouped data.

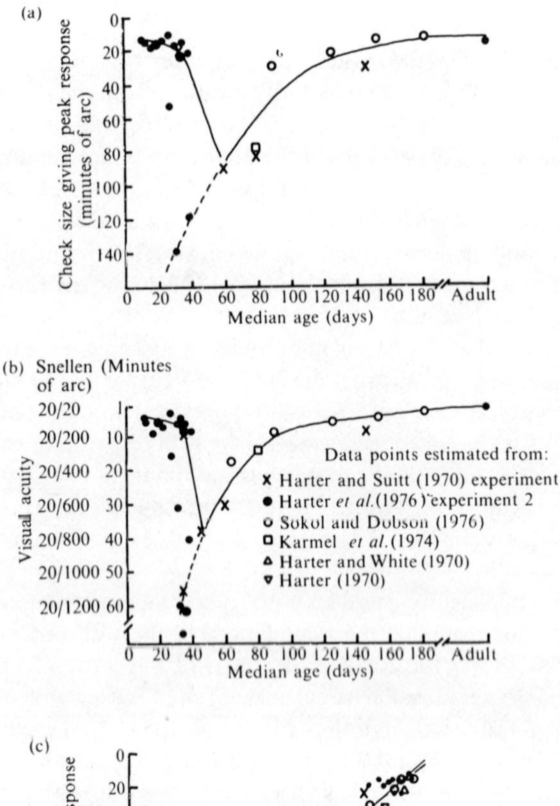

Fig. 17.10. (a), (b) Effects of age on the check size associated with the peak of the check size/VEP amplitude function (a) and the check-size threshold estimate of visual acuity (b). The points are from the data shown in Figs. 17.8 and 17.9. Visual acuity is expressed according to both the Snellen system and the visual angle subtended (minutes of arc). The solid line indicates the visually best-fit line. The dashed line is best fit through data points associated with the second mode of the VEP/check-size function in response to larger check sizes. (c) Scatter diagram and regression lines indicating the correlation between the peak amplitude and check-size threshold measures. The regression lines indicate the correlation of changes when the variation in these values was due to age alone (solid line) and age plus other factors (dashed line: eccentricity of retinal stimulation and induced refractive error) which influence visual acuity. Note: data from experiment 2 are plotted for both individual subjects (small dots) and the mean of the youngest and oldest 5 infants (large dots) in the left portion of the figure. Only individual data from experiment 2 were used in determining correlation coefficients.

Pattern visual evoked potentials in infants

VEP estimates of changes in visual acuity as a function of age (Figs. 17.9 and 17.10) indicate that the acuity temporarily declined from the first to the second month from approximately 20/117 to 20/760 and then improved in a negatively accelerated manner to 20/34 on about the 183rd day of life, approaching that of adults with normal vision. The drop in acuity from the first to second month was due to the disappearance of the first mode of the VEP functions. If estimates based on the second mode alone are considered, visual acuity improved in a negatively accelerated manner from about 20/1200 during the first month to 20/34 during the sixth month.

Estimates of visual acuity based on optokinetic nystagmus are reasonably consistent with those based on the first mode of the VEP amplitude functions. Dayton, Jones, Aiu, Rawson, Steele, and Rose (1964) obtained optokinetic nystagmus from 3-day-old infants with electro-oculograms (EOGs) in response to moving grids of different bar widths. Optokinetic nystagmus was obtained to 7·5′ bars, the smallest used, suggesting acuities better than 20/150. Gorman *et al.* (1967) used a similar procedure on infants less than 5 days old and estimated acuities of 20/350 or better.

Estimates of visual acuity based on visual preference techniques are reasonably consistent with those based on the second mode of the VEP amplitude functions. Fantz *et al.* (1962) using the criterion of preferring the pattern 75 per cent of the time found a minimum separable visual angle of 40′ (Snellen equivalent of 20/800) for both the first and second months which improved to 10′ (Snellen equivalent of 20/200) by the 6th month. Had they extrapolated the 50 per cent pattern-size threshold, these estimates would have been respectively 20/400 and 20/100 and would correspond with the changes from the second to sixth month in the VEP data. An extrapolated check-size threshold in the 1st month may be inferred from the percentage time fixated data of experiment 2 of 30′ (Snellen equivalent of 20/600) and from preference-of-looking data reported by other investigators not specifically concerned with visual acuity of 38′–60′ (Snellen equivalents ranging from 20/760 to 20/1200 (Brennan *et al.* 1966; Karmel 1969*b*; Miranda 1970; Horowitz, Tims, and McCluskey 1974).

In summary, the VEP data reviewed and synthesized here indicates visual acuities during the first 45 days ranging from 20/46 to 20/170 based on the first mode of the VEP amplitude function and about 20/1200 based on the second mode of the VEP amplitude functions. These two estimates correspond to some degree respectively to those based on optokinetic nystagmus (20/150 to 20/350) and on looking preference (20/400 to 20/1200). VEP estimates of visual acuity improved to 20/34 during the first 6 months.

Looking preferences in infants

Karmel (1969*b*) reviewed data by himself, Hershenson (1964), Brennan *et al.* (1966), and others on pattern-size preferences in infant looking behaviour at different ages. These studies indicated peak looking responses to pattern element sizes subtending approximately 480′ (newborns), 360′ (21 days), 120′ (56 days), 70′ (91 days), 45′ (140 days), and 23′ (older infants and adults). Harter and Suitt (1970) and Karmel *et al.* (1974) have suggested that the peak of the inverted-U-shaped function between VEP amplitude and pattern element size in infants correlated with the pattern size that the infants prefer to look at. The VEP data reviewed in the present study (Figs. 17.9 and 17.10) indicate the peak check size changed from 16′ or 160′ (first month), 90′ (second month), 50′ (third month), 20′ (fourth month), to 15′ (sixth month). Although somewhat smaller, these values are similar to those indicating size preference for corresponding ages, with the exception of infants less than 45 days of age. The functions between VEP amplitude and check size for infants less than 45 days of age tended to be bimodal. If the peak of the second mode (dashed line in Fig. 17.10) is compared to the preference data reviewed by Karmel (1969*b*), there is reasonable correspondence for the infants less than 45 days of age. Horowitz *et al.* (1974) also studied the relations between fixation time and check size, but did not express check sizes in minutes of arc. They found a bimodal response between visual preference and check size in infants from 3 weeks to 5 weeks old. Unfortunately, most eye-movements studies have not sampled a sufficient range of pattern sizes, particularly the small pattern sizes (20′ or less) with young infants, to assess the presence or absence of such bimodal functions.

Conclusion

What optical and neural factors underly the changes in the function between VEP amplitude and check size with age? The overall improvement in spatial resolution from 20/117 in the first to near 20/20 in the sixth month indicated by VEPs may be due to numerous factors related to visual development (Hershenson 1967; Scheie and Albert 1969, p. 105; Reese and Lipsitt, 1970, p. 35): decrease in refractive error (Duke-Elder 1963, p. 312), increase in the accommodative power of the lens (Haynes *et al.* 1965) and neural development, particularly of the macula and fovea (Walsh 1957, p. 348). More detailed data are required on these factors during the first 6 months of life before the relative contribution of each to the changes in VEPs may be isolated.

The apparent temporary drop in VEP estimates in acuity to 20/800 during the second month is more difficult to explain. One possibility is that it may be due to changes in pupillary size. The pupil is miotic during the first month (Scheie and Albert 1969, p. 105; Reese and Lipsitt 1970, pp. 34–6) which would increase depth of focus and reduce refractive error. As the pupil became more functional during the second month (more dilated since the VEP data were typically collected in darkness or dim illumination), the benefit of the small pupil would be lost and any refractive error would become manifest.

A second possible explanation is the differential development of the scotopic and photopic systems. In spite of considerable controversy, luminosity data suggest that the photopic system is more functional at birth but that the scotopic system develops rapidly during the first 2 months of life (Doris and Cooper 1966; Doris, Casper, and Poresky 1967; Trincker and Trincker 1967). One may speculate that the increased sensitivity to light and the contribution of the scotopic system to the VEP may result in the reduction in visual acuity and the development of the second mode in the VEP check size functions in the second month. Regan and Richards (1973) reported that VEPs to large checks reflect luminance effects.

The bimodal nature of the function between VEP amplitude and check size suggests additional neurophysiological explanations. It has been suggested that inverted-U-shaped functions between the pattern spatial frequency and (a) single-unit activity (Campbell *et al.* 1969), and (b) VEPs (Harter and White 1970; Harter 1970, 1971; Armington *et al.* 1971; Karmel *et al.* 1974) reflect the spatial tuning characteristics of the neurones activated. The peak of the function presumably reflects the modal optimal size or spatial frequency of the neural receptive fields activated and the check-size threshold reflects the smallest size or the highest spatial frequency of the receptive fields activated. For the present data, the bimodal functions would suggest activation of two aggregates of neurones tuned respectively to relatively high and low spatial frequencies. A likely explanation is that the first mode reflects the activity of subcortical cells and the second the activity of cortical cells. This interpretation is suggested by estimates of acuity based on optokinetic nystagmus as compared to visual preference techniques. Optokinetic nystagmus is presumably mediated by subcortical mechanisms, while visual preference techniques presumably involve the cerebral cortex and are thus indicants of perceptual processes (Fantz *et al.* 1962; Hershenson 1967; Linksz 1973). Estimates of visual acuity during the first month of life were 20/150 to 20/350 based on optokinetic nystagmus and 20/400 to 20/1200 based on visual preference, which correspond reasonably well with estimates based on the first (20/100–20/200) and second (20/1200) modes of VEP functions (bottom of Fig. 17.10). Therefore the first mode could well reflect the activity of subcortical neurones, which are relatively developed and tuned to high spatial frequencies at birth, while the second mode would reflect activity of the less developed cortical neurones, which are tuned to lower spatial frequencies at birth. If this hypothesis was correct, the apparent impairment of visual acuity reflected by the VEP functions in the second month reflects that point in maturation when the cortex became sufficiently functional to substitute for the subcortical activity.

Acknowledgements

Thanks are due to L. Salmon, Dr. K. Sharpless, G. Femrite, and G. Jackson for help in various aspects of these studies. The research was supported by the National Science Foundation under Grant GB-8053.

18. Hemispheric differences in the rhythmic responses to photic stimulation in human infants

D. H. CROWELL, L. E. KAPUNIAI, and J.A. GARBANATI

Department of Psychology, Pacific Biomedical Research Center, University of Hawaii, Honolulu

Recent studies on the cerebral development of human newborns has suggested a right-hemispheric specialization for rhythmic visual stimuli and also a relative lack of interhemispheric integration (Crowell, Jones, Kapuniai, and Nakagawa 1973). This was based on spectral analyses of VEPs which showed a significant right unilateral photic driving to bilateral repetitive visual stimulation, the driving being represented by a significant increase in spectral power at the stimulating frequency. These studies are relevant to problems of early brain organization, maturation, and function. In this chapter we attempt to define the developmental sequence of VEP to repetitive photic stimuli, to assess how newborns process such stimuli in the time-domain, and to determine the correlation between patterns of harmonic activity and hemisphere during maturation. Lastly, this chapter evaluates driving as a function of repeated exposure to the photic stimuli.

Method and procedure

Data were obtained from three groups of infants selected from Kapiolani Hospital, Honolulu and of heterogeneous racial backgrounds. Their participation was with the consent of both the attending physician and the mother. Groups 1 and 2 were clinically normal full-term infants seen at a mean age of 47 hours. Serial measurements were made on some of the subjects in group 1 at mean ages of approximately 3 months and 5 months of age. Longitudinal data for some group 1 subjects, supplemented with data from other normal full-term infants, comprised the two older-age categories. Group 3 was composed exclusively of low-birth-weight infants whose weight at birth was 2·5 kg or less. Since some of these infants were initially under intensive care, they were assessed at various ages. The low-birth-weight group includes both premature and small-for-date infants. Gestational ages (Dubowitz, Dubowitz, and Goldberg 1970) were estimated at the time of assessment for group 2 and 3 subjects.

Groups 1 and 3 were involved in a developmental psychophysiological programme

Visual evoked potentials in man: new developments (ed. J. E. Desmedt), pp. 353–62. Clarendon Press, Oxford 1977.

evaluating responsivity to auditory, visual, haptic, and nociceptive stimuli. Following these, 16 photic trials were presented; only these data will be considered here.

Stimulus frequency for groups 1 and 3 was 3 flashes per s with a stimulus duration of approximately 4 s. For group 2, two stimulus frequencies, 1·75 Hz and 3·60 Hz were used. Electrodes for groups 1 and 3 were O_1-A_2 and O_2-A_2. Group 2 placements were O_1-O_Z, O_2-O_Z (occipital montage) and O_1-T_5 and O_2-T_6 (temporal montage). In all these groups, electro-oculograms (EOG), left eye–A_2, and right eye–A_2 (Anders, Emde, and Parmelee 1971) were monitored on two additional channels. Group 2 infants were given a total of 24 trials in 4 blocks of 6 trials. Each block consisted of one frequency at one montage. These blocks were counterbalanced for frequency and montage.

After the electrodes were attached, the head was wrapped with gauze bandage to reduce artifacts. The infants were swaddled and then buckled in a plastic infant seat, adjusted at an angle of approximately 45°. The stroboscope lamp was aligned so that the centre was perpendicular to the frontal plane of the face and directed midway between the eyes. The experimental room was semi-dark. Attempts were made to initiate photic stimulation only when the babies were quiet with eyes closed.

Photic stimuli were presented with a Grass PS-2 photostimulator, intensity setting 8 on a scale of 1–16, at a distance of 46 cm from the eyes, directly in the line of vision (groups 1 and 2). In group 3, 42 out of the total subjects had the lamp 62 cm from the eyes. The EEG and EOG signals were monitored, simultaneously digitized at the rate of 30 samples per s and 5 samples per s respectively, and recorded on an incremental digital tape-recorder. Instrumentation details are found in Crowell *et al.* (1973).

Two types of analyses of the photic response were conducted; one in the frequency- and the other in the time-domain. All trials presented were not used in the analysis; the method of screening for artifact was described in Crowell *et al.* (1973). The test for photic driving and harmonics in the frequency-domain determined whether the estimated spectra for the pre-stimulus and the stimulus periods were the same or different. The differences of the logarithms of the estimated spectra were then summed over trials. An application of this statistical method is shown in Fig. 18.1, which illustrates bilateral driving and harmonic activity in a 2-day-old neonate.

The time-domain test for detecting change was based on an auto-regressive time-series model (Jones, Crowell, and Kapuniai 1969; 1970). The test was applied to the photic trials of the group 1 2-day-old data. In this model, a test for a response was made at each time-point and yielded a test-statistic t with the appropriate degrees of freedom. This t is a standardized variable which shows the direction and relative amount of change in the infant's EEG for each trial. The ts at each time-point were averaged across trials for each baby to determine the photic response for the individual and then across subjects to yield group responses. Examples of the

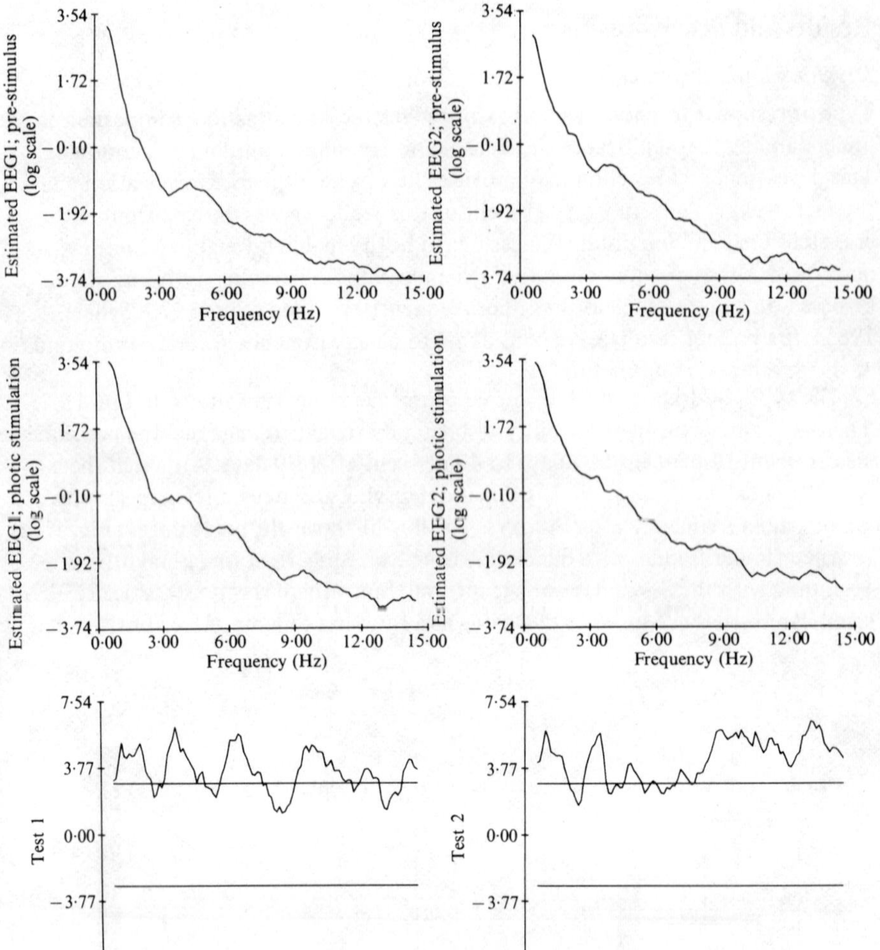

Fig. 18.1. Bilateral photic driving to a 3 Hz stimulus in a clinically normal 2-day-old full-term newborn infant. The EEG1 (O_2-A_2) and EEG2 (O_1-A_2) graphs are the logarithmic estimated spectra for 4 s of pre-stimulus data and 4 s of photic stimulation. Bilateral driving is indicated in the Test 1 and Test 2 graphs, where the test statistics exceed the 95 per cent confidence limits at 3 Hz and the harmonics.

group responses appear in Fig. 18.4. The 99 per cent confidence limits established the time and relative magnitude of these statistically significant averaged responses.

Results and discussion

Developmental sequence

Type of response to photic stimuli as an age-related phenomenon is important in understanding the significance of hemispheric asymmetry and brain functioning. This developmental function may provide clues to hemispheric organization and the factors which govern it. Assessment of this sequence was derived from both cross-sectional and longitudinal measures of both low-birth-weight and term newborns. Although more definitive generalizations concerning ontogeny should be based on a design such as the cohort-sequential method (Buss 1973; Schaie 1965), the present results were considered to be a reasonably accurate approximation of the developmental function.

The types of driving which occurred across age groups are shown in Fig. 18.2. There was an increasing probability of bilateral driving with age, i.e. the percentage shifted from 12 per cent at 2 days to 48 per cent after 30 days. Although there were more cases of right than left unilateral driving at 2 days, they appear with almost equal frequency after 30 days. The low-birth-weight percentages (Fig. 18.2) revealed similar trends, with bilateral driving exceeding right unilateral driving beginning with the 3–29 days-of-age interval. Since there was no statistically significant difference in types of driving as a function of lamp placement, χ-squared

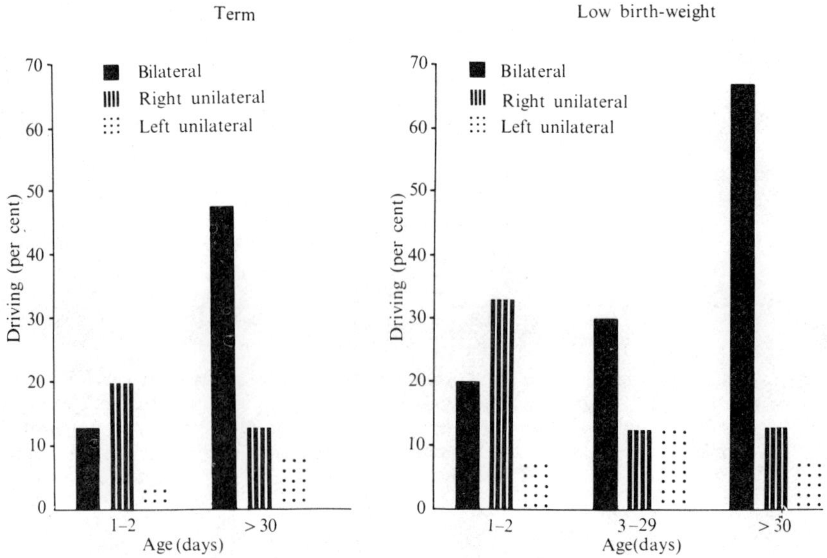

Fig. 18.2. Developmental sequence for types of driving to photic stimulation at 3 flashes per s for approximately 4 s in clinically normal full-term (group 1) and low-birth-weight infants (groups 3)

test, the two groups were collapsed for all analyses. Data were not available at 3–29 days to evaluate this pattern in group 1.

The information about gestational age for the low-birth-weight group was used to detect the earliest time when photic driving appeared in these data. The gestational age assessments, made within 14 days of birth, were available for 45 subjects. The percentage of subjects exhibiting driving was calculated for babies at 35–36 weeks, 37 weeks, and 38–39 weeks gestational age (Fig. 18.3). Since

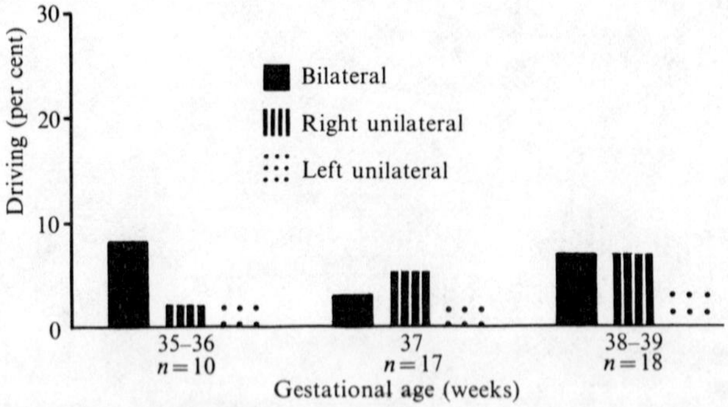

Fig. 18.3. Types of photic driving to 3 flashes per s for approximately 4 s stimulus as a function of gestational age in low-birth-weight infants less than 14 days of age (group 3).

the low-birth-weight group was composed of premature as well as small-for-date babies, this heterogeneity may have obscured any trends across these ages. It was evident that the percentage of driving was low, but all types of driving were detected as early as 35 weeks gestational age. The developmental sequence again showed that right unilateral driving occurred with greatest frequency for those subjects who exhibited driving at 2 days of age. Bilateral driving became the predominant response by 30 days of age. Larger sample sizes at the oldest age groups would make these conclusions more definitive. Since rapid changes occur in the visual system and brain (Conel 1939–59) during the first post-natal months, these may account for the shifts in type of driving. The bilateral response may be an early index of maturation. Since the commissures and especially the corpus callosum are reported to be incompletely developed at birth (Crelin 1973; Hewitt 1962), bilateral driving in these infants does not seem to coincide with the development of these structures and, therefore, may not necessarily reflect inter-hemispheric synergy. Gazzaniga (1970) hypothesizes that inter-hemispheric communication is reduced in the human newborn. At the same time, it should be recognized that synergy might be present at other subcortical levels (Trevarthen and Sperry 1973).

Although it is reasonable to consider the shift from a unilateral to bilateral response as a maturational phenomenon, asymmetry, as well as bilateral absence

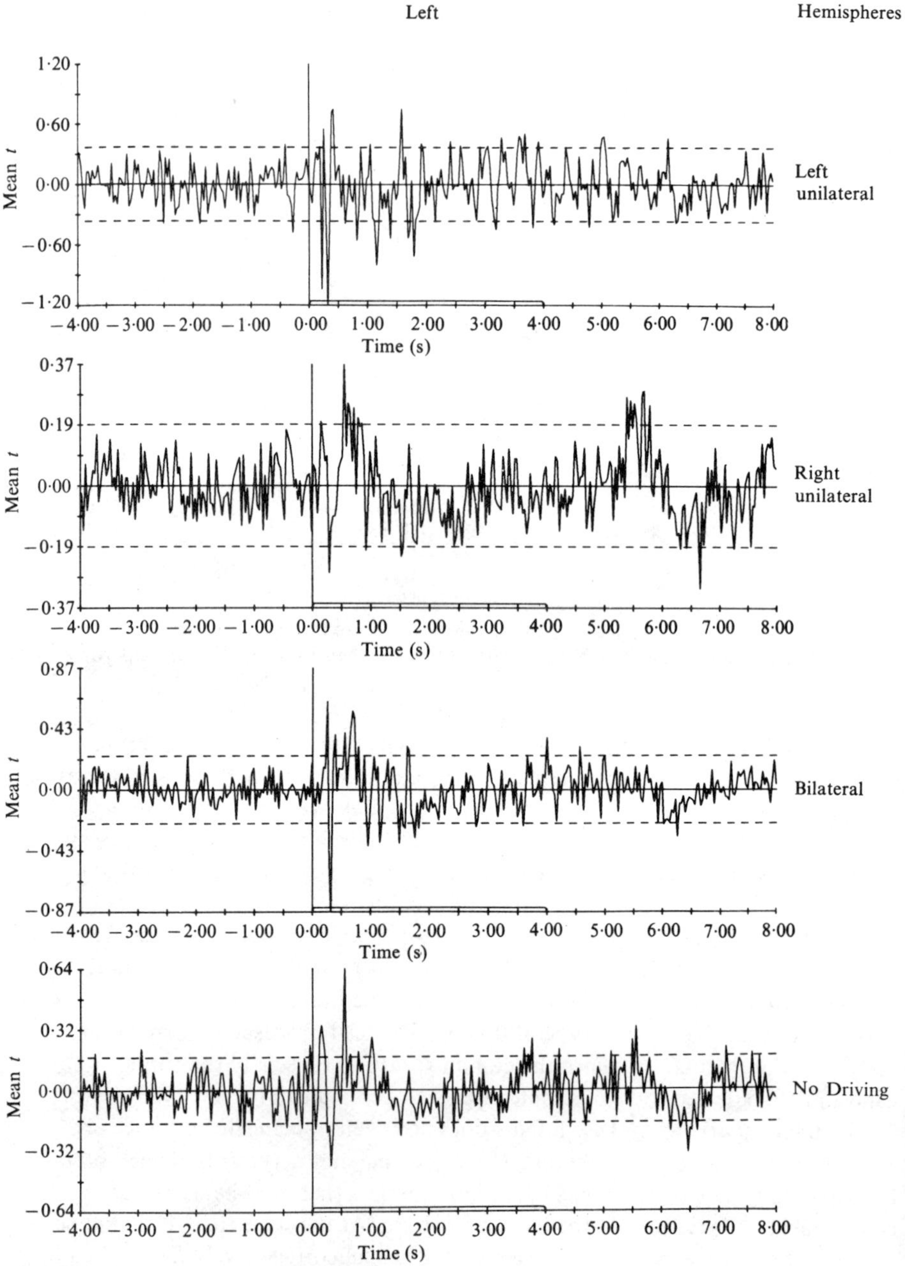

Fig. 18.4. Averaged (mean *t*) time-domain responses to photic stimulation (3 flashes per s for 4 s) of clinically normal full-term 2-day-old newborn infants with left (*N* = 3) or right unilateral (*N* = 19) photic driving, bilateral driving (*N* = 11) and a sample of those with no driving (*N* = 18) for both the right and left occipital regions (hemisphere).

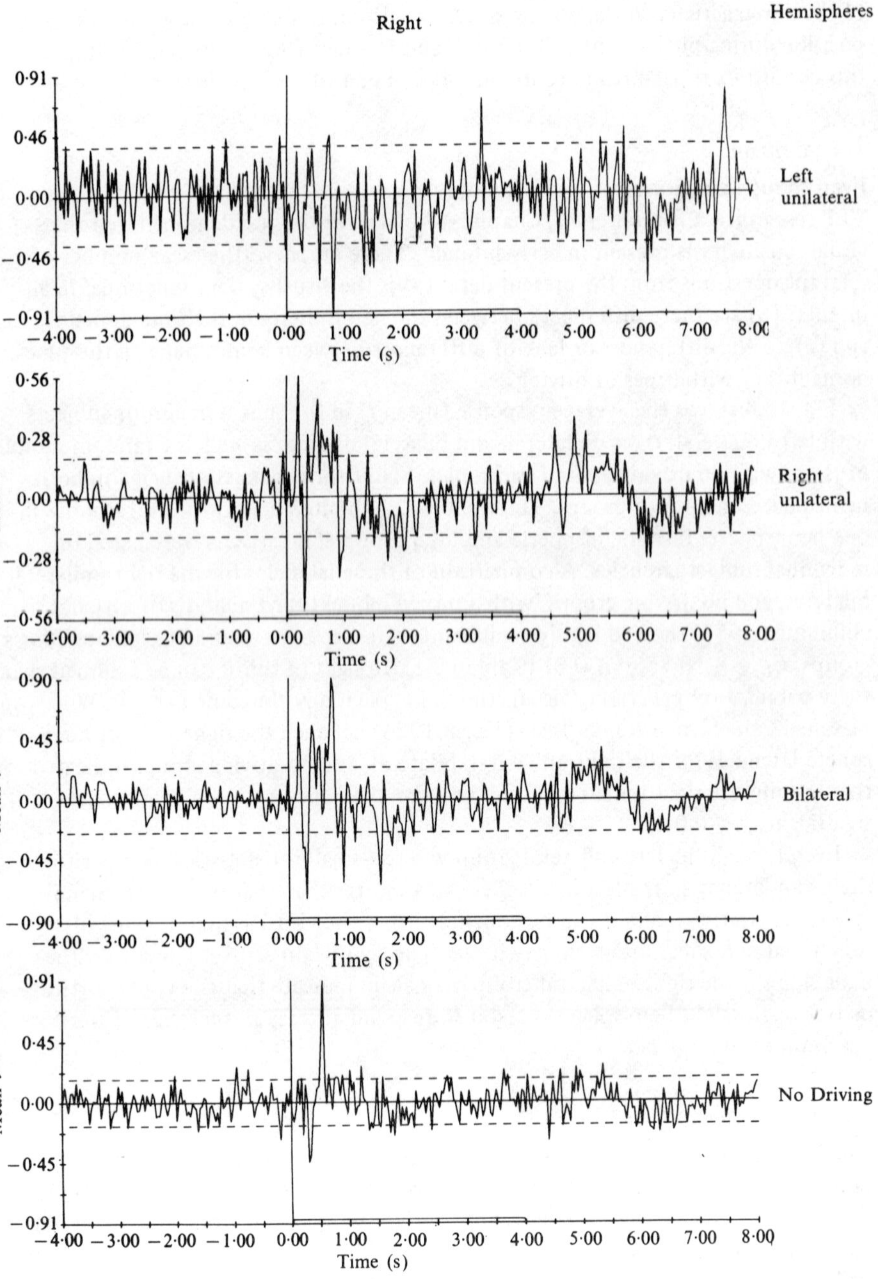
Right
Hemispheres
0·91
0·46
0·00
−0·46
−0·91
−4·00 −3·00 −2·00 −1·00 0·00 1·00 2·00 3·00 4·00 5·00 6·00 7·00 8·00
Time (s)
Left unilateral
0·56
0·28
0·00
−0·28
−0·56
−4·00 −3·00 −2·00 −1·00 0·00 1·00 2·00 3·00 4·00 5·00 6·00 7·00 8·00
Time (s)
Right unilateral
0·90
0·45
0·00
−0·45
−0·90
−4·00 −3·00 −2·00 −1·00 0·00 1·00 2·00 3·00 4·00 5·00 6·00 7·00 8·00
Time (s)
Bilateral
0·91
0·45
0·00
−0·45
−0·91
−4·00 −3·00 −2·00 −1·00 0·00 1·00 2·00 3·00 4·00 5·00 6·00 7·00 8·00
Time (s)
No Driving

of rhythmic activity in the resting state, has also been related to the infant's head position during birth (Churchill, Grisell, and Darnley 1966). The relationship of this condition at parturition to driving should be further investigated.

Time-domain

Even though a majority of the 2-day-old full-term infants did not exhibit driving, VEP research (cf. Harter *et al.*, Chapter 17 of this book) has demonstrated that visual sensitivity is present in early infancy. There are, nevertheless, a number of relevant questions from the present data: (a) is the visual system functional in all infants? (b) are there differences between the hemispheres in the time-domain? and (c) do the differences or lack of differences between hemispheres in the time-domain vary with types of driving?

Fig. 18.4 shows the average response (mean t) in the time-domain for subjects with left unilateral, right unilateral, and bilateral driving, as well as a random sample of those with no driving and no harmonics. Significant changes occurred in both hemispheres in all four groups. Three subjects exhibited no significant response in one hemisphere. Inter-hemispheric and inter-group comparisons were based on individual subject latencies. A comparison of these latencies for the right unilateral, bilateral, and no driving groups, with a mixed model type I analysis of variance (Lindquist 1953) showed highly significant differences between hemispheres across groups, $F_{1,\,40} = 10{\cdot}75$, $p < 0{\cdot}01$ (Table 18.1). In light of this it can be assumed that these babies were processing visual stimuli in essentially the same manner. Wilcoxon Matched-Pairs Signed-Ranks Tests (Siegel 1956) between the right and left hemisphere latencies for the right unilateral, bilateral, and no driving groups indicated that in only the right unilateral group was the difference between hemispheres significant, $p < 0{\cdot}01$.

Even though the left unilateral group was too small for statistical comparison, the mean latency in the left hemisphere was shorter than that in the right hemisphere. From these data it can be concluded that the visual system is generally functional in normal, full-term newborns. The significant shorter latency on the right side for the right unilateral group may again indicate that the visual cortical matrix of the right hemisphere is faster to respond at least at one stage of the developmental sequence.

Stimulus frequency

One important factor which may have an influence on hemispheric response to photic stimulation is stimulus frequency. The 11 babies of group 2 were tested at 1·75 Hz and 3·60 Hz. Suggestive trends were found. More bilateral and unilateral right driving occurred at 3·60 Hz. No subject exhibited a combination of bilateral and unilateral responses within a montage. In general, the left hemisphere never exhibited driving to a faster stimulus frequency than did the right hemisphere. In one subject, left hemisphere driving at 1·75 Hz did occur in conjunction with right unilateral driving at 3·60 Hz. Such evidence that the right hemisphere showed driving to a faster frequency than the left may provide additional support for the proposition that the right hemisphere is more mature (Carmon, Harishana, Lowinger, and Lavy 1972; Crowell *et al.* 1973; Giannitrapani 1967).

Rhythmic and harmonic activity

Besides the electrical activity at the driving frequency, some infants disclosed also activity at harmonics of the 3 Hz stimulating frequency. This has been analysed in detail.

For the term infants harmonics in both the right and left hemispheres increased with age. With left hemispheric driving and for those with no driving, harmonics seemed to become more prevalent around 30 days of age. Subharmonics were rarely present, and their occurrence diminished sharply with age. The same trends were apparent in the low-birth-weight infants who exhibited more harmonics and sub-harmonics than the term infants. This may have been a function of cohort differences or of decreased stimulus intensity which, in turn, may have been related to differences in lamp placement (Montagu 1967).

TABLE 18.1 *Mean latency (ms) to first significant average response for individual subjects in each hemisphere for group 1 term infants*

		Hemisphere	
	N	Right	Left
Type of driving			
Unilateral			
Left	3	447	250
Right	17	225	396
Bilateral	11	223	277
Absent†	15	295	383

† Data are presented only for 15 subjects with no driving and no harmonics.

It was generally true that more harmonics appeared in the right than left occipital region for the group 1 subjects at 2 days of age. This phenomenon was manifested to a greater extent in right unilateral and to a lesser extent in bilateral driving and non-driving subjects. Although the same trend was apparent for the infants older than 30 days, an additional pattern emerged which showed the increased occurrence of an equal number of harmonics in both hemispheres. These observations also held true for the low-birth-weight babies up to 29 days of age with the exception of the bilateral group. These infants consistently showed more harmonics in the right region. For babies older than 30 days, there were slightly more cases where the number of harmonics in the left exceeded that in the right. In 2-day-old term and low-birth-weight subjects, the higher harmonics usually occurred in the right hemisphere. There were too few cases of subharmonics to make any substantial statements, but it should be noted that the occurrence of left greater than right appeared to increase after 30 days.

In summary, the presence of harmonics increased with age. This fact along with the evidence of hemispheric differences in harmonic activity may reflect some maturational process, and a more advanced development of the right hemisphere. Why there are more and higher harmonics in the right hemisphere is a provocative question. Van der Tweel and Verduyn Lunel (1965) found that noise added to a signal frequency reduced harmonic activity. It might be postulated that 'neural noise' is reduced in the right hemisphere, and therefore, harmonics are more likely to be present.

Trial effects

The question whether the capacity for driving was present immediately or required repeated exposure to photic stimulation was tested by separating trials into subsets for the 32 group 1 2-day-old subjects who had provided sufficient data. These analyses showed that the probability of driving increased with the number of trials analysed. In the early trials, driving was as likely to appear in the right as the left hemisphere. Bilateral responses were not likely to occur early. The majority of subjects exhibited no driving during the first two trials analysed. Further analyses are warranted to determine if the driving response is more likely to appear on later trials or appears as a function of the number of trials analysed.

Conclusion

This chapter has presented evidence that hemispheres differ in certain parameters to rhythmic visual stimuli at birth. These differences are modified in infants older than 30 days. Whether these asymmetries are due to maturation or other variables as, for example, recovery from the birth process, is not known. Trends in the data favour the maturation hypothesis.

Acknowledgements

Research supported in part by the National Institute of Child Health and Human Development Grant HD 00869, the Grant Foundation, Social and Rehabilitation Service, HEW, Grant 56-P-45315/9, and the Developmental Disabilities Planning and Advisory Council of Hawaii, Department of Health, State of Hawaii.

19. The cerebral evoked potential: life-span changes and twin studies

R. E. DUSTMAN, T. SCHENKENBERG, E. G. LEWIS, and E.C. BECK
Veterans Administration Hospital and *University of Utah, Salt Lake City*

The experiments described in this chapter represent an effort to provide normative information and to describe changes in the VEP during development, ageing, and senescence. We report on VEPs recorded from 425 normal subjects, approximately equally divided between male and female, whose age distribution spans 85 years, and we also describe studies of monozygotic and dizygotic twins.

Methods

The subjects studied were normal, paid volunteers, all right-handed. Each subject was seated in a comfortable, padded chair in a sound-deadened and darkened room while electrodes were placed at F_3, F_4, C_3, C_4, O_1, O_2 according to the International '10–20' System. Recordings, which generally lasted less than an hour, were unipolar with linked earlobes as reference. Stimuli (flashes of light, clicks, or shocks) were triggered manually at 2–5 s intervals during artifact-free periods of the EEG. Brain waves amplified by an 8-channel Grass EEG machine were stored together with pulses accompanying the stimuli on a 7-channel magnetic data-recorder. Stored EEG was then played into either an analog–digital converter, and thence to a PDP-9 computer for averaging, summing, and computation or directly into a CAT. The sampling rate employed was 500 Hz for the computer and 400 Hz for the CAT.

The recording system was calibrated by series of 10-Hz sine waves, 50 μV peak to peak, amplified by a factor of 30 000 and stored on magnetic tape in the manner that brain waves were recorded. The sine waves were then played into the computer or CAT and measured. Gain settings were adjusted when necessary to insure that the amplitudes of sine waves on each channel were equal. Upper and lower frequency limits (half-amplitude), 110 Hz and 5 Hz, respectively, were determined from Bode plots.

Visual stimuli of 10 μs duration were generated by a photo-stimulator. With few exceptions the setting of the stimulator was 2 on a scale of 1 to 16. The stimulator lamp, enclosed in a fibre-glass and foam-rubber container to muffle clicks accompanying the flashes, was positioned behind and directly above the subject's

Visual evoked potentials in man: new developments (ed. J. E. Desmedt), pp. 363–77.
Clarendon Press, Oxford 1977.

head and aimed at the centre of a reflecting hemisphere 70 cm in diameter. This method ensured a relatively constant level of retinal illumination regardless of the direction of gaze of the subject. At a stimulator setting of 2 (on a scale 1–16) the measured luminance at the distance of the subject's eyes, 40 cm from the centre of the hemisphere, was 12 1x. Auditory stimuli were binaural clicks of 0·25 ms duration and 80 dB intensity with reference to 0·0002 μbar. Somatosensory stimuli of 0·25 ms electrical pulses were delivered to the index finger of the dominant hand through two silver clip electrodes. A copper cuff was placed on the forearm as a ground. Stimulus intensity for each subject was twice the subjective threshold determined by the method of ascending and descending limits.

VEPs and ageing

The VEP changes in both amplitude and peak delay of the various components seemed to follow certain developmental and ageing transitions. Fig. 19.1 illustrates typical VEPs in children, young adults, and aged subjects. When recorded from the occiput (O_1, O_2) the VEP shows a rapid increase in amplitude of most components during early childhood reaching a maximum in 6–8-year-old children. At this age, the mean amplitude of the VEP was more than twice as large as the VEP amplitude of older age groups. Following this increase there was a decline in amplitude associated with increasing age until ages 13–14 when an abrupt increase in amplitude appeared in components occurring in the first 200 ms. This surge in amplitude during the early teenage years was consistently observed. After that age, the amplitude of VEPs appeared to reduce and stabilize at about age 16. Fig. 19.2

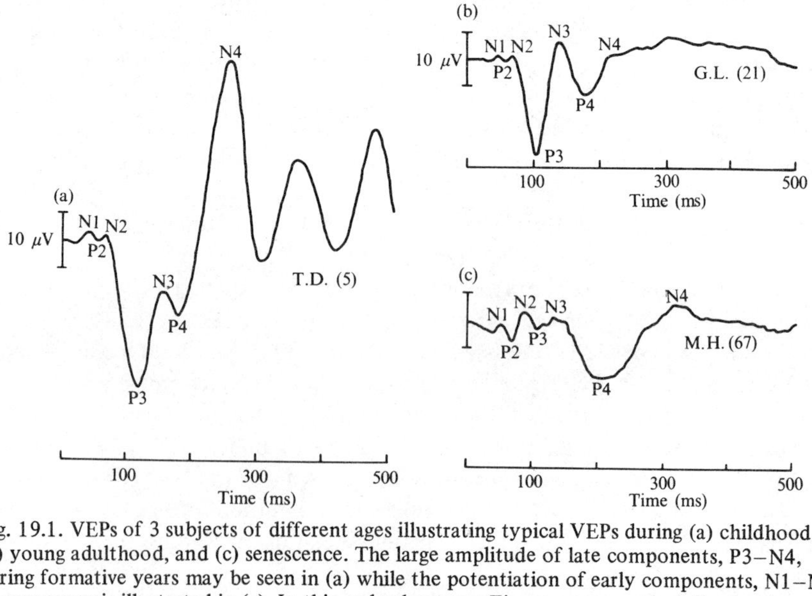

Fig. 19.1. VEPs of 3 subjects of different ages illustrating typical VEPs during (a) childhood, (b) young adulthood, and (c) senescence. The large amplitude of late components, P3–N4, during formative years may be seen in (a) while the potentiation of early components, N1–N2, in senescence is illustrated in (c). In this and subsequent Figures an upwards deflection is negative

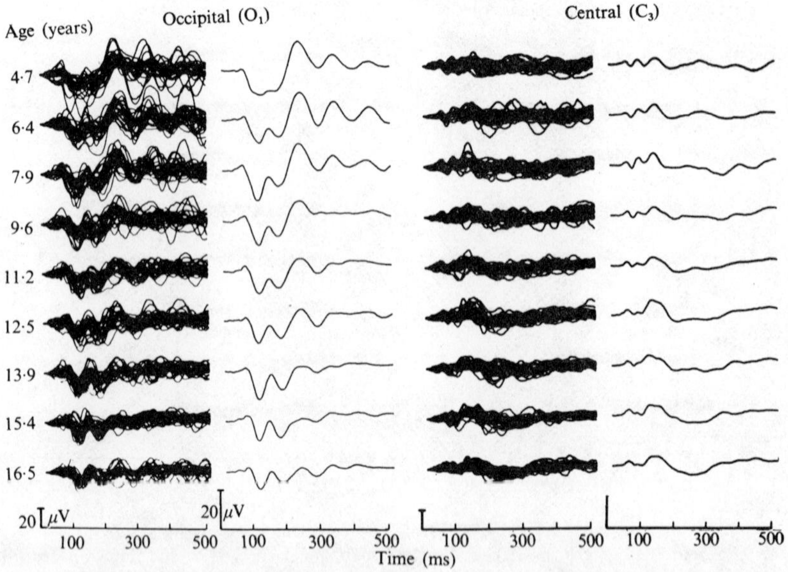

Fig. 19.2. VEP changes during maturation. VEPs of 225 individuals ranging in age from 4 years to 16 years. Each of the 9 age groups, designated by mean age at the left of the figure, is composed of 25 subjects roughly equally divided into boys and girls. Potentials are from occipital scalp (O_1) on the left and from central scalp (C_3) on the right. Both superimposed VEPs of individuals and group averages for each age level are depicted. The trend of decreasing amplitude of late components with increasing age is obvious in both the individual and in the group VEPs.

illustrates VEPs of 225 subjects ranging from 4 years to 16 years of age. These are divided into 9 age groups and the averaged group potential for each is plotted. Potentials recorded from both the occiput and central areas are shown. The trend of decreasing amplitude of late components during development is more clearly seen in recordings from the occipital area. Trends in early components do not emerge clearly in Fig. 19.2 because of small amplitude and individual variability, but they do appear in Fig. 19.1.

The progressive changes during ageing and senescence are illustrated in Fig. 19.3, which portrays VEPs of 200 individuals ranging in age from 17 years to 86 years. The 200 individuals have been divided into 8 groups of 25 age-related subjects. With older subjects, earlier components (designated N1, P2, N2 in Fig. 19.1) were consistently larger and arrived significantly later than did those of younger subjects. There is also a gradual attenuation of later components in the VEPs of ageing subjects. Although some changes in amplitude may be seen in potentials from central areas, these changes are minimal when compared to those recorded from the occiput. It should be noted that these reciprocal changes, namely, attenuation of late and potentiation of early components, may be seen as early as the fourth decade. The reader should note the transition from age 35 to 45 in Fig. 19.3.

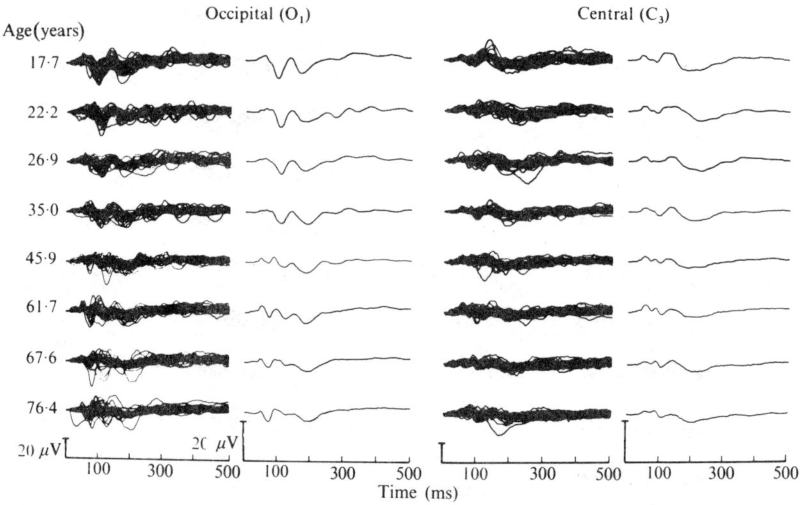

Fig. 19.3. VEP changes during ageing. VEPs of 200 individuals ranging in age from 17 years to 86 years. Each of the age groups, designated by mean age at the left of the figure, is comprised of 25 subjects rather equally divided, male and female. Superimposed individual VEPs and group averages are both displayed. Increasing amplitude of earlier components may be seen beginning at mean age 45·9 years.

To examine life-span changes in amplitude of various waves of the VEP, components were arbitrarily divided into those occurring during three different time-epochs: 0–100, 100–200, and 200–300 ms. The amplitude of components occurring in each epoch was measured by summing the absolute voltage values of all points within that time-interval (Fig. 19.4(a)). The VEP time-segments had previously been reduced to a zero baseline by subtracting the mean of the total epoch from each point. The rapid rise in amplitude during early childhood with an equally rapid decline after the age of 8 years, the surge of amplitude of some components during ages 13–14 years, and finally the increase in amplitude of early components in later life are shown clearly in Fig. 19.4(a).

Latency or peak delays of various components of VEPs also change with age. In general, peak delays of early components N1, P2, and N2 arrive significantly later in infancy, remain stable during childhood and young adulthood, and then gradually increase in latency in middle-age and throughout senescence. Mean peak delays and amplitudes with standard deviations of several recurring components of VEPs are provided in Tables 19.1 and 19.2 respectively. In an attempt to examine VEP similarities among subjects of similar ages, the VEPs of 25 subjects in 17 age groups were compared. The comparisons were made by intercorrelating the VEPs of all subjects in each group. This was done for VEPs from two scalp areas, occipital O_1 and central C_3. For example, the wave and phase relationship of VEPs for a group of 25 young children may be intercorrelated to note their degree of similarity.

TABLE 19.1 *Peaks delays (ms) of nine components of the VEP for 8 age groups. Left occipital scalp* (O_1)

Age range (years)	Mean age (nearest year)	Peaks																	
		P1		N1		P2		N2		P3		N3		P4		N4		P5	
		Mean	S.D.	Mean	S.D.	Mean	S.D.	Mean	S.D.	Mean	S.D.	Mean	S.D.	Mean	S.D.	Mean	S.D.	Mean	S.D.
4–6	5·0	28·1	4·3	44·3	7·8	55·3	6·7	71·4	6·4	111·2	11·0	143·8	20·1	173·1	12·5	236·8	10·8	292·0	21·2
6–8	7·0	28·5	2·9	39·0	3·8	50·6	7·2	68·2	8·3	111·4	10·6	145·9	13·4	175·3	13·3	229·8	13·9	284·6	19·9
8–10	9·0	27·9	3·3	41·1	4·6	50·7	7·4	69·1	7·8	106·2	10·0	142·2	10·4	172·3	12·2	229·9	12·3	274·9	16·9
10–12	11·0	27·8	4·4	40·4	5·2	50·9	6·0	66·1	6·1	106·5	5·7	138·4	8·9	168·4	10·9	227·5	19·0	274·8	17·2
13–20	17·0	27·8	3·6	44·8	7·1	49·7	9·3	71·0	9·2	100·7	9·6	133·6	7·6	174·4	11·1	229·6	21·2	268·7	24·1
35–48	41·0	29·9	3·5	49·0	3·8	64·5	7·0	85·4	8·7	109·9	7·6	142·0	12·5	184·1	15·3	243·4	16·1	281·1	25·4
60–70	66·0	30·1	5·8	52·2	4·9	70·6	7·8	93·1	8·4	123·8	9·3	149·9	9·8	188·6	16·2	244·3	20·9	286·0	29·6
70–86	77·0	31·0	3·7	53·1	5·8	72·3	6·3	92·5	5·4	118·9	9·1	151·9	13·6	191·0	14·7	267·1	20·6	303·0	25·3

Note. In Tables 19.1 and 19.2 there were 20 subjects in each age range, equally divided male and female.

TABLE 19.2 *Amplitudes (μV) of eight components of the VEP for 8 age groups. Left occipital scalp* (O_1)

Age range (year)	Mean age (nearest year)	N1		P2		N2		P3		N3		P4		N4		P5	
		Mean	S.D.	Mean	S.D.	Mean	S.D.	Mean	S.D.	Mean	S.D.	Mean	S.D.	Mean	S.D.	Mean	S.D.
4–6	5·0	2·0	1·3	2·0	1·4	3·3	2·5	18·2	6·4	8·4	5·7	5·4	5·4	25·1	13·9	16·7	11·9
6–8	7·0	2·0	1·4	2·2	1·6	4·6	3·2	18·0	5·3	12·0	8·5	9·3	10·3	25·1	12·9	20·4	11·4
8–10	9·0	2·6	1·6	1·8	1·0	3·6	2·5	17·6	6·3	15·0	7·7	12·4	7·9	26·1	10·3	14·7	8·6
10–12	11·0	2·7	1·7	2·0	1·3	4·3	1·8	18·8	6·9	12·5	9·1	9·3	7·5	20·8	8·5	12·2	4·9
13–20	17·0	3·3	2·4	3·6	2·6	4·5	2·0	14·3	5·8	14·6	7·8	13·6	7·3	11·6	5·3	6·7	3·6
35–48	41·0	2·9	1·4	3·2	1·9	4·8	3·2	9·3	4·5	9·1	5·4	10·7	4·9	8·8	4·7	4·7	2·6
60–70	66·0	2·9	1·6	5·7	5·1	7·9	4·8	9·9	3·2	7·2	4·5	6·6	1·9	7·4	3·5	3·9	3·2
70–86	77·0	3·2	2·4	6·1	4·2	9·3	5·8	11·0	7·1	7·7	4·6	7·0	7·3	8·4	4·4	2·6	1·4

Note. The amplitude of N_1 was computed as the voltage difference between the initial baseline and the peak of N_1. The amplitudes of succeeding waves were computed as the voltage difference between the wave in question and the preceding wave of opposite polarity.

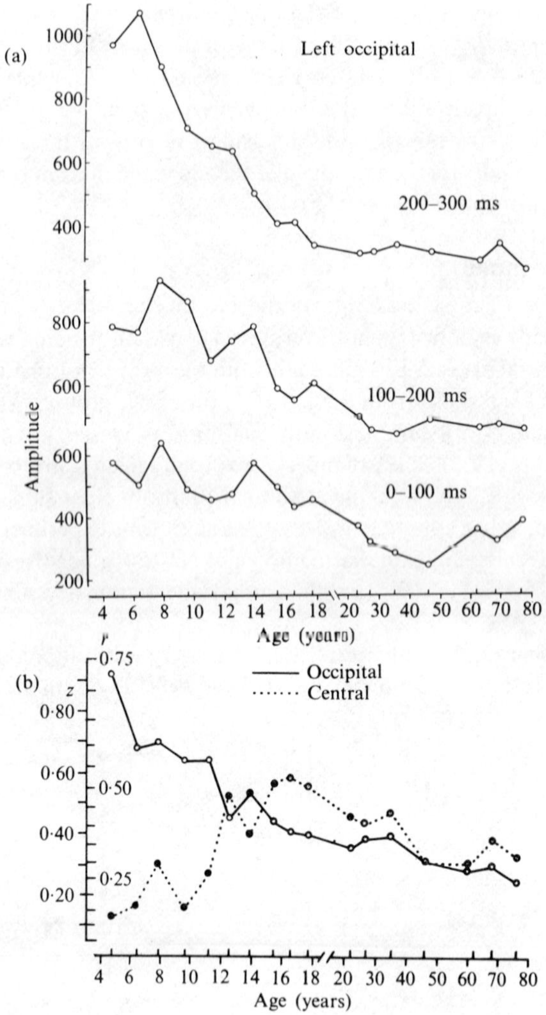

Fig. 19.4. (a) Changes in VEP amplitude of early and late components during maturation and increasing age. Three epochs were measured, the first 100 ms, from 100 ms to 200 ms, and from 200 ms to 300 ms. Amplitudes for each epoch were obtained by summing the absolute values of all points within that interval (arbitrary units). (b) Intercorrelations of VEPs recorded from occipital and central scalp at different age levels illustrating trends in group homogeneity with maturation and ageing. Each point on the graph is the intercorrelation of 25 subjects of a certain age range, i.e. the mean of 300 correlations. (Fig. 19.4(b)) is from Beck and Dustman 1975.)

That is, a VEP from child 1 may be correlated with a VEP from child 2, then with one from child 3, child 4, etc. Such a manoeuvre with 25 children will ultimately provide 300 correlations. A mean *r* of these will describe to some degree the similarity or *homogeneity* of the VEPs of the group. Thus VEPs recorded from the occipital scalp of 25 4-year-old children yield a mean *r* of 0·73, while those recorded from central scalp show little homogeneity with an *r* of 0·12 (Fig. 19.4(b)). The Figure illustrates how this relationship changes rapidly with increasing age, up to about age 12 years. From then on there is a gradual and continuous diminution of homogeneity throughout the older groups.

Hemispheric asymmetry

This was not seen with any consistency in the auditory or somato-sensory evoked potential. Amplitude asymmetry, however, was a consistent finding with the VEP recorded from central areas. VEPs recorded from the right hemisphere (C_4) were consistently larger than those from the left (C_3) for all age groups. While the difference was small, 1–5 μV in most individuals, it was consistent and was found at each age level (Fig. 19.5). The asymmetry was found mainly in a late component, a negative-going wave P3–N3 peaking at about 140 ms. In older subjects asymmetry was also seen in an earlier component, N2–P3. Subsequent experiments, not reported in these results, indicate that component N3–P4, a positive-going wave arriving around 175 ms (Fig. 19.5) exhibits amplitude asymmetry similar to those above.

Interestingly, we found that hemispheric asymmetry was not present with some subjects in other studies. No asymmetry was noted in VEPs of children with Down's

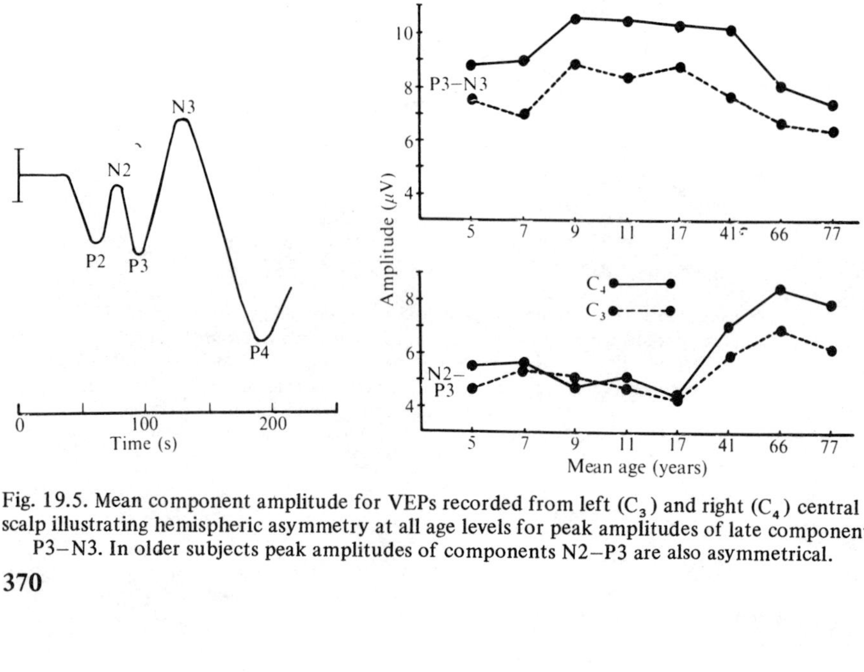

Fig. 19.5. Mean component amplitude for VEPs recorded from left (C_3) and right (C_4) central scalp illustrating hemispheric asymmetry at all age levels for peak amplitudes of late component P3–N3. In older subjects peak amplitudes of components N2–P3 are also asymmetrical.

syndrome (Bigum, Dustman, and Beck 1970) nor in those of mentally retarded children (Rhodes, Dustman,and Beck 1969), and asymmetry tended to disappear with moderate ingestion of alcohol in young adults (Lewis, Dustman, and Beck 1970).

Sex differences

In one study, 80 males and 80 females, ranging in age from 4 years to 86 years, were compared. During childhood the VEPs of males were reliably larger than those of females. The reverse characterized VEPs recorded during adolescence and adulthood, the female's potentials being consistently larger. These sex differences emerged as a general difference. Although they were seen more clearly in the VEP they were not specific to any particular sensory system, electrode placement or component.

Other sensory evoked potentials

While the major emphasis in our research has been the VEP, in one study three sensory systems were studied concomitantly. VEPs, auditory evoked potentials (AEPs), and somatosensory evoked potentials (SEPs) were recorded during

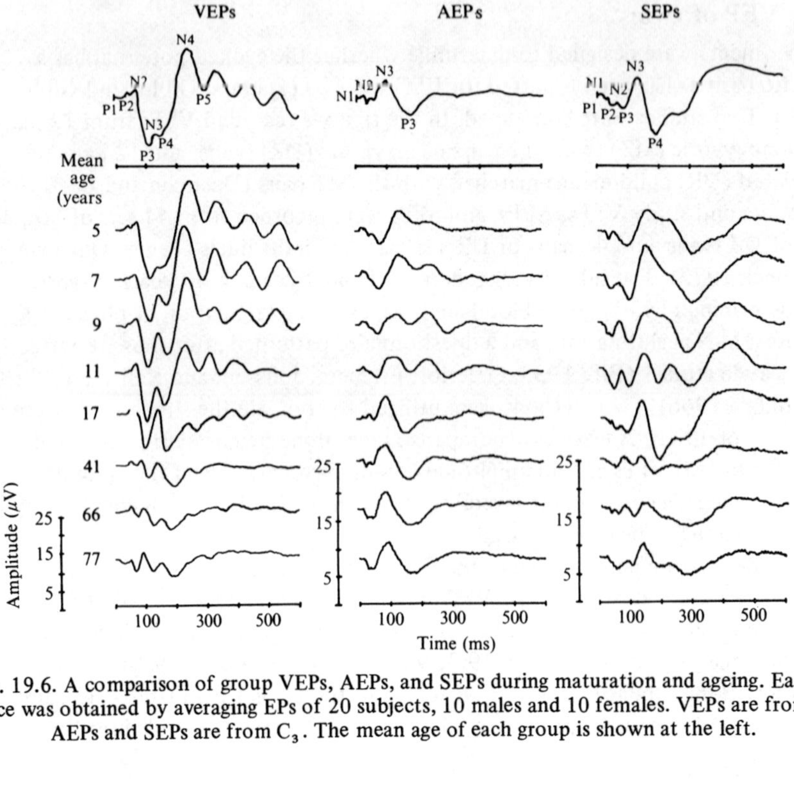

Fig. 19.6. A comparison of group VEPs, AEPs, and SEPs during maturation and ageing. Each trace was obtained by averaging EPs of 20 subjects, 10 males and 10 females. VEPs are from O_1, AEPs and SEPs are from C_3. The mean age of each group is shown at the left.

the same session in 160 normal subjects from 4 years to 86 years. These were divided into 8 age groups with 10 males and 10 females in each group. Post-primary portions of the SEP increase in amplitude from early childhood to adolescence then decrease in middle age and senescence, following a trend very similar to that of the VEP except that potentiation of early components during senescence does not occur with SEPs as it does with VEPs (Fig. 19.6). Peak delays of SEPs, like VEPs, gradually increase in middle-age and continue to increase through senescence. Changes in the AEPs are also illustrated in Fig. 19.6. The AEPs do not follow the same trend. Amplitude and latency of early components of AEPs change significantly from early childhood to adolescence but remain stable from then on. No changes were noted peculiar to senescence. Peak delays of various components decrease from childhood to adolescence but remain stable throughout the rest of life. Fig. 19.6 shows an interesting change in AEP configuration from childhood to adolescence. A late component, a negative wave following P3 by 50 ms or more, is present in groups whose mean ages are 7, 9, and 11 years; it disappears completely in late adolescence. A study of the maturation of the early components of the SEP from birth has recently appeared (Desmedt, Brunko, and Debecker 1976).

The VEP of twins

Experiments were designed to determine whether the evoked potential has a genetic basis as has been reported for EEG tracings (Lennox, Gibbs, and Gibbs 1945). Two studies were conducted. In the first we recorded VEPs from 12 pairs of monozygotic (MZ) twins, 11 pairs of dizygotic (DZ) twins, and 12 pairs of unrelated (UR) children age-matched with the MZ pairs (Dustman and Beck 1965). In the second study VEPs, AEPs, and SEPs were recorded from 44 sets of MZ, 46 sets of DZ twins, and 46 pairs of UR age-matched individuals (Lewis, Dustman and Beck 1972). The subjects ranged in age from 4 years to 40 years. Zygosity was determined by extensive blood analysis, careful examination of physical features, M-N agglutination, and a questionnaire patterned after those reported in earlier twin studies (Rife 1933; Cederlöf, Frieberg, Jonsson, and Kaij 1961; Nichols and Bilbro 1966). Two methods were utilized to compare the similarity between pairs of potentials. A waveform comparison was done by correlating digitized portions of two VEPs and an amplitude comparison determined the amount of voltage change occurring over several time-epochs of the EPs. Each epoch analysed contained a major peak and trough.

The most prominent finding of the first study, in which only the waveform comparisons were done, was that the VEP of MZ pairs exhibited a consistently higher degree of similarity than those of the DZ or the UR groups. This high degree of concordance may be seen in Fig. 19.7, where the VEPs of 5 sets of identical twins show a striking similarity between the pairs. In the second twin study, the same high degree of concordance was found between MZ subjects for all three sense

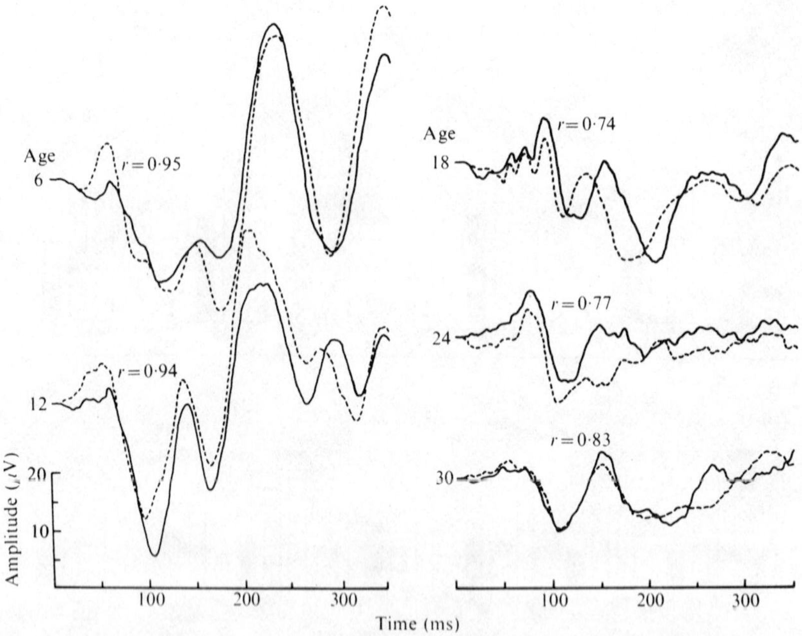

Fig. 19.7. The VEPs of twins illustrating the individuality and similarity of EP of 5 sets of identical twins.

modalities, VEPs, AEPs, and SEPs, regardless of the area of scalp from which the record was taken or the method used to determine similarity between responses. Fig. 19.8(a) is a comparison of waveform similarities of VEPs, and AEPs of MZ, DZ, and UR individuals. While SEPs are not included in the figure, these also showed the same relationships. Time-epochs were divided differently in (a) and (b) of Fig. 19.8. In (a) the waveform configuration of both VEPs and AEPs was broken into two time segments: 0–88 ms and 90–300 ms, on the assumption that early and late components derive from different sources and hence should be compared separately. In (b) of Fig. 19.8, which portrays the results from amplitude measures, both VEPs and AEPs were broken into different time-segments determined by prominent waves that occurred during different time-epochs, hence different divisions or time segments for VEPs and AEPs. It should be noted that essentially the same relationship holds regardless of the measure used. Thus the results indicated a considerable genetic component in waveform and amplitude characteristics of EPs.

Discussion

If EPs are to become a truly effective research and diagnostic tool, their limitations as well as their advantages must be evaluated. The present studies provide descriptive

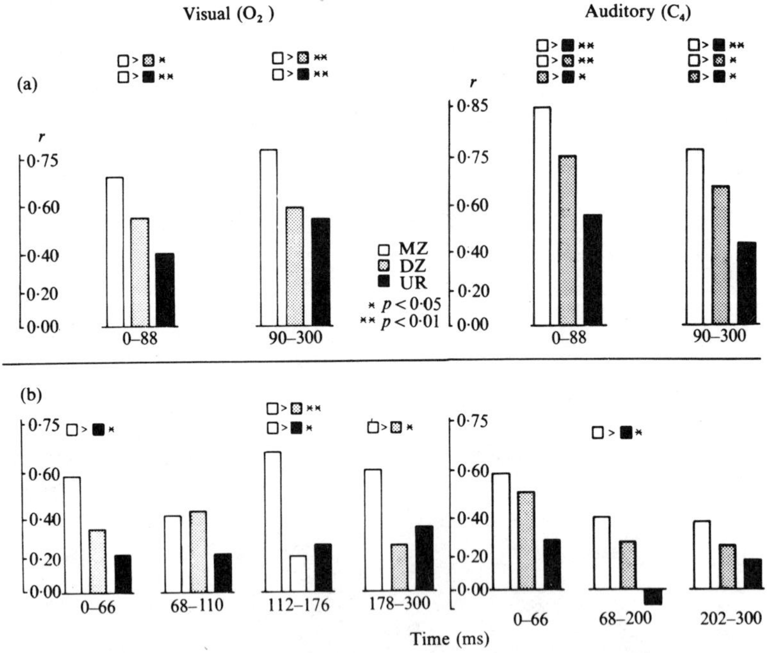

Fig. 19.8. A comparison of waveform (a) and amplitude (b) similarities of EPs of MZ, DZ, and UR individuals. Mean correlations were derived from waveform and amplitude comparisons of VEPs and AEPs for each of the 3 groups of subjects. Pairs of EPs were intercorrelated and then averaged for each group. In (a) the VEPs and AEPs are divided into two time-segments, providin comparison of early and late components. In (b), VEPs and AEPs were divided into different time-segments determined by occurrence of prominent waves for each modality.

information regarding changes in EPs throughout the life-span. There are obvious changes in amplitude. Some EP components of children are 2–3 times the amplitude of those of adults. There are marked changes in latency. The latency of some late components may differ by 50 ms or more at different ages. One EP component could easily be confused with another as one compares subjects of different age (Figs. 19.1–19.4) and such background data are important for clinical applications of EPs. The techniques used were calculated to be simple and straightforward, in order to be easily adapted by other laboratories. While the International '10–20' electrode system does not always provide the best EP data, it is an acceptab standard procedure now rather universally adopted and allows for sensible recording from three sense modalities, visual, auditory, and somato-sensory. We favoured unipolar recordings to avoid the confusion regarding polarity. The stimulation techniques were designed to provide quick and straightforward practical methods for general application, particularly for unsophisticated subjects, children, ageing adults, and poorly cooperative patients.

Age-related changes in VEP amplitude (Fig. 19.4(a)) show four main transitions that may correlate with developmental transitions at different age levels. The first is a rapid increase in amplitude of late components in the early years reaching a peak amplitude at 6–8 years. The second is a surge of amplitude occurring during adolescence. The third is the emergence of a stabilized or adult pattern in the VEP during late teenage years. And finally there is an increase in amplitude of early components as contrasted to an attenuation of late components beginning at about age 40 and continuing throughout senility. The first change correlates interestingly with that period of maturation in which the child is considered to have sufficient development to enter school. The second developmental change may be related to pubescence or more trivially to increased levels of psychophysiological arousal. Teenage youngsters may be more self-conscious and hence more alert than others who participate in our experiments. This parameter has not been analysed quantitatively in this chapter. The emergence of the adult-like VEP pattern correlates interestingly with mental abilities which appear to reach a certain plateau. Most mental tests such as the Stanford–Binet and the Wechsler Adult Intelligence Scales are based on the assumption that a level of adult mental development is reached in middle or late teens.

Finally, with advancing age, peak latencies of early VEP components increase throughout senescence. With late components, the main effect of increasing age is a diminution or attenuation of amplitude. Changes in peripheral sense organs with increasing age cannot account to any appreciable degree for the loss of speed or the slowing of voluntary responses with encroaching age (Critchley 1956; Birren 1959; Magladery 1959; Weiss 1959). The logical alternative is to look to central nervous processes which could indeed be reflected in the late EP components, which were found to change significantly with increased age. What anatomical changes are occurring at this time? While the morphological changes which presumably take place in the ageing nervous system are poorly understood, atrophy is universally accepted to be a common feature of ageing. For example, an examination of over 3600 specimens indicated an almost 20 per cent reduction in brain weight by 80 years of age (Bürger 1952). Concomitant with the reduction in brain weight and volume is a decrease in the total number of brain cells based on microscopic studies of the brain and nervous system (Bondareff 1959; Yakovlev 1962). However, most pertinent to our data are those studies that indicate that different parts of the brain 'age' differentially. For instance, the reticular formation and certain parts of the thalamus shrink and contain fewer myelinated fibres with increasing age (Yakovlev and Lecours 1967). Returning now to the maturation data, the areas of the cortex that continue development throughout childhood are the association areas. Collaterals of the brain-stem reticular formation and pathways to unspecific nuclei of the thalamus also grow and continue myelination until late adolescence (Turner 1948; Yakovlev 1962; Yakovlev and LeCours 1967). Changes in these structures may contribute to changes in late VEP components during formative years. However, it is disturbing to note that changes in VEP amplitude during development are most clearly seen in recordings from occipital scalp and not from central and frontal areas.

It should be noted that the above rationale, which compares behavioural, morphological, and electrophysiological changes during maturation and ageing, does not, of course, indicate a causal relation. A serious concern is that, while VEPs follow such a chronology, AEPs and SEPs do not in some instances. Could some of the VEP changes noted be due to changes in the eye during development and ageing? With increasing age there is a change in the length of the eye as well as in lens accommodation and pupillary reflex. However, refraction with ± 3 dioptre had little effect on amplitude of VEPs to diffuse light as used in our experiments. VEPs to higher-intensity flashes were studied with 10 subjects and the amplitude of both early and late components increased concomitantly with intensity. This contrasts to the changes in older subjects, where there is a decrease in amplitude of late components but an increase in earlier ones.

In our twin studies the most striking finding is the consistency with which EPs of MZ twins show a greater degree of similarity than do responses recorded from DZ or UR pairs, regardless of the sense modality tested, the area of scalp from which the record is taken, or the method used to compare the EPs. It could be argued that factors other than neural processes in the brain may have influenced the twin findings. For example, head length, and width from ear to ear are known to be correlated highly in identical twins, $r = 0{\cdot}91$ (Lenz 1961). This possibility seems unlikely since there was little relationship ($r = -0{\cdot}04$) between cephalic index and EP similarity in 13 subjects whose cephalic index ranged from 0·78 to 0·84 (Dustman and Beck 1965). Lennox *et al.* (1945), after examining numerous twins, concluded that the EEG pattern was determined to a large degree by hereditary factors and this would also appear plausible for the VEP.

With respect to sex differences, the VEPs of males are larger than those of females during childhood, while the reverse is true during adolescence and adulthood, which seems to resolve some contradictory reports in the literature. It appears that those who found EP of males to be larger actually used children as subjects, while those who found the reverse used adults (Rodin, Grisell, Gudobba, and Zachory 1965; Shagass, Schwartz, and Straumanis 1966).

Regarding *cerebral asymmetry*, a majority of children and adults in our laboratory presented larger VEP amplitude in the minor or right hemisphere, particularly from central leads, C_4 larger than C_3 (Fig. 19.5). With the 'brain at rest' there are inherent asymmetries in the EEG. The EEG recorded from the left hemisphere of right-handed subjects typically exhibits a lower mean amplitude (Butler and Glass 1974). Alpha amplitude in MZ mirror-image twins, identical in every respect save for reversed laterality, was found to be greater in recordings from the nondominant hemisphere for each twin pair. Thus the left-handed twin exhibited larger amplitude alpha from his left hemisphere, while the opposite was true with his right-handed twin brother (Raney 1939). In view of these, and other studies, it should come as no surprise that there is asymmetry in some VEP measures (Rhodes *et al.* 1969; Bigum *et al.* 1970; Lewis *et al.* 1970; Richlin, Weisinger, Weinstein, Giannini, and Morganstern 1971; Robinson and Strandburg 1973; Callaway 1973).

What is surprising are those conditions wherein it is not present or disappears. We have not found it in children with Down's syndrome (Bigum *et al.* 1970) nor in retarded children (Rhodes, Dustman, and Beck 1969) and we have noted its disappearance with ingestion of alcohol in fairly small amounts (Lewis, Dustman, and Beck 1970). It is most pronounced in children with high I.Q. (Rhodes *et al.* 1969). When asymmetry is present it should be noted that it occurs mainly in right-handed subjects and it is seen whether the subjects are viewing plain field or patterned light with no mental task imposed upon them.

While we originally supposed that hemispheric asymmetry might indicate a more efficient nervous system, i.e. that asymmetry was more pronounced in bright, alert individuals and missing in retarded and Down's syndrome children and disappeared with ingestion of alcohol, we now feel there is an alternative explanation. The clue to the difference among groups lies in the fact that bright, alert people in an experimental situation in which no task is assigned do not put their brains to rest. In all probability they play a variety of mental games or engage in some sort of mentation. This results in different hemispheric functions and hence generates a hemispheric asymmetry of electrical activity. In contrast a less endowed individual, such as a Down's syndrome child or an individual who has ingested alcohol, is less alert, his brain is less active and less inclined to mentation, hence little or no asymmetry results.

Part 3 Clinical applications of visual evoked potentials, and pathophysiological studies

20. The assessment of visual function in patients with opacities: a new evoked-potential method using a laser interferometer

G. B. ARDEN and U. B. SHEOREY
Department of Visual Sciences, Institute of Ophthalmology and Electrodiagnostic Clinic, Moorfields Eye Hospital, London

The retinal and visual capabilities which remain available behind corneal opacities or cataracts are difficult, if not impossible, to assess by the usual clinical means. VEPs to flash are therefore of interest in spite of their now well-known limited significance for the genuine evaluation of visual function. VEPs to pattern have not as yet been obtainable in the presence of opacities. This chapter describes a new method whereby VEP to laser-generated retinal patterns can be averaged from the scalp under clinical conditions in patients with opacities, and it shows the practical usefulness of these results for prognosis and treatment.

We have used a low-power helium–neon laser to produce interference fringe patterns on the retina, by focusing a pair of coherent point sources in or near the pupil plane. Fringes are formed, even in the presence of considerable ocular scattering. The basis for using interference fringes and the techniques for formation of fringes on the retina are well known. They have often been used in combination with subjective assessments of contrast thresholds to measure the ocular transfer function (Campbell and Green 1965). There have also been several recent studies of cataractous eyes (Goldman 1972; Green and Cohen 1971; Maumenee 1971; Rassow and Wolf 1973) using subjective techniques. In clinical work, visual acuity has been assessed by determining the highest spatial frequency of fringes that the patient can see. This mode of analysis has several shortcomings. First, it is difficult to direct the attention of the patient to the fringes, and to get reliable results requires training. Secondly, the judgement to be made is difficult, because the laser fringes suffer from a variety of imperfections. Aberrations in the optical system and in the eye cause the set of fringes to appear broken, displaced, and 'speckled'. Laser speckle noise is also troublesome. Speckling is due to scatter of the laser beams in the media, and forms a random diffraction pattern, which in general has a very high contrast (Hopkins and Tiziani 1970; Lowenthal and Arsenault 1970) and a

Visual evoked potentials in man: new developments (ed. J. E. Desmedt), pp. 381–94. Clarendon Press, Oxford 1977.

high mean spatial frequency which is superimposed on the interference pattern.

Fine fringes are therefore severely masked (relative to lower spatial frequencies) and 'laser visual acuity' may seem to be reduced although the macular is normal. Moreover, if a fine fringe pattern is to be formed, the two foci in the pupil plane must be relatively far apart, and if the clear aperture of the eye is limited (by the opacity), high spatial frequency fringes cannot be transmitted.

For all these reasons we have used a different approach. VEPs to pattern-reversing interference fringes have been recorded, resulting in an objective test. The VEP amplitude is maximal for a coarse pattern of only a few cycles per degree, is markedly reduced when visual acuity falls due to retinal disease, and is predominantly generated by macular and paramacular retina. We can thus use coarse gratings of suprathreshold contrast to estimate visual acuity, using response amplitude as a criterion: the difficulties produced by the high-frequency 'noise' in the laser signal, troublesome with the psychophysical tests, are largely circumvented.

In this chapter we briefly describe the apparatus we have made and the essential results on a group of normal subjects and also on patients with various types of opacities. The results from the group of normal subjects using this technique are compared with those obtained from a checkerboard pattern (Arden 1973), a technique which has been proved over some years to be useful clinically for the diagnosis of a variety of ophthalmological disorders.

Methods

Optical apparatus

The optical apparatus is based on a 'polarization interferometer' (e.g. see Françon and Mallick (1971)) in which the reversal of the fringe pattern is achieved by modulating the phases of the two orthogonally polarized light beams which are derived from a single point source. The fringe spacing is determined by the angular shear between these two beams. The optical arrangement is shown schematically in Fig. 20.1. The light source is a helium–neon laser, 230 mm in length, with a

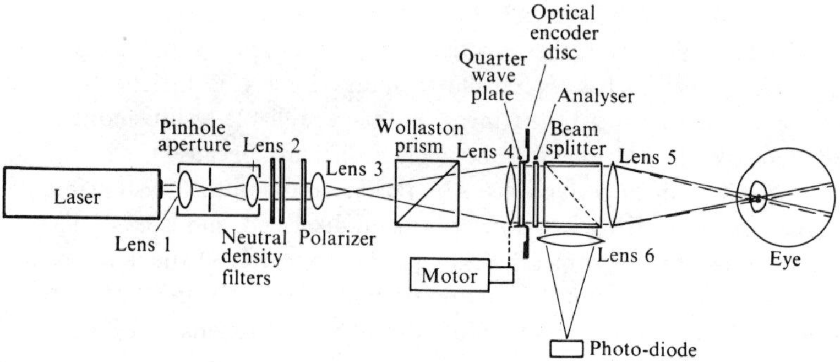

Fig. 20.1. Schematic arrangement of the laser interferometer used to produce pattern-reversing interference fringes at the retina.

nominal beam diameter of 1 mm and an output power of about 0·7 mW at the wavelength $\lambda = 0{\cdot}6328\ \mu m$. In order to produce a collimated, uniform distribution of intensity, the laser beam is passed through a pinhole spatial filter which consists of a 45 x, 0·65 NA microscope objective lens, 1, a 50 μm diameter pinhole aperture, and a 10 x, 0·17 NA microscope objective lens, 2. The emergent beam is about 4 mm in diameter and is attenuated and polarized by the neutral density filters and the polarizer. To produce the interference fringes, a Wollaston prism is placed between a point source, produced by the 5 x microscope objective, lens 3, and a collimator, lens 4. This lens is followed by an analyser. The prism can be moved along the axis of the optical system so as to produce a variable angular shear and thereby vary the spatial frequency of the pattern. The collimated beam is focused into the pupil plane by lens 5. Lenses 4 and 5 are biconvex doublets, of 100 mm focal length and 25 mm in diameter. All the lenses and the non-polarizing optical components were selected for low scatter and low residual birefringence.

The reversal of the fringe pattern is accomplished by modulating the phases of the two orthogonally polarized beams emerging from the Wollaston prism. This is done by rotating the quarter wave plate. When the polarizing axes of the polarizer and the analyser are set at 45° to the principal axes of the Wollaston prism, rotation of the quarter wave plate produces an increase in the intensity of one of the two beams while the other beam decreases in intensity by an equal amount. Hence there is no net luminance change but the light and dark bands of the interference fringe pattern phase-reverse by exactly half the fringe separation. A beam-splitter is included in between the lenses 4 and 5 so that the stimulus intensity may be monitored continuously. Thus any luminance modulation which might occur (e.g. arising from alterations in the birefringence of the Wollaston prism with temperature) can be detected and compensated for by a slight rotation of the analyser. The quarter-wave plate is mounted in a ball-race and driven through a reduction gear by a d.c. servo-controlled motor. The stimulation rate can be continuously varied over the range 6–25 Hz. The gear-reduction ratios and the motor speed are chosen such that there is no simple relationship to the pattern-reversal rate and consequently any residual audio noise and vibration are not synchronized to the visual evoked response. An optical encoder disc is mounted coaxially with the quarter-wave plate so that square-wave reference waveforms and trigger pulses can be derived for a signal averager and a phase-sensitive detector.

The Wollaston prism used in our apparatus produces a shear of 1° 2′ and consists of two 45° right-angled quartz prisms joined together to form a 20 mm cube. This enables a spatial frequency range of 0–40 cycles per degree to be covered. The total angular subtense of the fringes is about $\frac{1}{5}$ rad. The Wollaston prism is mounted on a dovetail slide carrier and is moved along the optical axis by means of a hand-operated rack and pinion mechanism. It is oriented to produce fringes which are inclined at 10° to the vertical. This was done to reduce any tendency of the patient to follow fringe motion with his eyes. The distance between the successive maxima of the fringes on the retina is given by the expression

$$d = \lambda/\alpha,$$

where d is the fringe separation, λ is the wavelength of light, and α is the angular shear between the two beams incident on the pupil. The angle α is given by

$$\alpha = \beta z/f$$

where β is the angular shear produced by the Wollaston prism, z is the distance from the point source to the prism, and f is the focal length of the collimator lens (Welford 1969). This relation was checked by measuring the spacing of the fringes projected onto a semi-transparent millimetre grid. The grid was placed a known distance behind a microscope lens of 17 mm focal length, which was itself placed along the optical axis and in the focal plane of the lens 5.

The unattenuated laser power, measured in the plane of the pupil, was 22 μW. For the optical arrangement described above, taking the transmission factor for the ocular media as 75 per cent, the retinal intensity would be of the order of 2 W m^{-2}. However, during viewing and the VEP recordings, the beam was further attenuated by neutral density filters in the range 2–5 density. For routine clinical evaluation on clear eyes, a 3·0 neutral density filter was used. In cases of dense opacities, the intensity was increased 10 times.

Appearance of fringes

The appearance of the interference fringes to the normal eye is somewhat disconcerting, the most prominent features being the following.

(a) The fringes are mixed with speckles and diffraction rings as a result of the optical aberrations and dust particles at the various optical surfaces. This occurs because of the use of coherent light.

(b) The intensity distribution across the field of view is non-uniform, being high along the axis and decreasing with increasing radius. This is due to the Gaussian distribution of the TEM mode pattern of the laser beam.

(c) The fringes appear to be mottled and have ragged edges. This is due to scatter in one's own eye.

(d) The bright fringes appear to be significantly broader than the dark fringes at the centre of the field of view. Towards the periphery the reverse appears true. This is of subjective origin, as was determined by measuring the luminance profile of the fringes. This profile showed an insignificant departure from the expected sinusoidal distribution and had a high contrast ratio, greater than 0·95.

Reducing the intensity of the laser source, superimposing a uniform green background field, or using a rotating scatter disc in the light path (Lowenthal and Joyeux 1971) all helped to improve the subjective appearance of the fringes but did not significantly increase the amplitude of the VEP. As satisfactory VEPs could be obtained from a range of patients, these additional features were not incorporated in the basic instrument. Furthermore, in the preliminary evaluations of this technique on normal subjects, it was noted that the distractions due to these and simulated optical distortions could largely be ignored while concentrating on the reversal of the fringes.

VEP recordings

The arrangement used for recording and processing is shown in Fig. 20.2. The

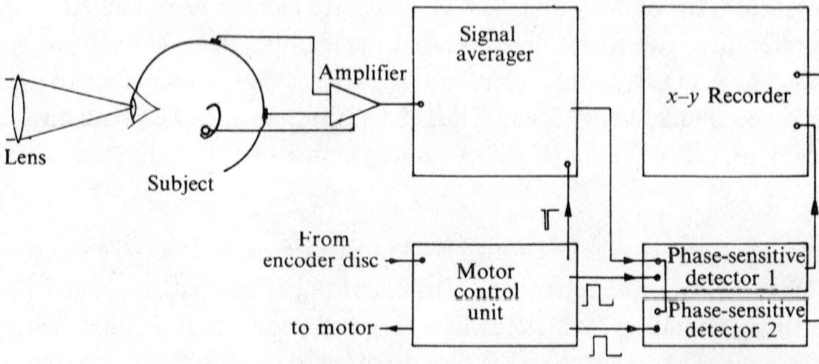

Fig. 20.2. Schematic arrangement for the recording and processing of VEP.

optical equipment (Fig. 20.1) was mounted on a slit-lamp table. The patient sat on a comfortable chair, and placed his head in the head and chin rest of the slit lamp. The operator moved the interferometer with the slit-lamp joystick so as to position the laser beams through a suitable part of the dilated pupil. In subdued lighting, the back-scatter from the focused laser beams was visible to the observers. The eye not being tested was covered with an occluder.

A fixation target was provided during the initial trials, either by placing a cross-wire in the light path to the left of the lens 4, by an illuminated target via the beam-splitter, or by a small red adjustable lamp for the other eye. Subjects with clear media have no difficulty in fixating along the optical axis. There is no obvious difference in VEP whether or not the subject maintains accurate fixation. However, patients who are elderly, who suffer from binocular disparity, or who have lenticular disorders or a severely limited field of view have great difficulty in seeing a target. Thus everyone was instructed simply to minimize their head and eye movements during the recordings and to look at the stimulus, keeping the maximum brightness in the centre of the field. The VEPs were recorded differentially by two Ag–AgCl electrodes, 10 mm in diameter, one placed on the midline 2·5 mm above the inion and the other on the vertex, the earlobe being earthed. A good contact was facilitated by de-greasing the skin and using a conducting electrode gel. A signal averager (Medelec MS6) was used for most of the measurements. One revolution of the quarter-wave plate corresponds to 4 cycles of the evoked response and one sweep of the averager. The sweep duration was adjusted so as to display between 3 and 4 cycles of response. Thus trigger-locked artifacts or alpha entrainment could be recognized at an early stage of the recording. Also it was easy to compare successive responses and to determine if adequate signal enhancement had been achieved. For normal subjects, 100 sweeps were averaged without a break, while for patients, particularly the elderly patients and those with severe opacities, larger samples were often required. The averager was temporarily halted if the patient lost the view of the fringes or required a rest.

In addition, the output signal from the pre-amplifier was led to two phase-sensitive detectors (Brookdeal, models 411 and 9412) which were locked to the quadrature reference waveforms derived from the encoder disc. The output signals from the two phase-sensitive detectors were fed to a $x-y$ recorder so as to obtain a polar display of the detected signal. Thus the amplitude and the phase angle of the fundamental component of the evoked response could be directly measured.

Subjects

The normal subjects were persons aged 18–35 years employed in the Department or the Clinic, and all were familiar with VEP recordings. The patients, aged 13–84 years, were those attending Moorfields Eye Hospital and were unfamiliar with the techniques.

Results

VEPs from normal subjects

When the quarter-wave plate revolves at more than 1·5 Hz (the lowest rate we have investigated), the VEP recorded is approximately sinusoidal, with a frequency 4 times that of the rotating plate. This comes about because for every 90° of rotation of the plate, the fringes reverse phase, and this appears to be the effective stimulus. Maladjustments of the polarizing optics produce luminance changes in the stimulus at half the frequency of pattern reversal: under these conditions a luminance VEP is produced, and mixed with the contrast VEP.

A typical VEP is shown in Fig. 20.3, which also shows the VEP to a black–white checkerboard pattern. The VEPs to both types of stimuli are sinusoidal but the one to the fringes is only about 25 per cent of that to the checkerboard pattern. This reduction is to be expected since the fringe pattern lacks several features present in the checkerboard. The fringe pattern does not contain, for example, sharp edges and corners; it is monochromatic and essentially uniharmonic.

Fig. 20.4 shows how the VEP amplitude of two young, normal observers alters as the spatial frequency of the stimulus is changed. The reversal rate for the solid symbols was 12 Hz. The VEP amplitude decreases as the spatial frequency of the pattern increases. It is possible to join the experimental points and extrapolate to determine the spatial frequency at which the VEP amplitude would be zero. However, it can be seen that this occurs at very different spatial frequencies for our two subjects, both of whom have 6/6 (normal) vision. Therefore, it is probably not possible to predict the visual acuity from graphs such as these. Note, too, that

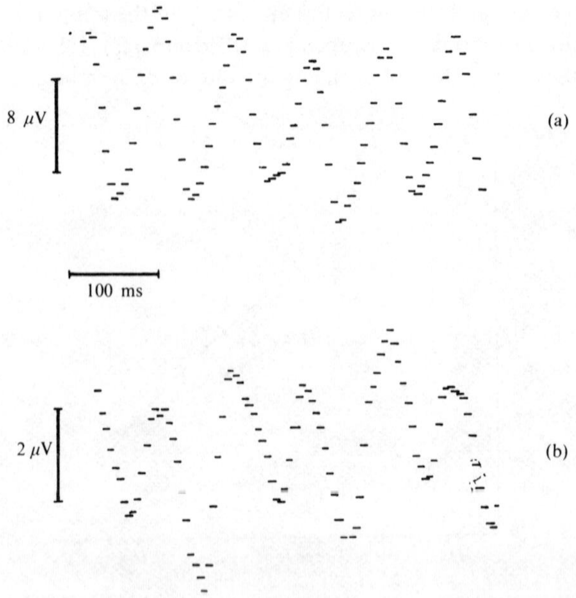

Fig. 20.3. Comparison of the averaged evoked response from (a) a pattern reversing black white checkerboard, at 1·25 cycles per degree, (b) laser interference fringes, 1 cycle per degree, both presented uni-ocularly to the right eye of a normal subject, at a reversal rate of 12 Hz. Subject D.J.F.

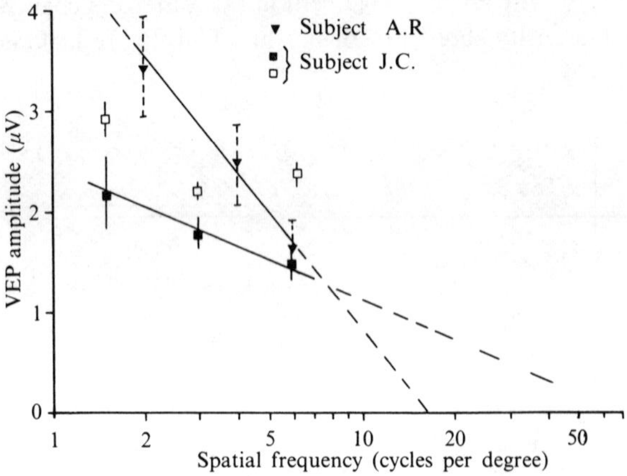

Fig. 20.4. The amplitude (peak-to-peak) of the averaged evoked response to the pattern-reversing laser interference fringes as a function of the spatial frequency. The results shown were obtained from two normal subjects, at a reversal rate of 12 Hz. The averaged responses evoked by a slower reversal rate of 8 Hz are also shown for comparison for one of the subjects.

the slope of the lines and the intercept depends upon the temporal frequency. This is illustrated for one observer (the open and filled squares).

Fig. 20.5 shows the effect of changing the rate of pattern reversal on the VEP

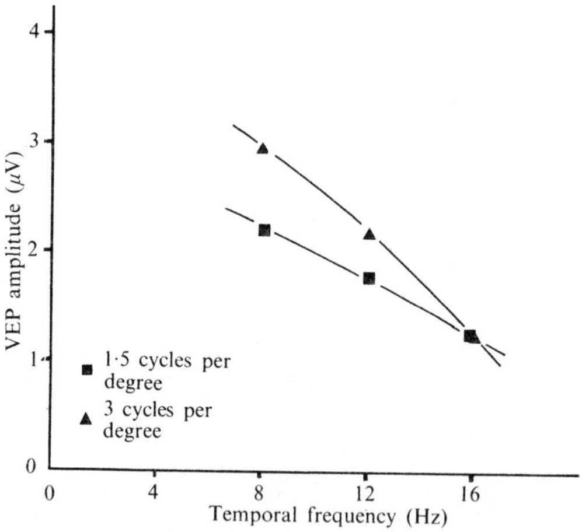

Fig. 20.5. The amplitude (peak-to-peak) of the averaged evoked response to the laser interference fringes as a function of the reversal rate, at two different spatial frequencies Subject J.C.

amplitude for two different spatial frequencies. The signal amplitude decreases rapidly with increasing reversal rate for finer fringes.

Fig. 20.6 shows the very small dependence of VEP on retinal illumination, namely, a change of only about 50 per cent in the VEP for a change of say, two orders of retinal intensity about a median value. Thus the retinal intensity used in

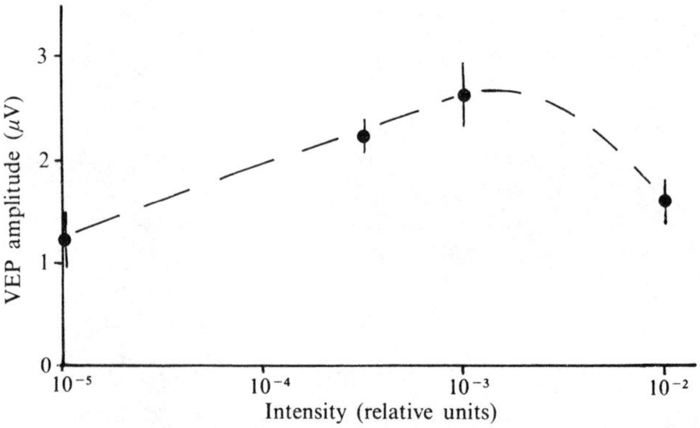

Fig. 20.6. The amplitude (peak-to-peak) of the averaged evoked response as a function of the retinal intensity. The retinal intensity is referred to 22 μW of laser power ($\lambda = 0{\cdot}6328\ \mu m$) incident at the pupil plane. Subject U.B.S.; 2 cycles per degree; 8 Hz.

almost all of the measurements on normal eyes was around this value, by using neutral density filters of 2·5 or 3·0 density in the path of the laser beam.

Fig. 20.7 shows the amplitudes of VEPs recorded separately from the right and

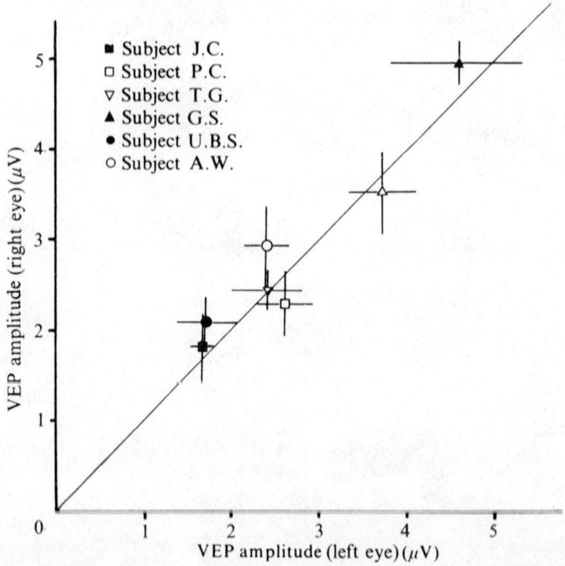

Fig. 20.7. Amplitudes of the evoked responses (peak-to-peak) from the right eyes plotted against those evoked from the left eyes of a set of normal subjects, for pattern-reversing laser interference fringes, at 2 cycles per degree and a reversal rate of 8 Hz.

left eyes of a group of normal subjects. Although the amplitudes vary considerably between the different subjects, the VEPs from the two eyes of the same subject are similar. We have also noted that there is no significant difference in the VEP for entry of the laser signal through various parts of the pupil.

In all these respects, VEPs generated by the fringes are similar to those produced by the checkerboard stimulator. Since the VEP from the two eyes of a normal subject are similar in amplitude, in patients it is possible to determine whether there is a uni-ocular lesion by comparing the VEPs from their two eyes. Further, it was decided that, to minimize the effects of disturbances such as eye movements and scatter, a relatively coarse pattern of 2 cycles per degree be used and a stimulation rate of 8 Hz was selected to balance between the requirements of having a large response, a large number of averaging samples, and a short analysis time, while avoiding the entrainment of alpha activity in patients.

A phase-sensitive detector has also been used to measure the amplitude and the phase angle of the fundamental component of the VEP. Fig. 20.8 illustrates the output of this system. The recording began a few seconds after the subject began to view the fringes and continued for 50 s. The length of the line drawn by the pen from the origin represents the root-mean-square (r.m.s.) value of the VEP, and the direction of the line gives the phase angle of the response.

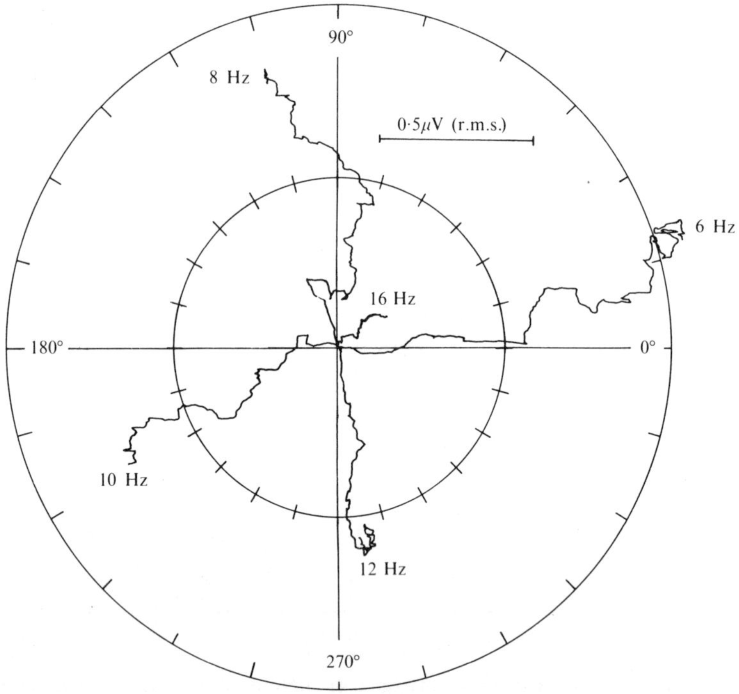

Fig. 20.8. Polar display of the evoked response to laser interference fringes at different reversal rates. Each trace records the build-up of the signal during the first 50 s of viewing. Note that the zero of phase angle is arbitrary. Subject U.B.S.; 2 cycles per degree; phase-sensitive detector time-constant: 30 s.

In analysing patients' responses we have not used the phase-sensitive detector extensively. There are several reasons. The phase information given is of little use, for, while VEP amplitude is not intensity dependent, the phase angle changes with intensity, and this must alter considerably in the presence of opacities. Secondly, the signal from our patients cortices is not stationary; one reason for this is loss of fringes, due to slight eye motions, but there are other factors involved. In our simple phase-sensitive-detector system, we cannot stop data acquisition during such periods of loss of stimulus. Also, we are forced to use large time-constants in the phase-sensitive detector, which destroys its main clinical advantage over a signal averager. Thus, the results that are described in the following section were obtained using a signal averager which is equipped with the necessary interrupt facility.

Results on patients (see Table 20.1)

We have investigated patients with opacities of the cornea, the lens, and the vitreous. The VEP amplitudes obtained were smaller than in our normal subjects.

This is due first to the much greater age of the patients, and secondly to the fact that they suffered from a variety of disabilities, e.g. spinal arthritis, so that they were unable to sit comfortably at the slit lamp. Thus head and eye movements, with loss of fringes and temporary halts, occurred during the data-averaging periods. Usually 150–300 averager sweeps were required to characterize the signal, taken in groups of 50–100 sweeps. For comparison, young normal subjects gave large, clear responses after 50–100 sweeps. In patients, the spatial frequency was 2 cycles per degree and the reversal rate was 8 Hz. Several records were obtained in order to ensure that the voltage recorded was a repeatable phenomenon. In patients with poor vision, it is possible to get a very large alpha rhythm which can be entrained with the stimulus. We recognize this phenomenon by incorporating almost 4 cycles of response on each sweep of the averager and by recording with slightly different presentation rates.

TABLE 20.1 *Table of cataract patients*

Types of cases tested	Number of patients
Senile cataracts	5
Traumatic cataracts	6
Cataracts caused by systemic disease	3
Congenital cataracts	1
Results	
No evoked response in the affected eye or a response very much less than other eye	4
Visual acuity of affected eye less than or equal to c.f.†	4
Cataract caused by systemic disease	1
Traumatic cataract	2
Congenital cataract	1
Amplitude of VEP in affected eye less than or equal to that of the other eye	10
Visual acuity of affected eye less than or equal to that of c.f.†	8
Visual acuity of affected eye less than or equal to that of 6/60	1
Visual acuity of affected eye less than or equal to that of 3/36	1
Senile cataract	4
Traumatic cataract	4
Cataract caused by systemic disease	2
No response in either eye	1
Visual acuity of affected eye c.f.†	
Senile cataract	

15 patients were seen in all. Ages: 13–84

† c.f. stands for compatible only with counting fingers (low acuity)

The assessment of visual function in patients with opacities

Patients with cataracts form the largest proportion of the series. Only in one patient of the series was it impossible to obtain reliable VEPs. In 4 cases, the VEP from the cataractous eye was reduced or absent, while in 10 others, it was equal or of greater amplitude than the response from the non-cataractous eye. The results are suggestive, for in the 4 cases where the VEP was reduced, it is likely that retinal or cortical disease coexists: thus one patient has a congenital cataract and therefore would have an amblyopic type of pattern VEP, even if the retina had no other disease. In 2 more cases, the cataract was produced by trauma and in one it was associated with diabetes.

It should be emphasized that all these cases had dense opacities, of the sort that prevent the psychophysical assessment of visual acuity with fine patterns. This is true even for the patient whose acuity was 3/36 with a pinhole: in this case, there was a very small 'clear area' and the spatial separation of the two beams required for fringes of high spatial frequency would not be obtainable unless one penetrated a denser scattering area. Further, as noted earlier, the patients had great difficulty in recognizing the speckled fringes above 10 cycles per degree, even with the better eye. Since with these patients the psychophysical tests had given disappointing results, the fact that the VEP to coarse fringes was not reduced is encouraging.

Fig. 20.9 also shows some individual records of other patients' opacities. We have obtained VEPs from 6 patients with vitreous haemorrhages and 3 cases with corneal opacities. The vitreous haemorrhages were due to diabetic retinopathies and were so dense that the patients had very little perception of light or vision. Most had bilateral disease. The VEPs obtained in most cases were very small and there was no 'normal' eye for comparison. However, in the case shown in Fig. 20.9, a VEP to laser was generated, although VEPs to the checkerboard pattern in such subjects would of course be absent. The absorption of deep red light by blood is low, so there is a particular advantage in using the red laser light. Further, because the light is coherent, interference fringes of adequate contrast can still be formed, despite considerable scattering. However, when the scattering is so severe that fringes cannot be distinguished, the patient's subjective response as to the apparent size and number of speckles in the central region can still give a useful indication of the foveal function (cf. Ehrich's method for observing the foveal field using focused diascleral illumination for mature cataracts) (Goldman 1972).

The traces in Fig. 20.9(c) are from a young man with a unilateral corneal opacity. The VEPs from the two eyes are very similar although the vision with the affected eye is extremely poor. It is this type of condition, where the opacity, though extremely dense, is localized to a thin layer, that promises to give the best results. This patient's corneal lesion was due to a failed corneal graft, itself required after injury to the eye. As a result of the inflammatory process around the graft, a secondary glaucoma had developed. Visual function was very poor, but the VEP is larger than in the fellow eye with an acuity of 6/6. It is in such cases where the assessment of probable visual function is of most importance in deciding if further surgical intervention is justified. In simple cataracts, on the other hand, it is

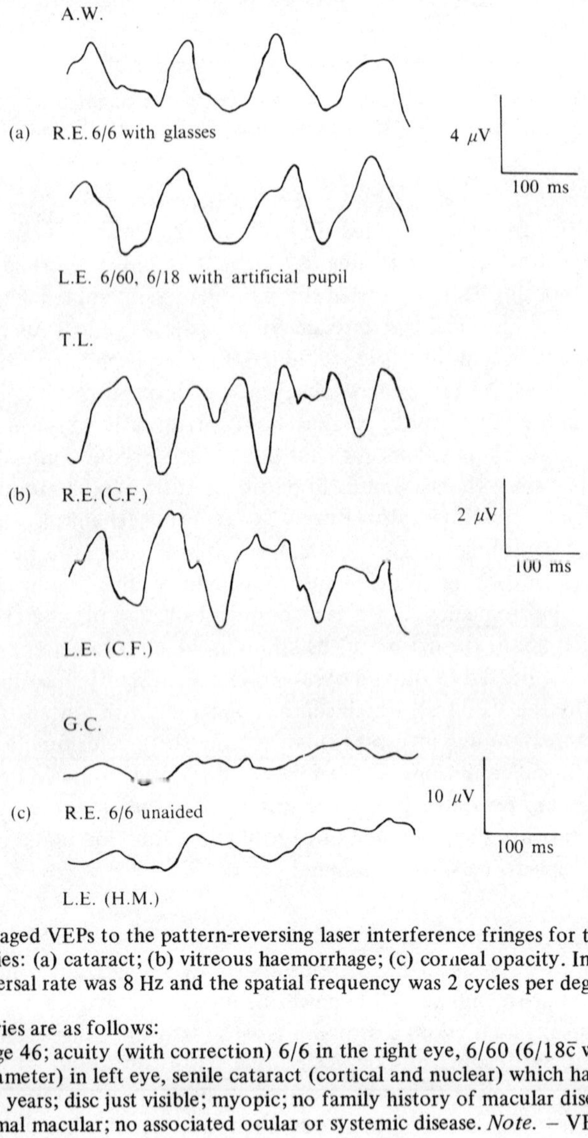

Fig. 20.9. Averaged VEPs to the pattern-reversing laser interference fringes for three typical cases of opacities: (a) cataract; (b) vitreous haemorrhage; (c) corneal opacity. In each case, the reversal rate was 8 Hz and the spatial frequency was 2 cycles per degree.

Patients' histories are as follows:

(a) A.W., age 46; acuity (with correction) 6/6 in the right eye, 6/60 (6/18c̄ with artificial pupil 1 mm diameter) in left eye, senile cataract (cortical and nuclear) which has developed over the past 3 years; disc just visible; myopic; no family history of macular disease; right eye clear with normal macular; no associated ocular or systemic disease. *Note.* – VEP amplitudes are equal in right and left eye.

(b) T.L., age 52; diabetic, for $6\frac{3}{4}$ years; retinopathy repeatedly treated by light coagulation since 1971; July 1972 vitreous haemorrhage in left eye, visual acuity reduced to counting fingers; Right eye, hand movements only. Fundus, no view left or right. *Note* – characteristic VEP response is present in each eye.

(c) G.C., age 22; March 1968, laceration of both corneas by car windscreen in a road traffic accident; July 1968, left linear extraction and division of anterior synechiae; November 1971, left corneal graft; developed intermittent secondary glaucoma; August 1972, cyclo-dialysis of left eye; developed secondary divergent squint in left eye; January 1973, left medial rectus resection of 5 mm, lateral rectus resection of 7 mm performed and cyclo-animization of the insertions of both muscles; February 1974, cornea opaque with an opaque central oedematous graft; there are many areas of deep vessels; large medial and lateral areas of scleral thinning; intra-ocular tension in left eye was 134 mm and would not respond to treatment. Vision H.M. (able to detect hand movements) only. No view of fundus. Right eye – media clear, nothing abnormal detected. *Note* – low sensitivity of amplifiers and larger VEP in affected eye.

desirable to attempt extraction, even if subsequently the visual acuity is not very high: the patient will be grateful for the improvement.

Discussion

The VEPs resulting from our stimulus are small in normal subjects compared with the VEPs to the checkerboard stimulus. Although it would be possible to produce large VEPs by choosing a stimulus with sharp borders (containing higher spatial frequencies; cf. the sinusoidal interference fringes), these would be preferentially degraded by opacities, and therefore would be of no use in the assessment of our patients. In this investigation, we have always used fringes of maximum possible contrast ratio. In the presence of opacities, the contrast ratio will be decreased, in an uncontrollable manner. This does not prevent the production of VEPs, which is understandable, since the maximum amplitude is known to be produced with patterns having a low contrast ratio (Regan 1972). The mechanisms whereby we perceive high spatial frequencies are not simply explicable in terms of the known activities of single cortical neurones. Thus, to recognize a fine grating against a background of high-frequency 'noise' is a complex task, and in general is eased by prior information about the nature of the stimulus which is to be recognized. This is why patients (compared to trained observers) have difficulty in seeing fine gratings, and why the VEP test, which can be concerned with low spatial frequencies is advantageous. A thorough investigation of the ocular transfer function is not practicable in clinical conditions. This applies to both psychophysical and VEP techniques. The very restricted procedure employed in the series reported here seems likely to provide a useful index of central visual function under conditions which prevent other forms of measurement.

Summary

Pattern-reversing interference fringes are produced by a polarization interferometer using a Wollaston prism and a red low-power helium–neon laser light source. The optical apparatus is mounted on a slit-lamp table so that the fringes can be manually positioned to project through any relatively clear part of the pupil. Fringes of low spatial frequency, 2 cycles per degree, are used to assess the visual function in three types of opacities: corneal and lenticular cataracts and vitreous haemorrhage. The stimulus is presented uniocularly to the patient by focusing the image of the source in the pupil plane. The VEPs from the two eyes are recorded separately and compared. Even in the cases of dense and mature opacities, it is possible to obtain a useful VEP and thus an indication of visual function.

Acknowledgements

Thanks are due to Mr. G. Mould for the construction of the optical apparatus; to Mr. D. J. Faulkner for assistance with the motor servo-control electronics; to Miss A. Williams for clinical assistance with VEP measurements; and to Mr. I. M. Chisholm for clinical examination of the patients prior to VEP tests.

21. Visual potentials evoked by gratings in normal and astigmatic subjects

L. MAFFEI
Laboratory of Neurophysiology, CNR, Pisa

The electrophysiological studies of Hubel and Wiesel have shown that visual cortical neurones are practically insensitive to flashes of diffuse light, but very responsive to bars of appropriate orientation and width. Our approach to the analysis of the human visual system has been to study VEPs evoked by a grating which is modulated in contrast while its space-average luminance is kept constant (Campbell and Maffei 1970). The photic stimuli were generated electronically on the face of an oscilloscope (pattern of dark and luminous bars with a sinusoidal luminance profile). It is then possible to investigate the mechanisms responsible for the transmission of spatial information in isolation from complicating factors such as light and dark adaptation. This method proved very convenient and allowed in several cases a strict correlation between the psychophysical experience of the subject and his VEPs, which disclose after suitable filtering a simple and characteristic waveform (Fig. 21.1(a)).

VEP and subjective contrast threshold

For each spatial frequency of the grating the VEP amplitude was linearly related to the logarithm of the contrast of the grating (Fig. 21.1(b)). In the graph the straight lines were fitted by the least-squares method and their dotted section is the extrapolation to the zero voltage point. The psychophysical contrast thresholds (arrows) agree very well with the zero-voltage VEP extrapolations. Fig. 21.2(a) assembles the results obtained at many spatial frequencies and shows a good agreement between the contrast values obtained by extrapolating VEP to zero voltage position and the psychophysical thresholds (Campbell and Maffei 1970).

Subsequently Fiorentini and I, by using psychophysical techniques, found that there is a linear relation between the apparent contrast and the logarithm of the objective contrast, i.e. the same relation found between the amplitude of the human VEP evoked by gratings and the grating contrast. Experiments were then performed on the cat to investigate whether a linear relationship would also be found between the logarithm of stimulus contrast and the amplitude of VEP. The answer was positive at each tested spatial frequency (Fig. 21.2, (b)–(e)).

Visual evoked potentials in man: new developments (ed. J. E. Desmedt), pp. 395–400. Clarendon Press, Oxford 1977.

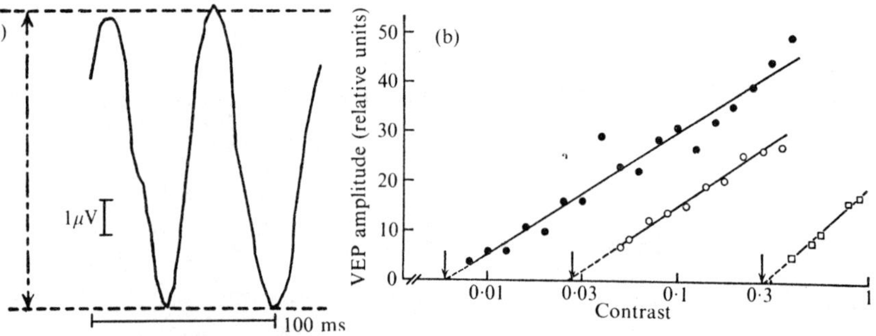

Fig. 21.1. (a) VEP resulting from 1000 averages obtained with a grating of 4 cycles per degree and a contrast of 1 log unit above the psychophysical threshold. The duration of the record is 125 ms. The amplitude was gauged by eye shown with the dotted lines. (From Campbell and Maffei 1970.) (b) The three sets of VEP results were obtained at spatial frequencies of 3·5 cycles per degree, 9 cycles per degree, and 18 cycles per degree from left to right respectively. The arrows indicate the psychophysical threshold obtained at each frequency. The VEP amplitude is plotted in relative units on the ordinate. (From Campbell and Maffei (1970). © 1970 American Association for the Advancement of Science.)

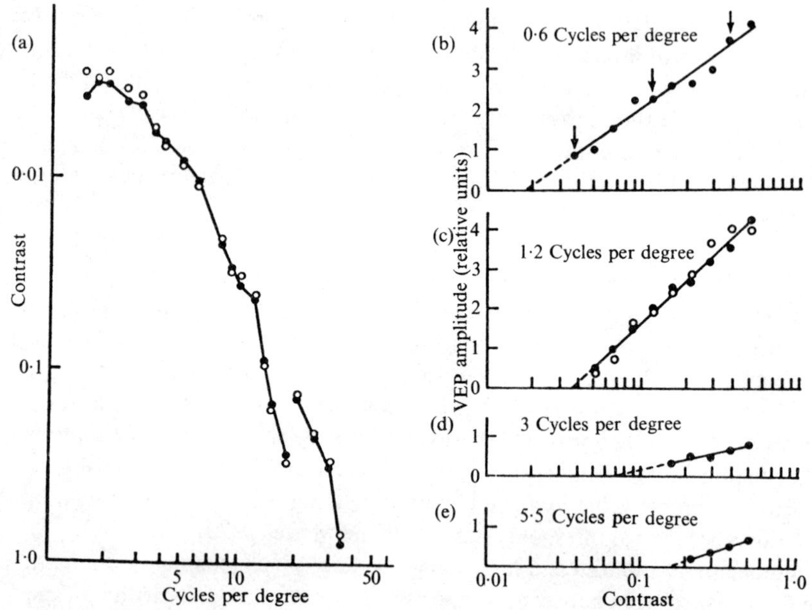

Fig. 21.2. (a) Human data; the straight lines join the contrast values (filled circles) obtained by extrapolating to zero amplitude for a number of spatial frequencies which are indicated in cycles per degree on the abscissa. The open circles represent the psychophysical contrast threshold. The main curve to the left was obtained at a luminance of 9 cd m^{-2} and the results to the right were obtained at a luminance of 21 cd m^{-2}. (From Campbell and Maffei 1970.) (b)–(e) Cat data, four examples of the relation between the voltage evoked by gratings at different contrast levels and at four spatial frequencies. Ordinate, VEP amplitude in relative units. In (c) the experiment was repeated twice to show the reliability of the data. (From Campbell, Maffei, and Piccolino 1973.)

We then investigated whether in the cat's visual system there is a relation between the contrast of the stimulus and the amplitude of VEP. We systematically investigated single-unit responses at the level of the retinal ganglion cells, lateral geniculate body, and simple and complex cells of striate visual cortex. The results are summarized in Figs. 21.3 and 21.4. It will be noted that only for the simple

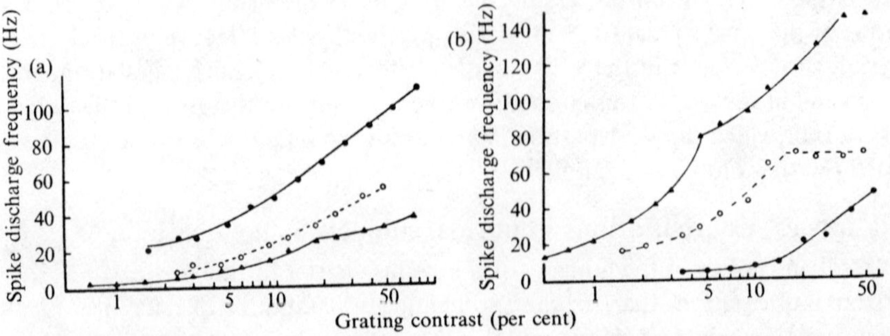

Fig. 21.3. Spike discharge frequency in the response of cat's retinal ganglion cells and of lateral geniculate nucleus cells to a grating as a function of grating contrast (indicated on the abscissa). (a) Retinal ganglion cells: on-centre cell, type Y, diameter of receptive field centre 1·3° (filled circles); on-centre cell, type X, diameter of receptive field centre 0·5° (open cicuits); on-centre cell, type X, diameter of receptive field centre 5° (triangles). (b) Lateral geniculate nucleus cells: on-centre cell, type Y, diameter of receptive field centre 1° (triangles); on-centre cell, type X, diameter of receptive field centre 0·3° (open circles); off-centre cell, type Y, diameter of receptive field centre 1·3° (filled circles). (From Maffei and Fiorentini 1973.)

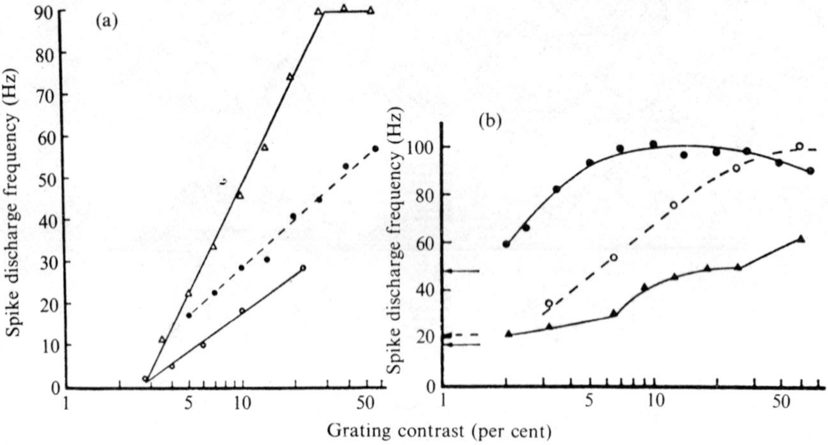

Fig. 21.4. Spike discharge frequency in single neurones of the cat's striate cortex as a function of grating contrast. The grating is continuously moving across the cell receptive field (indicated in per cent on the abscissa). (a) Simple neurones. Size of receptive field: 2° (triangles), 1° (filled circles), 1° (open circles). (b) Complex neurones. Size of receptive field: 2·5° (dots), 5° (circles), 4° (triangles). The arrows indicate the average discharge of each cell for zero contrast. (From Maffei and Fiorentini 1973.)

cells of the visual cortex (Fig. 21.4(a)) did a linear relation apply between the spike discharge used as an index of amplitude of response and the log contrast. Therefore one might tentatively conclude that, in the cat, the property of cortical VEP under consideration reflects mainly the behaviour of the simple cells in the visual cortex.

Another observation along this line is offered by the changes of VEP during adaptation to gratings. Blakemore and Campbell (1969) showed that prolonged observation of a high-contrast grating greatly reduces the visibility of a low-contrast grating of the same spatial frequency. This psychophysical effect finds its electro-physiological correlate in the VEP recorded before and after such adaptation, both in man and in the cat. In this context we recently found in the cat that the only class of cells which show adaptation to gratings is the simple cells of the striate cortex (Maffei, Fiorentini, and Bisti 1973).

VEP in various orientations in normal subjects

The resolving power of the human visual system is better for the vertical and horizontal orientations than for the two oblique orientations (for references see Howard and Templeton (1966)), and it is known that the effect is not caused by the optics of the eye. For example, the contrast threshold in the 45° meridian is greater by a factor of 2 than that in the vertical and horizontal meridians. Maffei and Campbell (1970) found a neural correlate of this phenomenon by recording VEP in response to gratings of various orientations. As shown in Fig. 21.5, the

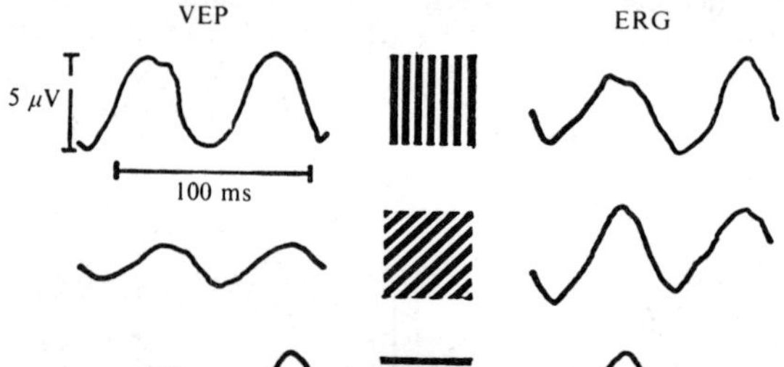

Fig. 21.5. VEP recorded from the scalp occipital area (*left*) and from the eyeball (*right*). The orientation of the gratings is as indicated. The upper six records were obtained with a grating contrast 1·3 log units (x 20) above the psychophysical threshold. The lower set of four records (control experiments) were obtained with lower contrast levels; the first row was obtained with a grating 1·15 log units (x 14) and the second row with a grating 1·0 log unit (x 10) above the psychophysical threshold. (From Maffei and Campbell 1969.)

amplitude and waveform of the VEP obtained when the grating was oriented vertically and horizontally were very similar. However, when the grating was presented obliquely, there was a decrease in cortical VEP amplitude but not in the simultaneously recorded ERG. Thus the neural mechanism for the specialization of the vertical and horizontal meridians must be located between the retina and the visual cortex. Two observations suggest that the visual cortex is the neural locus mainly involved: first, the cells of the visual cortex are the only ones sensitive to the orientation of the stimulus (Fig. 21.4(a)), and secondly, Mansfield (1974) recently found in the monkey that the proportion of the cells of the visual cortex selectively sensitive in the vertical and horizontal coordinates is much greater than those for the oblique orientations.

VEP in various orientations in astigmatic subjects

Freeman and Thibos (1973) and Fiorentini and Maffei (1974) have used VEP to find electrophysiological evidence of the nervous alterations caused by ocular astigmatism. It is well known that subjects with high degree of astigmatism may have a visual acuity lower than normal even if accurately corrected, especially if the correction was not started early in childhood. In astigmatic eyes the contours having different orientations cannot be focused together on the retina. According to the type of astigmatism and the viewing distance, lines can be focused that are oriented parallel to one or the other of the two perpendicular planes of symmetry of the astigmatic eye. All other contours are more or less blurred, depending upon their orientation and the degree of astigmatism. In some cases of severe astigmatism the subject accommodates preferentially for lines of one orientation, so that detailed visual information on the opposite orientation is largely lost.

Some astigmats show a difference in visual acuity in the two principal meridians even after full optical correction. Recent findings have shown that in some astigmatic subjects the contrast threshold for a grating is higher in one meridian than in the opposite one, even if the threshold is measured by a method which bypasses the optics of the eye (Freeman, Mitchell, and Millodot 1972; Mitchell, Freeman, Millodot, and Haegerstrom 1973). This suggests that the impairment of visual acuity has a neural origin, one working hypothesis being that the partial deprivation of visual information in one meridian affects some of the neurons which should respond preferentially to that orientation in the visual field.

We examined 23 astigmatic subjects. Each subject was accurately refracted and corrected for both spherical ametropia and astigmatism. Sixteen subjects had a degree of astigmatism of 0·5–1·5 dioptre in one or both eyes. The remaining 7 subjects had a total astigmatism of 3–4 dioptre in both eyes. VEPs were evoked by sine-wave gratings of 3 cycles per degree and of moderate contrast for various orientations.

The subjects with a high degree of astigmatism showed a marked asymmetry in the VEP amplitude according to pattern orientation. The VEP was larger in one of

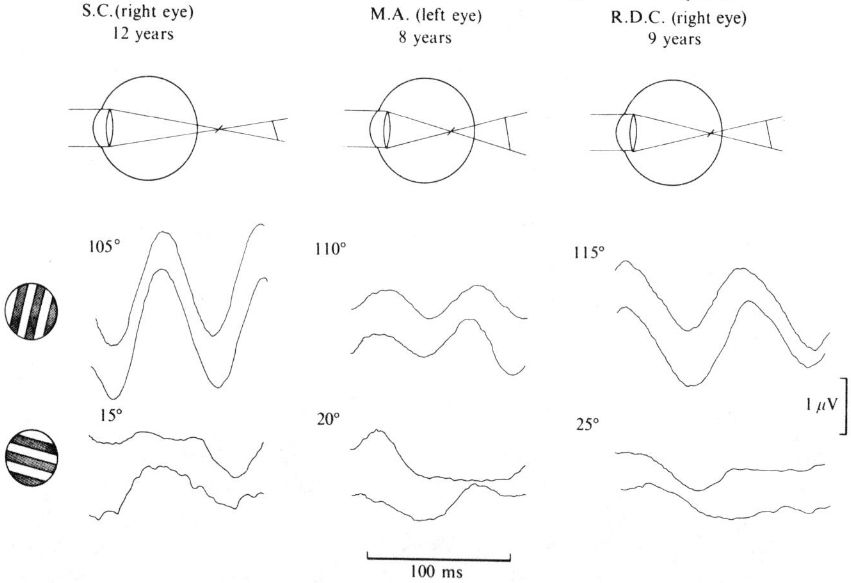

Fig. 21.6. VEP of 3 astigmatic subjects in response to an alternating grating oriented parallel to the two planes of symmetry of the astigmatic eye. *Top*, position of the two focal lines in the uncorrected astigmatic eye accommodated at infinity. *Bottom*, VEP for the two orientations of the grating. Patient S.C., right-eye visual acuity 10/10 with full correction (sph + 1·55 cyl + 3, 105°). Patient M.A., left eye, visual acuity 9/10 with full correction (sph – 1·5 cyl + 4, 110°). Patient R.D.C., atropinized right-eye visual acuity 7/10 with full correction (sph – 0·75, cyl + 4 115°). (From Fiorentini and Maffei 1973.)

the two principal meridians of the astigmatic eye and much smaller (or even not significantly different from zero) in the other meridian. Examples for three subjects are reported in Fig. 21.6. In the subjects with a small degree of astigmatism no significant difference was found for the amplitude of the VEP between the two orientations of the stimulus pattern parallel to the two principal meridians of the astigmatic eye. Strangely enough, however, for most (14) of these subjects, we could not detect the small but significant difference in the VEP amplitude for patterns oriented at ± 45° from the vertical which had been observed in normal subjects (Maffei and Campbell 1970).

22. The use of visual evoked potentials in optometry

M. MILLODOT

Department of Optometry, University of Wales Institute of Science and Technology, Cardiff

Optometry is principally the measurement of the components of the eye and how these relate to visual functions. It endeavours to estimate the focusing of the eye and the monocular and binocular (taking into consideration the oculomotor balance) visual acuity. These various measurements are carried out mainly by subjective methods and, to a lesser extent by objective methods. Objective techniques are useful to the practitioner and they are indispensable in cases of malingerers, young infants, mentally disturbed deaf and dumb patients, elderly people who cannot cooperate, and conscripts to the Armed Forces.

The classical objective methods of refraction are retinoscopy (or skiascopy) and refractometry, which have been used around the world for about a century (Millodot 1973). These methods suffer from one drawback: the assessment they provide is not as good as that obtained subjectively, although the discrepancy is slightly less than half a dioptre on average. Therefore these objective instruments usually serve only as a guide to the final prescription, and refraction is precise only when psychophysically determined. Likewise it is important, in the class of patients mentioned above, to be able to measure visual acuity objectively. The techniques used at present are based on inducing eye movements, either optokinetic nystagmus (e.g. Lewkonia 1969), pendular eye movements (Millodot, Miller, and Jernigan 1973), or galvanic skin response (Pearson 1970). But none of these methods is very accurate, although they do provide approximate information on the visual acuity of the patient.

The advent of VEP techniques to estimate the refraction and visual acuity of the eye objectively is an important development in optometry. These methods are more valid than those used previously, since the VEP depends upon the same receptive processes as visual perception. In retinoscopy, on the other hand, it is assumed that light is reflected from a layer different than that of the receptors (Glickstein and Millodot 1970); there is always a small but systematic error in the determination of refraction (Emsley 1963) which is related to other factors besides the choice of site of light reflection. In any case this discrepancy is greater the

Visual evoked potentials in man: new developments (ed. J. E. Desmedt), pp. 401–409. Clarendon Press, Oxford 1977.

smaller the eye, such as in infants (Millodot 1972) or in animals (Meyer and Schwassmann 1970; Millodot 1971; Moser and Krueger 1972; Sivak 1974).

Another advantage of the VEP technique over retinoscopy and refractometry is that the whole visual pathway is implicated. The presence of a normal VEP indicates an intact visual pathway. Retinoscopy or refractometry evaluate only the quality of the focusing power of the eyeball. Blindness caused by a lesion along the pathway or in the visual cortex would remain undetected by the latter techniques in a human or animal unable to respond verbally, but would affect the VEP.

VEP and refraction

Copenhaver and Perry (1964) noted a slight effect of the refractive state of the eye on the VEP. Spehlmann (1965) found a marked effect of the focusing of the eye upon the VEP using a +10 dioptre lens to degrade the retinal image. Similar observations were made by Spekreijse (1966), Rietveld, Tordoir, Hagenouw, Lubbers, and Spoor (1967), and Cobb *et al.* (1967). Harter and White (1968) refined the previous findings and demonstrated that it was possible to measure refraction systematically by recording VEP. Thus the method became clinically feasible.

Harter and White (1968) stimulated the subject's eye at a rate of 1 Hz by flashing for 10 μs on a bright checkerboard target, leaving the eye in the dark. They found a correlation between the VEP amplitude at two latencies (a negative component at 90–100 ms and a positive component at 180–200 ms) and changes in target clarity induced by lenses of varying power. With this technique, a large portion of the VEP is attributable to light intensity and various ways must be found of separating out the response due to the state of refraction. White (1969), Duffy and Rengstorff (1971), and Ludlam and Meyers (1972) used an electronic subtraction technique in which the VEP to non-patterned light stimulus was subtracted from the VEP to the patterned light.

Another very effective method uses the pattern-reversal stimulus in which the average luminance remains constant (Spekreijse 1966; Cobb *et al.* 1967; Riggs and Sternheim 1969; Maffei and Campbell 1970; Freeman and Thibos 1973; McCormack and Marg 1973; Regan, Chapter 11 of this book). Millodot and Riggs (1970) employed this technique in human subjects to measure the effect of lenses of varying dioptric power placed in front of the eye to reduce errors of refraction.

Experimental methods

The stimulus was either a checkerboard or a grating. The former yielded a greater VEP response than the latter, possibly because it has more contours and because the VEP reflects the photopic visual system which is specialized in form discrimination. Thus I used as a stimulus a checkerboard pattern in which the dark squares were substituted for clear squares and vice versa in a sinusoidal fashion. The total amount of light remained nearly constant but the frequency of the pattern-reversal stimulation could be varied. The frequency was chosen above or below 8–12 Hz to minimize EEG alpha contamination. Millodot and Riggs (1970) used 12 Hz and 15 Hz, depending on the subject. Lately, Regan (1973*c*) has noted that VEP are larger at 6–7 Hz than at 12 Hz. McCormack and Marg (1973) also adopted 7 Hz in their measurement of refraction.

Although most investigators have used high-contrast patterns it is preferable to use a contrast below 40 per cent in order to avoid complications due to saturation (Spekreijse 1966; Regan 1973*c*; Ronchi and Castellini 1973).

The subject was seated 85 cm from the pattern because of the constrictions imposed by the apparatus. Longer distances between target and subject may be used to minimize accommodation and convergence effects (Duffy and Rengstorff 1971; Ludlam and Meyers 1972; McCormack and Marg 1973; Regan 1973*c*). To assess the refractive state of the eye a given pattern with a constant size element is used. The optimum VEP is obtained for a check or bar size subtending an angle of 10–20′ at the subject's eye, while using larger checks might lead to substantial errors (Regan and Richards 1973). Millodot and Riggs used a target with individual squares of 14′and the overall target subtended an angle of 9·5°, sufficient to stimulate the macular area that mostly affects the VEP. The subject was requested to fixate a dot in the centre of the field. The VEP was recorded either with bipolar electrodes (Millodot and Riggs 1970; McCormack and Marg 1973) or monopolar electrode (Harter and White 1968; Ludlam and Meyers 1972; Regan 1973*c*). The experimental set-up is shown in Fig. 22.1. The subject viewed the checkerboard reflected on a mirror. Lenses of various powers were placed in front of the viewing eye (monocular measurement) and the VEP plotted on the *x–y* recorder for each lens.

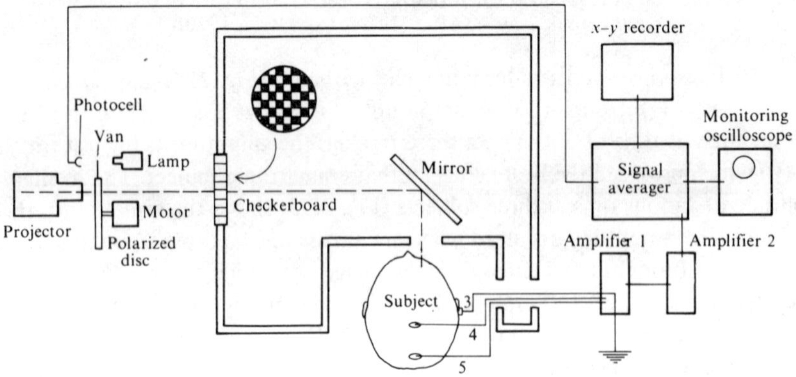

Fig. 22.1. Apparatus used to stimulate and record VEPs. The polarized disc is rotated by the motor; a van on the disc interrupts light from trigger source. A lamp illuminates the photocell used to provide a synchronized pulse to the signal averaging computer. The mirror reflects light from checkerboard to the right eye. 3, 4, and 5 are recording electrodes on the scalp, and amplifiers 1 and 2 supply the signal averaging computer. (Modified from Millodot and Riggs 1970.)

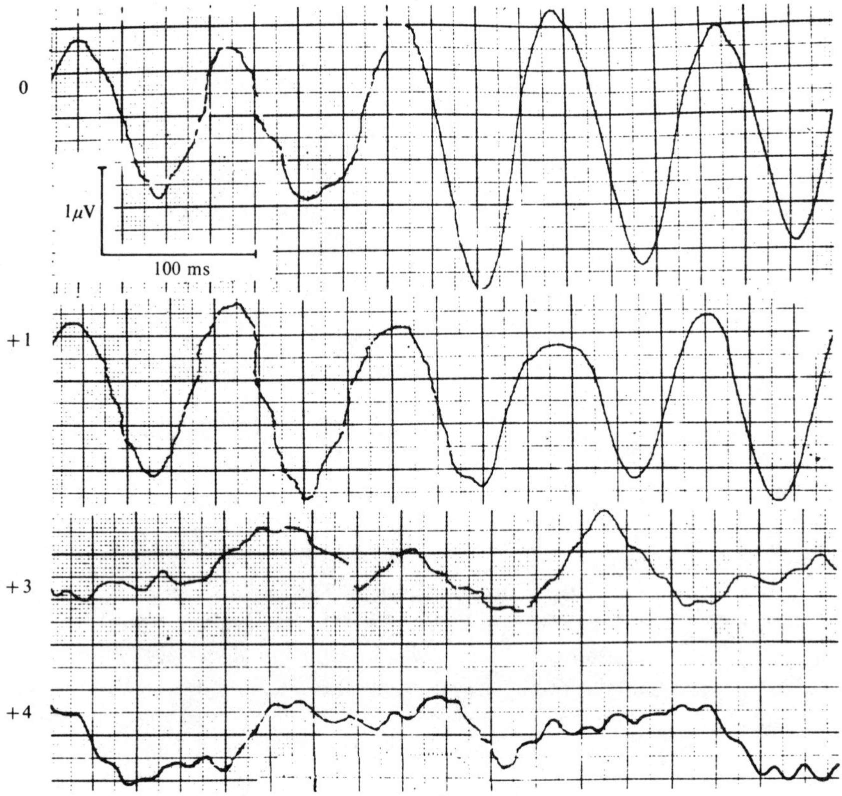

Fig. 22.2. Tracings of VEP obtained when viewing a checkerboard pattern through several ophthalmic lenses. (After Millodot and Riggs 1970.)

The VEP responses to the alternating checkerboard (Fig. 22.2) appear as a series of waves. The trough-to-peak amplitude of each was measured on the record using an analysis time of 500 ms. In these tracings the amplitude is highest for the lens (0) which provided the best acuity in that emmetropic subject. The median amplitude of various runs in three subjects (Fig. 22.3) shows the same trend: the maximum VEP amplitude occurred when the image was reported to be in perfect focus. The VEP amplitude decreased as the image was degraded by either positive or negative lenses. The VEP is quite sensitive to de-focusing and under optimum conditions a difference is noted for 0·25 dioptre if accommodation was relaxed. Certainly the response amplitude was appreciably lower for 0·5 dioptre degradation These results have since been confirmed by McCormack and Marg (1973) and Regan (1973) using a similar technique to the one described here (Millodot and Riggs 1970; Millodot 1971*b*). Duffy and Rengstorff (1971), Ludlam and Meyers (1972), Dawson *et al.* (1972) have obtained similar results using a different stimulus technique.

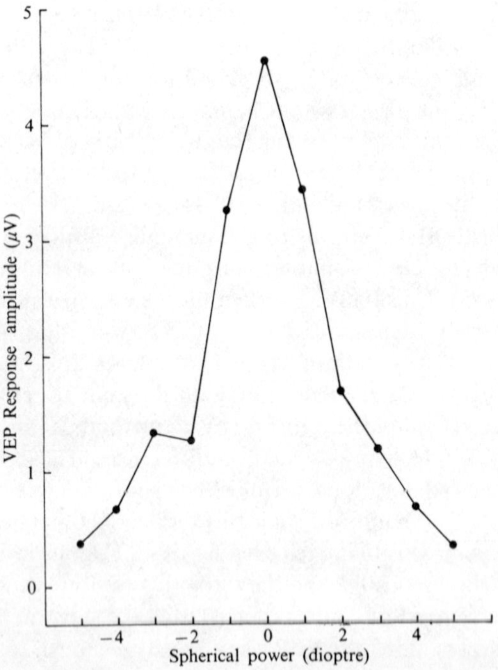

Fig. 22.3. VEP response amplitude as a function of the lens used in viewing a 14′ check stimulus. Each data point is the mean of three subjects.

This method is in principle valid because it is dependent upon the same initial physiological processes in the retina as vision itself. And indeed most VEP measurements of visual functions have been shown to be in good accord with the psychophysical determinations (Riggs and Wooten 1973). In our own measurements the comparison between VEP and subjective findings did not differ by any more than ± 0·25 dioptre, but such sensitivity has yet to be substantiated in the clinic with a greater variety of patients. In any case, the VEP does not afford a greater sensitivity than retinoscopy and refractometry when accommodation is relaxed. The VEP is, like retinoscopy, an excellent guide towards the final evaluation of the refractive state of the eye and as such it is useful in people who cannot be tested subjectively.

VEP determination of astigmatism

Ludlam and Meyers (1972) and McCormack and Marg (1973) measured the astigmatism of the eye by VEP elicited by a grating which was rotated to various angles. If the eye was affected by astigmatism the VEP would be larger in one direction of the bars of the grating than in another. However, the use of a grating affects the sensitivity since the signal-to-noise ratio is diminished. None the less Ludlam and Meyers (1972) and McCormack and Marg (1973) determined the cylinder power and axis in that fashion. The latter investigators arrived at a sensitivity of about 1 dioptre on cylinder power and ± 10° with regard to the axis, whereas Ludlam and Meyers (1972) got cylindrical corrections within 0·5 dioptre and within ± 10° for the axis. Regan (Chapter 24 of this book) improved these measurements of astigmatism by having the subject view a checkerboard pattern through a rotating stenopeic slit. He had a VEP estimate of refractive correction within 0·5 dioptre for power and within 10° for the axis. The VEP was treated by Fourier analysis instead of averaging to give an on-line display of the instantaneous VEP amplitude which thus continuously informed of the result of a change in the refractive corrections. Thus the VEP refraction can be performed in less than 2 minutes with relatively good sensitivity (Regan, Chapter 24 of this book). The use of a slit and a checkerboard pattern has two advantages: first it gives a larger amplitude VEP; secondly, since the rotating slit does not affect the orientation of the checkerboard pattern on the retina this VEP method does not confound the astigmatism of the eye with any orientation differences in acuity encountered when a grating is placed in various meridians even in fully corrected astigmats (Freeman *et al.* 1972) or in normal subjects (Maffei and Campbell 1970).

In spite of the good sensitivity achieved by this technique it is not yet equal to that obtained psychophysically. And the refraction measured subjectively represents, as it were, the last court of appeal, that is the correction which is most likely to be prescribed. Moreover VEP is not sensitive enough to be a good clinical test of the axis of astigmatism, although the accuracy depends on the power of the cylinder. The rapidity of the examination is comparable to the other objective methods of refraction. For clinical practice the VEP technique is indeed painless, but it can be somewhat awkward for the patient as skin electrodes have to be attached to the scalp and ear and the paste has to be washed away after the recording session. The technique should gain popularity if thin needle electrodes were used. In the VEP method the patient's cooperation is very important since the patient must maintain his or her gaze on the centre of the stimulus field for a certain period of time, and avoid eye movements or head movements which would spoil the VEP.

A definite advantage of VEP method is the measurement of an infant's visual system. In this case retinoscopy can assess only the quality of the focusing of the eye, whereas a lesion along the visual pathway can be discovered by VEP. VEP techniques may also be useful in older patients with whom communication is so difficult as to make subjective testing very tedious. In these patients the ocular media are quite opaque so that retinoscopy or refractometry is impossible, especially as the pupils of these subjects are usually very tiny. Although retinoscopy will remain the favourite objective tool, it is expected that many eye hospitals will establish VEP laboratories for dealing with particular patients. The demand of the general public for visual care is increasing and future researches in the VEP area will be aimed at increasing the sensitivity even further, at minimizing the complexity of the apparatus, at devising simpler electrodes, and at reducing the cost of the operation.

After the monocular testing of refraction has been carried out it is also essential to carry out some binocular tests of refraction in order to obtain a correction which is not only adequate to each eye separately but to both eyes working together, especially as a different state of relaxation of accommodation might have prevailed while one eye was being tested and the other occluded. This area of binocular refraction still needs further research (cf. White and Bonelli 1970; Harter *et al.* 1973).

The aim of binocular refraction is to achieve equal visual acuity in the two eyes, which is relatively simple if the two eyes are about the same optically. It is recommended (Giles 1960) that a pair of 0·25 dioptre lenses be placed in front of the eyes and to add this value to the correction if vision is not reduced by these lenses. One of the established rules of optometry is to prescribe the maximum positive lenses and the minimum negative lenses that give optimum visual acuity, so as to minimize the accommodative effort for distance vision whilst convergence remains at a minimum. Another consideration arises when one eye is dominant. Some authors recommend correcting the eyes in order to obtain equal visual acuity; others prefer to preserve a better acuity for the dominant eye, so as not to upset the normal dominance by giving a better acuity to the non-dominant eye (Giles 1960; Borish 1970). Such testing is done subjectively and has not yet been explored by means of VEPs. The VEP technique would be a most valid objective technique, since large VEPs are obtained when the two eyes are stimulated (e.g. Harter *et al.* 1973) and the VEP has been shown to correlate well with perceptual phenomena.

VEP and visual acuity

Visual acuity, or the ability of the eye to resolve fine details of an object, is tested optometrically in order to indicate whether a person's eyes are correctly focused or require a different correction. This test guides the practitioner in the final stage of prescribing lenses. Visual acuity depends on a multiplicity of factors (see Riggs 1965; Le Grand 1956). The subjective measurement as done in the clinic with the Snellen letters which have been in constant use since 1862 is simple to accomplish but complex to interpret. In many cases an objective measurement of visual acuity is necessary. Numerous attempts at measuring visual acuity objectively have been made over the last 40 years (see e.g. Pearson 1966) with varying degrees of success. The methods so far employed have been difficult to use with patients: they are not sufficiently accurate in cases with very bad or very good acuity (Millodot *et al.* 1973), and also they are time-consuming and require a certain amount of cooperation from the patient. The possibility of using VEP to assess visual acuity is a welcome addition to the present objective techniques.

Rietveld *et al.* (1967) measured VEP over a large range of check sizes varying from 3′24″ to 4°1′. They found a maximum VEP response for a check-size pattern of 10–20′. As the pattern became finer the response amplitude dropped sharply.

Yet they obtained a different VEP response with the smallest check size they used (3′24″) from that of a blank. Harter and White (1970) extended the study by varying visual acuity with ophthalmic lenses placed in front of the subject's eyes and were able to get appreciably different VEP with a check size of 5′ as compared to a blank. The VEP was maximum between 10′ and 20′ when the eye was in perfect focus, but there was some difference in the peak amplitude according to which wave was analysed. The surface-negative component N100 (latency 95–110 ms) was maximum with a check size of about 20′ whereas the surface-positive P180 (latency 170–200 ms) peaked around 12′. Regan and Richards (1973) obtained a peak between 10′ and 15′ check size over a large range of contrast. Harter and White (1970) also showed that with 1 dioptre de-focusing the VEP was reduced for all sizes of the check; with 3 dioptre it was further diminished – and in fact for the 5′ and 10′ check size it was hardly larger than that induced by a blank; only for a check size larger than 30′ was there an appreciable VEP. This was to be expected, as 3 dioptre de-focusing produces a visual acuity of less than 0·1, or 20/200 (see Sloan 1957). Thus it is necessary to present a much larger size of the checkerboard in order to elicit a significant VEP, as would be predicted psychophysically. With 5 dioptre of de-focusing the VEP is of practically the same size as that induced by a blank and in this condition it is not until the size of the check reaches 50′ that a significant VEP can be recorded. These results confirm at least qualitatively the well-known relationship between visual acuity and dioptre of induced de-focusing or refraction. And when the visual acuity is greatly reduced, as in amblyopia, the VEP is very affected or absent (Dawson *et al.* 1972). Campbell and Maffei (1970) showed that there is a good correlation between contrast threshold and VEP amplitude, and Regan and Richards (1973) found that blurring the retinal image with a +1 dioptre lens reduced the amplitude by about 30 per cent for a 3′ check size.

The clinical measurement of visual acuity consists in determining the threshold of resolution of the smallest optotypes. Basically it should suffice to record a VEP with the smallest possible check size such that it is just appreciably or significantly different from the VEP to a blank; but this has not yet been done. The validity of such a VEP measurement of acuity would be achieved by correlating this value with the psychophysical determination of visual acuity under the same stimulating conditions and not with Snellen letters. Moreover, to be of clinical application it would be necessary to carry out a normative study with improved signal-to-noise ratio in order to obtain a VEP for the smallest possible pattern which the visual system can resolve. The studies so far reported suggest that the method of measuring visual acuity threshold in the clinical context is feasible.

Conclusion

The relative newness of VEP application to optometry gives rise to various shortcomings. First, the VEP has been used to assess only a few visual functions, such as the refractive state of the eye, the effect of image degradation, and, lately, the

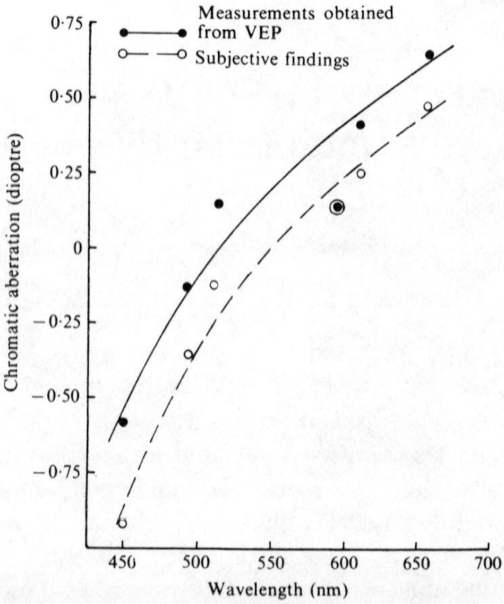

Fig. 22.4. Chromatic aberration of the eye as a function of wavelength. Each data point is the mean of three subjects. (After Ronchi and Millodot 1974.)

measurement of the chromatic aberration of the eye (Regan 1973*a*; Ronchi and Millodot 1974). Measurements of the chromatic aberration of the eye by VEP are shown in Fig. 22.4 together with the psychophysical determinations made in the same conditions. The two sets of results are well correlated and within 0·5 dioptre of each other, with the objective measurements shifted towards hyperopia. The VEP has also proved useful in the field of binocular vision and even orthoptics.

Secondly, instrumentation and data analysis still place some limitations on the wider clinical application of the VEP. But the advances have been so rapid that it is conceivable that soon in the future VEP will be a rapid, simple, and accurate means of measuring visual functions. Routine optometric examination may then make use of VEP. However, in the present state of development the technique is more a special examination carried out in some eye clinics only.

Thirdly, the information so far provided by the VEP is about the same as that obtained more easily and more quickly by other methods, except in testing the visual system of newborn infants or unconscious or totally uncommunicative patients, where the potential for the application of VEPs to clinical practice is great indeed. A VEP tests the whole visual pathway to the brain while the other objective methods are merely providing a window to the eyeball.

Acknowledgements

Fig. 22.4 is by permission of the *American Journal of Optometry* and Fig. 22.2 by permission of the authors.

23. Visual evoked potentials to checkerboard pattern stimuli in strabismic amblyopia

S. SOKOL

Department of Ophthalmology, Tufts-New England Medical Center Hospital, Boston

It has been only in the past few years that VEPs to patterned stimuli have been investigated in patients with visual disorders. The study of pattern VEPs in amblyopia, which appears to involve a defect in spatial vision, is of particular interest because it may clarify the mechanisms underlying amblyopia and provide a more effective tool for early detection and treatment. VEP studies can be complex even when trained subjects are used, and in clinical studies of the VEP and amblyopia, the testing of naïve subjects can pose additional problems, particularly if the subjects are children. Children can be reliably tested for only short periods of time and the experimenter cannot easily vary stimulus parameters and recording conditions for each subject. While this makes detailed investigation of the mechanisms underlying amblyopia in children difficult, it does not rule out VEP studies of childhood amblyopia. Children can be tested periodically under a narrow range of conditions to determine if there is any correlation between changes in visual acuity and the objective measures of the VEP. Also, the VEP may be of value in measuring visual acuity of very young amblyopes whose eye-chart reading is unreliable. The limitations of testing children can be circumvented by careful study of adults with well-established patterns of amblyopia. Such studies require adult amblyopes who are able to cooperate for long experimental sessions in which variations in luminance, field size, check size, retinal location and electrode placements can be systematically analysed.

Methods

The patterned stimulus used in children and adults is a polaroid checkerboard vectograph. All of the checks transmit light, but alternate squares are polarized in orthogonal planes. A sheet of polaroid is rotated between a tungsten–halogen light source and the vectograph resulting a sinusoidal alternation of the checks. While one-half of the checks increase to a maximum luminance level the other half are decreasing, and the total luminance flux remains constant. The rate of alternation of the checks is 12 Hz; the total luminance of the screen is 75 ft-L, and the contrast ratio of the checks is 0·89. The subject sits at a fixed distance (75 cm)

Visual evoked potentials in man: new developments (ed. J. E. Desmedt), pp. 410–17. Clarendon Press, Oxford 1977.

from the vectograph and is optically corrected. Check size can be varied by changing the vectograph print. Five sizes are available, subtending 7·5′, 15′, 30′, 60′, and 90′ at the retina. The VEPs are recorded either from a single electrode 2·5 cm above the inion along the midline with the two ears linked or from two electrodes 2·5 cm and 7 cm above the inion along the midline with one ear serving as ground. The electrical signals are lead to an a.c.-coupled amplifier with a band pass of 1–35 Hz and stored on an FM tape-recorder. From the tape-recorder the signals are lead through an 'active' narrow-bandpass filter (*Q* 10) locked to the stimulus frequency of 12 Hz and averaged on a computer of average transients (CAT). Fig. 23.1 shows signals before and after such filtering which has its

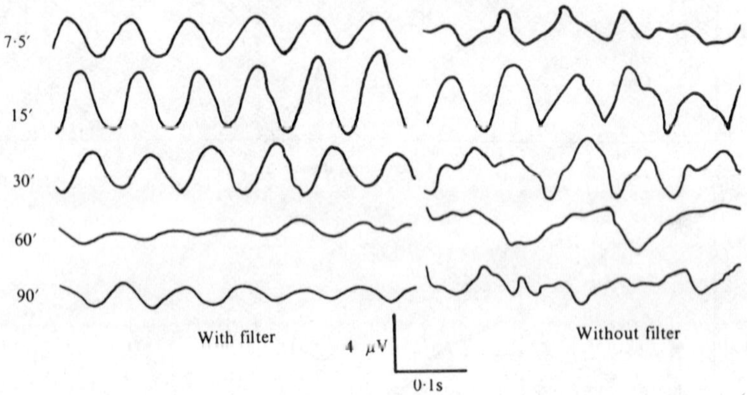

Fig. 23.1. Checkerboard pattern VEPs for five check sizes with and without the use of a narrow-bandpass filter. Normal adult subject. The size of the checkerboard field was 12° and 32 responses were averaged.

greatest effect under those conditions where the signal-to-noise ratio is small, in this case with large checks, i.e. 30′, 60′, and 90′. This technique can be especially helpful to improve the signal-to-noise ratio when testing children.

The VEP in adult amblyopia

One adult amblyope, a 62-year-old female with a right esotropia of 10 dioptre, was tested weekly for over 6 months. Line visual acuity was 20/20 in the normal eye and 20/400 in the amblyopic eye. The amblyopic eye improved to 20/200 when tested with separate letters. The refractive error was + 1·50 + 2·50 CX 90° in the amblyopic eye and + 1·0 + 1·0 CX 90° for the normal eye. Fixation in the amblyopic eye was unsteady. On some occasions it was central and on others it was eccentric. The degree of eccentricity was never greater than 30′. The subject had harmonious abnormal retinal correspondence and some stereopsis on the synoptophor.

Figs. 23.2 and 23.3 show the amplitude variations of the pattern VEP as a

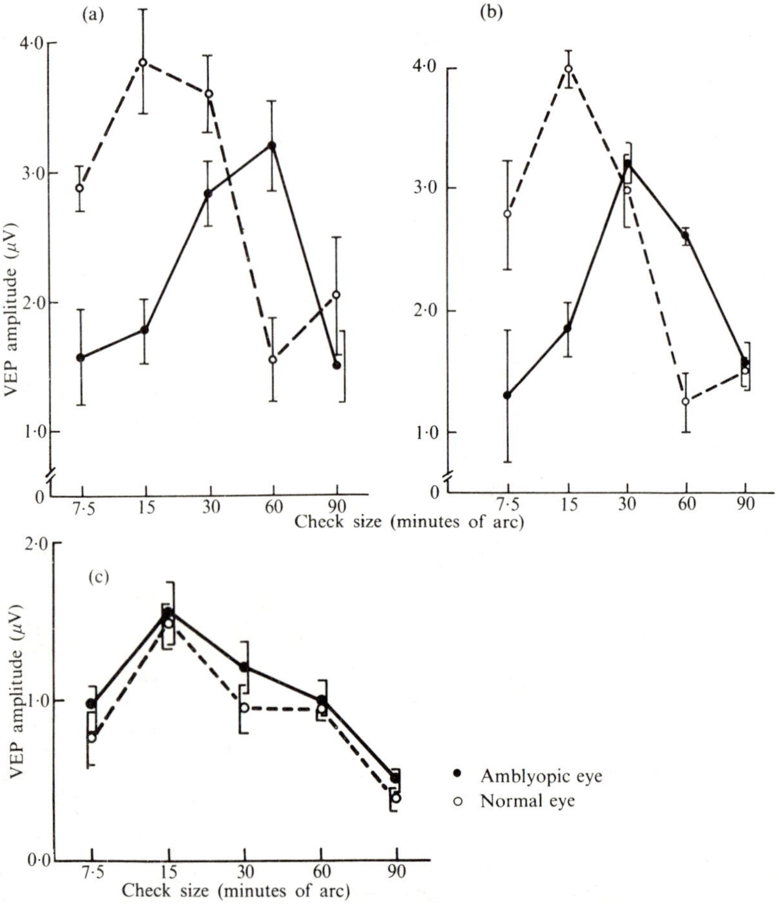

Fig. 23.2. Amplitude of pattern VEP as a function of check size for stimulation of the normal eye and of the amblyopic eye of an adult amblyope (see text for further details). (a) 12° field. (b) 6° field. (c) 3° field.

function of check size for each eye, for a series of different field sizes. In each graph the data points represent the mean amplitude for eight separate recording sessions and the vertical bars are the standard error of the mean. For the 12° field (Fig. 23.2(a)) the normal eye showed a maximum amplitude with 15′ checks, which is in agreement with other reports from normals when an emmetropic eye is tested (Harter and White 1970; Armington *et al.* 1971). The amblyopic eye showed a maximum amplitude at the 60′ check size. In addition to a shift in the peak amplitude for the amblyopic eye there was a significantly larger signal at 60′ from the amblyopic eye than from the normal eye. For a 6° field (Fig. 23.2(b)) the normal eye also peaks at 15′. Amplitudes for the small checks (7·5′ and 15′)

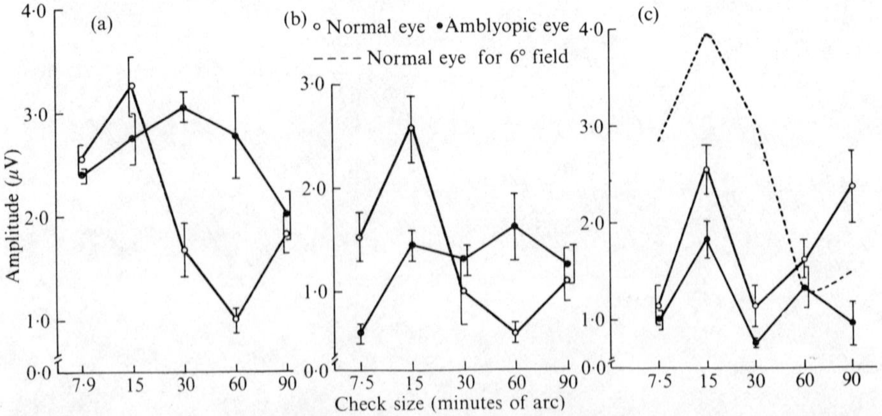

Fig. 23.3. Amplitude of checkerboard pattern VEP as a function of check size for stimulation of the normal eye and amblyopic eye. (a) 12° field with the central 3° removed. (b) 6° field with the central 3° removed. (c) 12° field with the central 6° removed. Dashed line is the VEP of the normal eye for a 6° field.

remained unchanged as the field size decreased but there was a drop in amplitude for the large checks. For the amblyopic eye the maximum amplitude occurred at 30′ but this appeared to be due more to the drop in amplitude for the 60′ checks with the decrease in field size rather than to an increase in the absolute amplitude of the 30′-check-size signal. The amblyopic eye continued to evoke a larger signal at 60′ than did the normal eye.

For a 3° field (Fig. 23.2(c)) both the normal and amblyopic eyes showed a maximum amplitude VEP for a check size of 15′ and there was no difference in amplitude between eyes at other check sizes. This would seem to indicate that the increase of VEP amplitude in response to large checks in the amblyopic eye for the 12° and 6° field was the result of a greater contribution to the VEP from the peri-fovea of the amblyopic eye than from the peri-fovea of the normal eye. This conclusion is supported by the results shown in Fig. 23.3. When a 12° field with the central 3° blanked out was presented the amblyopic eye made a greater contribution to the VEP for the 30′ and 60′ checks outside the central 3° than did the normal eye (Fig. 23.3(a)). When a 6° field with the central 3° blanked out was presented the amblyopic eye again showed a greater contribution outside the central 3° for the 60′ checks (Fig. 23.3(b)). Finally, to determine if regions outside the central 6° of the amblyopic eye showed any increase in their contribution for large check sizes, a 12° field with the central 6° blanked out was presented to each eye. With the central 6° blanked out (Fig. 23.3(c)) there was a large drop in the signals from the normal eye especially for small checks. In the amblyopic eye there was a drop in the signals obtained for the large checks.

We conclude that regions outside the central 6° are essentially similar for the normal and amblyopic eye. Therefore, the electrical signals arising from the

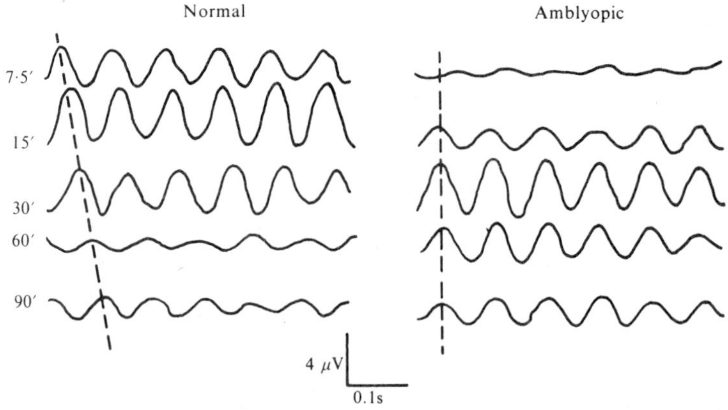

Fig. 23.4. VEP waveforms for 6° pattern field stimulation of the normal (a) and amblyopic (b) eyes. Check sizes are indicated in minutes of arc.

amblyopic eye receive their greatest contribution from a retinal region that lies outside the central 3° but within the central 6°. This corresponds to a retinal region with an inside diameter of 1·5° and an outside diameter of 3°. Fig. 23.4 shows the records obtained from each eye for the 6° field. For the normal eye there was a consistent phase shift as check size increased, but for the amblyopic eye there was no change in phase as the checks became larger. This phase relationship held for the 3° and 12° fields as well, indicating that amplitude alone was not solely responsible for the visual acuity of the amblyopic eye.

It has been previously reported that with large fields (greater than 12°) the amplitude of the pattern VEPs from the amblyopic eye were reduced (Lombroso *et al.* 1969; Dawson *et al.* 1972; Sokol and Bloom 1973; Sokol and Shaterian 1976; Yinon, Jakobovitz, and Auerbach 1974). When small fields were used in an adult subject,the normal and amblyopic eyes elicited equal amplitude responses, and the peri-fovea of the amblyopic eye elicited greater amplitude signals than the peri-fovea of the normal eye. Arden (1973) recently reported that when an anisometropic amblyope was presented with small-field spatially alternating checkerboard stimuli there was no differece in amplitude between the normal and amblyopic eye. Moreover, when only the periphery of the emblyopic eye was stimulated it evoked larger signals than the normal eye pheripheral responses. Spekreijse *et al.* (1972) also tested an anisometropic amblyope and found, unlike Arden and the present study, that the reversal of a 3° pattern field elicited larger signals from the normal eye than from the amblyopic eye for check sizes ranging from 2·5′ to 90′. The patterned stimulus used by Spekreijse *et al.* (1972) was presented as a low-contrast square-wave pattern reversal, while Arden's stimuli as well as ours consisted of sinusoidal modulation of high-contrast checks. Clearly, careful attention must be given to the design and interpretation of pattern VEP experiments in relation to the stimuli used (see Chapter 1 of this book).

Visual evoked potentials to checkerboard pattern stimuli in strabismic amblyopia

The amblyopic eye of our subject elicited a different VEP amplitude check-size function than the normal eye. This is compatible with previous studies of amblyopia which used non-patterned stimuli. Psychophysical evidence (Flynn 1967; Miller 1954) indicated that the central receptive fields of the amblyopic eye were abnormal because of a defect in the mechanisms responsible for lateral inhibition. Lawwill *et al.* (1973) used the Westheimer paradigm to study the VEP and found that the amblyopic eye elicited less inhibition than the normal eye and that larger annular fields were necessary to exert maximum inhibition in the amblyopic eye than in the normal eye. The increase in VEP amplitude at the 60′ check size for the peri-fovea of the amblyopic eye of our subject may be due to the inability of the central 3° of the amblyopic eye to exert sufficient lateral inhibitory effects. When only the central 3° was stimulated the amblyopic eye acted very much like the normal eye but when the amblyopic eye was presented with large patterned fields, which is more like the way the amblyope looks at the real world, the peri-foveal mechanisms dominated in sending electrical signals to the occipital cortex. Some amblyopes showed better acuity with separate-letter testing, perhaps because this may be analogous to presenting them with small-field stimulation. Also, the difference in temporal characteristics of the VEP of the normal and amblyopic eye suggest that the impulses are reaching the cortex at different times, thereby accounting for why the central 3° of the amblyopic eye is unable to attain the same visual acuity level as the normal eye.

The VEP in childhood amblyopia

As mentioned previously, children become impatient if the testing session is prolonged, and this results in an increase in artifacts. When testing children the experimenter remained with the child to monitor his behaviour and fixation; he could operate a remote-control switch to begin averaging when the child was quiet and comfortable. Averaging could be interrupted whenever the child became restless or refused to fixate. Sufficient records for each check size could be obtained with our narrow-bandpass filter in 25 s. A child can be tested with a series of 5 check sizes to each eye in a time of less than 30 min.

It has been well established that when checks of different visual angles are used, the maximum VEP in an emmetropic eye occurs with a check size of between 10′ and 20′ (Harter and White 1970; Armington *et al.* 1971; Regan and Richards 1973). The VEP amplitude is attenuated as the check size is made larger or smaller than 10–20′. Therefore, in those subjects with reduced acuity, even after optical correction, one might expect either a reduction in the VEP amplitude for checks subtending 10–20′ or a maximum VEP amplitude at a different check size.

Fig. 23.5 shows VEP–visual acuity functions determined with 12° fields from 3 strabismic amblyopes. All subjects had visual acuity of 20/20 in the normal eye. Subject S.C. (Fig. 23.5(a)) was a 10-year-old female with a right esotropia of 8 dioptre. Line acuity in the amblyopic eye was 20/100 and improved to 20/50 when tested with separate letters. The pattern VEP from the normal eye was maximum with a 15′ check size. In the amblyopic eye the maximum-amplitude VEP occurred at 30′ and the amplitude of the signals for the 30′, 60′, and 90′ checks were indeed larger than those obtained from the normal eye. Subject K.A. (Fig. 23.5(b)) was a 6-year-old male with a right esotropia of 10 dioptre. His line acuity was 20/50 in the amblyopic eye and improved to 20/30 with separate-letter testing. Maximum amplitude VEP occurred at 15′ with the normal eye and at 30′ for the amblyopic eye. Signals for the 30′, 60′, and 90′ checks were greater in amplitude for the amblyopic eye than from the normal eye. Subject A.C. (Fig. 23.5(c)) was a 9-year-old female with a left esotropia of 8 dioptre. Line acuity in the amblyopic eye was 20/100 and improved to 20/70 with separate letter testing. Maximum VEP amplitude was at 7·5′ in the normal eye and at 30′ in the amblyopic eye. This subject also had larger signals from the amblyopic eye at 30′ and 60′ checks than from the normal.

These three subjects have a number of things in common: (a) they are strabismic amblyopes with small angle esotropias, (b) they show better acuity when tested with separate letters, (c) their line acuity is between 20/50 and 20/100, and (d) the VEP–visual acuity functions from the amblyopic eye show a maximum amplitude pattern VEP at 30′. Thus there is a correlation between line visual acuity and the VEP amplitude/check-size function in the strabismic amblyope, which may help to measure visual acuity of a non-verbal patient.

Fig. 23.5(d) shows the results obtained when a 6-year-old male with mental retardation was tested. VEPs were measured binocularly for a 12° field using a retinoscopically determined correction. The pattern VEP showed a maximum amplitude at 30′ check size. Based on the data from the strabismic amblyopes one might cautiously estimate that the child had a visual acuity of somewhere between 20/50 and 20/100. This subject had a refractive error of + 2·00 – 2·00 CX 180° in the right eye and + 1·50 – 2·50 CX 180° in the left eye and had never worn glasses. Our results may therefore reflect a meridional amblyopia (Freeman and Thibos 1973). Also, as shown previously in the adult amblyope, there was an increase in VEP amplitude with checks larger than 30′ for the 12° (large) field, the result of a greater contribution from the peri-fovea of the amblyopic eye. Furthermore there was no difference in amplitude between the normal and amblyopic eye with a 3° (small) field. Therefore, the increase in visual acuity with separate letter testing found in the three strabismic amblyopes may be due to the fact that they are looking at each letter in a way that is roughly equivalent to a small-field pattern stimulus.

Summary

The patterned VEP can provide an effective tool for the study of amblyopia. The data collected from adult amblyopes help understand the physiological mechanisms underlying amblyopia and they provide a framework for the study of children with

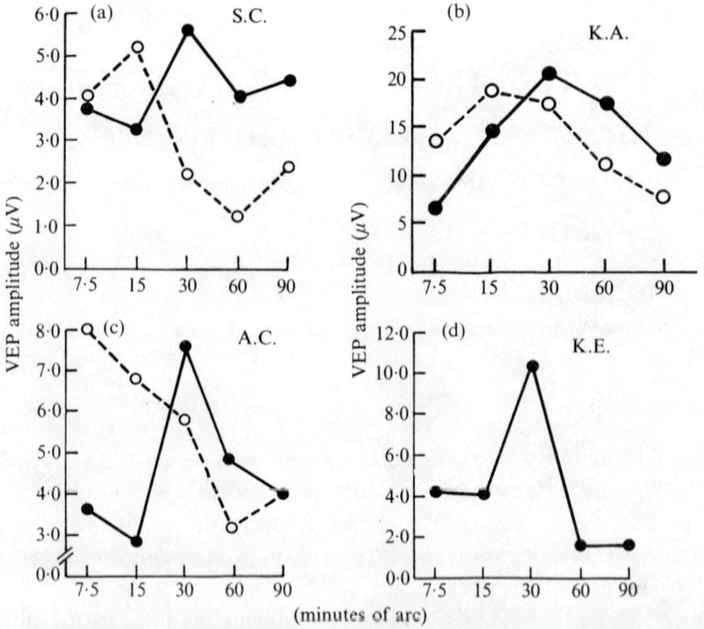

Fig. 23.5. Relation between amplitude of pattern VEP and the size of the checks in the checkerboard pattern stimulus. Open circles: normal eye. Filled circles: amblyopic eye. (a), (b), and (c): VEP results (12° field) from 3 children with strabismic amblyopia. (d) Results from a 6-year-old mentally retarded child, both eyes tested simultaneously (12° field).

amblyopia. By varying check size and measuring the VEP amplitude a VEP–visual acuity function is obtained which can then be used to estimate visual acuity of non-verbal patients. Before one can accurately and confidently estimate visual acuity using the patterned VEP, however, more normative data are needed both from amblyopes and from other patients with reductions in visual acuity resulting from pathological conditions of the macula.

Acknowledgements

Supported in part by National Eye Institute Research Grant EY 00926 and by a National Eye Institute Research Career Development Award EY 70275 and in part by a grant from the National Society for the Prevention of Blindness, Inc.

24. Rapid methods for refracting the eye and for assessing visual acuity in amblyopia, using steady-state visual evoked potentials

D. REGAN
Department of Communication, University of Keele

Slowness and variability are two major problems in applying VEPs to clinical problems. To some extent these problems are connected: increased speed may reduce the effect of variability. The clinical studies described below used speedy procedures based on the Fourier analysis method of recording VEPs (Regan 1966*a*, *b*, 1972; Chapter 4 of this book).

In all cases greater speed was 'bought' by reducing the information flow to the experimenter. The techniques were designed to provide the minimum information required. It was therefore essential to establish in preliminary experiments that the particular method was not blind to any important information. In that case the increase in speed was effectively 'cost-free'.

VEP refraction

There have been several reports of objective refraction using VEPs elicited by patterned stimuli (Harter and White 1968; Millodot and Riggs 1970; Duffey and Rengstorff 1971; Dawson *et al.* 1972; Ludlam and Meyers 1972; Millodot, Chapter 22 of this book). One report that considers the case when astigmatic and spherical errors are combined handles this problem by using a grating stimulus (Ludlam and Meyers 1972). This method is to record VEPs for each of a series of different orientations of the grating pattern. The orientations that give the largest and smallest VEPs are taken as the axes of astigmatism. Trial lenses are then inserted until maximum VEP amplitude is obtained for each of these two grating orientations.

Although this procedure can be greatly speeded by continuously rotating the grating pattern (Regan 1973*b*, 1974*b*), the method still retains drawbacks. One is that it fuses astigmatic defects of vision due to refractive errors with astigmatic defects of vision due to neural abnormalities (i.e. meridional amblyopia: Martin 1890; Mitchell *et al.* 1972). This latter effect is that if refractive astigmatism is

Visual evoked potentials in man: new developments (ed. J. E. Desmedt), pp. 418–26. Clarendon Press, Oxford 1977.

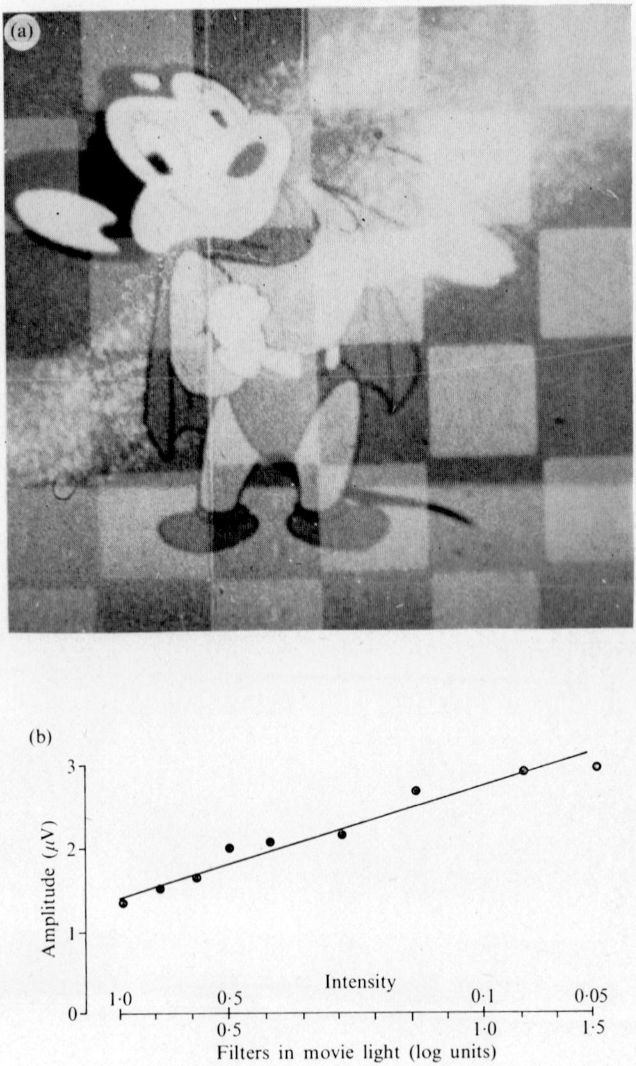

FIG. 24.6. (a) Subject's view of checkboard pattern superposed on movie cartoon. The picture subtends 4° when viewed at a distance of about 70 cm. (b) Effect of mean luminance of movie cartoon upon amplitude of pattern-reversal VEPs. Abscissa—neutral density filter placed in front of movie projector Relative intensities marked above abcissa. Check size 12 field size 8°. Bipolar recording between inion and P_z. Left mastoid grounded. Left eye occluded.

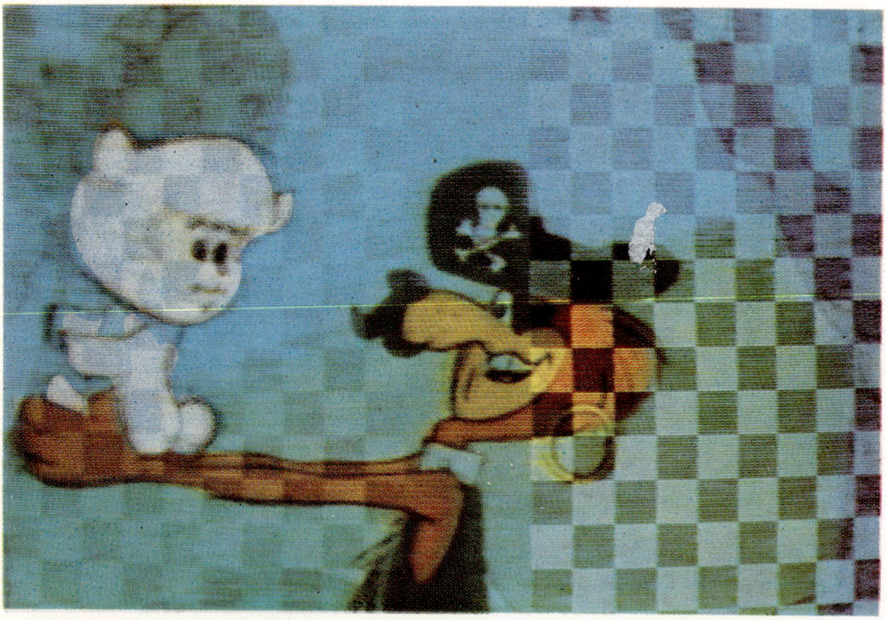

(a)

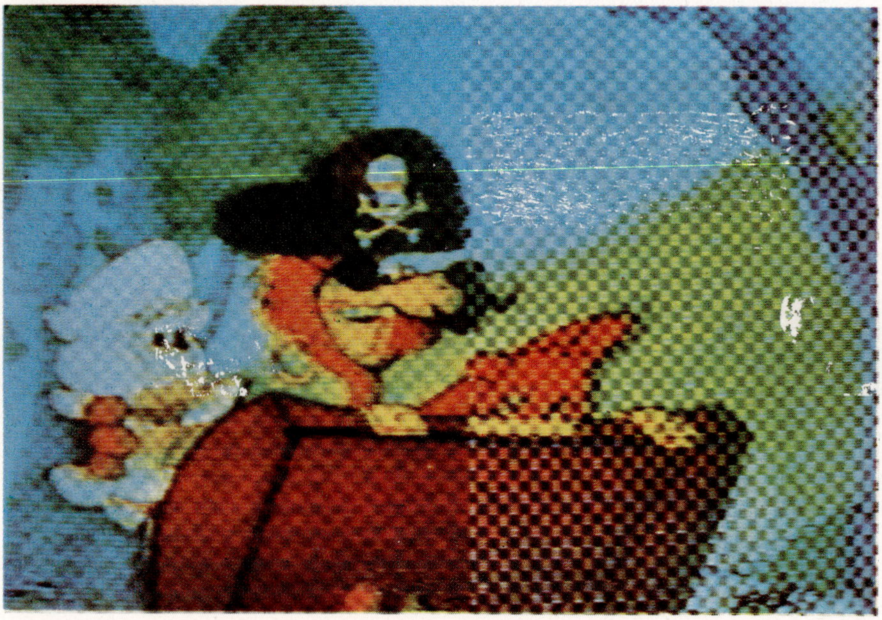

(b)

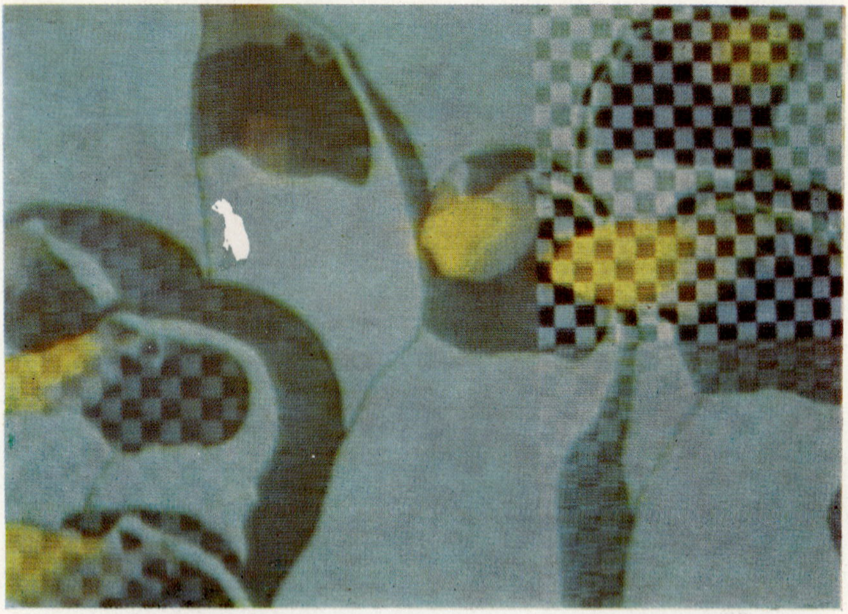

(c)

PLATE 3.1. Chequerboard patterns produced by a television technique

(a) The small squares subtend 11′ at a viewing distance of 1.5 m. The field is bipartite, with contrast ratios of 20 per cent on the left and 50 per cent on the right. (b) Bipartite field with larger squares (46′); the central vertical strip (3 squares) has been 'blanked'. (c) Field split into quadrants, square sizes 23′. A larger area of screen has been blanked. Contrast ratios 20 per cent and 50 per cent.

In each case, the chequerboard pattern signal has been mixed with the output from a cartridge video-recorder, and photographed with a 'frozen frame' technique which degrades picture quality. Note that mean luminance is independent of contrast, and the chequerboards vary in luminance and not in chrominance. It is equally possible to produce patterns which vary in chrominance.

(Plate by courtesy of Medelec, Ltd., Old Woking, Surrey.)

Erratum: In Plate 3.1, (a) and (b) have been transposed.

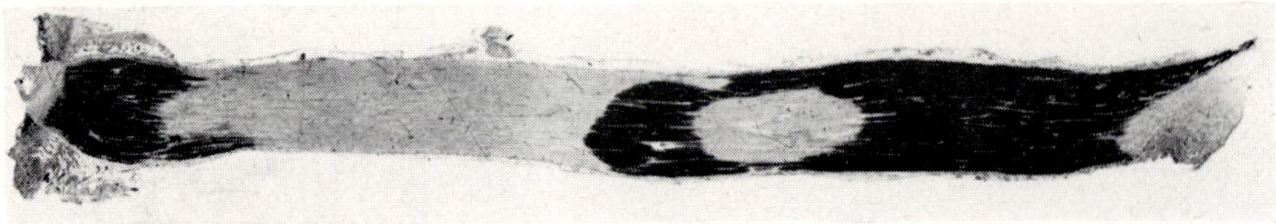

FIG. 25.1. Longitudinal section of the optic nerve of a patient dying with multiple sclerosis. Myelin preparation. (Greenfield, 1963).

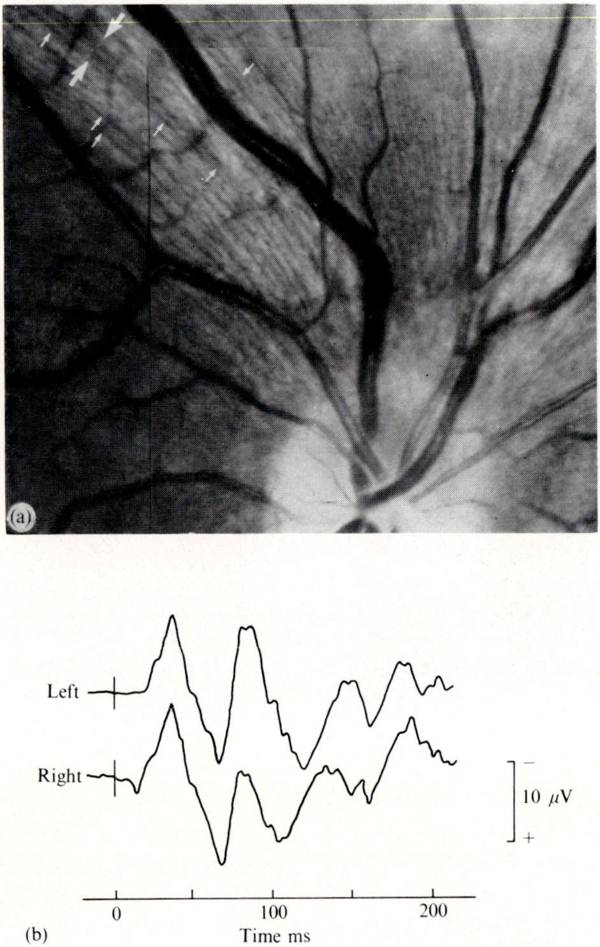

FIG. 28.1. (a) Fundus photograph of nerve-fibre layer in asymptomatic right eye of a patient with multiple sclerosis. Note multiple translucent slit-like defects (arrows) in the nerve-fibre layer. These represent retrograde degeneration of bundles of nerve fibres. The colour of the optic disc was normal. (b) Binocular flash-evoked-potentials recorded from the left and right occipital areas of a normal subject.

left uncorrected for too long, neural changes occur in the visual pathway such that the grating orientation that gave the most blurred retinal image gives both the smallest VEP (Fiorentini and Maffei 1973; Freeman and Thibos 1973; Regan 1973*b*, 1974*b*) and the poorest visual acuity (Martin 1890; Mitchell *et al.* 1972) even after refractive correction.

Stenopaeic slit method and running-average presentation of VEP data

The stenopaeic slit method of refraction is to view a stimulus pattern through a narrow slit placed immediately in front of the cornea (Duke-Elder 1970). The slit selects a narrow elongated area of cornea. If the cornea is spherical, the sharpness of the image will not depend on slit orientation. On the other hand, if the sharpness of the image does depend on slit orientation, then the cornea is not spherical, and this will result in an astigmatic retinal image. The slit angles that give the sharpest and the most blurred images respectively define the principal axes of the cornea.

An important feature of the stenopaeic slit method is that the pattern on the retina does not change orientation; it merely varies in sharpness as the slit rotates. Thus, this method does not confound optical astigmatism with meridional amblyopia. A second advantage of the stenopaeic slit method over the grating method is that a checkerboard stimulus may be used. This gives larger VEPs and therefore a more speedy procedure.

The Fourier analysis allows VEP amplitude to be presented as a running average, giving an approximation to instantaneous EP amplitude. Thus, the effect on VEPs of changing a stimulus parameter (e.g. a trial lens) can be seen immediately (Regan 1966*a*, 1973*b*, Chapter 4 of this book).

Results

Figs. 24.1–24.3 illustrate the speed obtained by using the running-average presentation of data in conjunction with a continuously changing stimulus.

In Fig. 24.1 the subject viewed a stimulus pattern via a 1 mm stenopaeic slit. The light and dark checks exchanged places 6 times per s. A small check size (20′) was chosen, since when large checks (e.g. 40′) are used, blurring can *increase* rather than attenuate VEP amplitude (Regan and Richards 1971, 1973). Fig. 24.1(a) shows VEP amplitude plotted versus slit orientation. Clearly, a slit orientation of 50° gave the largest VEPs; rotating the slit through 90° then gave the smallest VEPs. These two angles defined the axes of astigmatism. In Fig. 24.1(a) each point on the graph was recorded separately. Fig. 24.1(b) illustrates a quicker way of obtaining the same data. In Fig. 24.1(b) the slit was continuously rotated at a rate of one revolution every 18 s. The traces plot instantaneous VEP amplitude versus slit orientation. Two replications are shown. Each plot in Fig. 24.1(b) was obtained in 18 s as compared with about $1\frac{1}{2}$ hours for Fig. 24.1(a).

A more convenient way of displaying the data of Fig. 24.1 is illustrated in

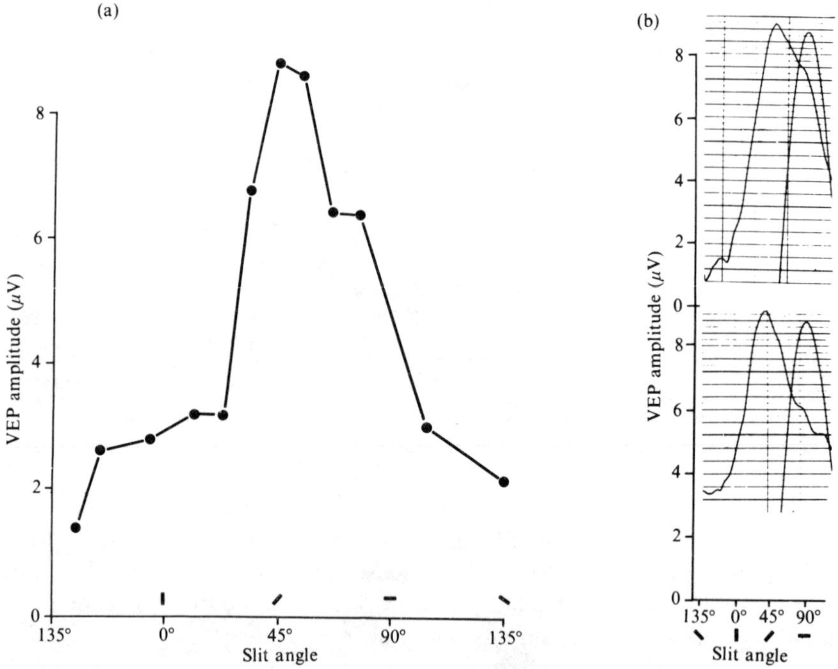

Fig. 24.1. Stenopaeic slit method of VEP refraction; determination of axes of astigmatism. The subject views a reversing checkerboard pattern through a narrow slit located immediately in front of the cornea. (a) The slit orientations giving maximum and minimum VEP amplitudes define the axes of astigmatism. (b) Two replications of this plot using a faster procedure where the slit rotated continuously. Each of the traces in (b) was recorded in 18 s. (From Regan 1973*b*.)

Fig. 24.2. The polar coordinate plot of Fig. 24.2 enables the directions of the axes of astigmatism to be read off more easily. The radial distance of any point from the origin gives VEP amplitude, while the orientation of the radius gives the orientation of the stenopaeic slit. Fig. 24.2(g) and (h) show how radial angle in the graphs (g) is related to slit orientation (h). Thus Fig. 24.2 shows how the directions of the axes of astigmatism can be found within 10 s recording time.

Refractive correction was obtained as shown in Fig. 24.3. The subject gazed at the checkerboard pattern through a stenopaeic slit oriented parallel to one axis of astigmatism. In front of the slit was a lens whose power was oscillated once every 18 s. Fig. 24.3 shows plots of instantaneous VEP amplitude versus instantaneous lens power. For one slit orientation, VEP amplitude was maximal for a power of −4·5 dioptre. When the slit was rotated through 90°, VEP amplitude was maximal for a power of −2·0 dioptre.

The required prescription lens is defined by the lens powers −4·5 dioptre and −2·0 dioptre plus the direction of the axes of astigmatism. The lens can be defined

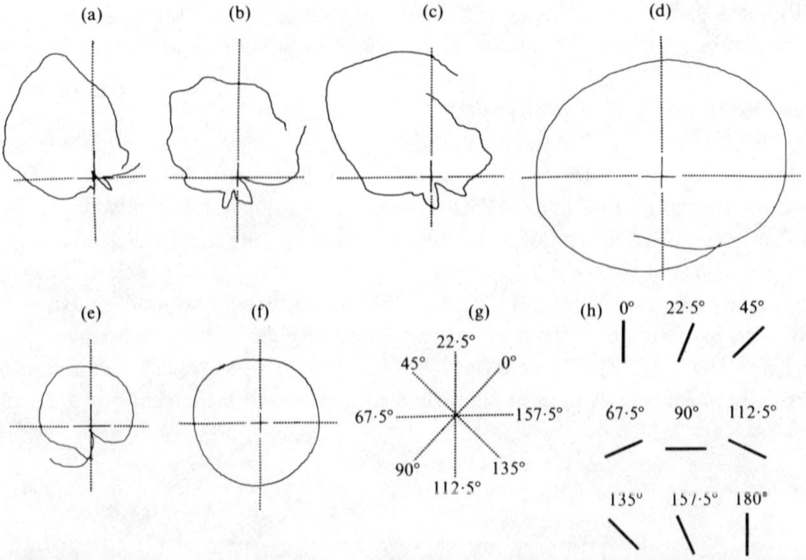

Fig. 24.2. Three replications of similar data to that of Fig. 1(b) are shown in the more convenient form of polar coordinates in (a), (b), and (c). Each plot took 18 s while the stenopaeic slit rotated through 180°. (e) Similar plot made in 10 s. (d) After astigmatism had been corrected. (f) 5 μV calibration. (g) Slit angles as plotted in (a)–(f). (h) Shows corresponding physical orientations of the slit. (a), (b), and (c) show maximum VEP amplitude for slit orientation of 30–50°, and near-zero VEP for slit orientations of 110–140°. (From Regan 1973*b*.)

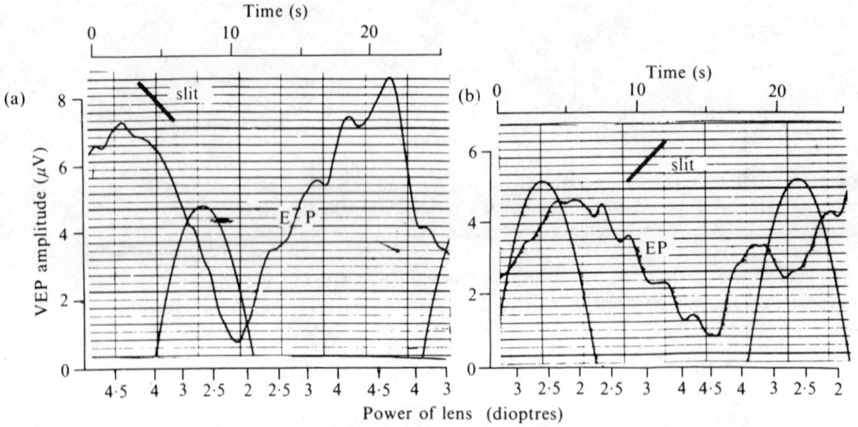

Fig. 24.3. Determination of cylindrical and spherical refractive corrections. The stimulus pattern was viewed through a stenopaeic slit set parallel to one axis of astigmatism in (a). A lens system was then placed in front of the lens and its optical power was continuously varied at a rate of one oscillation per 18 s. VEP amplitude varies as a function of lens power and is maximal for a power of –4·5 dioptre. In (b), the slit was turned through 90° and the experiment repeated. A power of –2·0 dioptre now gave maximum VEP amplitude. The two lens powers, with the direction of the astigmatic axes define the required prescription lens. (From Regan 1973*b*.)

within less than 1 min of recording time, a procedure about 100 times faster than a comparable point-by-point method using an averaging computer.

VEP assessment of visual acuity and amblyopia

It is well known that VEP to checkerboard pattern reversal are strongly influenced by blurring the retinal image (Spekreijse 1966; Cobb *et al.* 1967; Rietveld *et al.* 1967; Harter and White 1968, 1970). The effect of blur is not simply to attenuate VEP amplitude, since attenuation is more marked for the small check sizes (8–15′) that give mainly foveal VEPs (Spekreijse 1966) than for the larger check sizes that give mainly extrafoveal VEPs (Harter and White 1969). For larger check sizes (30–50′) moderate blurring may even enhance VEP amplitudes (Regan and Richards 1971, 1973). Thus a plot of VEP amplitude versus check size may change markedly in shape as well as in amplitude when the retinal image is blurred (see Fig. 24.4(a)).

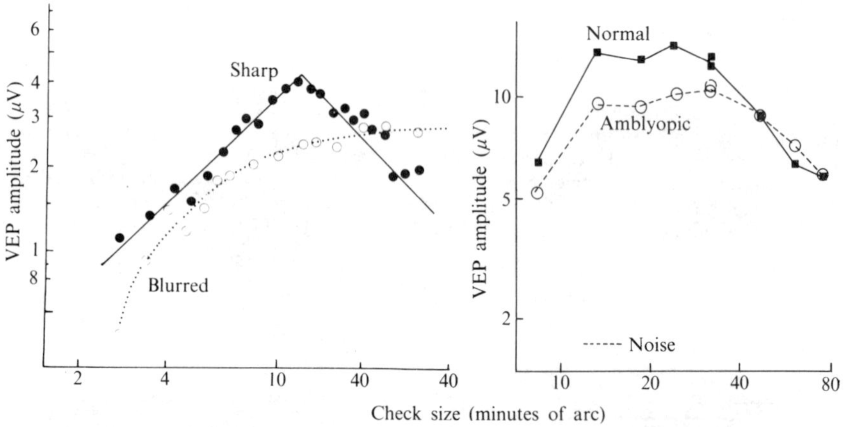

Fig. 24.4. (a) Effect of blurring the retinal image upon the plot of VEP amplitude versus check size. The stimulus was a 2° disc viewed binocularly at 175 cm. Open circles (continuous line) were recorded with the retinal image in sharp focus and filled circles (dotted line) with a + 1 dioptre lens placed before each eye. (Modified from Regan and Richards 1971.) (b) Pattern VEP in amblyopia. Amplitudes of pattern reversal VEPs from the amblyopic (6/18) and normal (6/6) eyes of a patient of 12 years who had previously suffered from squint. The 4° x 4° checkerboard pattern reversed with a frequency of 11 Hz; the 11 Hz component of the VEP was recorded. One electrode was on the inion and the other 9 cm ahead along the midline. The left mastoid was grounded.

This suggests that forms of amblyopia equivalent in their effect to a reduction of foveal visual acuity might be expected to result in an abnormally shaped plot of VEP amplitude versus check size and indeed the VEPs of Fig. 24.4(b)), recorded from an amblyopic subject, show exactly this feature. Fig. 24.4(b) confirms the report of Spekreijse, Khoe, and Van der Tweel (1972) that for a 3° stimulus field size the amplitude of VEPs from the amblyopic eye increased steadily with check size, whereas the normal eye gave maximum amplitude for checks of 10–20′ subtense. Spekreijse *et al.* also found that amblyopia attenuated parafoveal VEPs relatively less than foveal VEPs. Further to this, Arden (1973) and Sokol (Chapter 23 of this book) reported that extra-foveal VEPs were larger for the good eye than for the amblyopic eye.

These and other grounds suggest that pattern VEP might offer an objective index of amblyopia, and a means of detecting reduced acuity and of monitoring acuity changes. In particular, the shape of the VEP amplitude versus check size plot might be useful in assessing vision during occlusion therapy. It is important to avoid long recording sessions with children, since changes in fixation or accommodation can cause serious variability. This article describes a development of the Fourier analysis method tailored to the problem of rapidly measuring the shape of the required plot. The method is to average whole graphs rather than individual points.

Methods

A checkerboard pattern of black and white checks was photographed on microfilm using a high-resolution lens (Micro-Nikkor 55 mm). This was mounted on a Pye-Ling vibrator and abruptly oscillated through exactly one square's width so as to give *F* pattern reversals per s (*F* was usually between 3 and 7). The pattern was projected onto a rear-view screen by means of a 16 mm, 10:1 Angenieux zoom lens, carefully adjusted to give sharp focus throughout the zooming range (Fig. 24.5). The zoom lens was electronically driven so as to repetitively zoom up

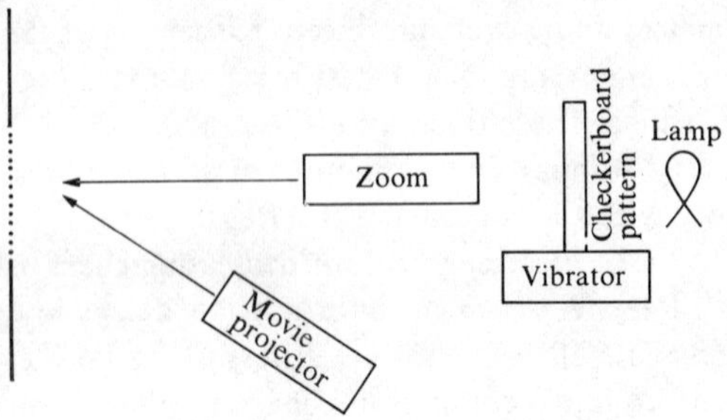

Fig. 24.5. Outline diagram of Zoom stimulator showing Pye-Ling vibrator, 10:1 zoom lens projecting checks onto rear-view screen, and a movie projector.

and down (the rate was usually between once every 10 s and once every 60 s). Accurate control of check size was ensured by feeding information as to the position of the zoom lens back to the a.c.-coupled servomotor that drove the lens. The triangular wave that drove the zoom lens could be shaped electronically so that the time-course of the zoom could be predetermined. In practice it was found convenient that log check size should change proportionally with time.

Unfortunately, when the lens zoomed so as to increase check size, the luminance of the pattern also changed so that the smallest checks were 100 times brighter than the largest checks. These luminance changes were eliminated as follows. A photocell sampled the total light flux falling on the screen. The photocell's output was fed to a second a.c.-coupled servomotor that drove the iris control of the zoom lens so as to maintain the photocell's output constant. The subject's view was as follows. He saw the screen covered by black and white checks (100 per cent contrast) that repetitively exchanged positions (e.g. 6 times per s). Check size slowly increased from 6 minutes of arc, reaching a maximum of 60′ in, for example, 15 s; check size then steadily decreased back to 6′ in a further 15 s.

With adult subjects there is little problem in maintaining the subject's gaze on the centre of the screen, at least until the onset of intolerable boredom. With children it was found helpful in maintaining gaze upon the screen to superpose a movie cartoon film upon the zooming check pattern.† Fig. 24.6(a) (see between pp. 418–19) gives an impression of the appearance of this stimulus. Fig. 24.6(b) shows the effect upon the amplitude of pattern VEPs of varying the mean luminance of the movie cartoon. The highest luminance used (intensity 1:0 in Fig. 24.6(b)) was equivalent to a uniform patch of light that reduced the pattern's contrast from 100 per cent to about 20–30 per cent and had little effect upon VEP amplitude, as would be anticipated because of VEP saturation (Spekreijse 1966). The main point is that the movie could be made sufficiently bright to see easily without seriously attenuating VEP amplitude.

An analog Fourier analyser recorded the *F* Hz component of the VEP elicited by *F* pattern reversals per s (Regan 1966*a*, *b*, 1972*a*; Chapter 4 of this book).

The Fourier analyser's output was the moment-to-moment running average of VEP amplitude. Each zooming cycle produced one sample of the required plot of VEP amplitude versus check size (Regan 1973*b*). Superposed on this trace were, of course, noise fluctuations. These fluctuations were reduced when several samples of the graph were summed by a computer of average transients (CAT) triggered synchronously with the zooming cycle (Regan 1975*b*). Records were obtained in this way both for increasing and for decreasing check sizes. This provided checks for VEP hysteresis and also for possible delays in the VEP trace caused by the time-constants of the smoothing filters in the Fourier analyser. In practice it was necessary to find a compromise between filter time-constants, length of zoom cycle, and number of sweeps averaged (Regan 1975*b*).

Advantages of averaging graphs rather than points

Averaging graphs rather than points has the advantages of speed and precision. The speed increase may be large, and though difficult to estimate quantitatively it may lie between 15 and 100 times. Increased precision can be understood as follows.

† A rather similar stratagem of interspersing patterns with cartoons has been proposed by Spekreijse and by Arden as a means of maintaining a child's gaze on their TV stimulators (see Chapters 1 and 3 of this book).

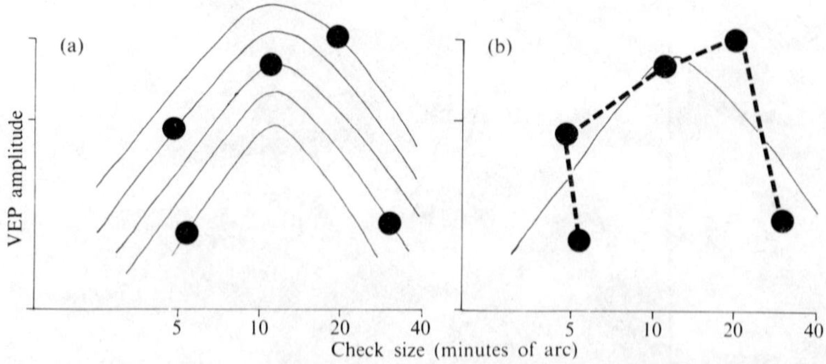

Fig. 24.7. Method of averaging graphs rather than points. Idealized plots of VEP amplitude versus check size. (a) Continuous lines show five idealized samples of graph taken at different times. Filled circles are averages of separate points. (b) Continuous line is the average of the five samples in (a). The dashed line joins the averaged points.

Note: this discussion is idealized for clarity. Imagine the *shape* of the plot of VEP amplitude versus check size remains constant with time but that, due to variability, the whole curve shifts bodily up and down. Fig. 24.7(a) illustrates an extreme form of this notion. The five continuous lines show the hypothetical relationships between VEP amplitude and check size at five points in time. This argument is restricted to the type of VEP variability shown in Fig. 24.7(a), so that each of the five lines can also be taken to represent a VEP trace fed into the CAT during the first half of a single zoom cycle. The continuous line in Fig. 24.7(b) is the average of the five samples in Fig. 24.7(a). The filled circles in Fig. 24.7(a) show VEP amplitudes obtained in the conventional way by five separate successive averages. In Fig. 24.7(b) the dashed line that joins these five points can be seen to give a poorer estimate of the VEP plot's shape than the continuous curve obtained by averaging rapidly-recorded samples of the whole plot.

Results

Preliminary checks were made to ensure that stimulus repetition frequency was in the correct range to give clear VEPs and that the luminance of the movie film was not so high that it appreciably attenuated VEP amplitude.

In Fig. 24.8 pattern reversal was at a frequency of 7 Hz. This frequency was selected by zooming the frequency up and down. In Fig. 24.8 check size zoomed from 60′ side length to 6′ side length and back every 60 s. Log check size was proportional to time. The stimulus field was a square of 4° side viewed at a distance of 250 cm with the left eye occluded. The running average of 7 Hz VEP component's amplitude was averaged on a CAT with a 60 s sweep time. Each of the traces is the average of four sweeps (i.e. four zoom cycles).

The two traces marked 'sharp' were recorded with the checks sharply accommodated. VEP amplitude peaked at a check size of 10–20′ for both increasing

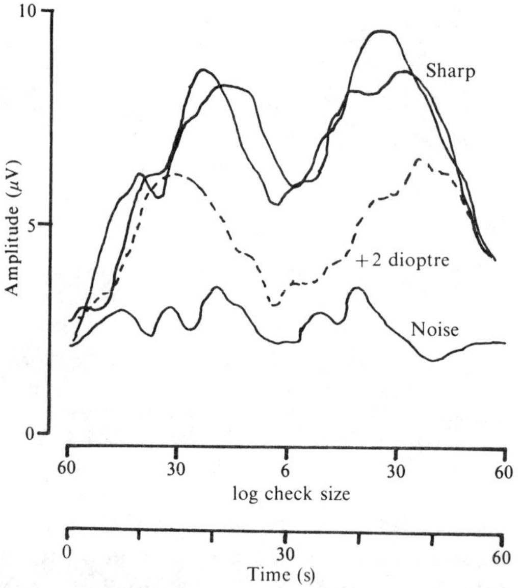

Fig. 24.8. Plots of VEP amplitude versus check size obtained by zooming. Pattern reverses at 7 Hz while the check size zoomed from 60′ to 6′and back every 60 s. Each of the upper two traces is the average of four sweeps. The dotted trace was recorded similarly, but with a + 2 dioptre lens before the eye. The noise trace was recorded with the stimulus occluded.

and decreasing check sizes. Thus hysteresis was not serious. Furthermore, these two traces were closely similar to curves obtained point-by-point in the conventional manner (not shown). Therefore, changing check size continuously did not of itself distort the curve to any great extent. Neither of these two points was self evident; VEPs in animals may show marked hysteresis and gross distortion in the dynamic situation (Regan, Schellart, Spekreijse, and Van den Berg 1975).

The trace marked 'blurred' was recorded with a +2 dioptre lens placed in front of the subject's eye. VEP amplitude was reduced and the peak was shifted to larger check sizes. The noise trace was recorded with the stimulus pattern occluded.

Acknowledgements

This work was supported by the Medical Research Council. Thanks are due to R. F. Cartwright and H. Wardell for technical support and to H. Henry for assistance in preparing this chapter.

25. Pathophysiology of conduction in central nerve fibres

W. I. McDONALD
Institute of Neurology, National Hospital, London

In this chapter I shall confine myself to an account of the effects of pathological processes on conduction in central nerve fibres, about which we now have precise information derived from experimental studies. I shall then consider the extent to which altered properties of nerve fibres themselves might contribute to the delays recorded in VEPs in human demyelinating diseases.

Pathology of central nerve fibres

There are two main classes of pathological process which affect nerve fibres: *axonal* or *Wallerian*-type degeneration, in which both axon and myelin disintegrate together, and *demyelination*, in which the myelin is destroyed but the axon remains in continuity through the lesion. Some demyelinated axons may show morphological alterations and not be completely disrupted (Lumsden 1955; Suzuki, Andrews, Waltz, and Terry 1969; McDonald and Sears 1970*a*). In the plaques of multiple sclerosis demyelination predominates, but a variable number of fibres may undergo axonal degeneration (Adams and Kubik 1952). Demyelinating lesions are commonly *focal*: it is usual for a limited region of myelin loss to be flanked by histologically normal nerve. This is illustrated in a myelin-stained longitudinal section through the optic nerve of a patient with multiple sclerosis (Fig. 25.1 see between pp. 418–19). There are several punched-out zones of myelin loss with normal myelin staining between. These lesions represent the end result of episodes of optic neuritis.

Physiological changes

Demyelination

From the physiological point of view there are three main questions about the effects of *demyelination* on conduction. (a) What happens to conduction at the margin of a demyelinating lesion? Does it continue or is it blocked? (b) If conduction continues is it normal or abnormal? (c) What are the properties of the histologically normal portions of the demyelinated fibres?

These questions have been examined experimentally in the focal lesion produced

Visual evoked potentials in man: new developments (ed. J. E. Desmedt), pp. 427–37.
Clarendon Press, Oxford 1977.

by the direct micro-injection of diphtheria toxin into the spinal cord of the cat (McDonald and Sears 1970*b*). Physiological studies were performed 2–4 weeks after the injection of toxin. The first step was to study conduction in large bilateral lesions affecting the whole of the posterior columns. In the terminal experiment, the posterior columns were functionally isolated by undercutting them, i.e. cutting away the rest of the spinal cord and leaving them as the only bridge connecting the rostral and caudal portions of the cord (Fig. 25.2). Stimulating electrodes were placed on the posterior columns rostral to the bridge and records were made at successively more distal sites caudal to it.

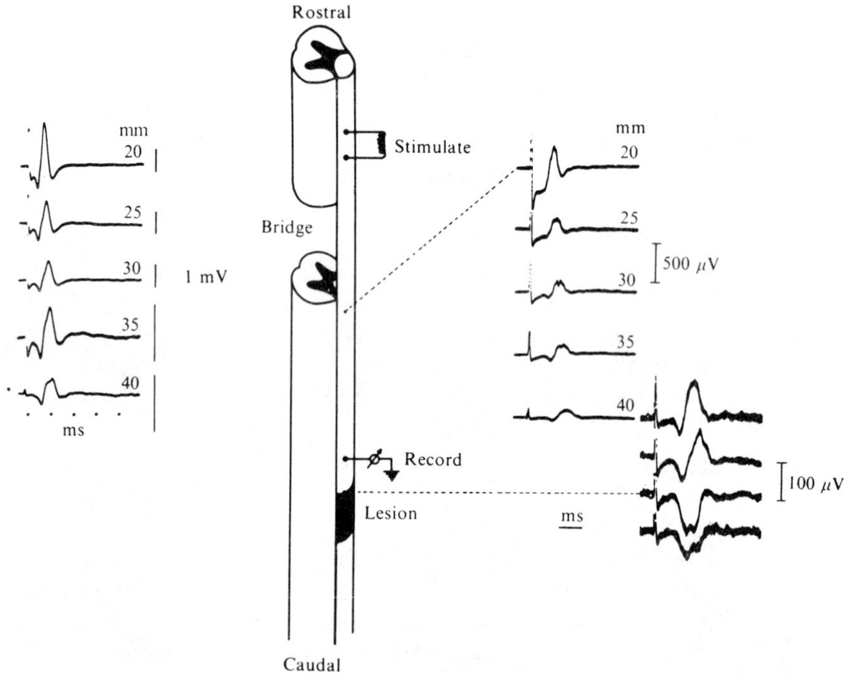

Fig. 25.2. Diagram to show the experimental arrangement used in examining the effects of a large demyelinating lesion on conduction in the spinal cord of a cat. *Left*: from a normal animal. *Right*: from an animal with a lesion involving the whole of both posterior columns. (after McDonald and Sears 1970*b*.)

On the left of Fig. 25.2 are shown typical triphasic compound action potentials recorded from a normal animal. On the right are comparable records from an animal with a large lesion in the posterior columns. The compound action potentials recorded from the histologically normal portions of the cord rostral to the lesion have a normal triphasic configuration, but at the margin of the lesion (42 mm) there is an abrupt loss of the negative component of the action potential and an increase in the positivity – the electrical signs of conduction block. Since the great majority of the fibres contributing to the action potential just rostral to the upper margin of the block are contributed by fibres with cell bodies caudal to the lesion, it is possible to draw two conclusions from this experiment. First, that large demyelinating lesions of central nerve fibres produce complete conduction block, and secondly that the portions of the nerve fibres distal to the block (with respect to the cell bodies) retain the ability to conduct impulses. Orthodromic conduction also persists up to the margin of the lesion. Measurement shows that the velocity is normal both rostral and caudal to the lesion in the histologically normal portions of the fibres.

In smaller lesions, conduction persists in many fibres. The properties of conduction in these circumstances have been examined in single fibres (McDonald and Sears 1970*b*). The technique used was developed by Sears and Stagg (1967) and depends on the fact that the intercostal muscles in the cat are supplied by tiny nerve filaments, each of which contains only two or three large afferent fibres. The fibres ascend for several segments in the posterior columns before synapsing. By recording from an intercostal muscle nerve filament after stimulation of the spinal cord with a shock of appropriate strength, it is possible to study conduction in single undissected nerve fibres. Using a series of electrodes at several sites above and below a demyelinating lesion in the cord it is possible to compare conduction in the demyelinated and normal parts of the same fibre.

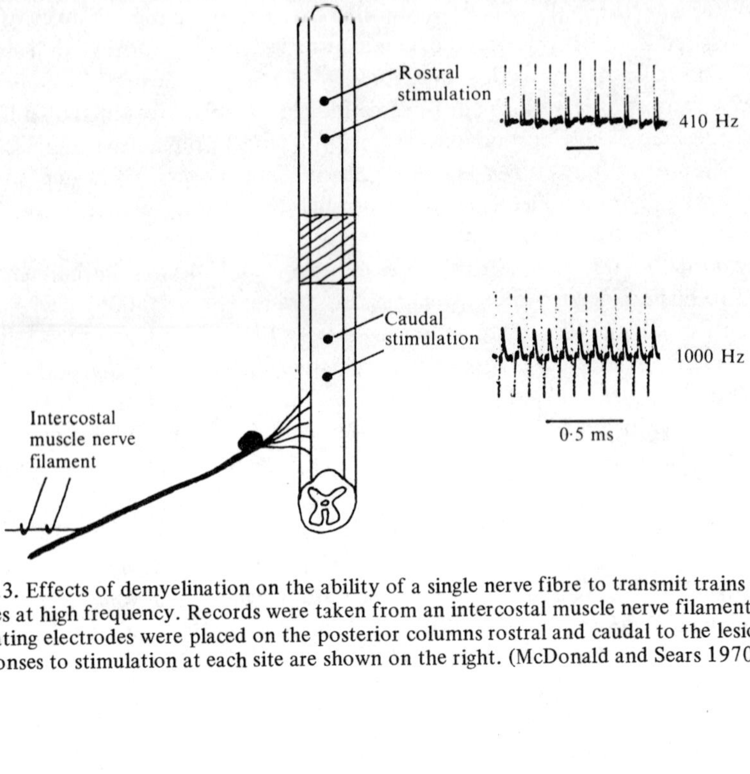

Fig. 25.3. Effects of demyelination on the ability of a single nerve fibre to transmit trains of impulses at high frequency. Records were taken from an intercostal muscle nerve filament. Stimulating electrodes were placed on the posterior columns rostral and caudal to the lesion. Responses to stimulation at each site are shown on the right. (McDonald and Sears 1970*b*.)

Transmission of trains of impulses

The ability to transmit trains of impulses was compared in demyelinated and normal parts of the same fibres. A typical experiment is illustrated in Fig. 25.3. The fibre followed every stimulus caudal to the lesion at 1000 Hz. When the same fibre was stimulated rostral to the lesion, transmission was intermittent at 410 Hz. These findings are in keeping with the prolongation of the refractory period of transmission of central demyelinated fibres (McDonald and Sears 1970*b*). This function provides a measure of the ability of an impulse *generated by a node* to traverse the damaged region, and is therefore particularly relevant to the behaviour of the fibres in the intact animal. Prolonged stimulation results in the accumulation of refractoriness of transmission producing periods of complete conduction block (McDonald and Sears 1970*b*).

We have not systematically explored the lower range of frequencies at which conduction fails, but in the course of other experiments we have observed failure at less than 70 Hz, which is well within the normal operating range for man (cf. Marsden, Meadows, and Merton 1971). Other evidence suggests that conduction is likely to fail at much lower frequencies than this in critically demyelinated fibres, and we have in fact observed failure in peripheral demyelinated fibres at less than 1 Hz (Gilliatt, McDonald, and Rudge, unpublished observations).

Conduction velocity

Observations on single fibres have established that the conduction velocity of an impulse is reduced as it traverses a demyelinating lesion, but is normal in histologically normal portions of the same fibres (McDonald and Sears 1970*b*). In Fig. 25.4 pairs of observations on the same individual fibres are joined by a line. Open circles represent the conduction velocity of fibres from normal animals, and triangles represent fibres traversing a focal demyelinated region (indicated diagrammatically by the shaded area). In normal fibres the difference in conduction velocity between two contiguous segments is $\ngtr 15$ m s^{-1} which is not significant ($p > 0{\cdot}05$). In abnormal fibres reductions of > 40 m s^{-1} occur across the demyelinated region – a highly significant difference ($p < 0{\cdot}005$). The sparing of occasional fibres is to be expected from the morphology of the lesion. The difference between the means of the velocities through the lesion and through the histologically normal portions of the same fibres is highly significant ($p < 0{\cdot}005$). There is no significant difference between the velocities of the normal portions of fibres from the two groups of animals ($p > 0{\cdot}1$) (McDonald and Sears 1970*b*).

Axonal degeneration

The reduction in conduction velocity which occurs through a demyelinating lesion contrasts with the situation in axonal degeneration. Conduction survives in the distal stumps of divided posterior column fibres for 1–6 days. During this time there is no reduction in conduction velocity (McDonald 1972, 1973). In animals

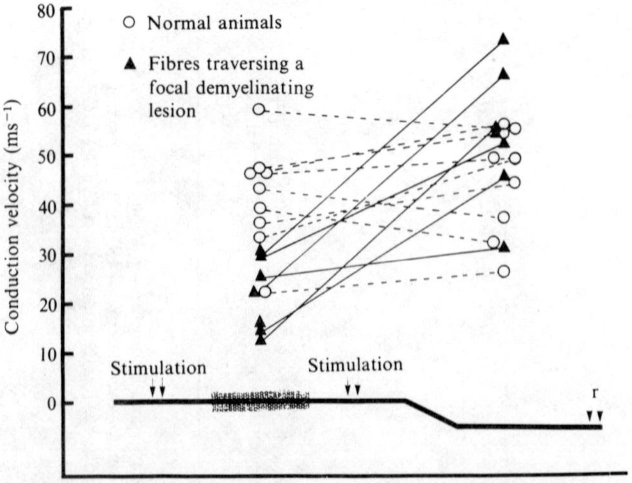

Fig. 25.4. Measurements of conduction velocity in contiguous segments of individual fibres. A single fibre is shown diagrammatically in the lower part of the figure. r = record
Pairs of observations for the same single fibre are joined by a line. (McDonald and Sears 1970*b*.)

with a diffuse but patchy axonal degeneration in the posterior column induced by tri-*o*-cresyl phosphate intoxication, the velocity of the surviving fibres remains normal (McDonald and Robertson 1972). This is illustrated in Fig. 25.5, in which

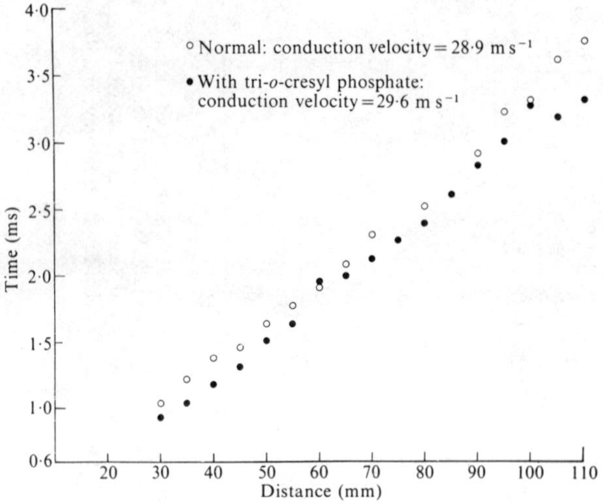

Fig. 25.5. Latency of response in the mid-thoracic to cervical posterior columns after single shock stimulation of the columns at the lower thoracic level plotted against conduction distance. Plotted for the normal animal, and for the animal with scattered axonal degeneration in the posterior columns due to chronic intoxication with tri-*o*-cresyl phosphate. (McDonald and Robertson 1972).

TABLE 25.1 *Conduction in myelinated nerve fibres*

Physiological process	Peripheral	Central
Saltatory conduction	+[1]	+[2,3]
Demyelination		
Conduction block	+[4,5]	+[6]
Conduction slowing	+[4,7,8]	+[9]
Ability to transmit trains of impulses	Impaired[10,11,12,13]	Impaired[9]
Wallerian degeneration		
Conduction velocity of degenerating fibres	Normal or decreased < 20 per cent[14,15,16]	Normal[17,21]
Conduction velocity of surviving fibres	Normal or decreased < 20 per cent[14,15,16]	Normal[17,21]
Time to conduction failure	1–9 days[14,16,18,19,20]	2–8 days[17]

1. Huxley and Stämpfli 1949. 2. Tasaki 1952. 3. Bement and Ranck 1969. 4. McDonald 1963. 5. Mayer and Denny-Brown 1964. 6. McDonald and Sears 1969. 7. McDonald 1962. 8. Hall 1967. 9. McDonald and Sears 1970*b*. 10. Lehmann, Lehmann and Tackmann 1971. 11. Lehmann and Tackmann 1970. 12. Rasminsky and Sears 1972. 13. Davis 1972. 14. Gutmann and Holubár 1950. 15. Kaeser and Lambert 1962. 16. Gilliatt and Hjorth 1972. 17. McDonald 1972. 18. Lissak, Dempsey, and Rosenbluth 1939. 19. Landau 1953. 20. Gilliatt and Taylor 1959. 21. McDonald and Robertson 1972.

the latency of the posterior column compound action potential is plotted against conduction distance. The open circles represent conduction in a normal animal, and the filled circles conduction in an animal with axonal degeneration in the posterior columns induced by chronic intoxication.

Limits of slowing in demyelination

How much slowing can occur in demyelinated fibres before conduction fails? In the central diphtheria toxin lesion we found focal reduction to less than one-sixth of the normal velocity in individual fibres. There is evidence from observations on peripheral demyelinated fibres to suggest that much greater slowing might occur. Before describing these results it is necessary to consider whether it is reasonable to apply data obtained from peripheral nerve to the interpretation of findings in the central nervous system, since there are important differences in the organization of central and peripheral myelin which might influence the characteristics of conduction (Bunge 1968). Table 25.1 summarizes the published data on conduction in normal pathological central and peripheral nerve fibres. It is clear that despite the morphological differences between the two types of fibres there are close similarities in the physiological features so far studied. As a working proposition therefore it is reasonable to conclude that, in principle, physiological information derived from the study of peripheral nerve fibres is relevant to the behaviour of central nerve fibres in comparable states.

Rasminsky and Sears (1972) have studied conduction within successive internodes in single undissected ventral root fibres in the rat. From the measurements on many hundreds of normal and demyelinated internodes they established that so long as conduction persists it remains saltatory. A wide range of internodal conduction times was found in different fibres and on the same fibre, presumably reflecting the histologically observed variation in extent of demyelination in different internodes. The maximum internodal conduction time observed was more than 25 times the mean normal value (Rasminsky and Sears 1972). Koles and Rasminsky's (1972) computer simulation of conduction in demyelinated nerve fibres is in good general agreement with the experimentally observed abnormalities.

Summary

Direct experiment shows that demyelination of central fibres results in complete or intermittent conduction block depending on the severity of the demyelination, and that when conduction does survive, it is slowed. In peripheral demyelinated fibres slowing may be by as much as 25 times in individual internodes.

Mechanism of delay in VEP

To what extent does the known pathophysiology of central nerve fibres provide an explanation for the delays observed in the VEP in human demyelinating disease? Since similar abnormalities of conduction in the peripheral nervous system have been observed in species as far apart as frog and man, and since there are close similarities between the effects of a given pathological process on conduction in the central and peripheral fibres, it seems certain that slowing of conduction contributes directly to the delays seen in the VEP in multiple sclerosis and optic neuritis. The delays observed in optic neuritis and multiple sclerosis range from 10 m s^{-1} to 100 m s^{-1} (Halliday *et al.* 1972, 1973*a*, *b*). It is of interest to enquire to what extent conduction slowing *per se* might contribute to the increased latencies. To answer this question we need to know something about the length of the plaques of demyelination in optic neuritis and multiple sclerosis, about the number of internodes that this corresponds with, and about the internodal conduction time in normal and abnormal fibres.

Sizes of plaques in demyelination

I have recently measured the length of 20 optic nerve plaques in 14 cases dying of multiple sclerosis. The length of individual plaques varied from 3 mm to 30 mm with a mean of 10·5 mm. In calculating the delay across a plaque I have considered a length of 1 cm.

Internodal length

There are only two published accounts of internodal length in the central nervous system and both refer to the spinal cord in experimental animals. Fig. 25.6 shows the relationship between internodal length and fibre diameter in the rat spinal cord (Yogendran and McDonald, unpublished observations). Similar results have been obtained for the rabbit (Hess and Young 1949) and the cat (McDonald and Ohlrich 1971). Measurements on a small sample of fibres ($N = 19$) from the cat

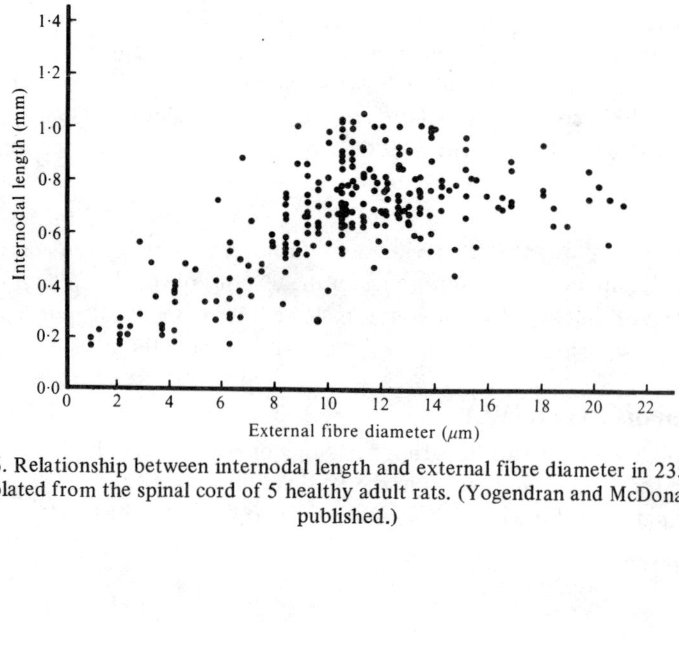

Fig. 25.6. Relationship between internodal length and external fibre diameter in 235 single fibres isolated from the spinal cord of 5 healthy adult rats. (Yogendran and McDonald, unpublished.)

optic chiasm have given comparable results (Gledhill, unpublished observations). In man 90 per cent of the optic nerve fibres have diameters of 3 μm or less (Chacko 1948). There are as yet no measurements of internodal length in man but if we accept that the dimensions are likely to be of the same order as in the cat, extrapolation of Gledhills' data suggests that the internodal length of the majority of fibres would be 200 μm or less. The assumption that the cat data is relevant to man is not unreasonable since the structure of corresponding parts of the nervous system is similar in different mammals; furthermore in the peripheral nervous system (where the relationship between internodal length and fibre diameter has been thoroughly studied) the results for cat, rabbit, guinea-pig, and man are closely similar (McDonald and Ohlrich 1971). On this basis it is likely that there are some five internodes per mm in the bulk of the fibres of the visual pathway in man. A demyelinated plaque of 1 cm would correspond with approximately 50 internodes.

Internodal conduction time

Again this has not been directly measured in man. The mean internodal conduction time in rat peripheral fibres of 10 μm diameter is 20 μs (Rasminsky and Sears 1972) and it is clear that it will be at least as long as this in a 3 μm fibre in the optic nerve. I have adopted a conservative approach in the calculation and accordingly have taken a value of 20 μs as applying to the optic nerve, although this is almost certainly a considerable underestimate. On this basis the time taken for an impulse to traverse 1 cm would be 1 ms. This would correspond with a conduction velocity of some 10 m s^{-1} which is of the same order as that obtained for the faster fibres in the monkey optic nerve (Ogden and Miller 1966).

Let us now return to the delay that might be introduced by slowing over 1 cm. If the findings in the peripheral nervous system apply to the central nervous system (as they do for the other aspects of conduction that have been described) then an increase of up to 25 times in internodal conduction time may be expected. This would give a figure of 25 ms to traverse 1 cm or an increased delay of 24 ms. Delays of this order are commonly seen in multiple sclerosis and optic neuritis (Halliday *et al.* 1972, 1973*a*, *b*; Asselman, Chadwick, and Marsden 1975).

There is thus a fair correspondence between the delays predicted from the known properties of demyelinated fibres and the VEP delays observed in human disease. It is important, however, to stress the limitations in the calculations. It is assumed that it is valid to transfer quantitative data from the peripheral nervous system to the central nervous system and from one species to another. I have argued that in broad terms this is reasonable. There are two further reservations. First, there is reason to suppose that conduction is likely to fail altogether where there is a succession of internodes with very long internodal conduction times (Koles and Rasminsky 1972). It is therefore possible that the theoretical maximum delay cannot be achieved *in vivo*. On the other hand, successive delays would be additive and it should be noted that multiple plaques in the optic nerves and posterior visual pathways are the rule at necropsy in multiple sclerosis.

The second reservation is that delays of the order of 25 ms have not been observed across focal experimental demyelinating lesions. Previous investigations have, however, been concerned with effects of demyelination on the larger fibres of the spinal cord and peripheral nerves, and there have been no studies of the effects of demyelination on conduction in very small myelinated fibres such as those seen in the optic nerve.

In summary, calculation suggests that delays approaching those seen in human VEP studies might be produced by focal slowing in the demyelinated region. The present evidence is, however, inadequate to justify the conclusion that slowing of conduction is the major source of delay in demyelinating disease.

Other factors contributing to delay

Whatever the direct contribution of conduction slowing to delays in the VEP, it is likely that other factors contribute. These include delays in the generation of the cortical response as a result of conduction block in many fibres or as a result of dispersion of the afferent volley from unequal slowing in different fibres. The possible role of such mechanisms has not yet been examined experimentally.

Another possibility is that some of the delay in the VEP is due to selective complete conduction block of the faster fibres, leaving only the slower fibres to mediate the response. It is unlikely that this is an important mechanism, at least in acute optic neuritis. The predominant affection in optic neuritis is of central vision and the fibres subserving this are generally agreed to be the slower, not the faster ones (Freund 1973). In our serial study of acute optic neuritis we found that the amplitude of the VEP was greatly reduced when the acuity was impaired but returned to normal as vision recovered, suggesting that conduction was restored in the majority of fibres. Nevertheless, the delay present when the response was reduced in amplitude persisted indefinitely after the amplitude recovered (see Halliday *et al.*, Chapter 26 of this book). The persistence of the delay in a response of normal amplitude and configuration in itself suggests an important contribution by slowing of conduction to the delay.

Finally, the possibility of a delay at retinal level must be considered. Recent work suggests that bundles of retinal nerve fibres commonly degenerate in optic neuritis and multiple sclerosis secondarily to the limited axonal degeneration which occurs in most plaques (Frisen and Hoyt 1974). If, as seems likely, the axonal loss is accompanied by loss of the corresponding ganglion cells, an alteration in retinal properties becomes a possibility. Electroretinographic evidence of retinal dysfunction in demyelinating disease is, however, conflicting (Halliday *et al.* 1972; Feinsod, Abramsky, and Auerbach 1973) and at present the question of a retinal contribution to delay in the VEP must remain open.

Conclusion

Experimental studies have shown that extensive demyelination of central nerve fibres results in complete conduction block. More restricted demyelination allows conduction to continue but the ability of the fibres to transmit trains of impulses at physiological frequencies is impaired and conduction velocity is reduced. This contrasts with the surviving conduction in axonal degeneration, where the velocity remains normal. While calculation suggests that the increase in latency across a demyelinated zone of appropriate length could be of the same order as that seen in the VEP in human optic neuritis, there are still too many uncertainties to be sure that this is a major mechanism of delay. It is likely that some of the increased latency is due to delays at the cortical level. The question of a retinal contribution remains open. What is needed now is precise data on two points in particular: first, we need to know the effects of lesions known to be associated with axonal degeneration and not demyelination on the VEP; and secondly, we need an analysis of the relative contribution of focal conduction slowing and of other factors to delays in the VEP produced by experimental demyelinating lesions in the visual pathways.

Acknowledgements

I am grateful to my colleagues for allowing me to quote from unpublished work.

26. Visual evoked potentials in patients with demyelinating disease

A. M. HALLIDAY, W. I. McDONALD, and J. MUSHIN
Institute of Neurology, National Hospital, Queen Square, London

Investigation of the somato-sensory response to electrical stimulation in patients with demyelinating disease has shown that the Rolandic response can be delayed in latency and altered in waveform in the presence of a plaque involving the dorsal column and medial lemniscal pathway (Halliday and Wakefield 1963; Namerow 1968, 1970; Baker, Larson, Sances, and White 1968; Tamura and Kuroiwa 1972; Desmedt and Noël 1973). A recent study by Small and Matthews at Oxford has extended this finding by demonstrating parallel changes in the early components of the response recorded from the spinal cord itself and suggests that this may be an even more sensitive index than the Rolandic response of the presence of demyelinating disease in the somato-sensory pathway (Matthews, Beauchamp, and Small 1974; Small, Beauchamp, and Matthews 1975).

A number of earlier attempts to detect similar changes of the occipital flash response in demyelinating disease of the visual pathways proved less rewarding. Changes in amplitude and latency of the VEP were recorded in some cases, but these were seldom sufficiently clear-cut or of large enough magnitude to allow a clear distinction between the normal and abnormal response in an individual subject (Richey, Kooi, and Tourtellotte 1971; Namerow and Enns 1972; Feinsod, Abramsky, and Auerbach 1973). Richey *et al.* (1971) for instance, reported significant delays in the mean latency of four of the first five occipital components, when comparing 50 patients with multiple sclerosis with 50 healthy controls. The mean delays for the whole group varied from 6 ms to 16 ms but the normal range of individual variability is hardly much less than this. Richey *et al.* attempted to set up a criterion for judging a patient's response to be abnormal, but the optimum measure allowed them to characterize the response of only 40 per cent of the multiple-sclerosis patients as abnormal, and, on the same test, 6 per cent of their healthy controls were also classified as abnormal.

This result illustrates the relative insensitivity of the flash VEP and the difficulty of using it clinically to assign any individual patient either to the normal or pathological group. However, recent work on the occipital VEP to a reversing black-and-white checkerboard pattern has shown it to be very much more useful

Visual evoked potentials in man: new developments (ed. J. E. Desmedt), pp. 438–49. Clarendon Press, Oxford 1977.

than the flash VEP as a clinical test. This is due both to the smaller variability in its waveform and latency in the healthy population and to its much greater sensitivity to lesions of the afferent visual pathways (Halliday *et al.* 1972; Behrman, Halliday, and McDonald 1972).

The VEP in acute unilateral optic neuritis

Halliday *et al.* (1972) compared the flash and pattern VEPs in a pilot study of 19 patients with acute unilateral optic neuritis. Normal values were first established on a control group of 17 healthy subjects. In the pattern VEP evoked by 100 complementary reversals of a 32° black-and-white checkerboard field, presented at a reversal rate of 2 Hz, there was a very consistent positive wave with a mean normal latency of 120·1 ms and a small S.D. (± 4·0 ms). This was some 15–20 ms longer than the pattern-reversal response recorded in an earlier study in which the stimulus was produced by alternately projecting a pattern and its negative by means of two projectors fitted with fast shutters (Halliday and Michael 1970; Michael and Halliday 1971). In the clinical study, because of the need for a large stimulus field, the pattern reversal was produced by rapidly moving the projected pattern sideways through one square. This was effected by back-projecting a patterned slide onto a translucent screen by way of a mirror which could be abruptly rotated through a small angle by means of an electro-mechanical transducer (see Chapter 1 of this book). Subsequent investigation showed that 15 ms of the latency value for the pattern VEP obtained by this method were an added instrumental artifact, due to the slowness of the mirror movement (about 35 ms). A subsequent test with a faster mirror (< 10 ms movement time) showed that the true latency is 103·9 ± 4·5 ms in a comparable group of normal subjects, which is virtually the same as the latency of the pattern response produced by the shutter method (see Halliday *et al.* 1973*a*).

Flash stimulation produced an occipital VEP with a positive component at about the same mean latency (102·3 ms) but the inter-subject variability was considerably larger (S.D. ± 13·7 ms: range 70–126 ms).

In the patient group, the VEPs from the unaffected eye were comparable in latency and amplitude to those obtained from the healthy subjects. The mean latency for the major positivity of the pattern VEP from the unaffected eye was 121·1 ± 5·9 ms. By contrast the mean latency of the VEP from the 18 affected eyes was 155·1 ± 20·0 ms. The nineteenth patient, who was recorded only in the acute phase, had no pattern VEP at the time, her visual acuity being reduced to the perception of hand movements. She never subsequently attended for follow-up. The pattern VEP from the affected eyes of the patients thus showed a mean delay of 35 ms. The range of values was large, but only one patient had a latency which overlapped with those obtained in the healthy group (Fig. 26.1).

In contrast to the pattern VEP, the VEP to flash in the affected eye of the same patients either showed no delay or an increase of only a few milliseconds, a

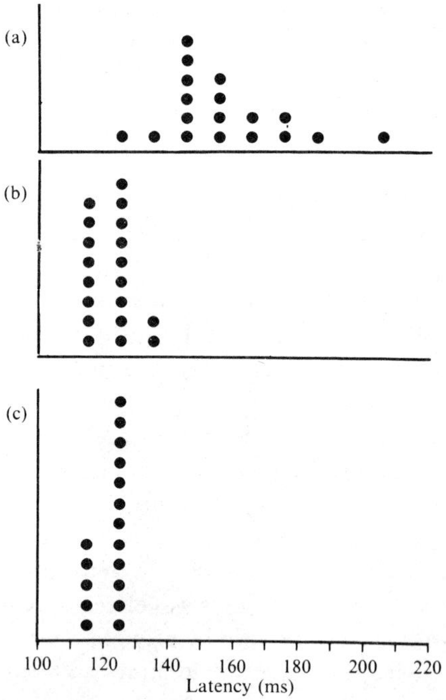

Fig. 26.1. Distribution of the peak latencies of the major positive component of the pattern VEP from the affected eye of 18 patients with unilateral optic neuritis (a), from the unaffected eye of 19 patients with unilateral optic neuritis (b), and from the right eye of 17 healthy subjects (c). No measurable VEP was recorded from the affected eye of 1 patient seen in the acute stage. (From Halliday *et al.* 1972.)

result similar to that reported by Richey *et al.* (1971). The flash test wholly failed to distinguish between the normal and abnormal response in an individual patient.

These results suggest that the pattern VEP is particularly sensitive to the effects of a demyelinating lesion of the optic nerves and that a pathologically delayed response will reliably identify those individuals who have suffered such a lesion in over 90 per cent of cases. Only one of the 18 patients in the trial gave an apparently normal pattern VEP – this is equivalent to a false negative rate of about 6 per cent.

Fig. 26.2 illustrates the pattern VEP to a checkerboard stimulus reversing at a frequency of 2 Hz from each eye of a patient recovering from acute optic neuritis of the right eye. This patient was not from the original study, and was recorded with the faster mirror stimulator. The pattern VEP from the unaffected left eye had a major positive component of normal latency with a mean peak amplitude of 16·7 μV at 106 ms. The VEP from the affected right eye was markedly delayed, with a peak positivity of 7·5 μV at 148 ms. An ERG of small amplitude and normal latency can be seen in response to pattern stimulation of each eye, under-

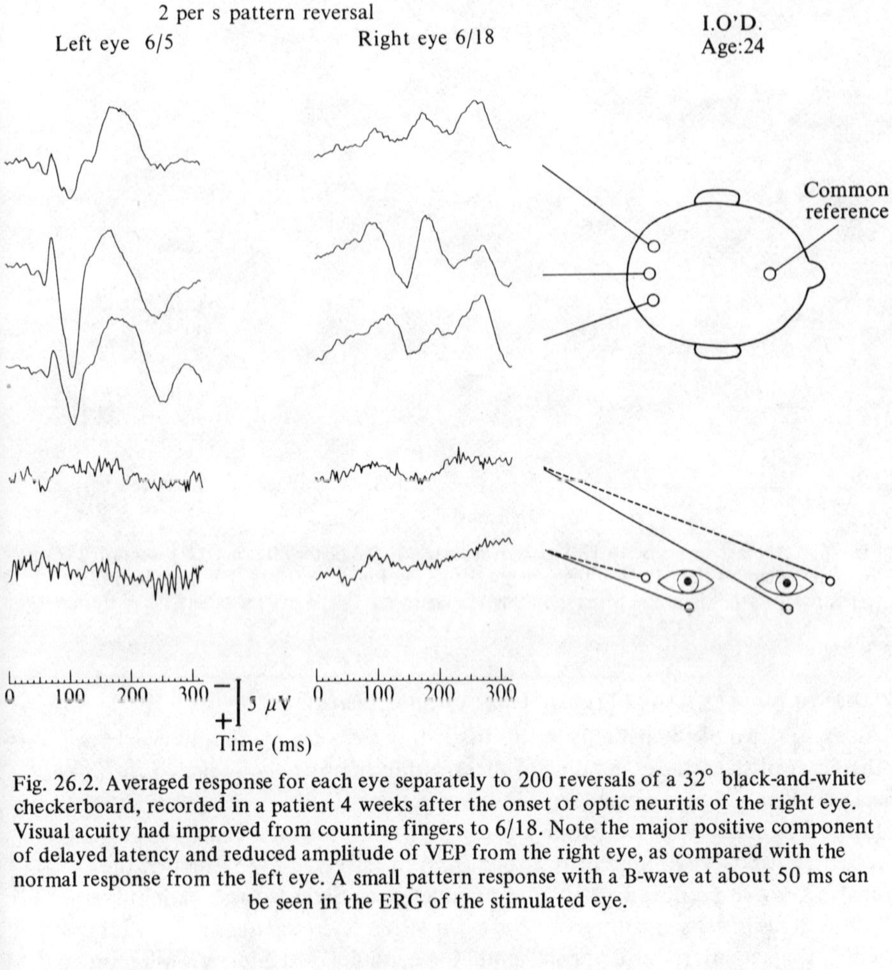

Fig. 26.2. Averaged response for each eye separately to 200 reversals of a 32° black-and-white checkerboard, recorded in a patient 4 weeks after the onset of optic neuritis of the right eye. Visual acuity had improved from counting fingers to 6/18. Note the major positive component of delayed latency and reduced amplitude of VEP from the right eye, as compared with the normal response from the left eye. A small pattern response with a B-wave at about 50 ms can be seen in the ERG of the stimulated eye.

lining the fact that the delay originates behind the retina. This delay in the occipital VEP to a 2 Hz pattern reversal is seen as a phase lag in the quasi-sinusoidal steady-state response to a 10 Hz pattern reversal (Fig. 26.3).

The VEPs to flash recorded in the same patient, are rather similar from each eye (Fig. 26.4). There is no latency shift in the response from the affected right eye comparable to that seen in the pattern VEP. An ERG of large amplitude and normal latency is recorded in response to the flash. The patient was seen four weeks after the onset of the attack. Vision in the right eye had initially been reduced to the ability to count fingers, but had gradually recovered to 6/18 at the time of the recording. There had been an afferent pupillary defect and a central scotoma in this eye. Vision in the left eye was 6/5.

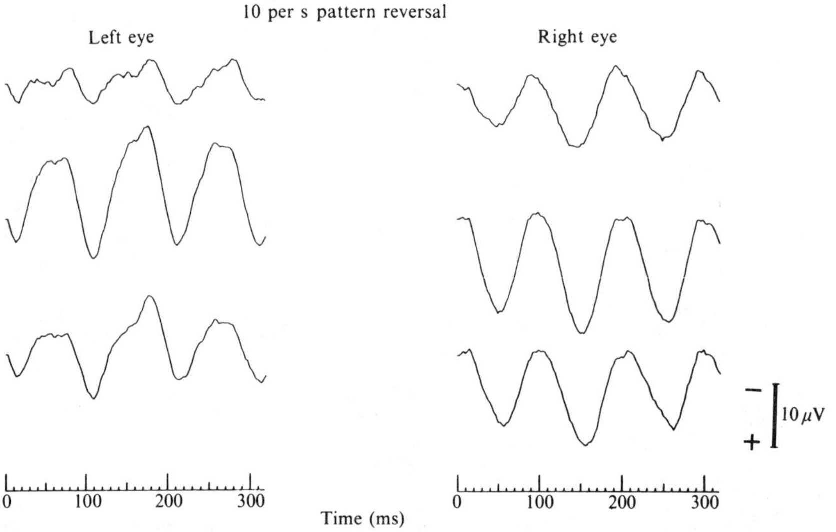

Fig. 26.3. Average response to 100 pattern reversals at the faster rate of 10 Hz, recorded from the same occipital electrodes in the same patient as in Fig. 26.2. Note the phase-lag in the response from the right eye, corresponding in magnitude to the delay in the 2 Hz pattern VEP shown in Fig. 26.2.

Loss of the VEP during the acute phase of optic neuritis

All except two of the patients in this first study were seen within 29 weeks of the onset of the attack, and nine of them within the first six weeks. In the initial stages where vision is greatly impaired, the pattern VEP may disappear altogether. In the 5 patients recorded within a fortnight of onset, whose acuity was 6/60 or less, no pattern VEP could be recorded from the affected eye, although the unaffected eye produced a VEP of normal latency. Four of these patients were followed up in subsequent recordings when vision had partially recovered, by which time a pattern VEP of small amplitude and delayed latency was recorded.

Changes in the VEP during the recovery phase following an attack

The recovery process was followed more carefully in a larger series of 53 patients following an attack of optic neuritis in one or both eyes, 8 of them being recorded on more than one occasion at different acuity levels and 8 having both eyes affected (Halliday *et al.* 1973*b*, 1974*a*). The recovery of VEP amplitude was not limited to the acute stage but continued, *pari passu* the improvement in acuity level, until, with the restoration of 6/6 vision, the amplitude of the pattern VEP returned to virtually normal levels. Fig. 26.5 shows the mean amplitude of the pattern VEP for the whole group plotted against the visual acuity at the time of the recording and indicates the progressive recovery. In the patients with most severely impaired acuity (6/60 or worse) the VEP was reduced to a third of its normal size, whereas

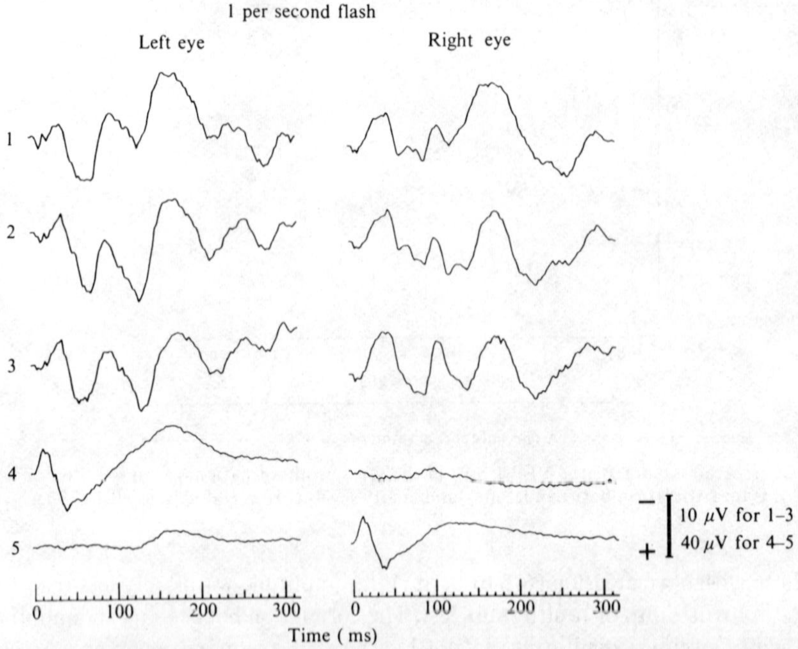

Fig. 26.4. The average response to 100 flash stimuli at 1 per second, recorded from the same patient as in Fig. 26.2 and 26.3. Note the absence of any delay in the flash VEP from the right eye comparable to that in the pattern VEP. The ERG to flash, which is of much larger amplitude than that to pattern, is shown at reduced gain. Electrodes the same as in Fig. 26.2.

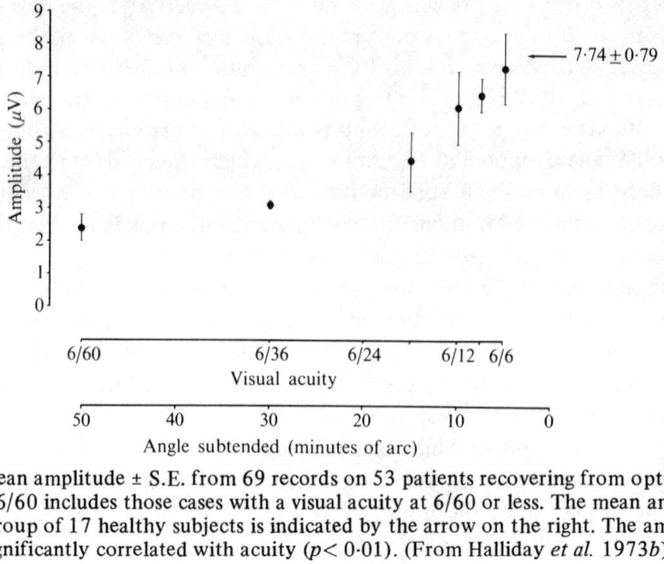

Fig. 26.5. Mean amplitude ± S.E. from 69 records on 53 patients recovering from optic neuritis. The data at 6/60 includes those cases with a visual acuity at 6/60 or less. The mean amplitude ± S.E. in a group of 17 healthy subjects is indicated by the arrow on the right. The amplitude is significantly correlated with acuity ($p < 0{\cdot}01$). (From Halliday *et al.* 1973*b*).

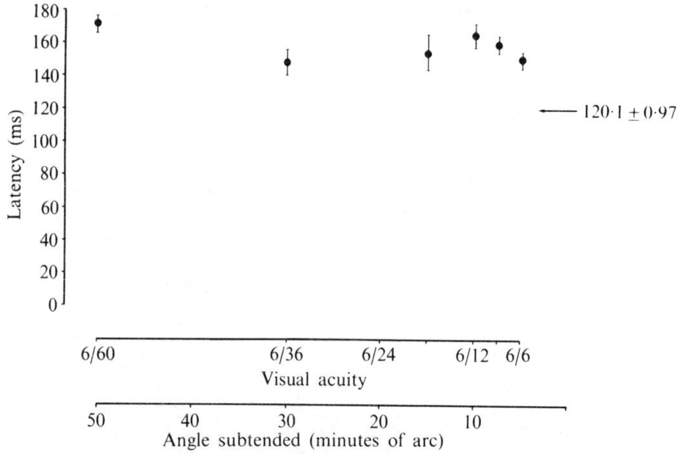

Fig. 26.6. Mean latency of the VEP ± S.E. in the same group of patients as in Fig. 26.5. There is no correlation between latency and acuity level. (From Halliday *et al.* 1973*b*.)

in those with normal vision (6/6 or better) the amplitude was hardly less than that in the control group of healthy subjects. The correlation between mean amplitude and acuity level was significant ($p < 0{\cdot}01$). This is all the more remarkable because the increased latency of the delayed VEPs did not return to normal. Fig. 26.6 shows the mean latency of the VEP for the same group of patients as in Fig. 26.5. There is no correlation between the acuity level and the magnitude of the delay, and the patients with normal vision are still markedly delayed.

We have recorded patients with delayed VEPs 15 years after the initial attack of optic neuritis. It appears that once present, the increase in latency is unaffected by the recovery process which leads to the restoration of normal amplitude. As in the original series of 19 patients with acute unilateral optic neuritis, there were a very few patients in the larger follow-up group who had latencies within the normal range. These amounted to 3 out of 53, which is very close to the original proportion of 1 out of 18. It appears, therefore, that about 5–6 per cent of patients with undoubted optic neuritis will have latency values for the pattern VEP overlapping the normal range.

Once established, the latency for a particular patient appears to be a stable phenomenon, unless a further attack of optic neuritis occurs which may increase the delay. This is to be contrasted with the processes associated with recovery of normal acuity levels, which may proceed over weeks or months, and appear to allow restoration of the response amplitude to levels approaching the normal value. This apparent anomaly may be explicable if the amount of delay depends on some fairly stable anatomical feature, such as the length of demyelinated fibres in the plaque, while the amplitude recovery may reflect the restoration of conduction in initially blocked nerve fibres. In the initial phase this no doubt parallels the subsiding oedema, but later the repair of the fibres by the development of an abnormally thin myelin layer might play a part (McDonald 1974). The normal latencies encountered in a small proportion of patients following typical clinical attacks of retrobulbar neuritis may well represent the minimal delays associated with unusually short plaques.

The VEP in multiple sclerosis

The overall incidence of plaques in the optic nerves in multiple sclerosis is unknown, but is certainly not limited to those patients with a past clinical history of optic neuritis. This is amply demonstrated by the incidence of pale discs in patients with no history of previous visual impairment. Since the pattern VEP is such a sensitive test of the presence of a demyelinating lesion in the optic nerve fibres, the incidence of delayed responses in patients with multiple sclerosis promises to provide the best test available of the presence of optic nerve plaques. For this reason the pattern VEP was recorded in the same way in a group of 73 patients, referred with suspected multiple sclerosis (Halliday *et al.* 1973*a*). Fifty-two (71 per cent) had delayed VEPs, but this certainly underestimates the incidence of delayed VEPs in this disease, as the group must have included a number of patients without demyelinating disease.

Adopting the more stringent diagnostic criteria proposed by McAlpine, Lumsden, and Acheson (1972), 34 out of the 73 patients could be classified as definite cases of multiple sclerosis, 5 as probable cases, and 12 as possible cases of this disease. Of this smaller total of 51 patients satisfying the diagnostic criteria, 49 had delayed VEPs in one or both eyes, whereas only 3 of the 22 other patients, who did not satisfy the diagnostic criteria, had delays. The criterion of delay adopted was rather a conservative one: a latency increased by more than $2\frac{1}{2}$ times the standard deviation of the normal mean latency. This means that only those patients with response latencies falling well outside the normal range qualify as delayed. Fig. 26.7 shows the range of increase of latency encountered in the more affected eye of the 51 patients with multiple sclerosis. The maximum delay of 100 ms is similar to that in the pilot study of acute optic neuritis, and the mean delay (43·3 ms, S.D. ± 20·1 ms) is only 8·3 ms longer. The group of 51 patients included 3 from the original optic neuritis study who had developed neurological signs elsewhere. The results suggest that (a) the incidence of optic nerve plaques is extremely high in patients with multiple sclerosis and (b) the pattern VEP is a reliable test for detecting their presence.

Correlation of VEP with clinical findings in multiple sclerosis

It is obviously interesting to know how these VEP results correlate with other clinical findings. Of the 51 patients with multiple sclerosis, 24 had a past history suggestive of optic neuritis in one or both eyes. All 24 proved to have delayed-pattern-evoked responses, confirming the results of the earlier study on optic

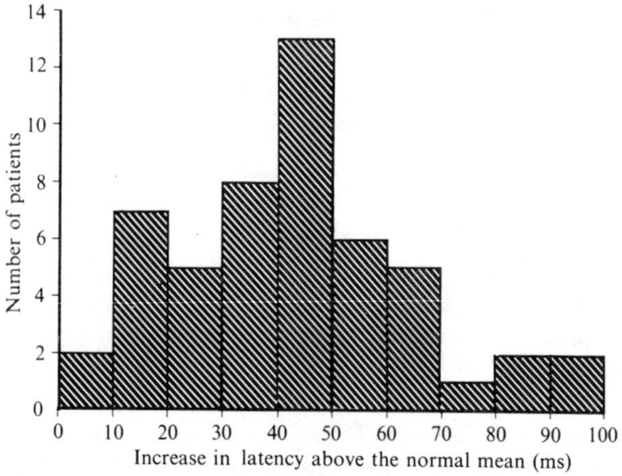

Fig. 26.7. Range of increase in latency of the major positivity of the pattern VEP recorded from the more affected of the two eyes in 51 patients with multiple sclerosis. (From Halliday *et al.* 1973*a*.)

neuritis. Twenty-seven other patients had no history of visual impairment, but of these no less than 25 turned out to have delayed pattern VEPs and there were only 2 individuals with normal responses in the whole group. On the basis of this data 96 per cent of patients with multiple sclerosis can be expected to have delayed-pattern VEPs and the expectation only falls to 93 per cent in those individuals with no clinical history of optic nerve involvement.

Delayed VEPs can thus be found in patients who have no history of visual impairment and in whom there is no disc pallor on examination of the fundi. Fig. 26.8 illustrates VEPs from a 48-year-old woman with 4 years' history of progressive inco-ordination of all her limbs, the right more than the left, accompanied by weakness of the right leg. Visual acuity was 6/6 in the right eye and 6/9 in the left eye with glasses, and there was no history to suggest previous optic neuritis. Colour vision was normal in both eyes on the HRR test. The pattern VEP showed a very delayed positivity of 6·7 μV at 140 ms from the right eye and 8·4 μV at 149 ms from the left eye (Fig. 26.8). Another example of a patient demonstrating delayed VEPs with no history of visual impairment is given by Halliday (1972, Fig. 4).

It is interesting to note that the incidence of binocular delays was higher in the group of patients with no visual history (Table 26.1). This may be related to the fact that those individuals presenting with a definite clinical history of visual impairment are more likely to be diagnosed early before the other eye is affected. It is nonetheless surprising to find that the incidence of bilateral involvement of the optic nerve is higher in the patients who deny any past visual impairment.

Temporal pallor of the optic discs is a common clinical sign in multiple sclerosis. How does the VEP compare with optic-disc pallor in identifying

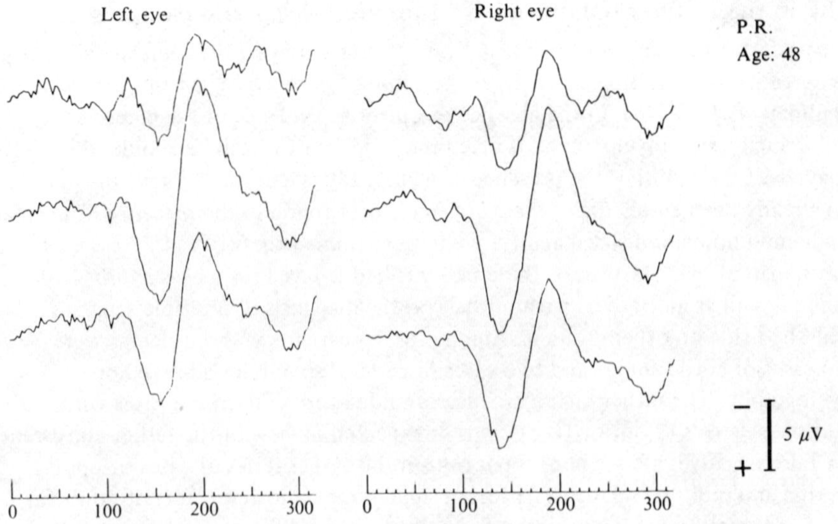

Fig. 26.8. VEPs to 2 Hz pattern reversal recorded from a 48-year-old female patient with probable multiple sclerosis, but no history of visual impairment. Note the markedly delayed VEPs from each eye. The same occipital electrodes as in Figs. 26.2–4.

patients with multiple sclerosis? Twenty-eight of the 51 patients in our series had definite pallor of one or both optic discs, and in every case this was associated with a delayed pattern VEP. Of the remaining 23 patients who had discs of normal appearance, no less than 21 had delayed responses. Twelve of these patients had no history of visual impairment and the delayed pattern response was the sole indicator of an optic nerve lesion. In a smaller group of patients it was confirmed that the pattern VEP could be delayed even in the presence of normal colour vision, fields, and pupils (see Halliday *et al.* 1973*a*).

TABLE 26.1 *Incidence of uniocular and binocular delays in 51 patients with multiple sclerosis*

	Normal VEP	Uniocular delay	Binocular delay	Total
No history of optic neuritis	2	3	22	27
History of optic neuritis	0	11	13	24
Total	2	14	35	51

VEP in the differential diagnosis of progressive spastic paraplegia

The pattern VEP may be of particular use in differentiating between spinal cord compression and multiple sclerosis as the cause of progressive spastic paraplegia (Halliday *et al.* 1974*b*). In the absence of objective evidence of a separate intracranial lesion myelography is often required, but this can be avoided if a delayed VEP establishes the presence of a clinically 'silent' optic nerve plaque. As has already been emphasized, these are frequently found in the presence of normal fundi and unimpaired visual acuity. We have examined the VEPs in 27 cases of spastic paraplegia. Thirteen of these patients had delayed responses and in 8 of these (as well as in 2 others without delays) the diagnosis of multiple sclerosis could be made on other grounds. Among the 14 patients without delays were two cases of cord tumour and two cases of cervical spondylosis proved by myelography. The rather high incidence of undelayed VEPs in the cases with multiple sclerosis (2 out of 10 cases) is unexpected in view of the rather consistent low false negative rate – about 6 per cent in the earlier series of cases of optic neuritis and multiple sclerosis. In such a small sample, however, it is of doubtful significance, although it could perhaps point to some difference in the overall distribution of demyelinating lesions in the group of cases presenting in this particular way.

Other conditions causing delayed pattern VEP

Multiple sclerosis is not the only cause of delayed pattern VEP and the test must be assessed in relation to the clinical picture as a whole. Among other conditions causing delay must be mentioned compressive lesions of the optic nerve. In a series of 16 such cases the VEP was delayed in 7, absent in another 3 and of altered waveform in 4. There may well be demyelination in some of these patients, occurring in association with pressure on the optic-nerve fibres, since recent experiments have shown that compression of central nerve fibres can produce selective destruction of myelin with survival of the axons (Gledhill, Harrison, and McDonald 1973). We have also recorded delayed VEPs in 2 of 3 patients with Friedreich's ataxia without visual symptoms.

More anterior disorders of the visual system appear to affect mainly the amplitude of the response without causing great changes in the latency of the major positivity. However, delays may occur on stimulating the affected area of the retina in glaucoma (Cappin and Nissim 1975) and the waveform of the positivity may be broadened with a somewhat delayed peak in cases with ischaemic optic neuropathy (Halliday, McDonald, and Mushin unpublished). Where acuity is 6/60 or worse, the VEP virtually disappears and no latency measurements can be taken. A few cases of multiple sclerosis have such gross visual impairment that it is not possible to ascertain whether the associated response is delayed or not, owing either to gross change in the waveform or to the reduction of the VEP amplitude to nearly the noise level. We have recorded three families with congenital optic atrophy, in whom it was only possible to record a pattern VEP of very small amplitude associated with the severe visual impairment.

Summary

Multiple sclerosis appears to be the most common cause of delayed VEPs and in our series over 90 per cent of patients with this diagnosis had delays. The pattern VEP may be particularly useful as a screening test for the early diagnosis of the disease or in the differential diagnosis of progressive spastic paraplegia. It can also be helpful to the clinician in distinguishing organic and functional sensory loss (Halliday 1972).

Acknowledgements

Fig. 26.7 is by permission of the *British Medical Journal* and Fig. 26.1 by permission of *The Lancet*.

27. Unilateral retrobulbar neuritis: a comparison of evoked potentials and psychophysical measurements

J. H. COOK and G. B. ARDEN

Department of Visual Science, Institute of Ophthalmology and *Electrodiagnostic Clinic, Moorfields Eye Hospital, London*

In patients with multiple sclerosis with evidence of retrobulbar neuritis, the cortical potentials evoked by pattern-reversing stimuli (pattern-reversal VEP) are abnormal. The abnormalities consist of a diminution in VEP amplitude in the acute phase of the disease, but even after recovery has advanced so that the usual clinical testing shows no abnormality of visual function, the culmination time of the VEP or the phase angle of the steady-state VEP are still increased (Halliday *et al.* 1972; Behrman *et al.* 1972; Halliday *et al.*, Chapter 26 of this book).

The increased 'delay' in the VEP is large. The normal VEP latency of about 120 ms may be extended by as much as 100 ms, although the average increase is about 30 ms. The reasons for such a delay are unknown. One plausible hypothesis (McDonald and Sears 1970*a* and *b*; McDonald, Chapter 24) is that demyelination decreases the conduction velocity in axons, by interfering with saltatory conduction in the nodes in a plaque. Although only very large plaques could produce delays of the magnitude found, there are additional possibilities: there could be multiple demyelinized foci, or the focus could cause retrograde degenerative changes.

Alternatively, the delay in the VEP might be a cortical phenomenon and demonstrate altered cortical activity, resulting from the changed sensory input. Yet another possibility would be selective damage to one of the types of axon in the optic pathway. It is known that these can be subdivided into two main types, called X and Y (Enroth-Cugell and Robson 1966). X-axons have smaller diameters and slower conduction rates (Fukada 1971). They are derived from retinal ganglion cells which have smaller receptive fields than Y-cells; an important distinction is that X-cells summate inhibition and excitation over their entire receptive field in a linear manner while Y-cells do not. Consequently, X-cells respond maximally when a contrasting border is placed precisely across the visual field, but may produce no response if the position of the border is shifted. Y-cells always respond, no matter what the position of the border. X-cells, at

Visual evoked potentials in man: new developments (ed. J. E. Desmedt), pp. 450–57. Clarendon Press, Oxford 1977.

least in the cat, are more common near the area centralis. These differences in organization can be plausibly related to visual function and it has been suggested that, while X-cells are specialized for signalling stationary detail, Y-cells are specialized for signalling change and movement (Ikeda and Wright 1972*b*). Cells whose function is determined by X- and Y-cells can be found in the lateral geniculate (Cleland, Dubin, and Levick 1971) and there is evidence in cat, that the cortical projection of the systems is different, only X-cells projecting to area 17, while X and Y both project to area 18 (Hoffman, Stone, and Shermon 1972). If selective damage to Y-fibres occurred in multiple sclerosis, the fastest conduction system would drop out, resulting in an increased conduction time. Additionally, there could be a change in the topography of cortical activity, so it is not possible to predict what effect such selective damage would have on the VEP.

Now, if there was only a non-specific conduction delay in the optic nerve, tract, or radiation, all measures of the delay, by psychophysical or VEP techniques, should give similar results. On the other hand, if there was selective damage, or if there were more complex reasons for the VEP delay, the value obtained might be dependent upon the technique of measurement. We have therefore measured stimulus-response intervals, using a variety of techniques, in a group of patients with mild unilateral retrobulbar neuritis. This chapter describes our preliminary findings.

In the first part, we describe experiments which show that a variety of techniques demonstrate a conduction delay of about 15 ms. However, uniquely, the delays found by pattern-reversing VEPs are approximately double this value. Thus either there is a special class of nerve fibres which generate the pattern VEP, or one of the alternative explanations mentioned above must explain the pattern VEP result. In the second part of the chapter we describe experiments designed to differentiate between these two hypotheses.

Methods

Patient selection

Patients presented to the Outpatients Department of Moorfields Eye Hospital. They all received thorough ophthalmological and neurological examination, and causes of retrobulbar neuritis, other than multiple sclerosis were excluded. No patient had anything but trivial history of symptoms suggesting multiple sclerosis. No patient had a previous attack of impairment of vision. No patients had any clinical signs (other than in the one eye). Only patients with mild symptoms in the one eye at the time of testing were included. The unaffected eyes of the patients had acuities 6/6 or better. The affected eyes had, at the time of investigation, acuities of 6/12 or better, and there were no scotomata. Thus we were able to compare the normal and abnormal eye in each patient.

Unilateral retrobulbar neuritis

Pattern-reversal VEP

The technique has been described previously (Behrmann *et al.* 1972; Arden 1973). The patient viewed a screen made of polaroid squares through an eye-piece which contained a rotating polaroid. The distance between patient and screen could be varied, and so could the area of the screen visible to the patient. Thus the stimulus could be made to fall on different portions of the retina, and the subtense of the squares in the pattern could be varied independently. Small squares (subtending 10′) produce a VEP which is derived from foveal and immediately parafoveal retina; larger squares test the responses of progressively more peripheral retina. The VEP amplitude is related to the contrast across the borders of the squares and it is significantly reduced by minor refractive errors.

Standard electrodes were placed on the scalp. The reference electrode was at the vertex and the ear was grounded. The active electrode was usually 2·5 cm above the inion: however, in some experiments, described on p. 455, the position was varied. Responses to stimulation of each eye were measured separately, and repeated to determine if consistent VEPs were recorded. Where the testing protocol was complex, the results were obtained in a semi-randomized sequence. Responses were recorded with a MEDELEC MS6 polygraph. Usually 100 repetitions of the averager were used, each containing 3 cycles of the stimulus presentation.

Latent period of sensation measured by a null method

This is an electronic version of the device used by Arden and Weale (1954). Two light-emitting diodes were mounted for dichoptic viewing in a modified stereo viewer. The light-emitting diodes were pulsed at approximately 0·7 Hz and produced 2 ms flashes. The retinal image subtended 1°, and the flux was 20 μJ (6385 A). The time-interval between the flashes could be varied by ± 200 ms by operating an accurately calibrated 10-turn potentiometer. The patient looked at the flashing LEDs, with the potentiometer off-set so that the flashes did not appear synchronous. He was asked to turn the potentiometer till he saw only a single flash. The experimenter read the potentiometer and off-set it once more, in the opposite direction, and the patient readjusted it. Four pairs of trials were made with this method of ascending and descending limits. With 16 normal subjects, there appeared to be a mean delay in sensation for the left eye of 1·7 ms (S.E. of mean, 0·58 ms). The apparatus as described above was modified in several ways.

(a) The LEDs were viewed against a luminous red background, and were rectangularly modulated, being bright for 100 ms and dim for the rest of the cycle. Patients were unable to make accurate judgements of simultaneity under these conditions.

(b) One of the LEDs was masked off, and the patient viewed the other. At the same time, the VEP to the flashes were recorded, using the same electrodes as had been used for the pattern-reversal VEP. VEPs were also recorded using the LEDs modified as under (a) above, but they were very small: in only three cases were the waveforms sufficiently well characterized for differences in culmination time to be measured with the necessary precision.

Visual latent period measured with EOG

Eye motion was recorded with a d.c. EOG technique, while the subjects gazed at a light moving in simple harmonic motion (period 2 s, angular deviation 50°). The moving light activated a trigger so that EOG records could be accumulated on a Biomac 1000 averager with overload rejection facilities. EOGs were recorded from each eye simultaneously but independently. Usually 16 cycles of eye motion were recorded. If the eye motions were exactly alike, the averager contents would be identical. However, if there was a difference in eye position, or if while tracking the light the eyes diverged or converged, there would be a phase-lag between the eyes. In fact, the patients reported that the light appeared to travel in an ellipse: thus the same phenomenon was observed as for the Pulfrich pendulum. The problem of eye motion and its effect upon subjective estimates of latency will be presented in detail elsewhere, and is included in this report for the sake of completeness (Reading and Bird, in preparation).

Results

Different estimations of VEP delay

Table 27.1 summarizes the results. The VEPs produced by the pattern-reversing stimuli to the affected eye peaked some 30 ms later than for the normal eye. This result is in good agreement with the work of Halliday (Chapter 26) and suggests that in our patients, as in Halliday's first series, patients with truly uni-ocular disease had been selected. It should be noted that the checkerboard squares used (15′) were considerably smaller than in Halliday's work, and the stimulus repetition rate higher. However, Halliday has shown that estimates of delay are unaffected by alteration in repetition rate.

All the other methods of estimating response delays in the affected eyes gave smaller values. The flashes of light from the light-emitting diode sources evoked VEPs with delays of *c.* 13 ms, i.e. approximately 50 per cent of those for pattern-reversing stimulus. The estimate of simultaneity with the light-emitting diode targets have an increased latent period of 16 ms, which is not significantly different from that for the flash VEPs.

Thus it appears that of all the methods used, only the pattern-reversal VEP gives anomalously long values for the delay. This conclusion is quite independent of whether our patients suffered from a single plaque in one optic nerve or whether the disease was multifocal and very asymmetric. In many conditions, there is a correspondence between changes in the pattern reversal VEP and sensation which

TABLE 27.1 *Latency differences between affected and unaffected eyes of patients with retrobulbar neuritis (all times in milliseconds)*

Patient no.	Pattern VEPs 70 cm full field	EOG	Light-emitting diode stimulus: Subjective, Black background	Subjective, Red background	Flash VEP, Black background	Flash VEP, Red background
4	34	12·1	17	15	29	21
5	9	15·8	5	4	4	4
1	42	24·0	20	5	32	3
6	23	8·6	12	5	–	–
7	25	16·9	12	8	19	–
8	28	6·0	21	25	17	–
9	60	1·9	25	30	27	–
Average	31†	13·0	16	11	21†	18
S.E. of mean	5·5	2·7	2·3	3·8	3·8	6·2

– Responses too small for reliable measurements.
† Significant at 0·05 level (*t*-test).

is considerably better than for other visual VEPs (Regan and Beverley 1973*c*). That this correlation should be reversed in multiple sclerosis is of considerable interest.

Mechanisms involved in VEP delays

In the first section (p. 453) it was shown that while several other methods of estimating the conduction delay in retrobulbar neuritis give estimates, in our group of patients, for whom the conduction delay was ~ 16 ms, the pattern-VEP delay apparently is *c*. 30 ms. There are several possible reasons: (a) that the extra duration results from specific slowing of those impulses which produce the pattern VEP; (b) that the VEP represents a stage of activity whose delay in appearance is not directly the result of an added conduction delay.

In order to try and distinguish between these hypotheses, we have recorded pattern-reversal VEPs under different conditions:

(i) The position of the active midline electrode was altered. If conduction delay was the cause of the delay in the VEP, then by recording from different cortical areas we might alter the absolute delay in VEP onset but not the difference between VEPs elicited from either eyes.

(ii) The retinal image was defocused. This should change the proportion of X- to Y-cells' discharge in the stimulus (Ikeda and Wright 1972*b*). Such a procedure could affect the relative delay between the two eyes in retrobulbar neuritis. For example, if Y-cells were preferentially affected, then the defocused stimulus should be more reduced in the affected eye.

(iii) The size of the stimulating squares was changed. This alters the retinal location from which the response can be evoked, and would alter the proportion of X- to Y-cells in the retinal area stimulated.

(iv) The central 3° of the retina, or the surrounding peripheral zone was stimulated: this procedure should show any alteration in VEP related to a local topographical damage due to demyelinization (should any exist).

The results of these measurements are shown in Table 27.2. Altering the parameters of the experiment may alter the apparent VEP delay but there is no systematic trend. It can be seen that the time-delays between VEPs elicited from either eyes of our patients can be affected by modifying any of the stimulus parameters in the ways listed above, although (iii) above produces little change. In this respect our results differ from those of Sokol (Chapter 23 of this book). However, there is no regularity to be observed in the results between different patients. This is illustrated by the VEPs obtained from three patients when the position of the active electrode is moved (Fig. 27.1). It can be seen that as the active electrode is moved rostrally along the midline, there is minimal change in patient 15 while the delay increases in patient 12 and decreases in patient 11.

Variable results can also be seen for other variations of stimulus parameters. They are inconsistent with the view that the time-delay in the appearance of the

TABLE 27.2 *Difference in peak times of VEPs elicited from normal and affected eyes*

Distance (cm)	Field	Distance of electrode from inion as percentage of nasion–inion distance	Added dioptres	Patient no.					
				10	11	12	13	14	15
120	Full	10 per cent above	0	27	22	12	12	20	16
120	Full	10 per cent above	+6	32	22	10		22	
70	Full	10 per cent above	+6	35	14	12		25	
70	Full	10 per cent below	0	24	36	4	22	18	19
70	Full	10 per cent above	0	27	20	10	16	17	16
70	Full	30 per cent above	0	7	12	16	2	10	14
70	Centre clear	10 per cent above	0	39	24	10	20	12·5	20
70	Centre black	10 per cent above	0	25	16	9	14	4·5	16

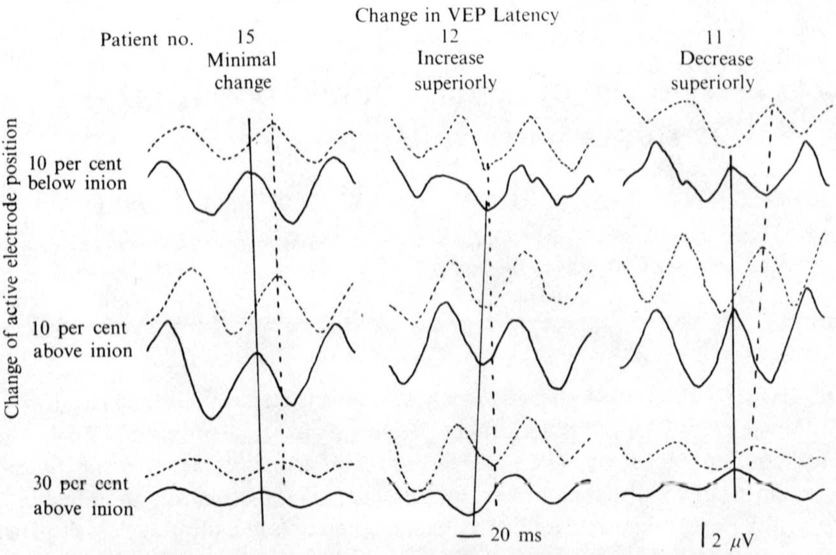

Fig. 27.1. The effect of change of electrode position on VEPs from three different patients. The recording from the affected eye is shown as a dotted line and that from the unaffected eye as a continuous line. The peaks are joined by straight lines as a guide to the reader's eye. It can be seen that as the active electrode is moved rostrally in the midline there is minimal change in patient 15, the delay increases in patient 12, and decreases in patient 11. Note that 10 per cent above inion is our standard electrode position.

pattern VEP is due to a simple, global increase of conduction time in all of the optic-nerve fibres subserving the central 15° of the visual field. They are also inconsistent with the view that one particular type of optic nerve fibre is selectively damaged in all our patients. It is more likely that in our tests, the pattern-reversing stimulus affects a large cortical region, which cannot be regarded as homogeneous with respect to its abstraction of information in the retinal input. The long and variable delay produced by the stimulus is produced either by changes in the cortical region generating the response, or by additional cortical delays which reflect the impaired data-processing consequent on a changed input from the radiation.

Heron, Regan, and Milner (1974) have also concluded that the delay in retrobulbar neuritis is not due only to impaired conduction in the optic nerve. Their results differ from ours for they found very large sensory delays, using an equipment somewhat similar to our light-emitting diode device, but which tested periphery against fovea. There is a strong likelihood that our two methods do not measure the same function, but it seems to be more direct to measure, as we have done, the sensation of simultaneity from one fovea to the other, the more so because this is what we do with the VEP. In our patients delays in sensation of more than a few milliseconds could not have occurred, since under these circumstances the illusion of the Pulfrich pendulum necessarily breaks down (Weale 1954).

28. The use of visual evoked potential in patients with multiple sclerosis

M. FEINSOD, W. F. HOYT, B. W. WILSON, and J. P. SPIRE

Neuro-Ophthalmology Unit, Department of Neurosurgery, University of California Medical Center, San Francisco

The diagnosis of multiple sclerosis requires documentation of multiple lesions (McAlpine *et al.* 1972). When a patient presents signs or symptoms of a single spinal cord or brain-stem lesion, the recognition of an additional, even subclinical, involvement of the visual pathways can help confirm the diagnosis. Examination of the ocular fundus may reveal focal axonal degeneration in multiple sclerosis patients, even in the absence of visual symptoms (Fig. 28.1 see between pp. 418–19). Such clinical finding correlates with the pathological (Greenfield and King 1936; Adams and Kubik 1952) and experimental (McDonald and Sears 1970*a, b*) evidence for combined axonal loss and demyelination foci, both of which may be insidious, as was also found in an epidemiological study by Kahana, Leibowitz, Fishback, and Alter (1973). The present study deals with VEP to flash in multiple sclerosis patients.

Methods

The 20 patients examined had the diagnosis of multiple sclerosis established at the neurology service of University of California Medical Center. No visual symptoms or signs were noted in 15 patients. The patients were examined with dilated pupils (Mydriacil 1 per cent) in a darkened room. Grass gold-plated electrodes were fixed with Grass electrode paste to the scalp. The flash VEP was recorded between on positions O_1 and O_2. Linked ears served as reference. The resistance between electrodes was kept at 2000–5000 Ω. The EEG signals were amplified by a Grass model VII electroencephalograph (bandwidth 1–70 Hz) and fed to a Mnemotron CAT 1000_B. A standard calibration pulse was averaged at the beginning of each test. A xenon discharge lamp activated by a Grass photostimulator PS-2 at intensity 4 on a scale of 1–16. The stimulus was 100 repetitive 1 per s flashes at 20 cm from the pupils. Each computer cycle was initiated 25 ms prior to the flash. Analysis

Visual evoked potentials in man: new developments (ed. J. E. Desmedt), pp. 458–60. Clardendon Press, Oxford 1977.

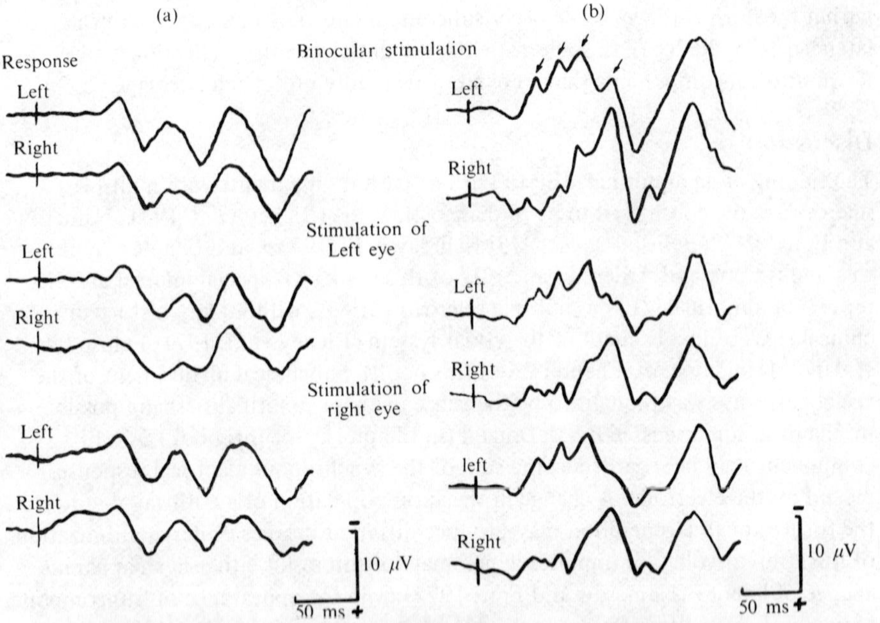

Fig. 28.2. (a) VEP to flash in multiple sclerosis patient. Note uniform prolongation of latencies of all components to binocular and monocular stimulations. (b) Binocular and monocular VEPs to flash in a multiple sclerosis patient, showing both delayed conduction and desynchronization of afferent volley. Latencies are markedly prolonged and the initial negative wave presents several subcomponents (arrows). Calibration 10 μV; 50 ms.

time was 250 ms. Auditory masking was not required. The VEPs to monocular and binocular stimulation were displayed on a Tektronix CRT 502 and photographed with a Polaroid camera.

Our normative data were found to be the same as reported by Kooi and Bagchi (1964) and by Richey *et al.* (1971).

Results

The normal flash VEP consists of an initial negative deflection with a peak latency of 40–50 ms, which is followed by a W-shaped wave (Fig. 28.1(b)). This chapter concerns changes occurring in this initial component. In all the 20 multiple sclerosis patients examined, the latency and the shape of the initial negative wave were affected, no matter whether the patients had ever had visual symptoms of their disease.

Two basic patterns of abnormal VEP to flash were found: (a) prolonged latency of all components, with the first negative deflection being delayed up to 80 ms (Fig. 28.2(a)); (b) breakdown of the initial negative wave into 'subcomponents', usually 2–4 in number. The latencies of some of these subcomponents may be within the normal range, while other subcomponents may be of delayed peak latencies (Fig. 28.2(b)). In some patients, the initial negative deflection broke down into subcomponents that were all of markedly prolonged latencies.

Discussion

The finding of an abnormal VEP to flash or pattern in patients with multiple sclerosis is now considered to be of diagnostic value (Richey *et al.* 1971; Namerow and Enns, 1972; Feinsod *et al.* 1973; Halliday *et al.* 1973*b*, and Chapter 26 of this book; Cook and Arden, Chapter 27 of this book). Of special interest are the reports of abnormal VEP in multiple sclerosis patients without any history or clinical signs of involvement of the visual system (Richey *et al.* 1971; Feinsod *et al.* 1973; Halliday *et al.* Chapter 26 of this book). Subclinical involvement of the visual pathways was thought to be the cause of these abnormalities; and possible mechanisms are discussed by McDonald (in Chapter 25 of this book). A VEP component may be regarded as the sum of the synchronous electrical responses picked by the electrode. A change in the axon population of a pathway due to the focal axonal degeneration may produce different degrees of desynchronization of the afferent volley of impulses which may in turn result either in an apparent change of latency (Namerow and Enns 1972) or in the appearance of 'subcomponents' as seen in Fig. 28.2(b). Demyelination in multiple sclerosis is not a uniform process but a disorder affecting different axons to different extent, thus producing a whole range of decreased conduction rates (McDonald and Sears 1970*b*; Davis and Schauf 1974) and distorting the normal organization of the afferent volley. These features must contribute significantly to the production of the VEP pattern seen in Fig. 28.2. The flash evoked potential thus appears, in our experience, to be a sensitive and reliable index for the diagnosis of multiple sclerosis.

Acknowledgement

Dr. Feinsod's fellowship in neuro-ophthalmology was supported by a grant from the Fight for Sight, Inc.

29. Slowing of visual signals in multiple sclerosis, measured psychophysically and by steady-state evoked potentials

D. REGAN, B. A. MILNER, and J. R. HERON
Department of Communication, University of Keele, and *North Staffordshire Hospital Centre*

Since VEP can indicate both slowing and attenuation of visual signals, it has attracted attention as a possible indicator of visual pathology caused by demyelinating disease and as a potential aid in the diagnosis of multiple sclerosis (Richey *et al.* 1971; Halliday *et al.* 1972, 1973*a*, *b*; Namerow and Enns 1972; Arden 1972; Cook and Arden, Chapter 27 of this book). Our work differs from previous studies in the use of the Fourier analysis method to record steady-state VEPs to repetitive stimulation (Regan 1966*a*, *b*, 1972, Chapter 4 of this book) which might provide different insights into the brain than the more familiar transient VEPs. Subjective delays in visual perception in retrobulbar neuritis and multiple sclerosis patients were also estimated by means of a 'delay campimeter'.

Equipment and method

Flicker elicits steady-state VEPs which, when analysed into their component harmonics by an analog Fourier method, appear to involve three types of component with different properties (Van der Tweel and Verduyn Lunel 1965; Spekreijse, 1966; Regan 1966*a*, 1972*b*); the frequency of one VEP component is in the range 8–12 Hz (Van der Tweel and Verduyn Lunel 1965; Spekreijse 1966; Regan 1966*a*), the second in the range 13–25 Hz (Regan 1968*a*, 1973*b*), and the third in the range 35–60 Hz (Fig. 29.1(b)) (Van der Tweel and Verduyn Lunel 1965; Spekreijse 1966; Regan 1968*c*). Each harmonic can be described by its amplitude A, and its phase ϕ (Fig. 29.1(c)). VEPs to pattern reversal have quite different properties to flicker VEPs (Spekreijse *et al.*, Chapter 2 of this book).

Steady-state VEPs to flicker and transient VEPs to pattern reversal were studied in 13 patients with classical retrobulbar neuritis, in a control group of 6 patients with unilateral retinal vascular lesions and in 6 normal subjects of similar age. VEPs were also recorded in 13 patients with spinal multiple sclerosis none of whom had a history of retrobulbar neuritis, and 6 of whom had no evidence of reduced acuity or disc pallor. Psychophysical measurements were made on 27 retrobulbar-neuritis patients, 19 spinal multiple-sclerosis patients, and 28 controls.

Visual evoked potentials in man: new developments (ed. J. E. Desmedt), pp. 461–69. Clarendon Press, Oxford 1977.

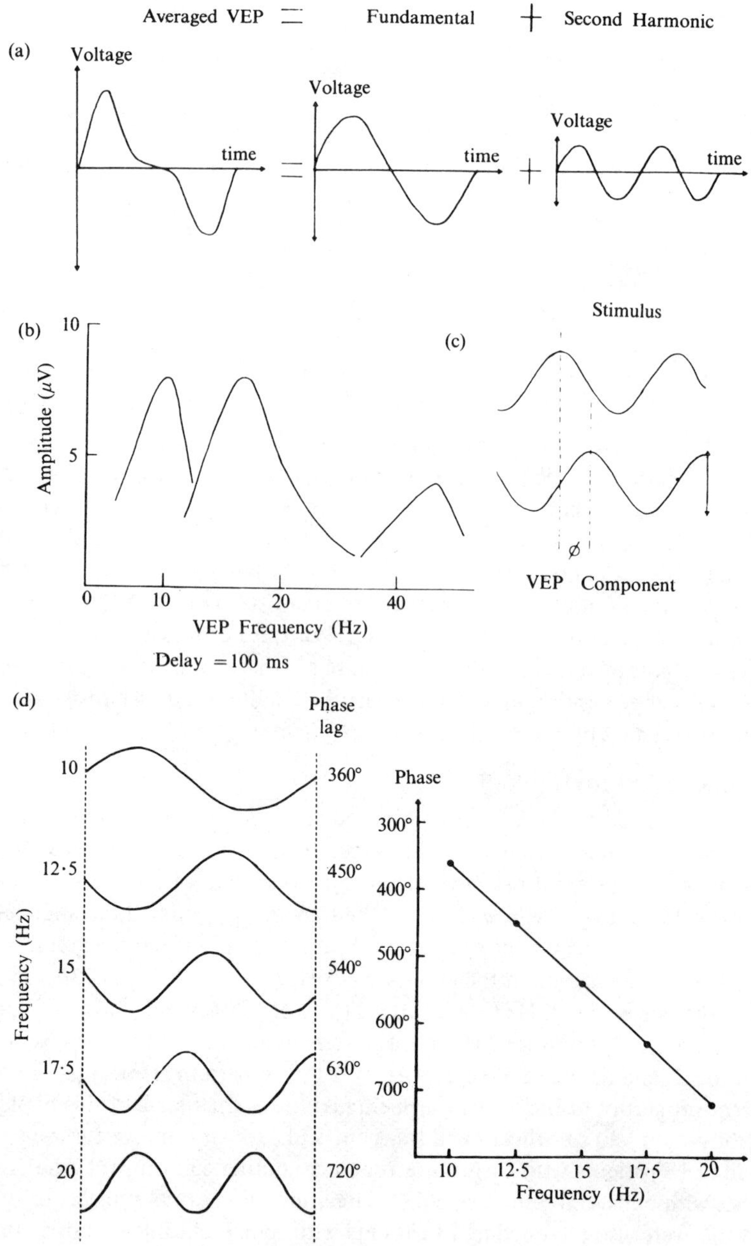

Fig. 29.1. (a) An example of the VEP elicited by flickering a light at F Hz. The waveform can be analysed into the two sine-wave harmonics as shown, a fundamental of F Hz and a second harmonic of $2F$ Hz. (b) Amplitudes of the fundamental components of steady-state VEPs to flicker of F Hz showing peaks near 10 Hz, 16 Hz, and 50 Hz. (c) Measurements on the fundamental VEP component of peak-to-peak amplitude A and phase lag ϕ. (d) The way in which a delay (here 100 ms) causes a phase lag between the VEP and the stimulus, and how this phase lag increases as stimulus frequency is increased. The plot of phase lag versus stimulus frequency is a straight line, the slope of which gives the delay (Regan 1969).

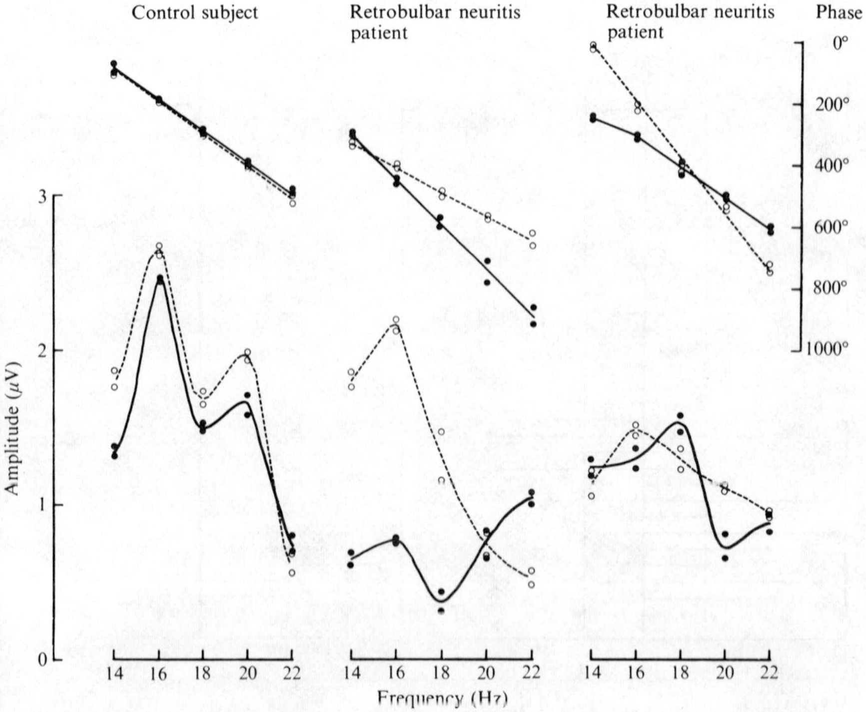

Fig. 29.2. Medium-frequency flicker VEPs in retrobulbar neuritis patients and control subjects. The control subject has similar amplitude and phase characteristics for each eye. The phase plot for the first retrobulbar-neuritis patient (left eye affected) shows an increased slope for the left eye corresponding to an increase in visual delay of 153 ms. The second retrobulbar-neuritis patient (right eye affected) shows an increased slope for the right eye corresponding to 116 ms increase in delay. (From Milner *et al.* 1974*a*.)

Results

Medium-frequency (13–25 Hz) flicker

Our main finding was that, in retrobulbar-neuritis patients, the phase versus frequency plot (Fig. 29.1(d)) was much steeper for the affected eye than for the unaffected eye (upper half of Fig. 29.2) (Milner, Regan, and Heron 1974*a*, *b*). The steepening of slope can be attributed to an increased delay (latency) in the affected eye, as explained in Fig. 29.1(d). All 13 patients with retrobulbar neuritis showed an increased delay in the affected eye. These delays were so large that they fell outside the range of the 12 control eyes and also outside the range for patients with retinal lesions. Thus the delay of medium-frequency flicker VEP is a test that can distinguish an *individual* patient with retrobulbar neuritis from these controls. The test is effective both in patients with poor acuity (counting

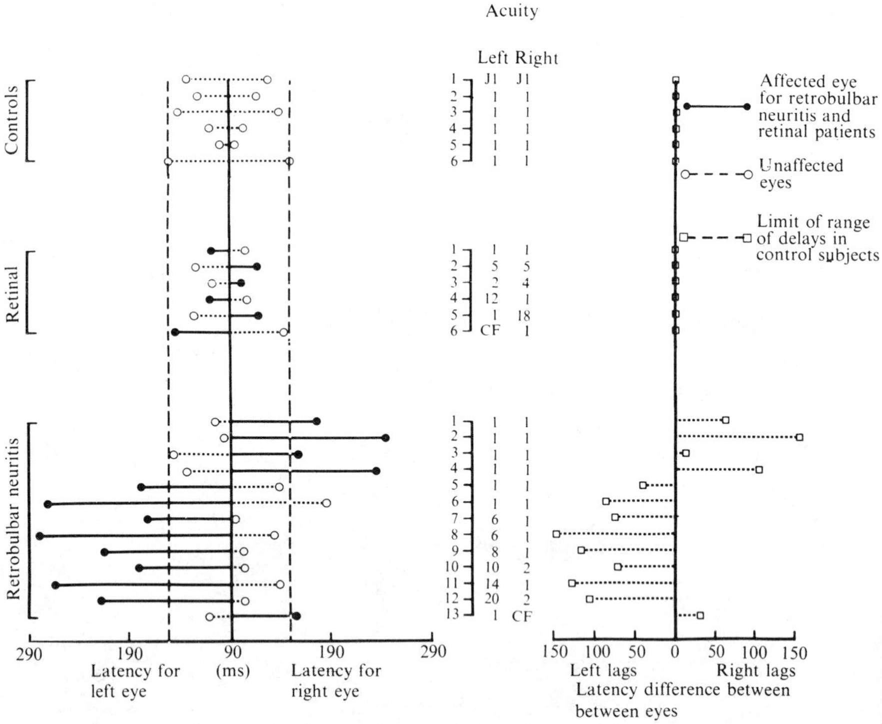

Fig. 29.3. Delays for medium-frequency flicker VEPs: results for all subjects. The lengths of the horizontal lines represent VEP delays. At the extreme right is shown the difference in delay between the left and right eyes in each individual subject. (From Milner *et al.* 1974*a*.)

fingers) and with J_1 acuity on the Jaeger scale. Increased delay persists long after an attack of retrobulbar neuritis, up to 12 years at least.

Fig. 29.3 shows the results of the medium-frequency flicker test for all subjects. A clear contrast is seen in the far right column which presents the difference between latencies for the left and right eyes by the length of the horizontal dotted line. The range of latencies for control subjects was only 8 ms. VEP amplitude was not a useful indicator of retrobulbar neuritis and it was reduced only in cases with poor visual acuity (Fig. 29.2).

High-frequency (35–60 Hz) flicker

High-frequency VEPs showed no difference in delays between the affected and unaffected eyes in retrobulbar-neuritis patients nor with respect to retinal patients and control subjects (Fig. 29.4). However, retrobulbar-neuritis patients differed in one curious manner from controls in that the phase plots for the two eyes were displaced bodily, by any angle from 0° to 180°, without change in slope (Fig. 29.4). The lack of change in slope meant that latencies were similar for the two eyes. We

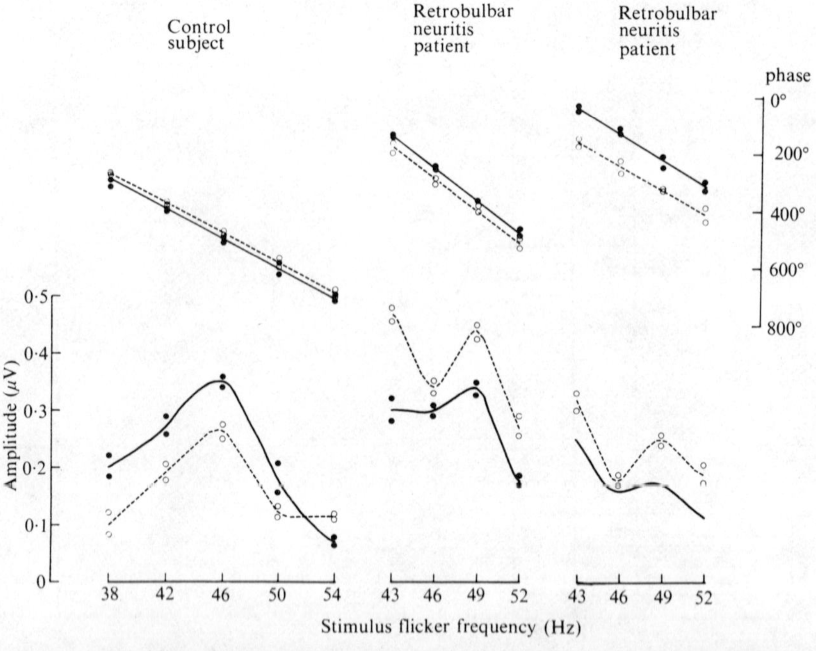

Fig. 29.4. High-frequency flicker VEPs in retrobulbar neuritis patients and control subjects. Continuous lines indicate the left eye, dotted lines the right. The right eye of each patient was affected by retrobulbar neuritis (and the slopes of the right eyes' phase plots were much increased for medium-frequency flicker VEPs), but for high-frequency VEPs the slopes of the phase plots are similar for left and right eyes. Hence, high frequency VEPs are not delayed by retrobulbar neuritis. However, the phase plot is displaced bodily in retrobulbar neuritis patients. (From Milner, Regan, and Heron 1974*a*.)

are not able to interpret this observation along the straightforward lines possible for 180° phase displacements (Regan 1973*a*, *c*).VEP amplitude was affected only when there were central scotoma.

Pattern-reversal VEPs

Pattern-reversal VEPs were recorded over a reversal frequency range from 4 Hz to 14 Hz for both small checks (14′, 4° field) and large checks (50′, 14° field) (see Fig. 29.5). For large checks, the left and right eyes of 10 retrobulbar-neuritis patients differed in latency so markedly that all patients fell outside the control range. Two other patients did not give measurable VEPs because of their poor visual acuities.

For small checks, 2 out of 8 retrobulbar-neuritis patients did not give abnormally delayed VEPs, even when left and right eyes were compared in individual patients. Furthermore, 3 patients did not give measurable VEPs.

Thus VEPs to large checks unequivocally indicate retrobulbar-neuritis patients, but in contrast to flicker they cannot be used when acuity is poor. VEPs to small

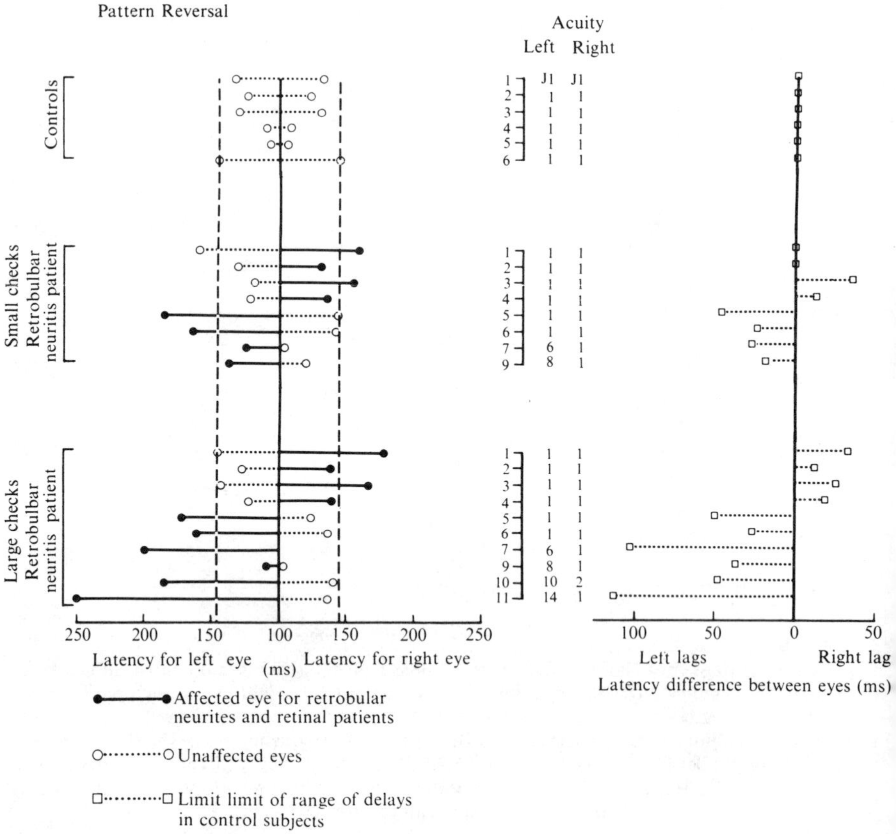

Fig. 29.5. Pattern VEP delays for all subjects. Patterns were small (14′) or large (50′) checks. Dashed lines represent the limits of the range of delays in control subjects for large and small checks. At the extreme right, differences in delays between the left and right eyes for each individual subject. These are abnormal for all retrobulbar-neuritis patients with large check stimulations, but for only 6 out of 8 retrobulbar-neuritis patients with small-check stimulation. (From Milner *et al.* 1974*a*.)

checks give some false negatives and seem less sure for retrobulbar neuritis than large-checks VEPs. This latter finding is surprising if one assumes that central vision is principally affected.

Comments

Medium-frequency flicker VEPs are delayed in retrobulbar-neuritis patients, whereas high-frequency flicker VEPs are not delayed. Medium- and high-frequency VEPs have quite different properties (Regan, see Chapters 2 and 4 of this book). Thus the above results might point to neural organizations within the visual pathway that are preferentially damaged by retrobulbar neuritis. More speculatively, since the visual signals leading to different types of flicker VEP may separate as early as retinal level (Spekreijse 1966), the different signals leading to medium- and high-frequency VEPs might travel in the optic nerve along axons with different susceptibilities to demyelinating disease.

Halliday *et al.* (1972, 1973*a*, *b*, and Chapter 26 of this book) found reliably abnormal transient VEPs to pattern in almost all retrobulbar-neuritis patients they studied. In practical terms our results are complementary, since the flicker test can be used in a patient whose acuity is so degraded that pattern VEPs cannot be measured.

However, Halliday *et al.* reported, like others, that VEPs to flash gave no reliable indication of retrobulbar-neuritis. The fact that we found retrobulbar neuritis to be reliably indicated by VEPs to both unpatterned and patterned stimuli may be due to the use of steady-state VEPs instead of transient VEPs.

Comparison between VEP delay and perceptual delay

We have found that visual perception is markedly delayed in retrobulbar-neuritis patients. One small light-spot (15′ diameter) was viewed by the left eye and a second one was viewed by the right eye. One light switched on before the other by an amount t ms that was varied until they appeared to the patient to switch on simultaneously. The time t ms then exactly compensated for his increased visual delay†. Every one of the 25 retrobulbar-neuritis patients studied was clearly outside the control range on this test (Heron *et al.* 1974). This group included 5 bilateral cases. We have found perceptual delays increased over 200 ms, though increases of 30–50 ms were most common. Since this subjective test is capable of detecting delays due to small 'islands' of demyelination it is not only simpler but it should in principle be more sensitive than the VEP tests which average over a comparatively large retinal area (Fig. 29.6). Nevertheless the VEP tests did give large latency increases that could reach 150 ms in some patients (Fig. 29.3, right). These large increases in delay observed in some patients are difficult to account for in terms of reduced axonal conduction speed due to demyelination (see Chapters 25 and 27 of this book).

Patients with spinal multiple sclerosis

Both medium-frequency flicker VEPs, large-check pattern VEPs, and abnormally delayed visual perception ('delay campimetry') were looked for in 13 patients suffering from spinal multiple sclerosis with no history of retrobulbar neuritis. One or the other of the three tests picked up a visual abnormality in 10 of the 13 spinal multiple-sclerosis patients who were examined with all three tests. While with retrobulbar-neuritis patients each of the three tests gave abnormal delays, only 2

†A subject's visual field can be mapped in terms of the perceptual delay at each point in the field. Such a 'delay field' (Fig. 29.6) is analogous to the conventional visual field for acuity as measured by perimetry or by Bjerrum screen campimetry.

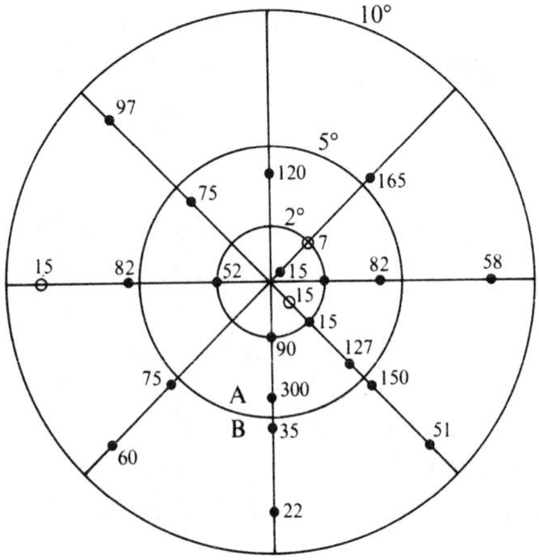

Fig. 29.6. Visual delay field for a multiple-sclerosis patient. The numbers are the delay of visual perception in milliseconds at different points in the right eye's visual field. Delays are measured relative to the left eye's fovea. The largest delay for control subjects is about 60 ms (limit of range). Note that very large delays (e.g. 300 ms, marked A) can be very localized and may be as close as 1° from a region of normal delay (marked B). Note also that the patchy areas of abnormal delay did not coincide with areas of reduced acuity.

of the spinal patients was abnormal on all three tests. These results can be compared with Halliday *et al.*, (Chapter 26 of this book).

In the spinal multiple-sclerosis patients the three tests used as a battery were much more effective than any one used singly. Although the numbers of patients studied are rather small, the VEP tests seemed to distinguish between the group of 7 patients with visual signs and the group of 6 patients without visual signs. Delayed pattern VEPs were recorded from almost all (6 out of 7) patients with visual signs, but from no patient without visual signs. In contrast, delayed flicker VEPs were recorded from only 1 (out of 7) patients with visual signs, but from 4 (out of 6) patients without visual signs. Perhaps this suggests that visual pathology was different in our spinal and retrobulbar-neuritis groups and, furthermore, that pattern and flicker VEPs evaluate different aspects of visual pathology. It was not surprising that our subjective test (delay campimetry) picked up 2 patients missed by the other two tests since, because of the small test stimulus (15′) used in delay campimetry, this test can detect small 'islands' of demyelination that would be insignificant with the large stimulus fields used in the other two tests (Fig. 29.6).

Thus measurements of visual delay by VEP recording or by psychophysical methods can aid the diagnosis of multiple sclerosis. Delayed flicker VEPs can be recorded even when there is no other evidence or history of visual pathology.

Multiple sclerosis patients need a markedly greater interval between two flashes of light in order to see then as double (13/14 patients at 0·01 level). This double flash measure is more sensitive than visual delay measured by either VEP or psychophysical means as an indicator of subclinical visual pathology (9/11 patients, at 0·01 level, with no history of retrobulbar neuritis and with normal fundi).

Apart from aiding diagnosis, the visual tests promise a means of monitoring the progress of demyelination and of aiding the assessment of experimental therapy. Elevating a patient's body temperature mimics increasing demyelination, while reducing body temperature improves axonal conduction. In some of our patients, double flash resolution was degraded when the body temperature rose and was improved when body temperature was reduced. Similarly, VEP delay increased as body temperature increased and decreased when the temperature was reduced.

Acknowledgements

This work was supported by the Medical Research Council. We thank F. Cartwright for technical support and H. Henry for assistance in preparing this chapter. We are grateful for the loan of a Delay Campimeter developed by Wilkinson Sword Research Ltd.

30. Visual evoked potential, electroretinogram, and electroencephalogram studies in progressive neurometabolic 'storage' diseases of childhood

A. HARDEN and G. PAMPIGLIONE
Department of Neurophysiology, Hospital for Sick Children, London

During this century an increasing number of neurometabolic 'storage' disorders which manifest themselves in infancy and childhood have been described. At first these were identified pathologically by the staining reactions of abnormally accumulating metabolites. More recently interest has centred on the biochemical structure of the stored material, and in some of these disorders the enzyme defect has already been identified. Enzyme studies offer the possibility of detection of carriers as well as recognition of the disease *in utero*.

Embryologically the eyes are part of the central nervous system, and it is hardly surprising that they should often share its fate in many of these neurometabolic diseases. Whenever such conditions are suspected our neurophysiological investigations have included not only electroencephalography (EEG), but also studies of the visual system by means of electroretinography (ERG), and cortical VEPs.

Over the last six years at the Hospital for Sick Children we have been using a simple technique for the combined recording of the non-corneal ERG, the VEP from the cortex, and the EEG to investigate children with a variety of suspected visual and cerebral disorders (Harden and Pampiglione 1970). The stimulus is a bright flash from a gas discharge lamp held close to the eyes. The averaged ERG is recorded from an electrode placed on the bridge of the nose between the eyes (summed response of both eyes unless one eye is covered during stimulation). The VEP is recorded from the mid-occipital region. In normal children over the age of 1 year the ERG and VEP recorded in this way show fairly consistent waveforms (Fig. 30.1). In the ERG there is a negative/positive complex ('a'- and 'b'-waves) with peak-to-peak amplitude varying from 11 μV to 45 μV provided the eyes are mostly open (Harden 1974). The VEP shows a consistent negative change with peak around 55 ms and amplitude ranging from 5 μV to 25 μV. This is usually preceded by a positive component with peak latency around 40 ms, which is of smaller amplitude

Visual evoked potentials in man: new developments (ed. J. E. Desmedt), pp. 470–80. Clarendon Press, Oxford 1977.

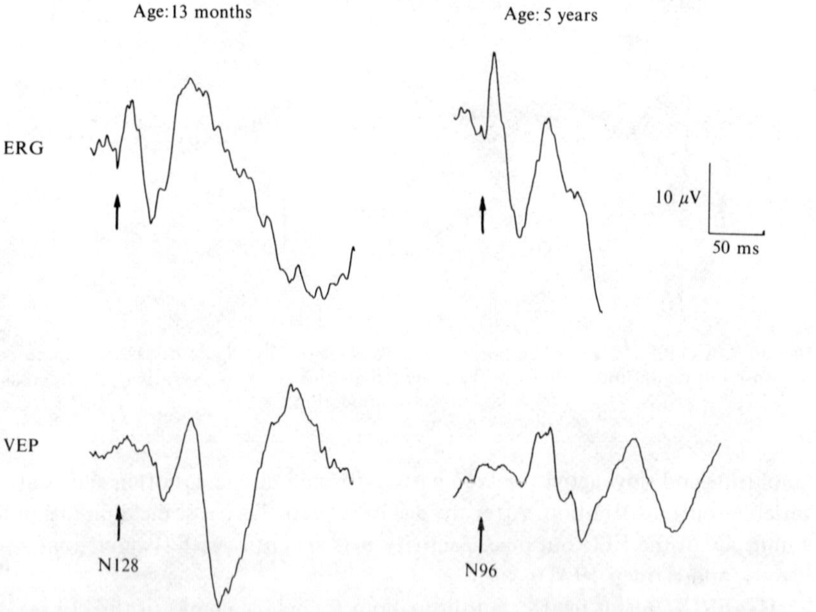

Fig. 30.1. ERG and VEP recorded from two restless and somewhat uncooperative normal children. For description of waveforms see text. A marked blink response is seen occurring after each retinal response. Stimulus at arrow. Negativity recorded as an upward deflection.

and not always easily recognizable. In our work greater importance is given to the VEP components occurring before 100 ms, which we refer to as the early components; the components occurring after 100 ms are more variable and seem to be altered by factors, such as attention, which are difficult to control in most young children.

Over 2000 such investigations have now been satisfactorily carried out during the waking state in babies as well as in active and retarded children without any sedation being necessary. Out of this total, 126 children have now been studied in whom a neurometabolic disorder has been verified histochemically and/or enzymatically. For the present study 82 cases have been selected because they could be grouped into one of the six distinct entities to be described below.

Tay–Sachs disease (17 cases)

The onset of clinical symptoms is usually in the first 6 months of life with progressive mental and motor regression and blindness. Death usually occurs at 3–4 years of age. There is intracellular storage of GM_2 ganglioside related to a deficiency of the enzyme hexosaminidase A.

The EEG shows relatively mild abnormalities during the first 12 months of life, even though the clinical signs are obvious before 1 year of age. Early in the second year the EEG deteriorates rapidly, with the appearance of irregular high

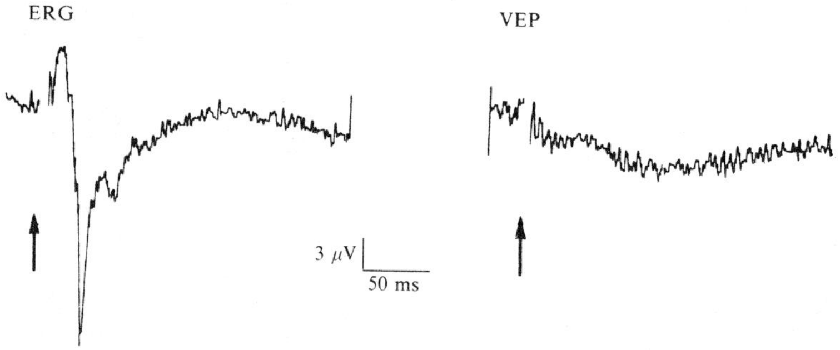

Fig. 30.2. A child of 2 years in a fairly advanced stage of Tay–Sachs disease with preserved ERG response but no definite VEP from the cortex. Stimulus at arrow. Negativity recorded as an upward deflection.

amplitude and slow activity mixed with ill-formed discharges often showing variable focal distribution. After the age of 2 years there is some diminution in amplitude of the EEG but phasic activity persists until death (Pampiglione, Privett, and Harden 1974).

The ERG remains unaffected throughout the whole course of the disease (Fig. 30.2), in keeping with the preservation of function of the outer retinal receptor elements (rods, cones, and bipolar cells), although the ganglion cell layer is grossly affected by storage material. The VEP is recordable in the early stages of the disease. However, the usual earlier components (before 100 ms) become poorly defined after 1 year and from 16 months of age the VEP is no longer detectable, suggesting that a complete loss of function of visual pathways and/or visual cortex has occurred.

Santavuori disease (5 cases)

This is a recently described form of 'neuronal ceroid lipofuscinosis' (Santavuori, Haltia, Rapola, and Raitta 1973). Clinically this disease begins soon after 12 months of age with rapid motor and mental regression so that by 3 years the children appear blind and are reduced to a vegetative state. These children may, however, survive many years. The storage material in the neurones is a lipofuscin-like substance but the enzyme defect is not yet known.

Soon after the onset of symptoms, a rapid deterioration of the EEG occurs with increasing slow activity which gradually decreases in amplitude. By the age of 3–4 years all phasic EEG activity disappears and the EEG remains equipotential throughout the remaining years of life (Santavuori 1973). The ERG and VEP decrease in amplitude parallel with the EEG deterioration, so that by the age of 4 years no retinal or cortical response is present (Fig. 30.3). These findings reflect the very rapid and severe cortical and retinal cellular loss while vital functions persist (Pampiglione and Harden 1974).

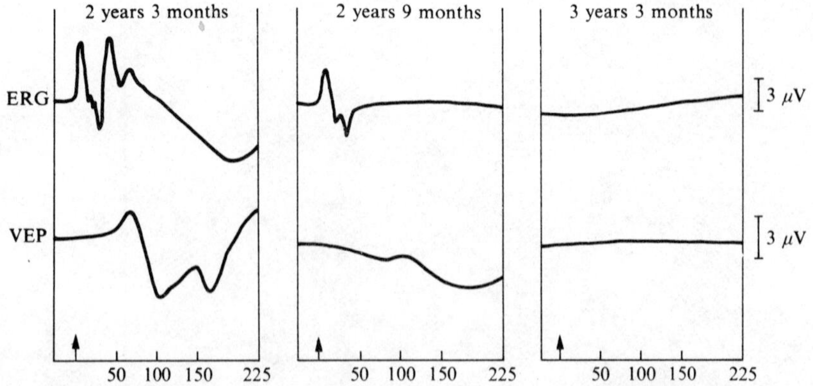

Fig. 30.3. Evolution of ERG and VEP in a child with Santavuori disease showing gradual disappearance of both ERG and VEP. The tracings have been smoothed to outline the main components. Analysis time 250 ms. Stimulus at arrow. Negativity recorded as an upward deflection.

Bielschowsky–Jansky disease (21 cases)

This is also called the late infantile form of amaurotic family idiocy, Batten's disease and neuronal ceroid lipofuscinosis. The clinical onset is at about 2–3 years of age with occasional seizures and motor and mental retardation, which progress with increasing myoclonic jerks. Death usually occurs at 6–7 years of age. There is neuronal storage of a lipofuscin-like substance, but the enzyme defect is not yet known.

From the early symptomatic phase the EEG shows a considerable abnormality with generalized large amplitude, irregular slow activity, and spikes or sharp waves of variable distribution. There is a distinctive EEG response to photic stimulation most obvious at low rates of flash (Fig. 30.4), with very large, polyphasic spikes, sometimes reaching 500 μV, most prominent posteriorly (Pampiglione and Harden 1973). The spikes related to each flash occur whether or not the child is jerking at the time.

These discharges are in fact grossly enlarged early components of the VEP, with latency and waveform comparable to the early components seen in normal children but with an amplitude some 12–20 times greater. In some patients there is an even earlier negative component than is observed in most normal children with a peak at about 35 ms. This grossly enlarged VEP is not altered with monocular stimulation (Fig. 30.5), in contrast with the more usual types of photosensitivity (Jeavons and Harding 1970). The ERG, however, is unrecordable from a fairly early phase of the disease, in keeping with the known progressive impairment of function of all retinal layers including rods and cones. This combination of ERG and VEP findings is even more remarkable because the characteristic enlarged VEP persists throughout the course of this progressive disease (Harden, Pampiglione,

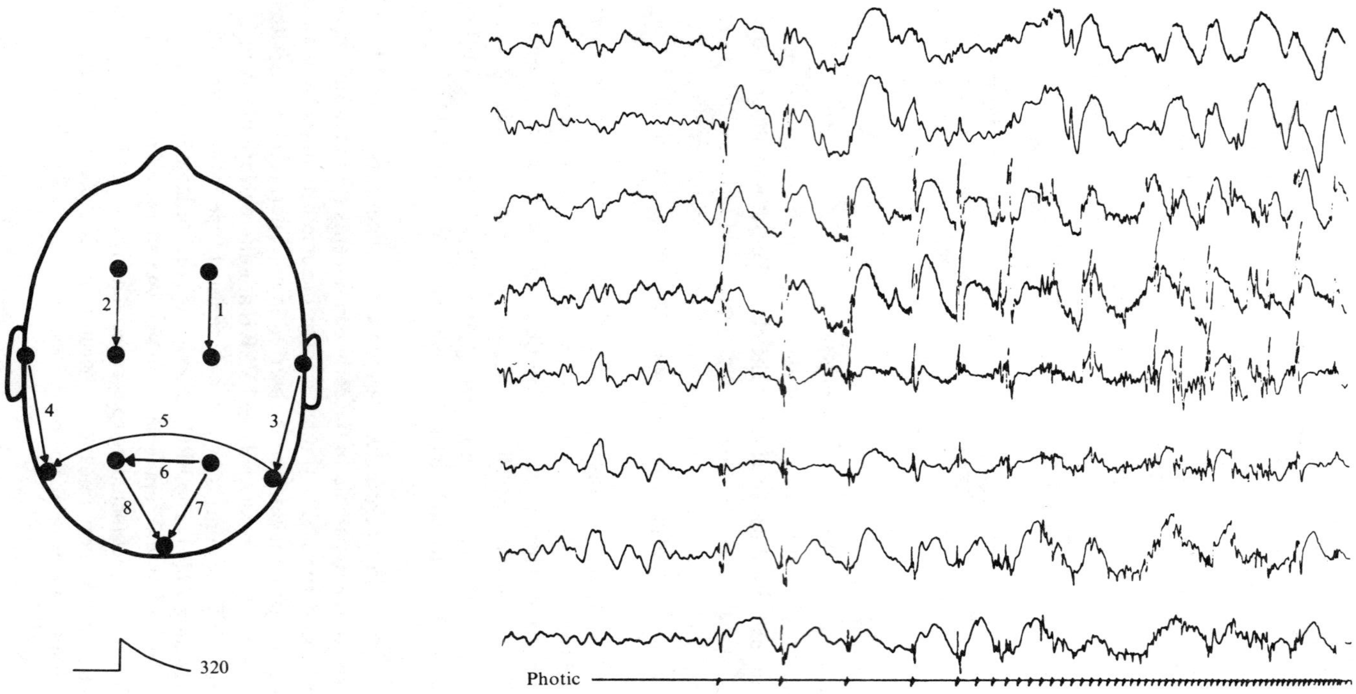

Fig. 30.4. EEG of a child aged $4\frac{3}{4}$ years with Bielschowsky–Jansky disease showing the spikes following each flash during photic stimulation, most obvious at low rates of stimulation.

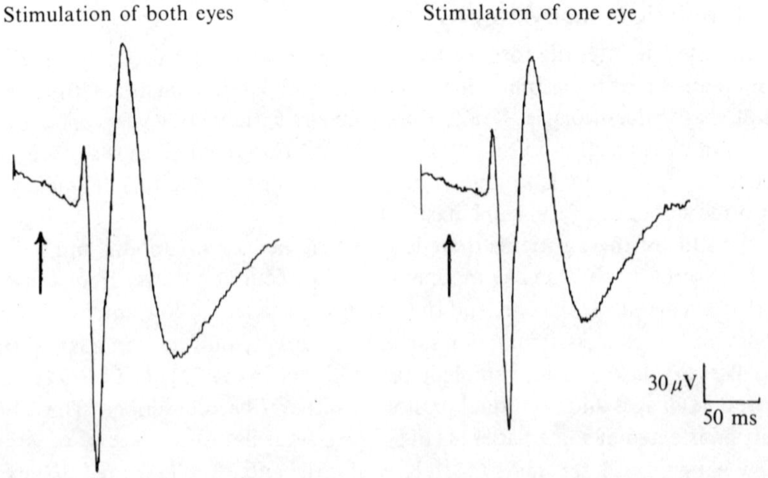

Fig. 30.5. A child of 5 years with Bielschowsky–Jansky disease showing grossly enlarged early components of the VEP (note size of calibration signal). This VEP is not reduced even if only one eye is stimulated. Stimulus at arrow. Negativity recorded as an upward deflection.

and Picton-Robinson 1973). Therefore, in spite of the early disappearance of the ERG, retinal function is presumably never completely lost. It must be remembered that the disappearance of the ERG, even when recorded from a corneal electrode, does not necessarily imply total loss of function of retinal receptors.

Spielmeyer-Vogt disease (5 cases)

This is also known as the juvenile form of amaurotic family idiocy, Batten's disease, neuronal ceroid lipofuscinosis, or neuronal lipidosis. The clinical symptomatology begins after 5–6 years of age with progressive visual loss and, later, mental deterioration and fits. Death usually occurs after the age of 15 years. The neuronal storage material is a lipofuscin-like substance but the enzyme defect is not known.

There is a slowly increasing abnormality in the EEG of these patients, with an excess of irregular slow activity and often prolonged somewhat rhythmic discharges of spike–wave complexes at a frequency of about 2/s (Pampiglione and Lehovsky 1968; Ellingson and Schain 1969). The ERG disappears at a fairly early phase of the disease, in keeping with the early retinal involvement of all layers, including the rods and cones. In some patients a small-amplitude VEP is still seen for some years, often with only ill-defined early components but in keeping with limited function of visual pathways to the brain. However, in the older patients the VEP is no longer recognizable, indicating a progressive and ultimately complete loss of function of visual pathways and/or visual cortex.

Metachromatic leucodystrophy (15 cases)

Clinically the late infantile form of the disease begins before thirty months of age, with increasing motor disability and hypotonia and, later, dementia with development of spastic quadriplegia. Death usually occurs within a few years. The juvenile form usually begins after 5 years with mental deterioration and runs a more prolonged course. There is storage of cerebroside sulphate due to a deficiency of cerebroside sulphatase (aryl sulphatase A).

In the EEG of these patients there is a gradual increase in amount and amplitude of fairly rhythmic components. These occur at a slower frequency than that expected for the age, and there is also an excess of low-amplitude fast components. Discharges are uncommon and are usually only seen at a late phase of the disease (Mastropaolo, Pampiglione, and Stephens 1971). The ERG is well preserved at all ages and no retinal pathology has ever been described. The VEP persists unaffected in some patients (Fig. 30.6), regardless of the age of onset, but in a few patients, at later stages (both late infantile and juvenile forms), the early components of the VEP become poorly formed and the response may even be absent. The reason why the cortical VEP should not be uniformly affected in all patients is not understood.

Mucopolysaccharidoses (19 cases)

At least 6 types have been recognized, each with characteristic clinical and enzymological features. There is storage of mucopolysaccharides and of gangliosides.

Only relatively minor EEG changes are seen in most patients with any type of mucopolysaccharidoses and there is no marked deterioration of the EEG features during the course of the disease (Hanefeld and Pampiglione 1972). No obvious abnormality of the ERG and VEP occurs in most of the children tested before 10 years of age (Fig. 30.7), although in some of our older patients there is a moderate reduction of amplitude of the ERG and sometimes the early components of the VEP. Gills, Hobson, Hanley, and McKusick (1965) have reported a subnormal ERG in many of their patients, some of whom were less than 10 years old. It would appear that the retina may well be progressively involved at least in some types of the mucopolysaccharidoses.

Discussion

Systematic studies of the ERG and VEP, as well as the EEG, are few for any of these neurometabolic disorders of childhood. While a single examination may be valuable, it is the evolution of these combined parameters that gives greatest information. Our studies show that there are combinations of neurophysiological features evolving in a particular way which are fairly characteristic for each neurometabolic disorder we have described (Table 30.1). Not only are the ERG–VEP–EEG features important in the differential diagnosis of each group of diseases

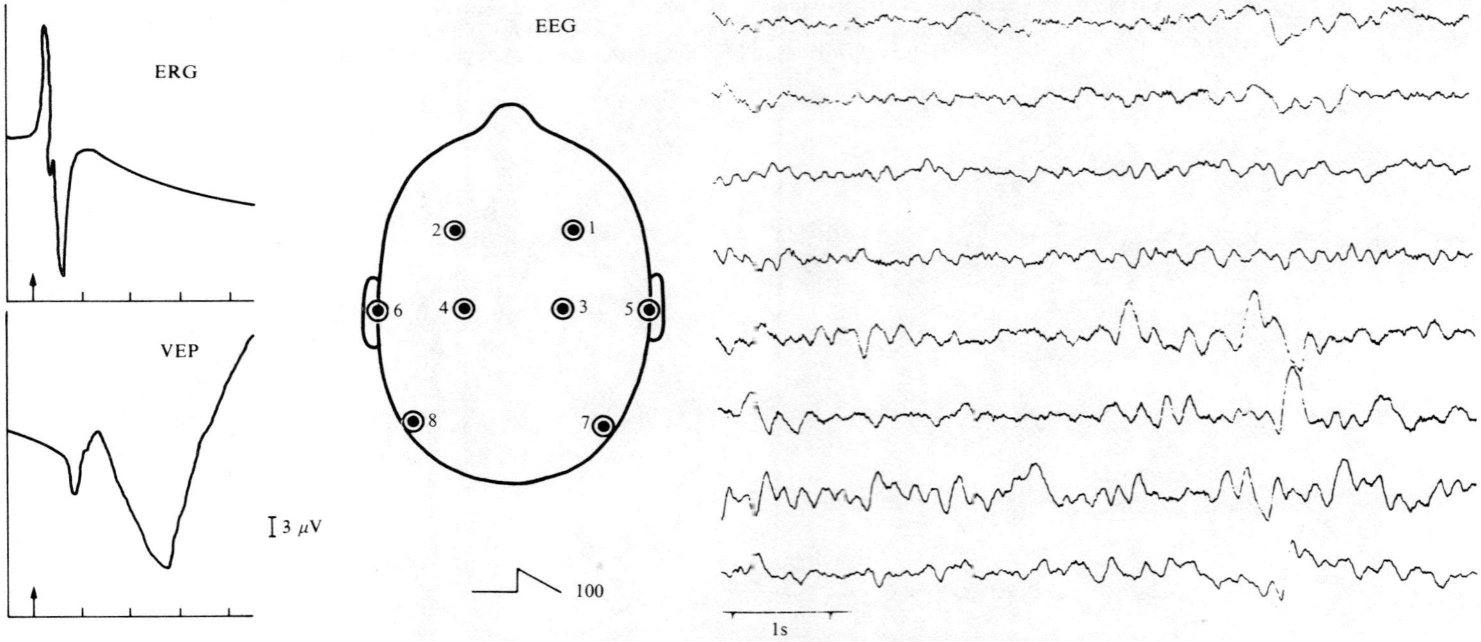

Fig. 30.6. The ERG and VEP are well preserved in this child of 3 years with metachromatic leucodystrophy, although the EEG shows an excess of rhythmic 4–6 Hz activity (child awake). Average reference recording. The tracings of the ERG and VEP have been smoothed to outline the main components. Analysis time of ERG and VEP is 250 ms. Stimulus at arrow. Negativity recorded as an upward deflection.

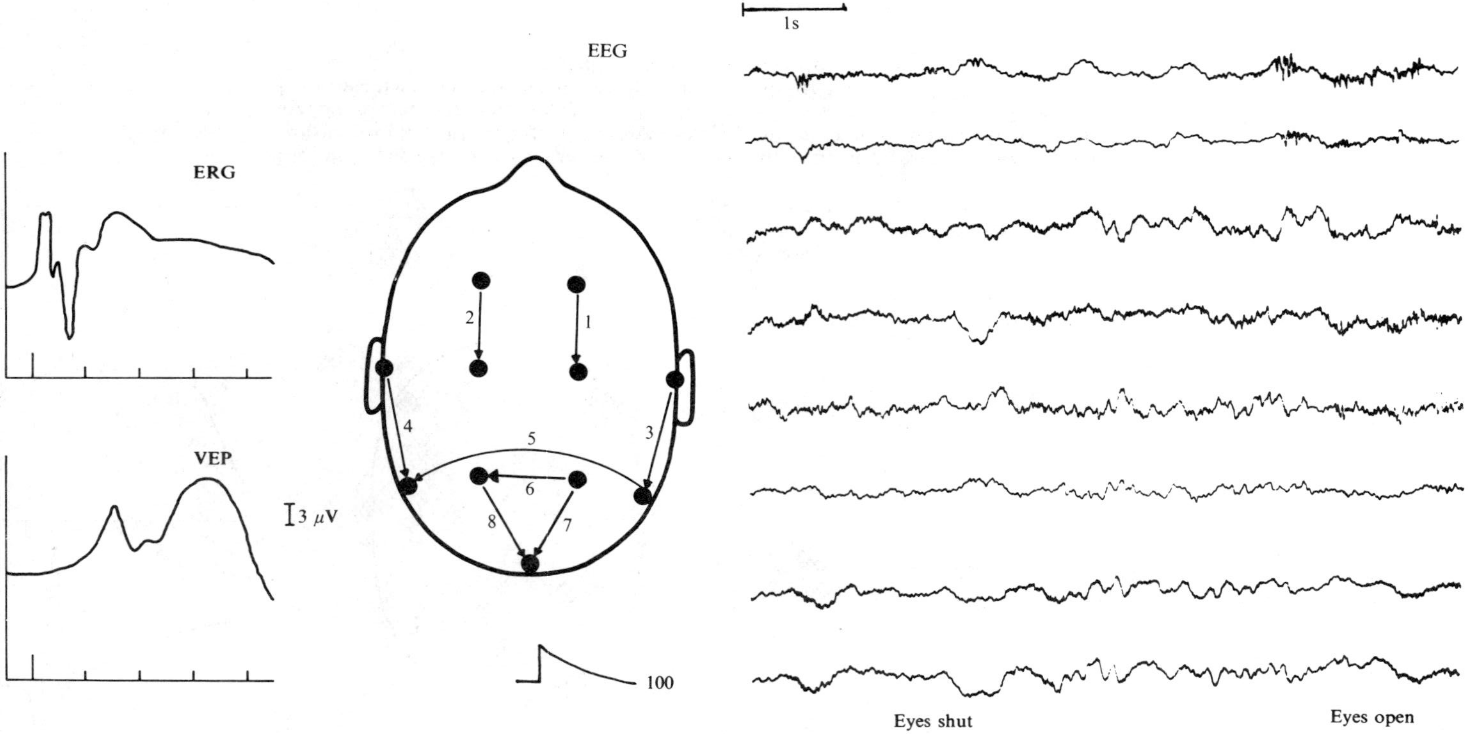

Fig. 30.7. In this child of 3 years with Hurler type of mucopolysaccharidosis, the ERG, VEP, and EEG show no gross abnormality. In the EEG the rhythmic activity produced by eye closure in the occipital region is in keeping with the child's chronological age (compare Fig. 30.6). The tracings of the ERG and VEP have been smoothed to outline the main components. Analysis time of ERG and VEP is 250 ms. Stimulus at arrow. Negativity recorded as an upward deflection.

TABLE 30.1 *Progressive neurometabolic 'storage' diseases of childhood*

Disorder	ERG	VEP
Tay–Sachs disease	Present	Present → poor → absent
Santavuori	Small → absent	Small → absent
Bielschowsky–Jansky	Small → absent	Grossly enlarged
Spielmeyer–Vogt	Small → absent	Present → poor → absent
Metachromatic leucodystrophy	Present	Present, poor, or absent
Mucopolysaccharidoses	Present or small	Present

but also in distinguishing them from other cerebral disorders of childhood which clinically may present in a similar way. An early diagnosis of these inherited diseases is important in relation to both prognostic and genetic implications.

Of particular interest are the groups of conditions described variously as Batten disease, neuronal ceroid lipofuscinosis, neuronal lipidosis, or amaurotic family idiocy, in which there is storage of a substance which resembles lipofuscin and/or ceroid. Some workers consider these conditions as a single disease entity with a variety of clinical expressions (Zeman and Dyken 1969). On neurophysiological grounds it appears that at least three distinct groups can be recognized (Santavuori, Bielschowsky–Jansky, and Spielmeyer–Vogt), each group showing a fairly homogeneous clinical picture. The only common neurophysiological finding is an early loss of the ERG after the onset of symptoms.

Moreover, we have also seen 12 other patients all with similar histochemical findings clinically called Batten's disease, in whom the ERG is also absent. However, their other neurophysiological features evolve differently from these three groups and therefore have not been included in this series. It is felt that these 'odd patients' probably represent even rarer, as yet unidentified, forms, each probably having its own particular neurometabolic-pathway disorder.

Although there are now sophisticated techniques for the recording of the VEP, particularly in relation to pattern stimulation, it must be stressed that any techniques involving the cooperation of the patient for fixation cannot be undertaken in young or retarded children. From a clinical point of view it is precisely in this type of patient that a neurophysiological approach has the greatest potential applications. Although the flash stimulus is regarded as crude, it is perhaps the best means of obtaining results with difficult children and from our experience the flash VEP gives reliable indications as to the integrity of the visual pathways to the brain. When this VEP is combined with the recording of the ERG and EEG, an even greater amount of information can be obtained, as has been shown in children with neurometabolic diseases. Such combined neurophysiological studies are not only helpful in relation to diagnosis, but also give the opportunity to study differentially the ways in which the retina, visual pathways, and various regions of the maturing brain are progressively involved in a number of disease processes.

31. Visual evoked potentials to flash in the clinical evaluation of the optic pathways

R. P. BORDA
Department of Neurophysiology, The Methodist Hospital and *Department of Physiology, Baylor College of Medicine, Houston*

There have been numerous reports in recent years of how the VEP may be altered in various disorders of the optic pathways, and much interest has been directed toward the use of patterned stimuli (see Chapters 23, 26, and 27 of this book). Pattern stimulation undoubtedly can be a valuable adjunct to clinical assessment of the visual system, but there are difficulties inherent in its application to routine screening. The main drawback to the use of patterned stimuli is that it requires the full cooperation of the subject; this precludes its use in infants, comatose patients or those under anesthesia, and malingerers. It also requires that the subject be able to focus the stimulus image properly, which demands that adequate refraction be employed and, in most cases, that cycloplegics are not administered.

Because of the difficulties noted above with using patterned visual stimuli, non-patterned (flash) stimuli appear to be the most practical for routine clinical use. The VEP to non-patterned flash possesses a rather high intra-subject variability in waveform, yet, as Vaughan and Katzman (1964) and Jacobson, Hirose, and Suzuke (1968) have pointed out, the VEPs to stimulation of each eye individually are, in any one subject, very similar in waveform and latency. There is also little difference in waveform and latency between responses recorded from homologous locations over the two hemispheres. Relatively slight hemispheric asymmetries of the occipital VEP, or discrepancies between monocularly evoked potentials, can be of diagnostic significance then, and are the basis for the routine clinical procedure used in this laboratory.

Methods

The routine clinical VEP procedure used in this laboratory involves the presentation of 75 flashes to each eye (the other eye is patched), followed by an additional 75 flashes with both eyes open. Electrodes are placed bilaterally over the occipital area, 3 cm from the midline and 2 cm above the inion. An additional electrode is placed at the vertex and all recordings are made with linked-ear reference electrodes. The lamp is placed 45 cm from the nasion but is moved closer if the

Visual evoked potentials in man: new developments (ed. J. E. Desmedt) pp. 481–89. Clarendon Press, Oxford 1977.

recordings must be made through closed eyelids. The flash stimuli are produced by a Grass photostimulator which contains a xenon flash tube and produces a bright, very brief (10 μs) blue–white flash. Where contamination by the auditory stimulation accompanying the light flash is considered to be a problem, masking noise is presented binaurally through lightweight earphones (Telex). Standard EEG amplifiers are employed and the signals are averaged over a 500 ms interval with a general-purpose digital computer (Digital Equipment Corporation PDP-12; digitizing bin width = 1 ms).

Normal VEP to flash

The occipital VEP generally presents five or more identifiable peaks (Fig. 31.1(a)). As previous authors have reported, the shortest-latency VEP component that can be identified in a high proportion of normals is a negative peak at about 40 ms. Using the nomenclature adopted at this symposium (polarity-mean latency), the components of the VEP illustrated in Fig. 31.1(a) are referred to as N40, P71, N91, P114, and N154. In this laboratory, the range of normal values for the latencies of these peaks is as follows: N40, 36–60 ms; P71, 50–80 ms; N91, 70–120 ms; P114, 95–155 ms; N154, 115–200 ms.

Certain features of the occipital VEP are fairly consistent across subjects and have proved to be useful in the assessment of visual function. Latencies of the early components, in particular, have been found sensitive to disorders of the optic nerves. In this laboratory, the latency of the early components carries much more weight than waveform or amplitude in the determination of 'normality'. The VEP

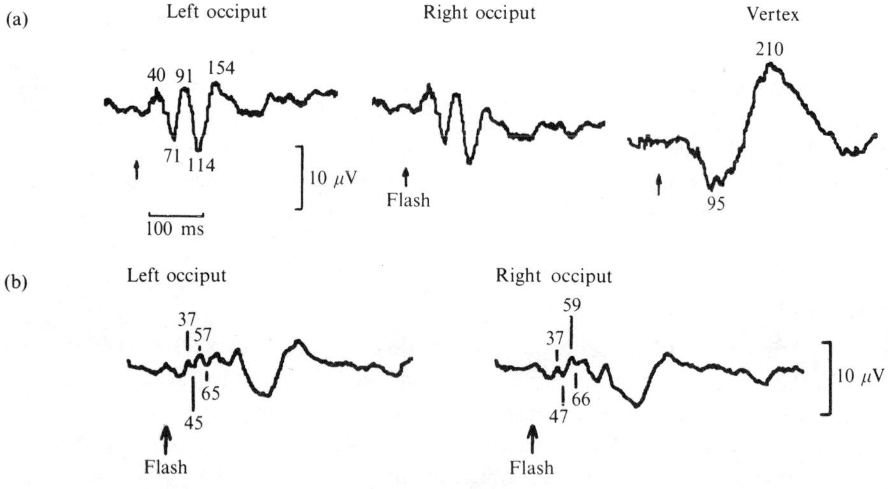

Fig. 31.1. (a) Normal VEPs to binocular flash stimulation, recorded over left and right occipital regions and from the vertex, all referred to linked-ear electrodes. In this and all subsequent figures, negativity at the active electrode is represented by an upward deflection. (b) Normal VEPs from left and right occipital regions in response to binocular flash stimulation.

of Fig. 31.1(b), for example, recorded from a subject with no disturbance of visual function, bears little resemblance to that shown in Fig. 31.1(a). Yet several peaks can be identified (N55, P70, N83, P105, N119) that fall within the above mentioned ranges. In the absence of significant hemispheric asymmetrics and marked differences in the VEPs to left and right monocular stimulation, these VEPs would be considered normal.

Lesions of the optic nerves and tracts

Valuable information for diagnosis results from the comparison of the VEPs to unilateral stimulation and the simultaneous analysis of hemispheric symmetry. For example, the patient in Fig. 31.2 with a 'patchy' loss of visual field in both

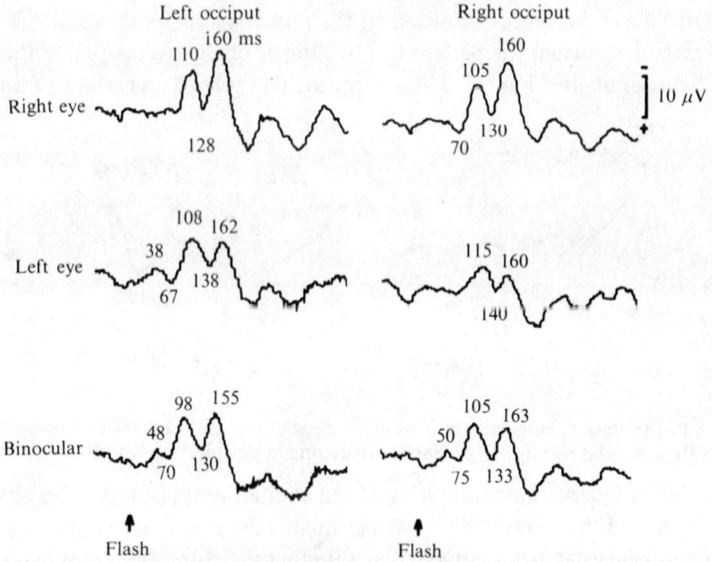

Fig. 31.2. VEPs to flash in a female patient of 65 years, with a tumour impinging upon the optic chiasm. Note the hemispheric asymmetries in the short-latency components with monocular stimulation.

eyes, had a normal electroretinogram (ERG) and a normal occipital VEP with binocular stimulation. Close comparison of the VEPs to stimulation of the left eye and of the right eye reveals clear-cut discrepancies, however. The evoked VEPs of the right eye are larger in amplitude and most of their peaks are of shorter latency. This alone would be indicative of a dysfunction of fibres in the left optic nerve. Another significant finding is the presence of short-latency components (less than 100 ms) over only the hemisphere ipsilateral to the stimulated eye. There is a small positive peak (P70) present in the VEP recorded from the right occipital area to stimulation of the right eye, but a comparable component is absent or greatly attenuated in the analogous left-occipital VEP. Similarly, with stimulation of the left eye, short-latency components (N38, P67) are evident over the left-occipital region but are absent over the right. There are also some slight differences in latency of homologous peaks, with those from the ipsilateral hemisphere having shorter latencies. All of these data suggest some interruption of crossing fibres in the region of the optic chiasm. The patient was eventually found to have a 4 x 6 cm supracellar meningioma lying over the optic chiasm. In our experience, recordable VEPs are usually present in lesions which affect the optic tract or nerves only secondarily through pressure on the fibres, but are not present in gliomas or other primary tumours of these pathways.

Lesions of the thalamocortical radiations or visual cortex

The VEP often can document disorders of the post-thalamic portions of the visual system, particularly when the patient is unwilling or unable to cooperate for tests of visual fields or acuity. Fig. 31.3 illustrates such a case, a 16-year-old victim of

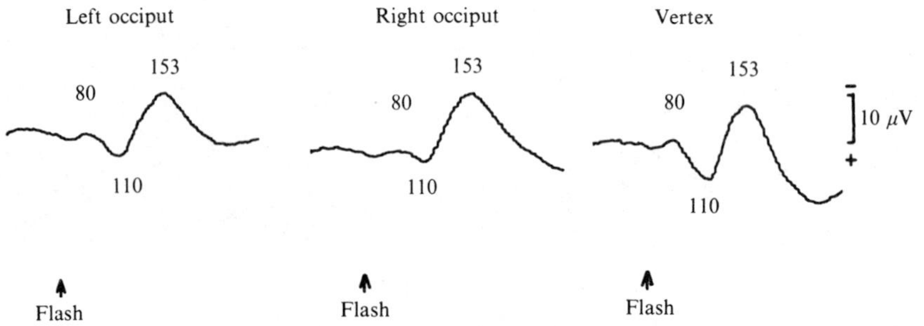

Fig. 31.3. VEPs to flash (binocular stimulation) in a patient of 16 years with a concussive injury to the occipital region. No potential originating in occipital cortex can be identified.

an automobile accident. Binocular stimulation elicited symmetrical VEPs at the occipital sites, and these might have been evaluated as relatively normal except for the lack of short-latency components, a finding that typically accompanies optic nerve disorders. A well-developed vertex response to photic stimulation was evident in this patient, however, suggesting that optic impulses were reaching at least the brain-stem centres. The vertex potential was similar in waveform and latency to the occipital VEPs but was of larger amplitude. This suggests that the 'occipital' VEPs recorded in this patient may have been volume-conducted posteriorly from the vertex region. Such potentials would, of course, have been greatly attenuated if a bipolar recording derivation had been used, and valuable information would have been lost. VEPs can be recorded from the vertex following stimulation in any sense modality and they have been called 'non-specific' potentials. Although there is, as yet, no agreement as to the mechanisms underlying the vertex potentials, they do appear to represent activation of pathways independent of the direct thalamic radiations to the occipital cortex.

The patient of Fig. 31.3 recovered visual function to an acuity of 20/50 within 10 months of the accident, yet his occipital VEPs were unchanged. It is not known whether this means that the macular region of the cortex had been premanently damaged or whether, as in other diseases, the EEG signs recover more slowly than the clinical symptoms.

Tumours or vascular lesions of the primary visual cortex or association areas are usually diagnosed by other techniques, but also produce abnormalities in the VEP. In Fig. 31.4 are shown VEPs recorded from a woman thought to have

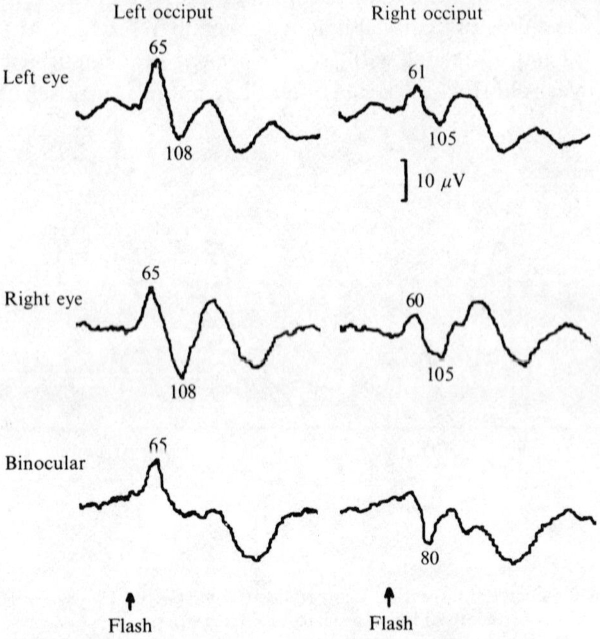

Fig. 31.4. Occipital VEPs to flash in a patient of 34 years with a meningioma of the right posterior-parietal region. Note the consistent hemispheric asymmetry.

symptoms of a primarily psychiatric origin. There is an obvious suppression of the EPs over the right-occipital region compared to those recorded from the contralateral occipital site. Amplitude differences as great as 50 per cent are not uncommon in normals, but the right-occipital VEP is almost always larger than the left. More striking in this patient is the disparity between monocular and binocular VEPs. In normals, binocular stimulation typically evokes a VEP of larger amplitude and slightly shorter latency than monocular stimulation. In this patient, the VEPs to binocular stimulation appear attenuated in comparison to the monocular VEPs. Radiographic contrast studies in this patient revealed the presence of a right posterior-parietal mass, which was eventually removed and identified as a meningioma. In retrospect, the VEP abnormality might have been related to functional interruption of visual association pathways.

Degenerative disorders of the central nervous system

The VEP in degenerative neurological disorders has proved to be useful primarily in documenting the progression of the disease rather than in aiding in its diagnosis. One exception to this may be the finding (Harden *et al.* 1973; Harden and Pampiglione, Chapter 30 of this book) that the VEP is useful in differentiating two subgroups of the type of neuronal lipidosis generally referred to as Batten's disease, the forms being associated with grossly elevated VEP amplitudes. One such patient, a 5-year-old (Fig. 31.5) had onset of symptoms (with seizures) at 3

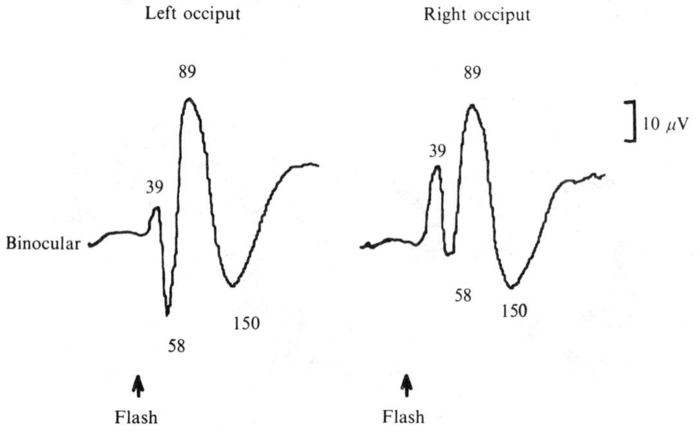

Fig. 31.5. Supranormal occipital potentials in a patient of 5 years with biopsy-confirmed juvenile cerebral lipidosis (Batten's disease).

years of age, and a cerebral biopsy confirmed the diagnosis of Batten's disease. One of his siblings, who had the same fluorescein pattern in the fundus, was also tested, but the VEP in this child (a 2-year-old) was of normal amplitude and latency. This child had not yet developed seizures or other clinical symptoms. It is not known whether such findings correspond to different disease entities or merely reflect a degenerative process with variable ontogeny and rate of progression.

The mucopolysaccharidoses, another type of metabolic storage disorder, have been studied in more detail in our laboratory. This disorder (with its six subcategories: the Hurler, Hunter, Sanfillipo, Morquio, Scheie, and Maroteaux–Lamy syndromes) is generally associated with marked VEP abnormalities which include increased latencies, attenuation of amplitude, and alteration of VEP topography, all no doubt reflecting gross disturbance of cerebral function. A 3-year-old child with a mild form of Hunter's disease (mucopolysaccharidosis type II) was tested serially (Fig. 31.6) while receiving treatment with purified plasma fractions of

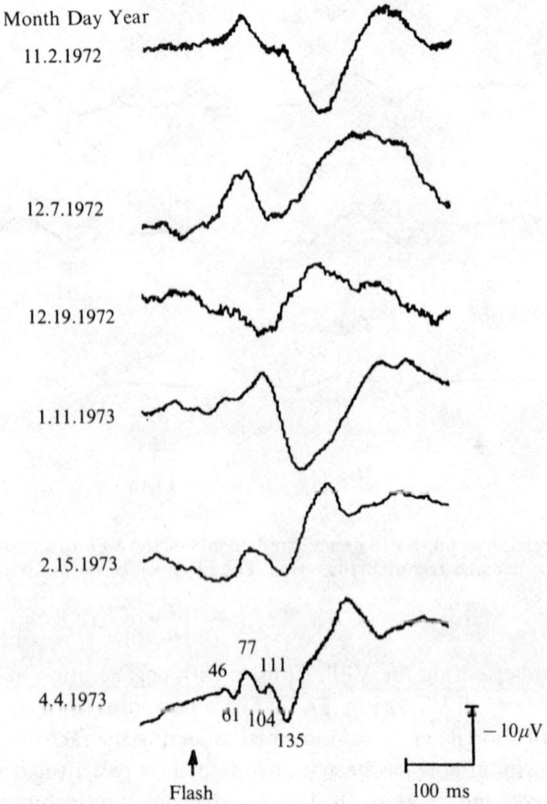

Fig. 31.6. Serial changes in the occipital VEP in a patient of 3 years with the mild form of Hunter's disease, undergoing treatment with purified plasma fractions.

normal serum (Coppa, Singh, Nichols, and Di Ferrante 1973) which theoretically corrects the enzymatic deficiency responsible for the abnormal protein metabolism. The patient's clinical and behavioural improvement with therapy was dramatic. The VEP was one of the few laboratory tests the changes of which seemed to parallel the child's clinical improvement. After more than one year of therapy, the VEP showed for the first time short-latency components that fell within the normal range. This case illustrates how VEP recordings can be of great value in assessing the efficacy of therapy.

Relationship to retinal function

The VEP is most commonly considered a test of neural function, but it obviously depends upon retinal function as well. The occipital VEP reflects activation of fibres arising primarily from the macular region (central 8–10°) of the retina. For this reason, any disorder affecting this portion of the retina may be expected to

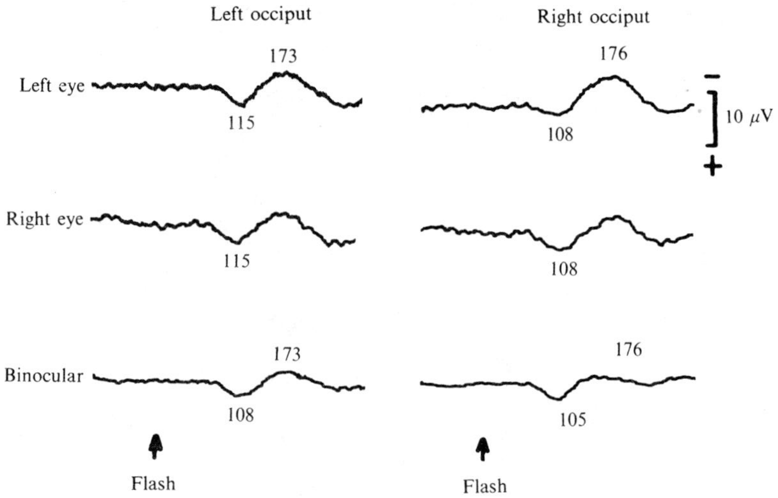

Fig. 31.7. Suppression of all short-latency components of the VEP in a patient with degeneration of the macular region of the retina. The ERG was of normal amplitude.

have a profound effect on the VEP. Patients with degeneration of the macula do, in fact, have abnormal VEPs (Fig. 31.7). These responses are characterized by a total absence of short-latency components, reflecting the fact that most of the input to the occipital pole has been interrupted. This patient had an ERG of normal amplitude, indicative of the lack of widespread retinal involvement. The converse is seen in retinitis pigmentosa, an inherited disorder with gross ERG abnormalities. The VEP in these patients may be essentially normal (Fig. 31.8) since the disease most commonly affects the periphery of the retina first, sparing the macula until the later stages of the degenerative process.

This independence of the ERG and VEP, pointed out by Schreinemachers and Henkes (1968), indicates how the two test procedures may be complementary (see also Harden and Pampiglione, Chapter 30 of this book). In the case of suspected retinal disease, the VEP can be of value in assessing the degree of macular involvement, and in the case of neurological disorders, the ERG can occasionally detect unsuspected retinal disorders.

Comments

The VEP to flash can be a very useful routine procedure in the evaluation of visual system disorders. Utilization of a diffuse stroboscopic flash as a stimulus, while in many cases not as informative as patterned stimuli, is applicable to patients of all ages, in all states of consciousness, and with varying degrees of patient cooperation. There will undoubtedly be marked advances made in the technique so that more

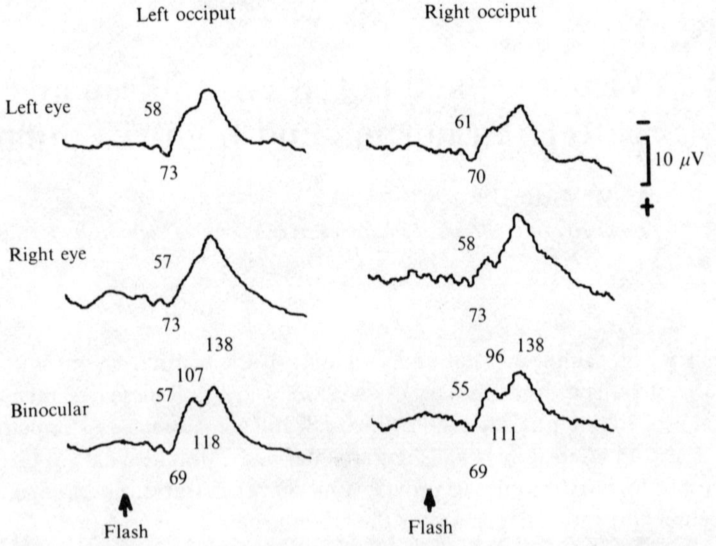

Fig. 31.8. VEPs of normal latency, recorded in a patient with retinitis pigmentosa; the ERG was non-recordable.

precise evaluations can be made. Indeed, recent work on sinusoidal intensity-modulation (flicker) (Spekreijse *et al.*, Chapter 2 of this book; Regan, Chapter 25 of this book) indicates that this mode of stimulation has a great potential as a diagnostic aid.

Acknowledgements

The work described in this chapter was supported in part by grant HL-05435 from the National Heart and Lung Institute, National Institute of Health, United States Public Health Service.

32. Visual evoked potentials to flash and pattern in normal and high-risk infants

M. M. MARCUS

University of California, San Francisco and *Sonoma State Hospital, Eldridge*

Efforts towards gaining a better understanding of the maturation of the central nervous system have used a variety of electrophysiological measures, including cerebral evoked potentials to auditory, visual, and somatosensory stimulation. There is also an interest in establishing well-defined, normative data in the first months of life, both in order to provide a means for detecting developmental or sensory impairment, and to monitor the effectiveness of intervention.

VEPs to flash

Dustman and Beck have studied waveform (1966) and amplitude changes (1969) from infancy to adulthood. The latency of VEP appeared significantly associated with both mental and motor scores at 8 months (Butler and Engel 1969) and verbal articulation skill at 3 years (Engel and Fay 1972), but no later measures of cognitive competence have been related up to the age of 7 (Engel and Henderson 1973; Henderson and Engel 1974). The infant occipital VEP to flash stimulation is larger in amplitude and simpler in waveform than that of the adult and it easily fatigues with repetitive stimulation (Ellingson 1968, 1970; Ellingson, Lathrop, Danahy, and Nelson 1973; Ellingson, Danahy, Nelson, and Lathrop 1974). Because of the great inter-individual variability of the waveform, the VEP to flash has been said to be unsuitable for making judgments about individual babies. Although different values of P2 component latency have been found, depending on the recording conditions, there is general agreement that latency decreases as a function of post-natal maturity, when maturity is based on gestational age.

In spite of marked inter-individual variability the VEP to flash in premature infants may be characterized as follows. Below 30 weeks gestational age a slow, high-voltage negative wave may be the only response. This subsequently begins to separate into two negative components (Hrbek, Karlberg, and Olsson 1973). Also, using an O_Z-P_Z derivation, Umezaki and Morrell (1970) report in the pre-term an initial negativity followed at about 32 weeks with a positive component and then another negativity. After 35 weeks post-term the common neonatal waveform is usually evident, though the P2 component is longer in

Visual evoked potentials in man: new developments (ed. J. E. Desmedt), pp. 490–99. Clarendon Press, Oxford 1977.

latency than that of the term infant. Latencies for this component at about 35 weeks range from 219 ms to somewhere around 275 ms (Umezaki and Morrell 1970). Ferris *et al.* (1967) show differences at term depending on weight (over 3 kg: 184 ms; under 2 kg: 219 ms). The occipital region is the source of both pre-term and full-term VEPs.

The presence of a known neurological impairment is not always reflected in an aberrant VEP to flash (Watanabe, Iwase, and Hara 1972; Ellingson 1968). Some brain-damaged infants do not produce any VEP at all in the first few days, and if they do, the latencies may be long with atypical waveforms (Hrbek and Mares 1964). Graziani, Weitzman, and Pineda (1972) did not detect abnormalities in the VEPs of their premature infants with respiratory distress unless hypoxaemia had occurred. When severe hypoxia persisted, the response tended to disappear but would reappear with the prompt application of resuscitation. Intracerebral haemorrhages were found at autopsy in infants who had abnormal evoked responses. Further studies are required to assess the suitability of VEPs for making clinical judgements on individual patients.

VEPs to pattern

That newborns attend selectively to pattern (Fantz 1963) indicates an innate human ability to perceive form. Clinically, it is particularly important to assess infant capacity for pattern processing, since it has been shown in behavioural studies that attention to pattern is reduced in neurologically compromised infants (Sigman, Kopp, Parmelee, and Jeffreys 1973). VEP to pattern and flash appear to be rather similar during infancy and become discrepant with increasing age. VEPs to pattern appear to reduce inter-individual differences (Marcus 1971).

Harter and Suitt (1970) carried out a longitudinal study of the VEP to checkerboard patterns in a normal infant from 21 days to 156 days and showed that size of checks influenced the amplitude of the infant's VEPs as an inverted U-shaped function. As the child grew older, progressively smaller check sizes evoked larger P2 components and by about 70 days the relationship became the characteristic U-shaped mature response (Harter and White 1968). These and more recent results are discussed in Chapter 17 of this book. Karmel, Hoffman and Fegy (1974) studied 13- and 20-week-old infants and showed, that the 'moving' inverted-U-shaped function, rather than being due to peripheral mechanisms, probably derives from maturation of central receptive field properties in the visual cortex. The increasing VEP amplitude to checks of smaller sizes paralleled behavioural measures of looking behaviour (Karmel 1969) and also appeared to be more closely related to chronological and neurological ages (P2-latency) than to gestational age. This latter observation suggests the significant role of environmental experience on central processing of form in development (Siegel, Coleman, and Riesen 1973).

Comparison of normal and high-risk infants

An investigation of P2 latencies of VEPs to flash and pattern was carried out on 101 infants at the Infant Development Research Laboratory in San Francisco's Children's Hospital. Those born at risk were placed in the intensive-care unit nursery or transferred there from another hospital. The control group consisted of 32 term or near-term infants (gestational ages from 260 days to 389 days) who were considered to be within normal limits by the attending staff. Most of these infants were discharged from the hospital 3–4 days after birth. Other normal infants at older ages were obtained through the well-baby clinic or referral. Four infants were returned for testing at later ages and their data is included, yielding a control group of 36.

The 62 high-risk babies were tested soon after they were released from their incubators or some short period thereafter (infants who were monitored in the recovery room were not kept in incubators but were available for testing only as long as it was determined that their condition would not be compromised). Three of these infants were brought back for testing at later periods, and this data is included. Each infant was assigned an Apgar value, rated on a scale of 1 to 10 (the optimum value), based on the infant's colour, pulse rate, response to stimulation, muscle tone, and respiration.

Each infant was brought to the testing room where a Beckman miniature Ag–AgCl electrode was pasted to the occipital scalp at the inion and approximately 2·5 cm to the right. Maximal VEPs to checks were obtained by recording at, rather than above, the inion. Furthermore, electrodes placed too close to the midline occasionally produced a negativity of the P2 component. By moving the electrode farther to the right, the P2 polarity reversed. A reference electrode was clipped to the right earlobe. No baby was tested unless the resistance proved to be less than 5000 Ω and eyes were open. The session was terminated if the baby appeared to be falling asleep and could not be awakened. Testing was often attempted again at a later point during the session but if this was unsuccessful the child was returned to the nursery.

The signals were fed into amplifiers set at 1–20 Hz with a 6 dB per octave roll-off (Bastin Associates, Hayward, California) then into a CAT (computer of average transients) 1000. This narrow bandpass was suggested by C. T. White (Harter and White 1968) since the 10–20 Hz range was rather sensitive and also tended to reduce contamination by movement artifact. Similar frequency limits were set by Harter and Suitt (3–35 Hz) and Karmel (2–30 Hz) with their infants. Preliminary testing indicated that setting the higher frequency limit at 20 Hz, rather than 30 Hz, had little, if any effect on the VEP.

The infant was tested in a shielded enclosure and was held at a distance of 30 cm to face a 20·3 x 28·0 cm (8 x 11 inch) window, which trans-illuminated black and white checkerboards with three check sizes (small = 4 mm, medium = 16 mm, or large = 48 mm). All checkerboards had equal amounts of black and white area. The clear flash was presented through an additional neutral density filter which reduced the luminance to equal that of the checkerboards. The light stimulus was provided by a Grass photostimulator set at a value of 8 (on a scale of 1–16) and triggered once per second. The CAT averaged 50 samples of 500 ms and a voltage calibrator wired in series with the occipital electrode provided a step recorded between 400 ms and 500 ms.

Fig. 32.1 illustrates read-outs from three high-risk infants at different ages. (Apgar ratings of 9, 5 min spent under each of four conditions: large checks, medium checks, and small checks (random order among infants) and flash.) Only the latency of the P2 component was identified. This was recorded independently by two assistants; data were discarded when the P2 component was poorly identifiable or when an infant fell asleep and could not be re-aroused. Thus all infants are not represented for all the VEP conditions.

A number of other measures were also taken into account for each infant: chronological age from birth; gestational age from the first day of the mother's last menses prior to conception; weight at birth and on the day of testing; and Apgar ratings at 1 min and at 5 min after birth.

The total group of subjects ranged in chronological age at testing from 2 days to 3 months of age. Table 32.1 summarizes the distribution by race, sex, and

TABLE 32.1 *Distribution of total sample by race, sex, and health status*

	Normal			High-risk			Total
	Caucasian	Black	Oriental	Caucasian	Black	Oriental	
Male	12	5	1	26	5	2	51
Female	10	8	0	13	15	4	50
Total	22	13	1	39	20	6	101

health status within the sample. The pathological conditions which determined risk varied both in kind and severity (Table 32.2). Table 32.3 reports the inter-correlations among all measures for all babies and appears to suggest that response latencies to patterns, but not to flash, correlate significantly with gestational age at birth and Apgar rating at 5 min after birth but not the 1 min score. (Apgar 5 and 1 respectively). Both flash and pattern latencies correlate highly with chronological age and body weight at testing. It is difficult to interpret the significance reached by the latency of only the small checks with birth weight, particularly since the latencies of the patterns seem to correlate more highly with one another than they do with the flash. This isolated association may be an

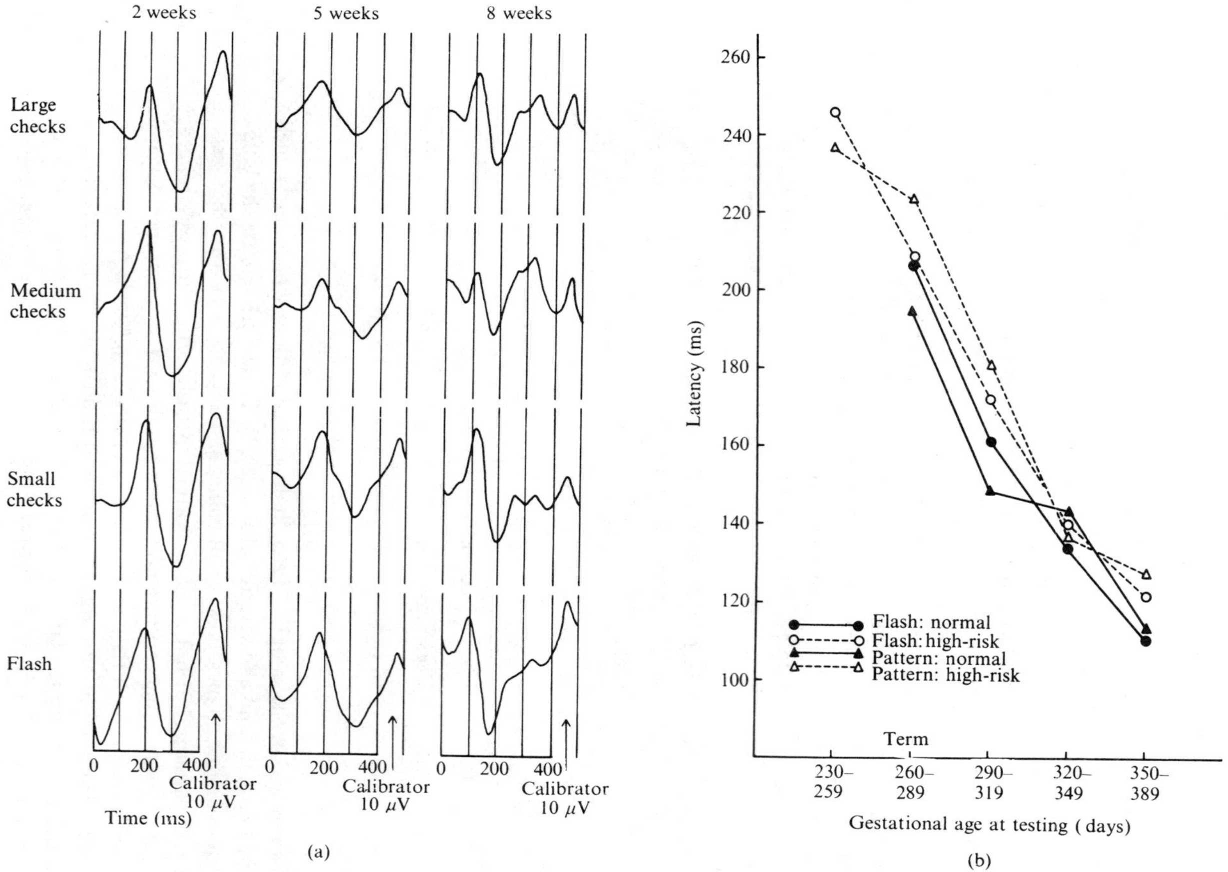

Fig. 32.1. (a) VEPs recorded from 3 infants at 2, 5, and 8 weeks of age. Though all 3 infants were born at risk, the VEP waveforms are essentially like those of normals. Positivity recorded upwards. (b) Mean latencies of VEPs to flash (circles) and to medium checks (triangles) at successive gestational ages in high-risk infants (open symbols) and in normal infants (filled

TABLE 32.2 *Kinds and frequencies of pathology among high-risk infants*

Pathology	*n*	Pathology	*n*
Hyperbilirubinaemia	16	Bilateral cortical atrophy	1
Hydrocephaly	3	Paralysis	2
Prematurity	14	Depression	3
Respiratory distress	14	Poor and inappropriate reflexes	3
Small for gestational age	9	Physical anomalies	2
Seizures	6	Heart murmurs	2
Heroin addiction	4	Meconium stained	10
Hypoxia due to cord about neck	10	Congestive heart failure	1
Pneumonia	3	Neurological malfunctions	2
Sepsis	1	Haematoma	3
Meningitis	2		

actual one or merely the chance significance that one expects to find among a large number of associational measures.

The relationship of gestational age at testing within each of the high-risk and normal groups was further carried out by means of a Pearson correlation. In addition, and within the normal group only, an effort was made to separate the effects of gestational age and weight (which tend to covary) on latency measures. Table 31.4 summarizes these results, and it may be seen that when the groups are separated the association between gestational age at testing and VEP latencies reaches high levels of significance and, for the normal group at least, is an almost monotonic function. When gestational age is held constant in the normal group, test weight has no association with the pattern latencies, but does significantly with the flash.

To confirm that selection of infants represented two separate sample groups an analysis of variance was carried out on the Apgar ratings. In order to determine whether there were differences between groups with respect to latency for flash and pattern irrespective of age of testing, an analysis of covariance was applied to the data. Because the latencies to all three check sizes tended to correlate so well with one another only the mean latency of the P2 to the medium checks was used.

The two groups differed significantly at both the 1 min and 5 min Apgar ratings. For these same groups significant differences were shown for P2 latency for pattern but not for flash (Table 32.5).

It seems clear then with this sample of babies that in normal infants P2 latency to flash has some bearing on maturity as measured by body weight, but this same relationship does not hold for pattern. Furthermore the P2 latency to flash does not separate the sick and well babies but the latency to pattern does. These two separate systems may perhaps be considered in terms of general physiological and general neurological development.

TABLE 32.3 *Intercorrelations among measures on normal and high-risk infants*

	1	2	3	4	5	6	7	8	9	10	11
1. Chronological age	1·00										
2. Gestational age at birth	–04	1·00									
3. Gestational age at test	88	44	1·00								
4. Birth weight	–10	70	25	1·00							
5. Test weight	78	36	86	41	1·00						
6. Apgar 1	–03	39	16	16	–03	1·00					
7. Apgar 5	19	31	32	15	24	60	1·00				
8. Small checks	–62	–38	–74	–23	–63	–12	–32	1·00			
9. Medium checks	–64	–37	–75	–15	–61	–13	–32	98	1·00		
10. Large checks	–61	–36	–74	–20	–62	–16	–31	97	97	1·00	
11. Flash	–56	–20	–61	–18	–58	04	–14	79	93	83	1·00

Correlations above ± 22: $p < 0{\cdot}05$
Correlations above ± 28: $p < 0{\cdot}01$

TABLE 32.4 *Pearson r correlations of body weight and gestational age at testing with VEP latencies*

	Gestational age (high-risk)	Gestational age (normal)	Body weight (normal only)	Gestational age (normal only). Body weight Constant	Body weight (normal only). Gestational age Constant
Small checks	−0·68†	−0·87†	−0·72†	−0·70†	+0·00
Medium checks	−0·70†	−0·87†	−0·74†	−0·67†	−0·08
Large checks	−0·67†	−0·87†	−0·71†	−0·69†	+0·05
Flash	−0·52†	−0·91†	−0·86†	−0·69†	−0·42‡

† $p < 0{\cdot}01$
‡ $p < 0{\cdot}05$

TABLE 32.5 *Variance analysis of Apgar ratings and VEP latencies (all measurements in milliseconds)*

	Apgar (1 min)		Apgar (5 min)		Medium checks		Flash	
	Mean	n	Mean	n	Mean	n	Mean	n
Pathology								
Normal	8·4	33	9·3	30	153	35	166	22
High-risk	7·2	50	8·5	39	189	51	184	38
Variance of Apgar ratings	$F = 15{\cdot}12$ $p = 0{\cdot}003$		$F = 7{\cdot}06$ $p = < 0{\cdot}01$					
Covariance of VEP latencies					$F = 3{\cdot}77$ $p = < 0{\cdot}05$		$F = 0{\cdot}397$ $p = 0{\cdot}53$	

It has been reported elsewhere (Marcus 1970) that flash and pattern waveform differences are not generally seen in infancy. In the course of a new study on developmental changes using a 3–20 Hz bandpass (24 dB roll-off) we obtained the records of Fig. 32.2 from an 84-day-old infant, which clearly indicates waveform differences. One may observe the slight latency shift at round 115 ms (P2) and the amplitude difference at 200 ms. In adults the differences between pattern and flash VEP waveforms occurs at least at 100 ms in the form of a polarity reversal and in some cases even earlier. One might presume various cortical structures to be related to such differences with age.

Discussion

The study of normal and high-risk infants appears to indicate that use of VEP to pattern at different ages may increase the clinical applicability of VEP testing: the wide inter-individual variability of the flash VEP reduces its effectiveness for predicting individual developmental outcome. The VEP to pattern seems to offer much greater possibilities but the question whether it will prove helpful in the clinical context of the individual patient and with only certain disorders is yet to be determined.

If one considers (a) that waveform differentiation between flash and pattern VEPs does not occur until later in infancy (Marcus 1971) and (b) that this differentiation occurs more in some forms of mental retardation than in others (Marcus 1970), one must conclude that the neurological maturation of higher cortical centres is quite relevant to the processing VEP to pattern. Whether the delay in latency of the pattern VEPs in high-risk infants compared to normals at the same gestational age is due to neurological immaturity or trauma affecting the development of these centres (Kayama 1974), or whether confinement in incubators

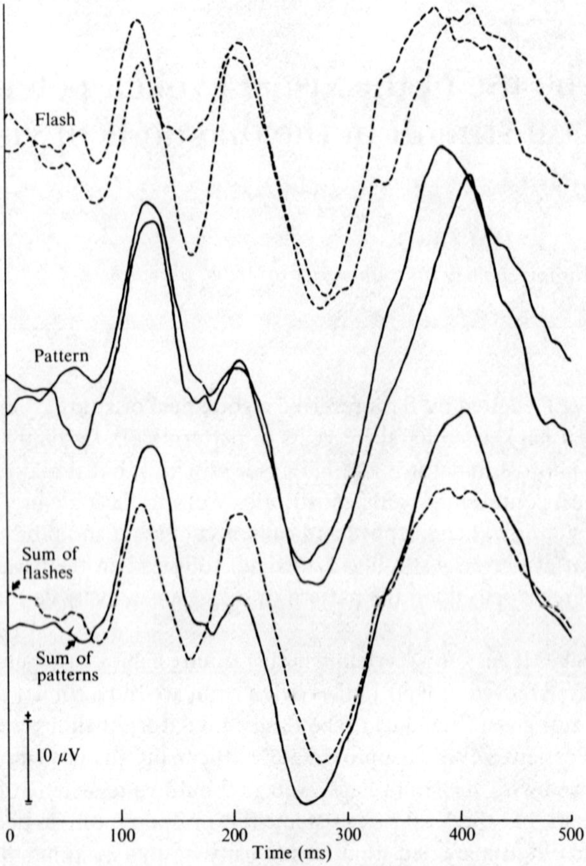

Fig. 32.2. VEPs to flash and to medium checks in an 84-day-old infant.

precludes adequate form stimulation leading to delays of receptive field development is unclear. In animals post-natal visual experience with contour can alter the firing pattern (Hirsch and Spinelli 1970) of single cortical cells.

Acknowledgements

The project reported in this paper was supported in part by grants from the Bureau of Maternal and Child Health, California State Department of Public Health, and NIH Grant 5 P01 HD 05317, NICHHD.

The author wishes to acknowledge the assistance of Dr. William Mallory in the statistical analysis of the data reported.

33. The use of the visual evoked potential to flash stimuli in the diagnosis of visual defects

G. F. A. HARDING
Neuropsychology Unit, University of Aston, Birmingham

Although the VEP elicited by flash received a good deal of study from early workers, interest has shifted in recent years to pattern VEP. Certainly the high-intensity flash photostimulator is a rather crude stimulus, but it may prove useful in certain clinical conditions as a diagnostic aid. VEPs to flash are useful when the patient is very young or handicapped and cannot cooperate and produce subjective responses. A pattern-reversal stimulus is difficult to use when the patient cannot or will not adequately focus upon the pattern or may even actively de-focus a pattern stimulus.

The VEP makes it easy to ascertain whether young babies have perception of light, the averaged record to light flashes being compared to a similar average when the stimulus is not given (Fig. 33.1). The flash stimulator is held by a technician in front of the patient's eyes at approximately 20 cm and the head and eye movement are followed with the lamp. Each average should be repeated at least 3 times in order to ascertain that the VEP is consistent. If no response can be obtained, further tests are carried out at increased stimulus intensity up to a maximum level of 483 nit per s. It is important to monitor the EEG simultaneously because frequently these children have suspected brain damage, and gross abnormality in the EEG may modify the VEP. Generalized bilateral symmetrical and synchronous discharges in the EEG may often affect the occipital regions to an equal degree, thereby obscuring the VEP (Fig. 33.2). Averaging sweeps with random intervals between the stimuli may provide evidence that an abnormal EEG background activity is being time-locked by the stimulus. On the other hand, localized anomalies of the occipital areas may affect the VEP, so that it appears to be reduced in amplitude and is not so clearly localized to the occipital electrodes. The monitored EEG, however, will reveal the localized abnormality and help evaluate the VEP (Fig. 33.3). Generalized or localized lesions are not always expected, and indeed the clinical history may give no suggestion of the possibility of such abnormalities. The child frequently does not have a reported clinical history of convulsions,

Visual evoked potentials in man: new developments (ed. J. E. Desmedt), pp. 500–508. Clarendon Press, Oxford 1977.

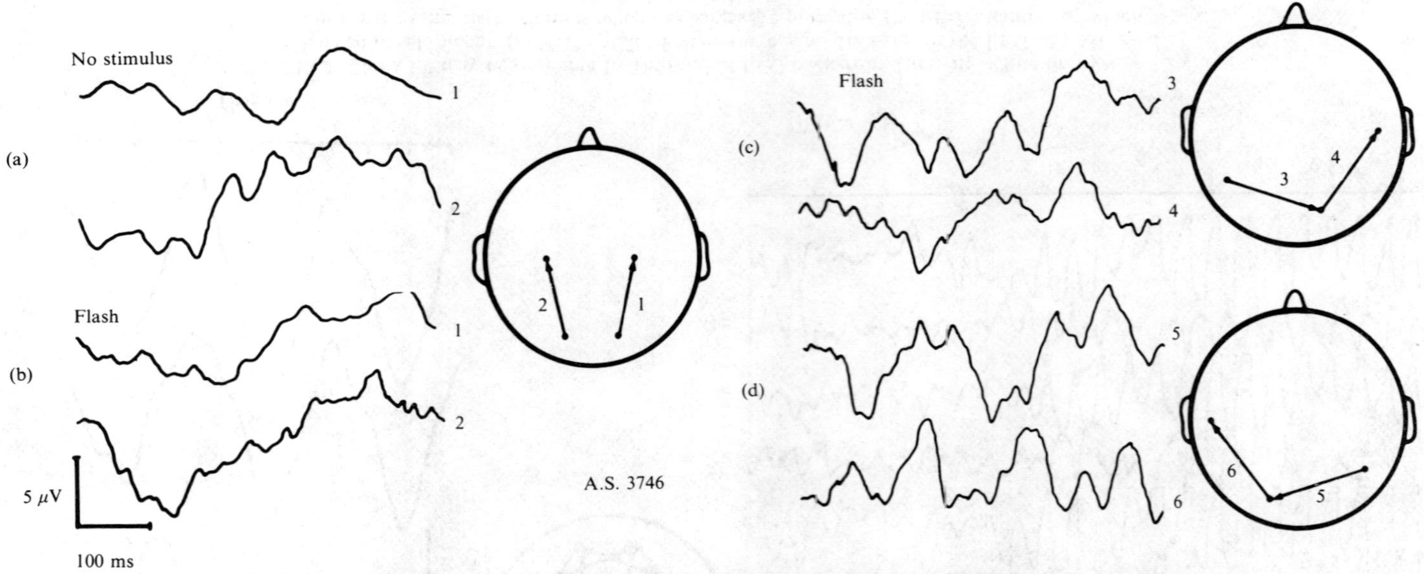

Fig. 33.1. VEP to flash in a child of 1 year and 7 months with suspected blindness. (a) averaged write-out from the right occipital–right central derivation (channel 1) and the left occipital–left central derivation (channel 2) when no stimulus is given. (b), (c), and (d) Averaged write-out when a bright flash stimulus (3939 nit) is given. In (c), channels 3 and 4 have the right occipital electrode in common. (d) As for (c) for channels 5 and 6 with the left occipital electrode. No clear response can be identified in any channels and there is no phase reversal. Negativity at grid 1 (tail of arrow) records upwards in this and following figures. (From Harding 1974.)

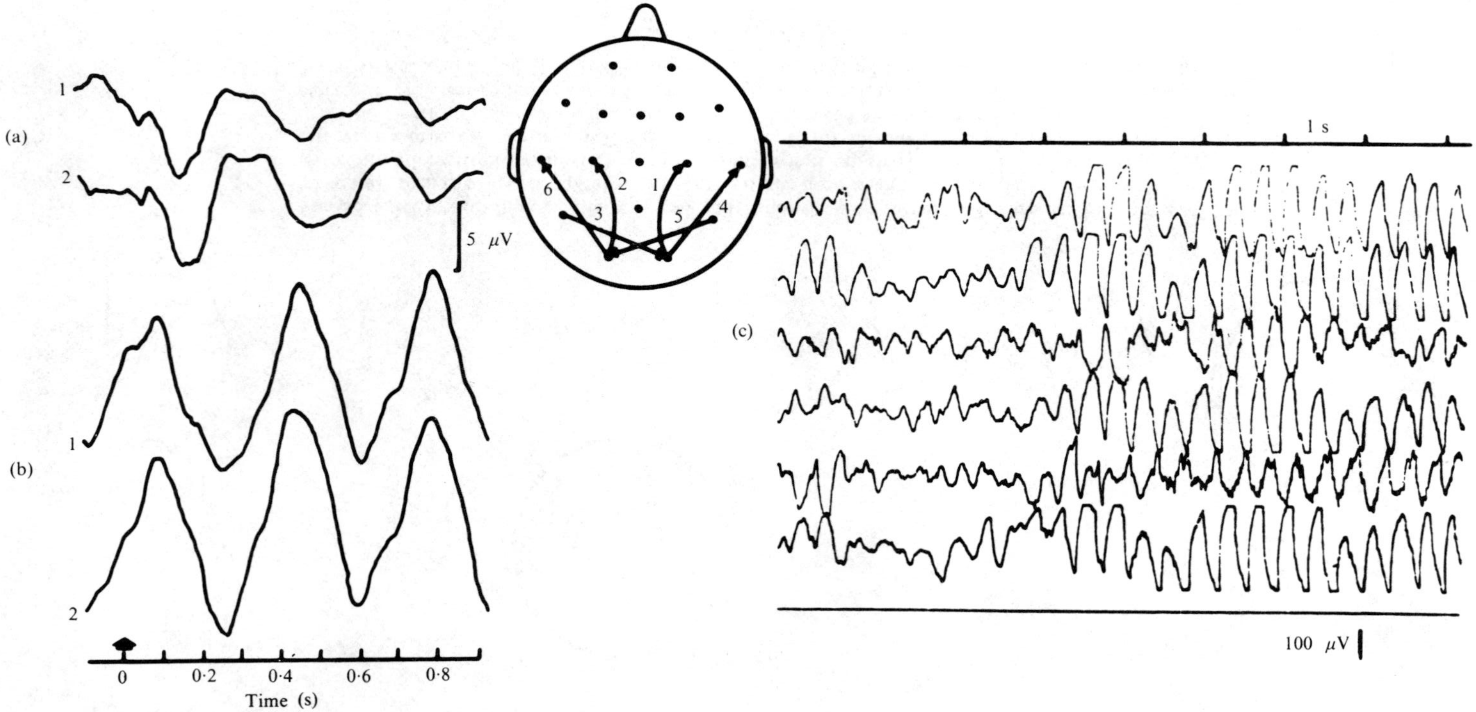

Fig. 33.2. The VEP may be obscured by rhythmical EEG background activity. Child of 5 years with delayed development. (a) VEP obtained when there is no discharge in the EEG. (b) Averaged write-out for the same flash stimulus when discharges are present in the EEG, a sample of which is shown in (c).

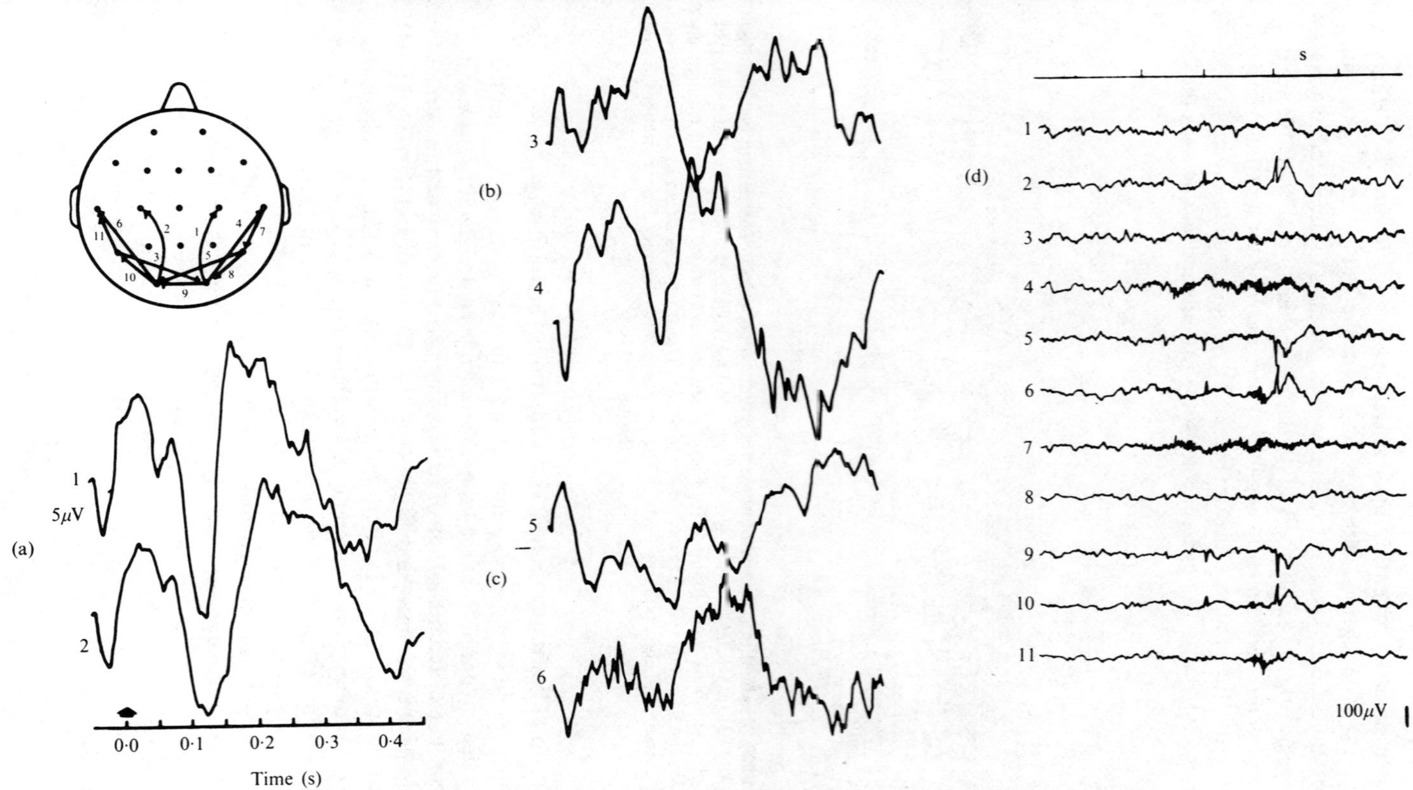

Fig. 33.3. Effect of a left occipital epileptogenic focal EEG abnormality on the VEP in a child of 6 years. In the EEG in (d), single spikes and waves may be observed in the left occipital derivations; they show phase reversal for the left occipital electrode (see channels 5 and 6 and 9 and 10). The VEP in (a)–(c) show some slight asymmetry in channels 1 and 2, but in channels 5 and 6 there is no phase reversal of the VEP components.

Psychogenic blindness

On some occasions the patient's subjective responses during routine ophthalmological investigation may be regarded with suspicion. Since the VEP technique does not require patient cooperation, it is frequently of use in cases of suspected blindness of psychogenic origin. Usually the VEP to flash is within normal limits for age in these patients, and it is frequently possible to alter the VEP by superimposing a grid pattern over the photostimulator (Fig. 33.4). Such change to superimposed patterns may not always be apparent since some patients actively defocus the pattern.

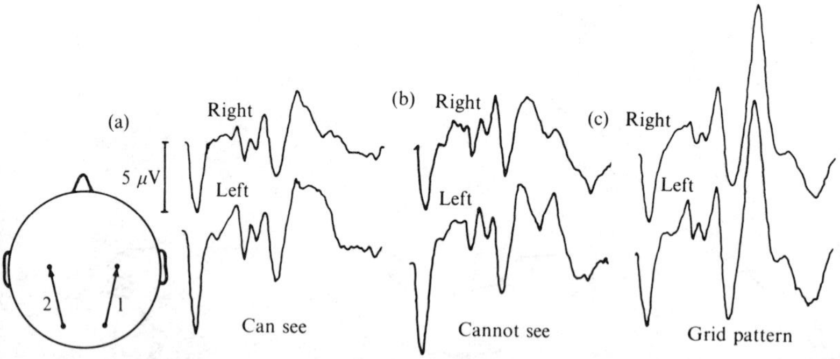

Fig. 33.4. VEPs obtained in a case of blindness of psychogenic origin. The patient claimed that she could only see very bright lights. (a) With a high-intensity flash stimulus she could observe the light and a clear VEP was obtained. (b) Flash of reduced intensity. The patient claimed she could not see the light but the VEP was very similar. (c) The superimposition of a grid pattern (which the patient said she could not see) on the photostimulus produced clear changes in the VEP. (From Harding 1974.)

Homonymous hemianopia in lesions of the optic pathway

Cohn (1963) found asymmetry of the VEP with homonymous hemianopia, the amplitude being reduced from the occipital electrode contralateral to the visual field defect. In a differential study of hemianopic patients compared to normal controls Vaughan, Katzman, and Taylor (1963) and Vaughan and Katzman (1964) found that the asymmetry was often confined to component P50. They suggested that a 50 per cent amplitude difference between the two sides was an appropriate criterium of asymmetry since none of the normals had more than 50 per cent asymmetry while 64 per cent of the hemianopic patients had an asymmetry greater than 50 per cent. Creutzfeldt and Kuhnt (1967) only found asymmetries in VEP when clear changes were already present in the EEG. Oosterhuis, Ponsen, Jonkman, and Magnus (1969) did not find asymmetry of the early components as suggested by Vaughan *et al.*, but did find asymmetry of component N80. Harding, Thompson, and Panayiopoulos (1970) found that differences in symmetrically recorded VEPs were not sufficiently exclusive to separate patients from control subjects completely. Neither conventional bipolar nor reference recording overcame this difficulty, and the further the reference electrode was from the occiputs, the more severe the problem became. Other authors have also commented on the problems of relatively distant reference electrodes (Oosterhuis *et al.* 1969). Vaughan *et al.* (1963) suggested a number of technical and theoretical reasons for these difficulties. Even when any inequality in electrode distance or resistance on the two sides was excluded, there was still difficulty resulting from the anatomical orientation of the visual cortices (macula representation) in depth.

In spite of these difficulties, which should be appreciated, the simple EEG technique of phase reversal in series bipolar recordings can be used to improve the localization of VEP to flash recorded from the right and left side of the occiput. Fig. 33.5(b) shows essentially the VEP of the right side, because the left occipital

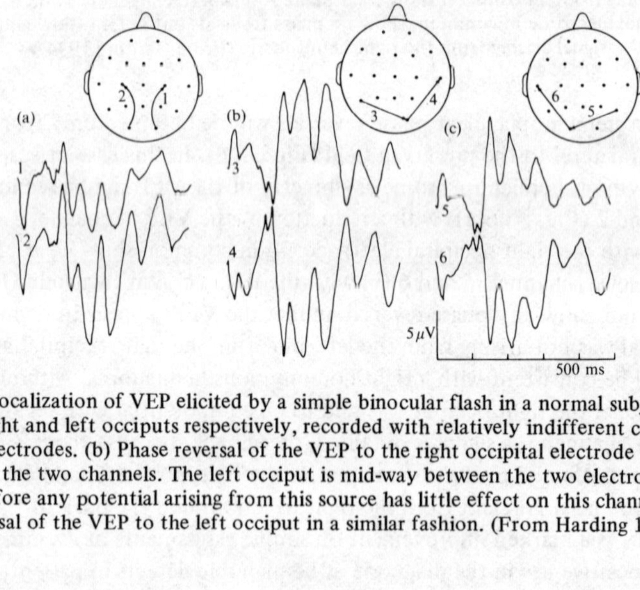

Fig. 33.5. Localization of VEP elicited by a simple binocular flash in a normal subject. (a) VEP from the right and left occiputs respectively, recorded with relatively indifferent central reference electrodes. (b) Phase reversal of the VEP to the right occipital electrode which is common to the two channels. The left occiput is mid-way between the two electrodes of channel 3 and therefore any potential arising from this source has little effect on this channel. (c) Phase reversal of the VEP to the left occiput in a similar fashion. (From Harding 1974.)

projection is about half way between electrodes T_5 and O_2 (using the international 10–20 nomenclature for EEG electrodes for channels 3 (left post-temporal electrode T_5 v. right occipital electrode O_2) and 4 (with O_2 v. right mid-temporal electrode T_4). The channel 3 should thus be approximately equipotential with respect to signals arising in the left projection. Any signal arising from the right projection will affect electrode O_2 which is common to channels 4 and 3, and lead to a phase-reversal between these channels (Fig. 33.5(b)). The same argument can be repeated for channels 5 and 6 in relation to the left projection (Fig. 32.5(c)).

Under these recording conditions, normal subjects without gross visual field defects show VEPs to flash with less than a 50 per cent asymmetry in amplitude and clear phase-reversal are observed for each occipital electrode. In patients with

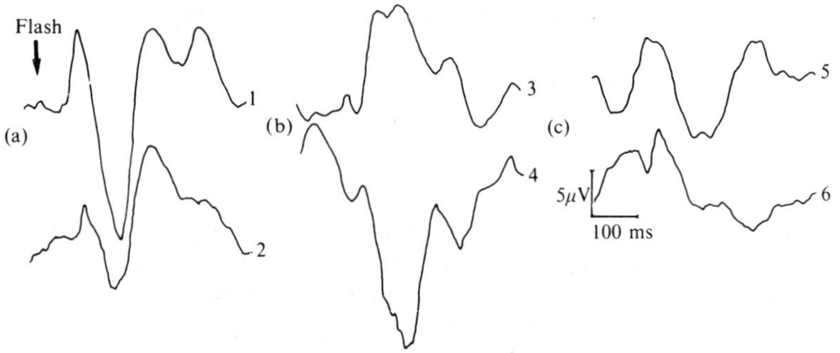

Fig. 33.6. VEP elicited by a binocular flash in a young child with suspected right homonymous hemianopia. Same electrode montage and labels as in Fig. 32.5. (a) VEP from the right occipital electrode is of greater amplitude than that from the left. (b) Channels 3 and 4 which have the right occipital electrode in common show clear phase reversal. (c) Channels 5 and 6, which have the left occipital electrode in common, show no phase reversals but in fact show an in-phase signal arising from the right hemisphere. (From Harding 1974.)

homonymous hemianopia, clear phase reversals will be obtained only from the occiput contralateral to the preserved field (Fig. 33.6). In this case of suspected right homonymous hemianopia some asymmetry of the VEP can be seen in channels 1 and 2 (Fig. 33.6(a)) with a reduction of the VEP in channel 2. Channels 3 and 4 (b) with the right occipital electrode O_2 in common show clear phase reversal. However, channels 5 and 6 (c) with the left occipital electrode O_1 in common do not show any phase-reversal; in fact the VEPs appear to be in phase as if the signal was not arising from the left, but from the right occipital area, which would be consistent with a right homonymous hemianopia. Although on a simplified model the right occiput was said to be equipotential with regard to the electrodes of channel 5, a signal *is* obtained, presumably because the left occipital electrode is not affected to the same extent as the right post-temporal electrode in view of the potential gradient from the right to left around the back of the head. The technique is a marked improvement on simple assessments of asymmetry and is certainly of positive use in the diagnosis of hemianopic defects in patients, in whom pattern-reversal techniques are inappropriate.

Macular diseases

VEPs tend to be affected by macular function to a greater extent than by homonymous hemianopia, but little work has been published on the use of VEP in macular diseases (Grader and Heller 1964; Fishman and Copenhaver 1967; Adams, Arden, and Behrman 1969). The few reports available seem to give equivocal results, and the type of macular degeneration is not always specified. A systematic study of patients with macular degeneration has been carried out at the Neuropsychology Unit in Birmingham. The majority of the patients had unilateral macular degeneration, and the VEP elicited by monocular flash to their normal eye was similar to the VEP elicited by a binocular flash. When the affected eye was stimulated, apart from a generally reduced amplitude, the P100 wave was markedly reduced. The phase-reversal technique discussed above proved of great use to indicate any asymmetry of the disciform degeneration, phase reversal being obtained only from the visual cortex related to the preserved retina (Fig. 33.7(a)).

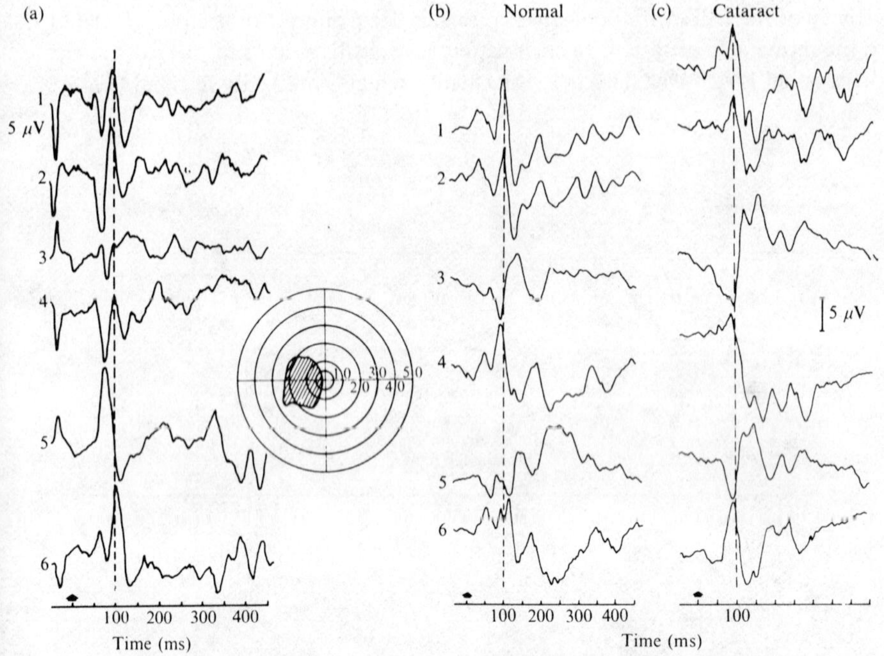

Fig. 33.7. VEP elicited by flash in a patient with localized scotoma disclosed in Goldman field chart. Same electrode montage and labels as in Fig. 33.5. Vertical interrupted line 100 ms after the flash. The VEP in channel 1 is of slightly lower amplitude than that in channel 2, and channels 3 and 4 do not show clear phase reversal. Channels 5 and 6 show relatively clear phase reversal in all components. (b) Patient with monocular cataract. Monocular flash stimulation of the normal eye. (c) Stimulation of the cataract eye in the same patient. Although the cataract was dense, the VEP obtained in (c) was similar to that in (b). After the cataract was removed the patient had good visual acuity and a normal fundus was observed.

Cataracts

The techniques have also been used in patients with developed cataracts. Under these conditions, observation of the retina is not practicable and therefore the outcome of an operation to remove the cataract is difficult to predict. By stimulating with diffused light flashes, it is possible to equate the VEPs from the normal eye with that from the eye with the cataract (Fig. 33.7(b) and (c)). The presence of the cataract appears to have little effect upon the amplitude or shape of the VEP to flash. Indeed even dense calcified cataracts appear to only slightly reduce the amplitude of the VEP and can usually be compensated by an increase in intensity of the flash from 53–68 nit per s.

The pre-operative VEP recorded with the cataract present is very similar to that obtained post-operatively after the cataract has been removed. If, however, retinal degeneration involving the macula has occurred, the VEP is markedly reduced in amplitude and the components become obscured by the background activity of the EEG with poor phase reversals occurring at the occiput(s) related to the retinal degeneration. In such patients no change occurs in the VEP when the cataract is removed, and the visual acuity remains markedly reduced (Fig. 33.8).

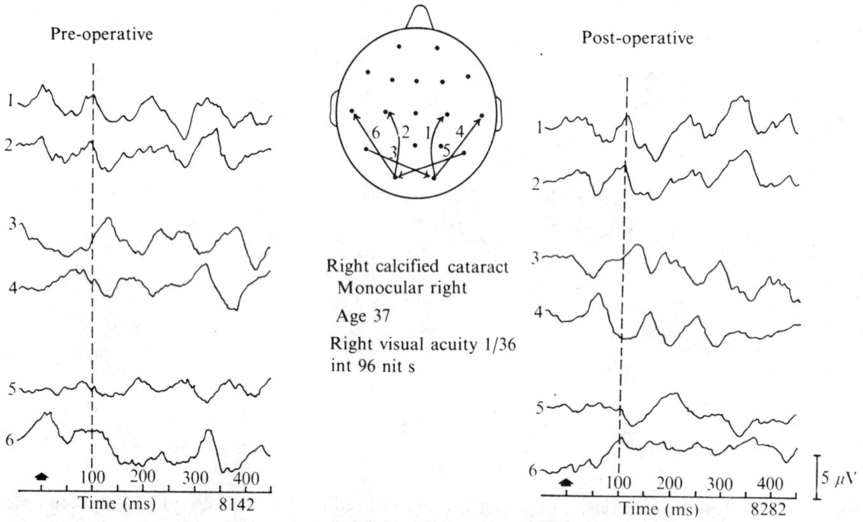

Fig. 33.8. VEPs to monocular right flash recorded pre-operatively and post-operatively in a patient with dense calcified cataract of the right eye. The pre-operative VEP was poorly defined and inconsistent phase reversals were seen, suggesting retinal degeneration. Following the removal of the cataract the VEP remained similar and the patient's visual acuity was still very poor.

Conclusion

From these and other results it appears likely that the flash-evoked VEP can function as an effective diagnostic aid in various ophthalmological conditions in which more common clinical investigations cannot be carried out.

Acknowledgements

I am indebted to Miss Cherry Thompson for her cooperation in many of these studies. Figs. 33.1, 33.4, 33.5, and 33.6 are by permission of S. Karger AG, Basel.

34. The visual evoked potential in photosensitive epilepsy

G. F. A. HARDING and M. DIMITRAKOUDI
Neuropsychology Unit, University of Aston, Birmingham

Patients with photosensitive epilepsy suffer recurrent convulsions in the presence of flickering light. Many of them never have convulsions at other times and usually have a normal resting EEG. The condition occurs in only approximately one in 10 000 of the population. Precipitants are sunlight reflected off water and sunlight seen through an avenue of trees, through railings, reflected off snow, or the flicker of the television set ('television epilepsy').

All our patients have routine EEG investigations with intermittent photic stimulation using a high-intensity photostimulator flickering at 16–25 Hz. In this situation photosensitive patients produce a photoconvulsive response in the EEG (Fig. 34.1(a)) which is generalized, involving both anterior and posterior regions, and often consists of spike and wave activity around 3 Hz. If the stimulation is continued the patient may jerk and, ultimately, a tonic–clonic convulsion may be precipitated. However, in some patients with photosensitive epilepsy, low flash rates between 5 Hz and 10 Hz may evoke focal occipital abnormalities such as localized spike and wave, usually at the same rate as the flashes (Fig. 34.1(b)), which may on some occasions precede the photoconvulsive response. These negative occipital spikes can be induced by either single, double, or trains of flashes and it has been suggested that they correspond to enhanced components of the VEP, occurring at a latency of either 45 ms (3 cases) or 88 ms (3 other cases) (Hishikawa, Yamamoto, Furuya, Yamada, Miyazaki, and Kanedo 1967). Panayiotopoulos, Jeavons, and Harding (1972) observed negative occipital spikes similar to those described by Hishikawa *et al.* (1967) but found that the latency of the negative occipital spike was similar to the positive P100 wave of the VEP. This seems to contradict the view that the negative occipital spike is a simple enhancement of the VEP, since the VEP of the patients of Hirshikawa *et al.* (1967) presented no negative component at the same latency.

In this initial study occipital spikes could be evoked in most of the patients only by relatively high flash rates, exceeding 8 Hz which frequently precipitated a generalized photoconvulsive response. In a later study (Jeavons, Harding, Panayiotopoulos, and Drasdo 1972) a grid pattern in which the squares subtended a visual

Visual evoked potentials in man: new developments (ed. J. E. Desmedt), pp. 509–13. Clarendon Press, Oxford 1977.

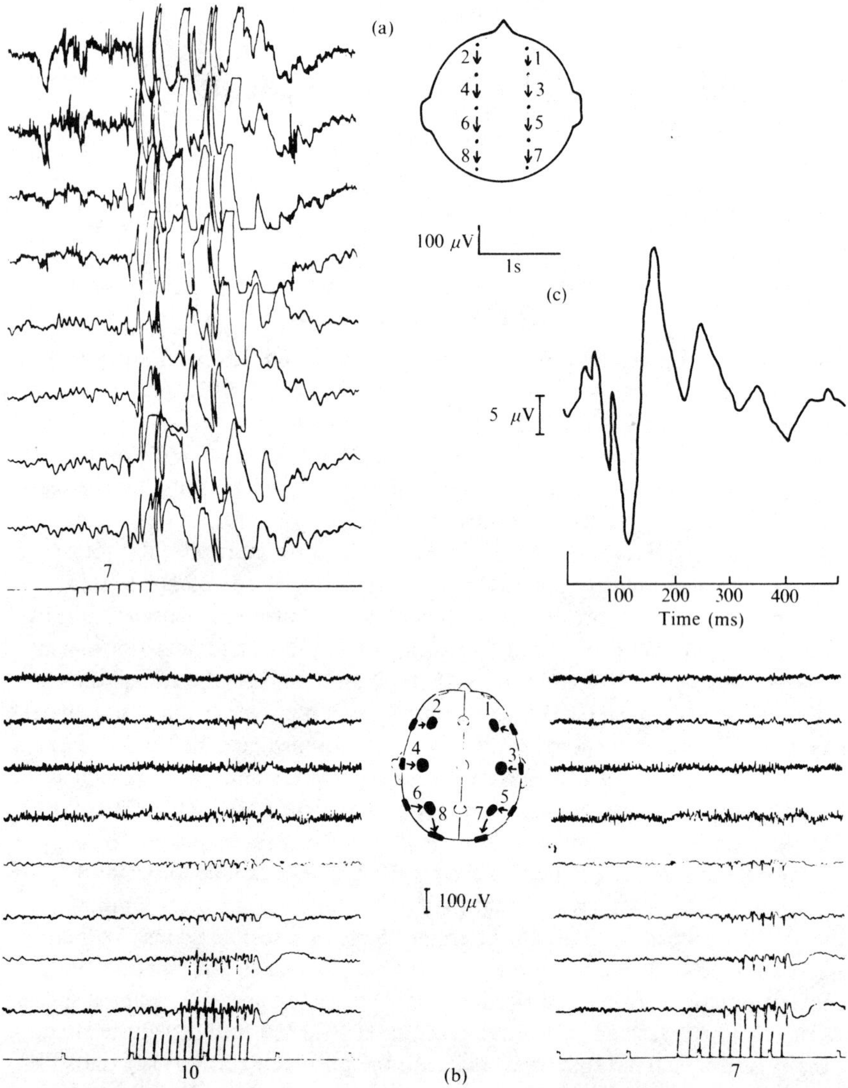

Fig. 34.1. (a) Photoconvulsive response to intermittent photic flash stimulation at 7 Hz. The flashes are indicated on the bottom trace and it can be seen that only 1 s of stimulation at this flash rate produced a generalized bilaterally symmetrical and synchronous discharge. (From Jeavons 1972.) (b) Focal occipital spikes evoked by flashes of 10 Hz and 7 Hz. The spikes occur in the posterior regions at the same rate as the flash and are maximal in the occipital derivations. (From Jeavons and Harding 1971.) (c) VEP of a patient with photosensitive epilepsy to photostimulator fitted with the grid pattern. The negative occipital spikes can be clearly seen on the descending portion of the type P100 wave. Negativity at grid 1 records upwards. Recording electrodes $O_2 - C_4$.

angle of 22′ was superimposed on the Grass photostimulator to investigate 46 patients, 21 with a history of photosensitive epilepsy, 15 with both photosensitive epilepsy and spontaneous attacks, and 8 with spontaneous attacks alone (but having proved sensitive to intermittent photic stimulation when tested in the laboratory). The remaining two patients had no history of epileptic attacks, but both produced photoconvulsive responses to intermittent photic stimulation. One of these patients was the identical twin of a photosensitive patient and the other patient had a history of migraine. The intensity of the photostimulator was set at 68 nit per s. The EEG was recorded on a 12-channel machine and the right or left occipito-central derivation (O_2-C_4, O_1-C_3) was averaged with a computor of average transients (CAT) externally triggered by a photocell through an amplitude discriminator. The overall time-constant of the system was 0·3 s and the high-frequency response was 6 dB down at 150 Hz.

All the patients were investigated under the following conditions: (a) binocular stimulation with diffuser fitted to photostimulator; (b) binocular stimulation with the photostimulator fitted with the grid; (c) monocular stimulation with the photostimulator fitted with the grid. When photic stimulation was given in the binocular state without a grid and only with a diffuser, occipital spikes were seen in the basic EEG of 7 of the 46 patients. Using averaging, a further 5 of the 46 patients showed occipital spikes in the VEP. In half of these patients the occipital spike was evoked at a frequency of 1 Hz. When the grid was added to the photostimulator 31 of the patients showed occipital spikes in the EEG, and 42 of the 46 patients showed occipital spikes in the VEP. In 26 patients the occipital spikes were evoked at 1 Hz. In 4 of the 46 patients no occipital spikes could be observed in either EEG or VEP. In one patient photoconvulsive responses were present at 1 Hz and this phenomena markedly affected the VEP. In the 3 other patients no explanation could be found for the absence of occipital spikes, although it is interesting that they all produced bilaterally symmetrical and synchronous 3 Hz spike-and-waves in response to intermittent photic stimulation.

With flash stimulation, there was a constant relationship between the negative occipital spike and the P100 component of the VEP, the negative occipital spike appearing generally on the descending portion of P100 (Fig. 34.1(c)). The mean latency of the occipital spike for all patients was 91 ± 3·5 ms (S.D.). The mean latency of the N60 component of the VEP was 58 ± 3·4 ms. The P100 component of the VEP showed constant latencies in each individual, irrespective of the flash rates used.

With the grid pattern present the occipital spike appeared at lower flash rates and showed increasing amplitude with increase of flash rate. In some patients, as the flash rate was increased the occipital spike appeared to replace the P100 component and to dominate the VEP. When the grid was removed at low flicker rates the occipital spike was much reduced or disappeared (Fig. 34.2).

In a number of the patients stimulated at increasing flash frequencies in the critical range the occipital spikes preceded the photoconvulsive response. This

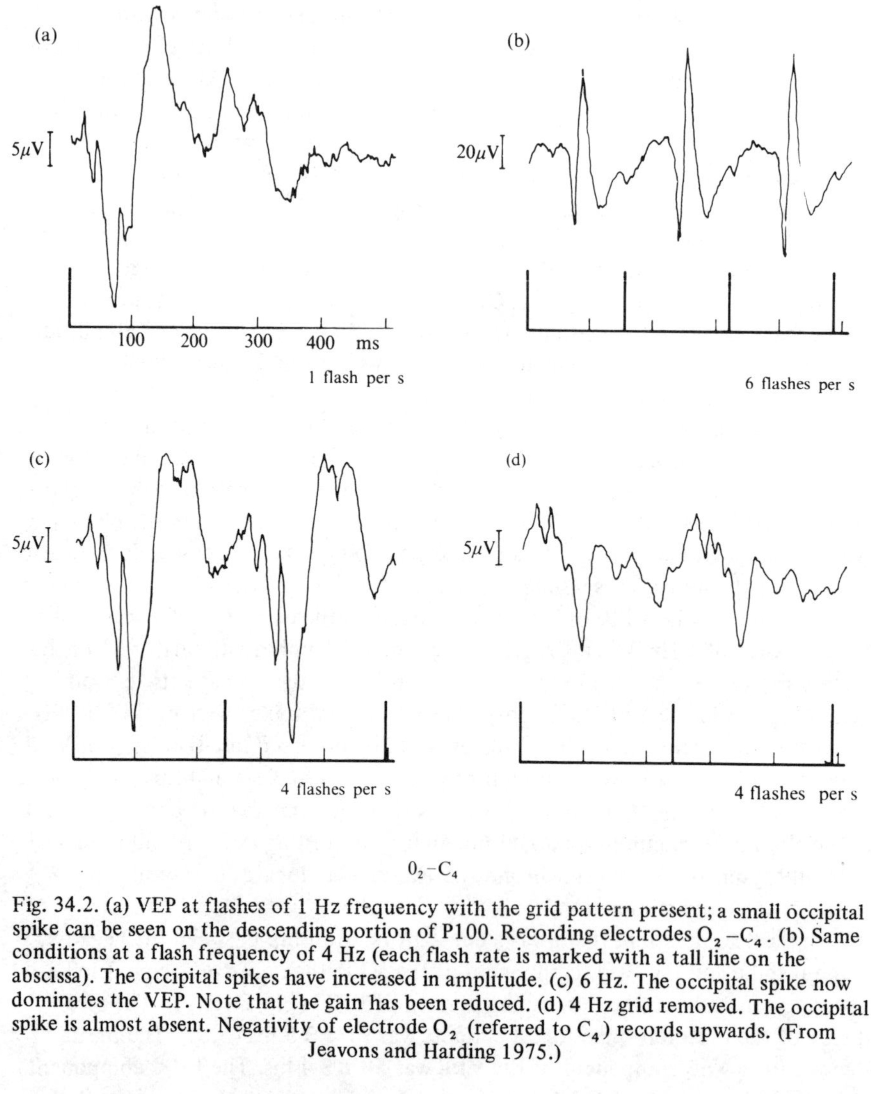

Fig. 34.2. (a) VEP at flashes of 1 Hz frequency with the grid pattern present; a small occipital spike can be seen on the descending portion of P100. Recording electrodes $O_2 - C_4$. (b) Same conditions at a flash frequency of 4 Hz (each flash rate is marked with a tall line on the abscissa). The occipital spikes have increased in amplitude. (c) 6 Hz. The occipital spike now dominates the VEP. Note that the gain has been reduced. (d) 4 Hz grid removed. The occipital spike is almost absent. Negativity of electrode O_2 (referred to C_4) records upwards. (From Jeavons and Harding 1975.)

finding was apparent only in patients with a history of photosensitive epilepsy. Whereas on binocular stimulation the occipital spike was clearly apparent in both basic EEG and VEP, on monocular stimulation the negative occipital spike was markedly reduced in the VEP and was often no longer apparent in the EEG (Fig. 34.3).

It is apparent from these results that the negative occipital spike is intimately related to the P100 mechanism of the VEP, and that the presence of the occipital spike is a consistent phenomenon in the VEPs of nearly all photosensitive patients.

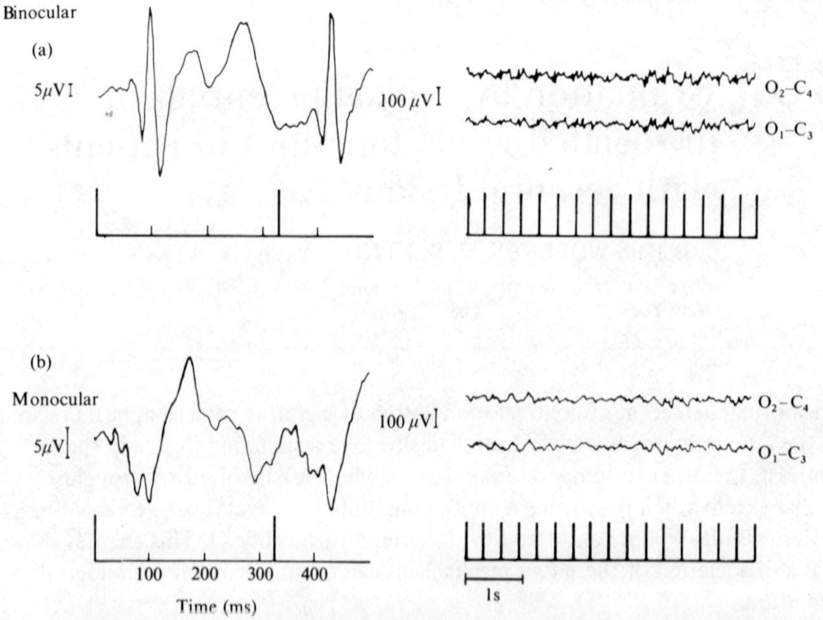

Fig. 34.3. (a) With binocular stimulation occipital spikes can be seen in the EEG (right) and are of high amplitude in the VEP. Recording electrodes O_2 $-C_4$. (b) With monocular stimulation occipital spikes are not observed in the EEG and are only present as a P100 wave in the VEP. (From Jeavons and Harding 1975.)

The suggestion that the negative occipital spike is of visual-cortex origin is supported by its increased amplitude with pattern stimuli and its decreased amplitude with diffuse flash and monocular stimulations. Therefore the occurrence of the occipital spike may reflect an abnormal reaction of the visual cortex to a massive stimulus and this focal abnormality may then trigger a secondary generalized discharge.

Acknowledgements

We wish to thank Dr. P. M. Jeavons who allowed us to study his patients.

35. Evaluation by evoked potentials of dissociated visual functions in patients with cerebral lesions

I. BODIS-WOLLNER, C. D. HENDLEY, and A. ATKIN

Departments of Neurology and Physiology, Mount Sinai School of Medicine, New York

The normal detection of contrast modulation of a grating pattern appears related to the interaction of two neural mechanisms, one responding to steady spatial contrast, the other to temporal modulation, which are involved to a roughly similar extent when presenting a contrast-modulated 6 cycles per degree grating pattern (Bodis-Wollner and Hendley, Chapter 9 of this book). This chapter shows that a dissociation of these two mechanisms can occur in certain pathological conditions.

Blurred vision frequently occurs in patients who do not have ocular pathology nor any eye-movement disorders. Such patients often complain of indistinct vision even though conventional methods fail to demonstrate any central scotoma or acuity loss. Over the last 4 years we have been investigating spatial contrast-sensitivity functions in patients with indistinct vision and cerebral lesions (Bodis-Wollner 1972; Bodis-Wollner and Diamond 1973). Vertical sinusoidal grating patterns of variable spatial frequency and contrast were used as a stimulus. The minimum contrast required for detection of such a pattern at each spatial frequency has been used to chart the 'contrast-sensitivity curve' of the subjects. The angular size of the bars in the finest detectable grating pattern at 100 per cent contrast is a measure of visual acuity. This spatial cut-off frequency is generally in fair agreement with the visual-acuity measurement established by conventional methods (Green 1970; Bodis-Wollner and Diamond 1973). A simple explanation of this is that in a patient with the clinically tested visual acuity reduced to 20/40, (which means that at a given distance the smallest detectable image must be twice as large as for the normal) the finest detectable grating should have bars twice as wide, thus with half the spatial frequency. But there could be different explanations, depending upon the particular model of visual-system organization postulated to underlie the human contrast-sensitivity curve. The fact is that there is no established theory for predicting the contrast-sensitivity curves of patients with cerebral lesions from their visual acuities since different relationships between conventional acuity measures and grating detection might be expected.

Visual evoked potentials in man: new developments (ed. J. E. Desmedt), pp. 514–24. Clarendon Press, Oxford 1977.

A patient's contrast-sensitivity curve must therefore be evaluated directly. Our method is based on the ratios of his contrast sensitivity to those of a normal person at any spatial frequency. These ratios, expressed in decibels, refer to the threshold contrast elevation and can be plotted at a number of spatial frequencies to establish a 'visuogram' (in analogy to the audiogram). Patients with similar visual acuities can have quite differently shaped visuograms. We found three major types of visuograms. The first and most common type shows a pronounced high-frequency drop, indicating a relatively greater loss in contrast sensitivity with increasing spatial frequency. The second type is fairly flat, indicating a level loss. The third and rarest type shows a selective loss over a narrow range of frequencies (Bodis-Wollner 1972). To gain some understanding of the mechanisms underlying abnormal visuograms, we undertook an investigation of the detection of contrast *modulation* of low- and mid-frequency gratings by patients with cerebral lesions. We reasoned that if spatial contrast and local luminance changes are processed in parallel in the human visual system, a simple grating-detection task would not reveal whether a given dysfunction involved the luminance mechanism, the contrast mechanism, or their interaction. We therefore tested both psychophysical responses and VEPs to contrast-modulated gratings as in normals (see Chapter 9), in spite of the extensive time and effort required both from the patient and from the experimenter to complete a single test. As a result of these investigations we suggest for clinical applications a simplified test utilizing VEPs which is of diagnostic interest.

Method

Hospitalized patients from the neurology wards were studied. Patients with gross aphasia or organic mental syndrome were excluded. Participation was voluntary and test procedures were carefully explained in advance. It was helpful in obtaining cooperation in these tedious studies that one of us (I. B.-W.) was well known to most of the patients as his or her personal physician. The patients were selected on the basis of either a history of indistinct vision or poor performance on simple clinical tests of visual functions, usually reading or picture recognition. We have also examined a number of hospitalized patients without visual problems. All patients had a complete neurological examination, including evaluation of retinal and oculomotor functions. Visual fields and visual acuity (Snellen charts) were obtained in each case. The neurological diagnostic procedures included EEG, brain scan, and often special X-ray studies.

Stimuli were vertical sinusoidal gratings produced on an oscilloscope, as described by Bodis-Wollner and Hendley in Chapter 9. A short horizontal fixation line was used. To establish the contrast-sensitivity curve, patients were seated comfortably in an armchair at 2·9 m from the grating, and at half this distance for the contrast-modulation tests. On–off presentations at a rate of 0·5 Hz were used for measuring contrast sensitivity. Contrast modulation using a square-wave modulating waveform was at the rate of 8 Hz. Usually four or five data-gathering sessions were devoted to a single patient. If there were any acuity or subjective differences in vision between the two eyes, they were tested separately. Otherwise only the eye contralateral to the lesion was used. Psychophysical thresholds were taken from frequency-of-seeing curves based on at least 20 decisions. Sometimes replicate measurements were obtained after several days or a few weeks. Procedures for establishing contrast-modulation functions as well as recording of VEP are described in Chapter 9. Occasionally we used a 5-electrode montage with one electrode placed on the forehead, 2 posterior temporal, and 2 occipital electrodes.

Results

VEPs were studied in 24 patients. Some of the patients found it difficult to complete all the tests, especially the psychophysical measures of contrast modulation. The data of five well-studied patients are presented in detail. All had cerebral pathology: 3 complained of blurred vision and 2 had normal central vision.

V.M., a 53-year-old man, complained of a feeling of 'fluttering' in the right eye, difficulty in reading, and loss of depth perception. He also had episodes of giddiness, of blurred vision, and of sensations of flashing light in his right field of vision. The neurological examination showed no deficits in mentation, power, co-ordination, or sensory functions. There was no nystagmus or dystaxia. He had a right homonymous hemiamblyopia and dyschromatopsia, with the inferior quadrant more affected. He performed poorly in reaching for objects in the vertical meridian as well as in his right field of vision. Visual acuity was 20/20 (both eyes tested together). A left parieto-occipital vascular tumour was demonstrated by angiograms.

The visuogram was similar for the two eyes, showing a 'level' loss between 10 dB and 16 dB with a somewhat greater drop at around 9 cycles per degree in the right eye (Fig. 35.1(a)). The contrast-modulation curve obtained at 6 cycles per degree had a slope of 0·8, which is significantly steeper than the slope in normal subjects (Fig. 35.1(b)). This indicates that the modulation sensitivity was not simply decreased together with loss in contrast sensitivity, but rather that there was a specific change in the modulation function. The slope is not consistent with a normal balance of interaction between spatial contrast and local luminance detector (Bodis-Wollner and Hendley, Chapter 9 of this book). The VEPs (Fig. 35.2) and psychophysical thresholds were comparable. At 0·4 mean contrast they were respectively 20 dB and 23 dB below full modulation. At 0·13 contrast they were both 15 dB. Regression lines for VEP amplitude at different mean contrasts as a function of modulation depth have similar slopes (Fig. 35.3(a)). The same data are plotted as a function of the change in contrast ΔC in Fig. 35.3(b) and a single line may be fitted to all the data irrespective of mean spatial contrast. In this patient, therefore, VEP amplitude is apparently determined by detectors which respond to local luminance changes but are barely sensitive to the spatial

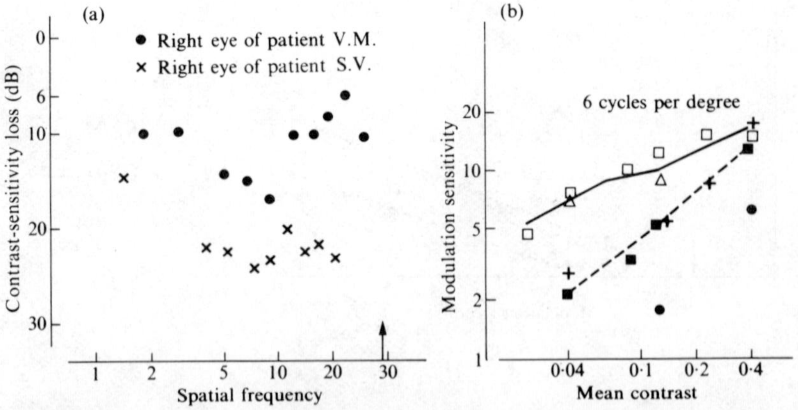

Fig. 35.1. (a) Visuogram or plot of the ratio of the contrast-sensitivity loss for a patient, compared to a normal at corresponding spatial frequencies. The right eye of patient V.M. shows a level loss with a dip at 9 cycles per degree. The arrow at the lower right indicates the cut-off frequency. The right eye of S.V. shows a gradient of 8 dB from 1·7 cycles per degree to 4·0 cycles per degree. From this spatial frequency on, there is a 'level' loss. The visuograms were similar for both eyes. (b) Contrast-modulation functions of 5 patients with cerebral lesions, compared with the average for 4 normal subjects (solid line, average slope, 0·47). The stimulus was a 6 cycles per degree sinusoidal grating. Filled symbols refer to patients with visual complaints, open symbols to those without impairment of central vision. The dashed line, slope 0·8, fits the data of patient V.M. (filled squares). Open squares, M.F. Triangles, S.R. Crosses, S.V. Filled squares, V.M. Filled circles, F.C.

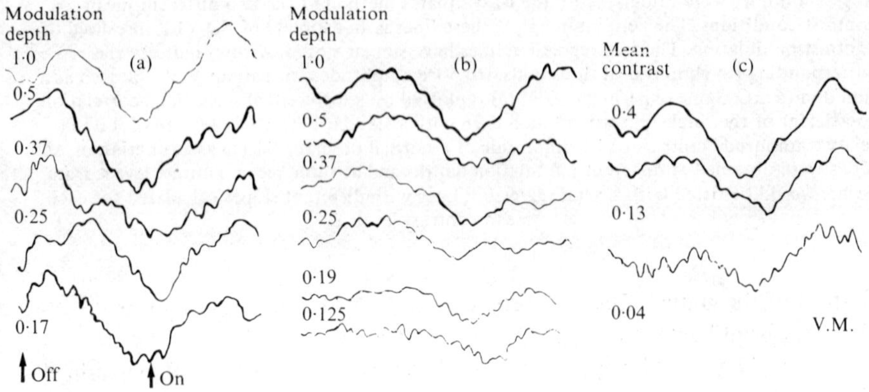

Fig. 35.2. VEPs of V.M. at different modulation depths. (a) Mean contrast level 0·4. The amplitude measured as half the average peak-to-peak amplitude decreases with decreasing modulation depth. Gain was doubled for the bottom two traces. (b) Mean contrast 0·13. (c) 100 per cent modulation of the contrast, shown for three different mean contrasts (indicated at right of each trace). Remember that 100 per cent modulation of the contrast is the same as on–off presentation of the grating. The gain was doubled for the lowest trace. Each trace represents an average of 512 responses. The sweep time is 125 ms.

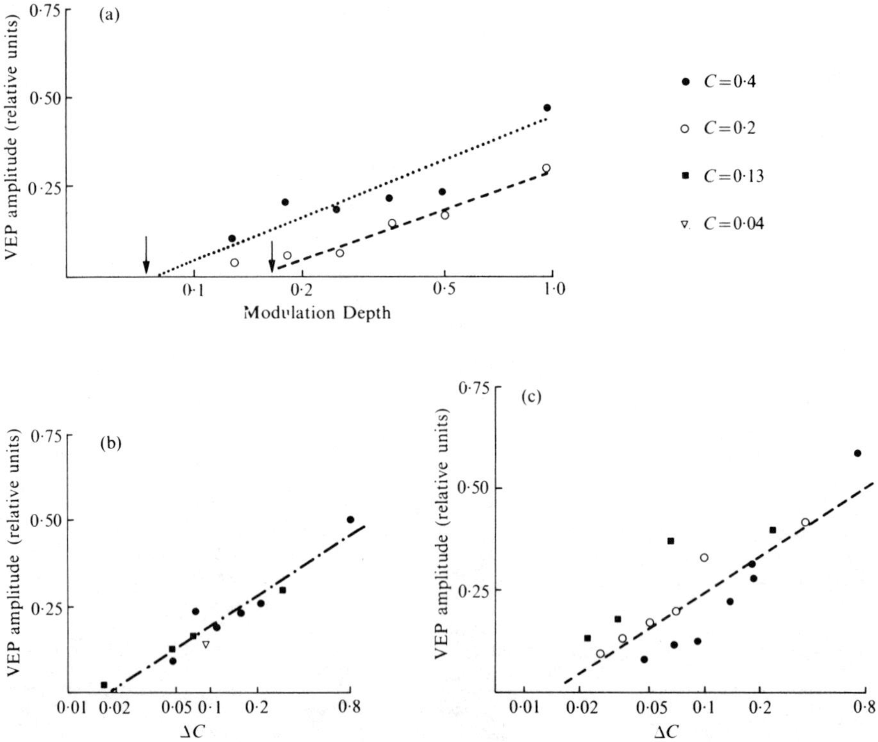

Fig. 35.3. (a) VEP amplitudes for patient V.M., plotted as a function of modulation depth. Regression lines were calculated by the least-squares method at the two different mean contrast conditions. The zero intercept of these lines is an estimate of the VEP threshold of contrast modulation. The two regression lines have similar slopes. Arrows indicate the corresponding psychophysical thresholds. (b) VEP amplitudes for patient V.M., plotted as a function of ΔC. Same experiment as in (a) replotted on a different abscissa. The correlation coefficient of the single regression line is 0·96 with a standard error of estimate of 0·07 in relative amplitude units. (c) VEP amplitude of a normal observer (M.L.) as a function of ΔC. VEPs were obtained at different modulation depths and at three mean contrast levels. Data points would be fitted with several regression lines with different slopes calculated for each mean contrast level.

contrast of the grating. This is different from the VEP functions of normal observers (see Chapter 5).

F.C., an 18-year-old man, was admitted because of headaches and increasingly blurred vision. At the time of admission the neurological examination was negative except for a 2 mm pupillary size difference. During hospitalization he developed transient diplopia and also episodic tinnitus in both ears. The mental functions were not disturbed. He was diagnosed as having a malignant liver tumour with metastasis to the brain and was submitted to radiation therapy. An electro-nystagmogram revealed no abnormalities of ocular motility. He had hypoactive

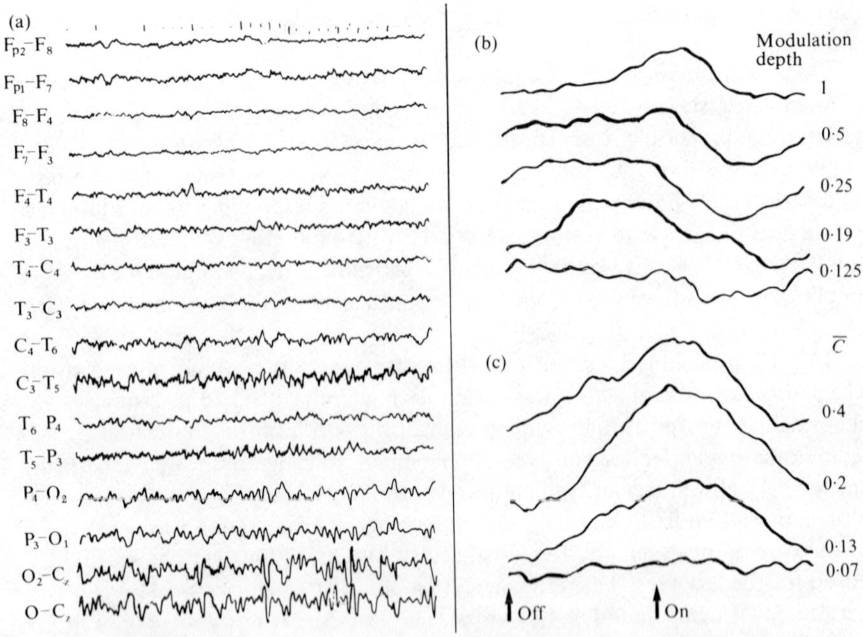

Fig. 35.4 (a) EEG of patient F.C. In both occipital leads presence of slow waves which appeared to be independent at times. They blocked with eye opening (not shown). (b) VEPs of F.C. at five different modulation depths. Mean contrast $\overline{C}$ was 0·4. The 'single hump' VEP response can also occur in some normal subjects. (c) VEPs of F.C. to 100 per cent modulation of contrast, for four different mean contrasts. The gain was halved for the uppermost trace. Note the flat response at 0·07 mean contrast. The triggering delay differed from that in (b). The total sweep time in (b) and (c) was 125 ms.

labyrinthine response on the left. The audiogram, which showed a 15–20 dB level loss, was interpreted as being within normal limits. Speech detection and masking results were also normal. The EEG revealed slow-wave foci most prominent in the left and right occipital scalp derivations (Fig. 35.4(a)). They appeared independent at times and blocked with eye opening.

An ophthalmological consultation found no evidence of ocular or retinal pathology. Visual acuity with best correction was 20/20 for the right eye and 20/30 + for the left eye. There was a superior temporal field defect for the left eye. Right homonymous field defects developed subsequently.

The visuograms of F.C. were flat and similar in the two eyes, with a 10–16 dB level loss. The cut-off frequencies of the VEP visuogram were 32 cycles per degree for the right eye and 24 cycles per degree for the left eye, corresponding to Snellen acuities of 20/19 and 20/25, thus very close to the acuities as measured by eye chart. The contrast-modulation functions at 6 cycles per degree had a slope of 1·0. This suggests that, in this patient, modulation was detected by mechanism sensitive only to local luminance changes and not to the spatial contrast of the pattern.

VEPs to different depths of contrast modulation (Fig. 35.4(b)) and over a range of mean contrasts (Fig. 35.4(c)) are shown. There was satisfactory agreement between the psychophysical (16 dB) and the extrapolated VEP threshold (18 dB). In line with the above interpretation of the psychophysical responses to contrast modulation the VEP appears to depend on detectors responding to local luminance changes, since a single regression line fits the VEP data rather well (correlation coefficient 0·91, with a standard error of 7 per cent of the maximum VEP amplitude). As we have shown, VEPs of the normal subjects cannot be fitted with a single regression line (Fig. 35.5).

S.V., 19-year-old girl, complained of headaches and increasingly blurred vision. The neurological examination was within normal limits. She had persistently abnormal cerebrospinal fluid findings compatible with a chronic intracranial (granulomatous) infectious process. A pneumoencephalogram showed a markedly enlarged lateral ventricular system but no definite etiological diagnosis of an obstructive lesion has been made. Ophthalmological examination was negative. There were no field defects. The visual acuity was 20/40 for the right eye and 20/30 for the left eye. The grating-detection cut-off frequencies were 24 cycles per degree OU, corresponding to a visual acuity of 20/25. The visuogram was fairly flat, with a slight drop from 1·8 cycles per degree to 4 cycles per degree (Fig. 35.1(b)). At 6 cycles per degree, the contrast-modulation function had a slope of 0·71, which is higher than the normal range (slope less than 0·5) (see Fig. 35.1(b)), and points to an altered balance of local luminance and pattern detectors. The VEP threshold (22 dB) was similar to the psychophysical threshold (18 dB) at 0·4 mean contrast. The VEP amplitudes plotted as a function of ΔC were fitted by a regression line with a lower correlation coefficient (0·85) than in the previous two patients. Nevertheless, this single function gives a better fit than two regression lines computed from her VEP amplitudes as a function of modulation depth at two separate mean contrast conditions. Unlike corresponding data in normals, the two lines have similar slopes.

S.R., 24-year-old man, was admitted for focal seizures on the left side. He had headaches but no visual symptoms. Neurological examination revealed poor co-ordination and loss of cortical sensory functions in the left hand. His mental status and the rest of the examination were normal. An angiogram demonstrated a cystic tumour on the right hemisphere, involving predominantly the inferior frontal and parietal lobes. The visual acuity and contrast sensitivity were normal. The slope of the contrast-modulation function at 6 cycles per degree was 0·53, which is within normal range. VEPs were plotted for several modulation depths and two mean contrast levels and gave closely fitting (correlation coefficient 0·99) regression lines, with significantly different slopes at the different mean contrast levels. The correlation coefficient of a single regression line fitted to the same data as a function of ΔC was 0·94 with a standard error of estimate of 18 per cent. Thus both his psychophysical and VEP data show the effect of pattern detectors, and are therefore more in line with the results in normals.

M.F., 62-year-old lady, developed discoordination of her left side and difficulty walking. She could not see well to her left side. The neurological examination disclosed a left hemisensory and mild hemimotor deficit. She had an abnormal EEG, brain scan, and angiographic study which demonstrated a right parieto-occipital intracerebral neoplasm. There was also a left homonymous field defect with macular sparing. The visual acuity with best correction was 20/30 OU. The grating acuity was 32 cycles per degree, corresponding to a Snellen acuity of 20/19. The visuogram was flat at about 5–7 dB thus well within the normal range. The contrast-modulation functions had a slope of 0·65 at 3 cycles per degree and of 0·53 at 6 cycles per degree (Fig. 35.1(b)), which is in the normal range. The VEP amplitude as a function of modulation depth had correlation coefficients of 0·97 and 0·95 for the two mean contrast levels, whereas the correlation coefficient was 0·93 for the ΔC function. Furthermore, the two regression lines fitted at the two mean contrast levels had significantly different slopes. The standard errors for these modulation functions were 9 per cent and 7 per cent, but 11 per cent for the luminance function. Thus the data are better fitted with two regression lines instead of one, and both the VEP and psychophysical functions express a contribution of pattern detectors.

Discussion

Syndromes of dissociated sensory loss of vibration, position sense, touch, pain, or temperature are well recognized in the somato-sensory modality. However dissociated disorders of visual functions have not received enough attention. Riddoch (1917) was one of the first to recognize that, in a patient with a blind field, vision may be preserved for the detection of motion although not of form. Subsequently Bender (1964) amply confirmed different degrees of impairment for the detection of different stimulus attributes in the 'blind' fields. Unfortunately, it is still common to speak of hemianopia in cases of cerebral lesions, even though these do not always cause hemiblindness for all possible stimulus attributes. Dissociated visual functions of central (foveal) vision have only recently been investigated, partly as a result of physiological (Enroth-Cugell and Robson 1966) and anatomical (Potts, Hodges, Shelman, Fritz, Levy, and Mangnall 1972) evidence of parallel pathways subserving central vision. Dissociation of these functions is suggested by studies of patients with demyelinating diseases (see Chapters 26, 27, and 29 of this book) and of amblyopes (Spekreijse, Khoe and Van der Tweel 1972; Chapters 23 and 24 of this book).

We studied patients with cerebral lesions who complained of blurred vision, and in a number of cases found a dissociation in the detection of spatial contrast and local luminance changes of 6 cycles/° grating pattern. The dissociation was demonstrated both by psychophysical and by VEP investigations. We have interpreted this dissociation using the conclusions reached from investigations of normal observers. Bodis-Wollner *et al.* (1972) suggested that responses to gratings in man normally involve a balance of detectors of pattern and local luminance changes. There may be an analogy between these detectors and the transient and sustained cells of the cat, respectively (Bodis-Wollner and Hendley, Chapter 9 of this book). A cellular dichotomy in the human visual system was also suggested by Tolhurst (1973) and Kulikowski and Tolhurst (1973). It was also suggested that the human VEP expresses the functions of both sustained and transient detectors (Kulikowski, Chapter 8 of this book).

There is evidence for sustained and transient neurones in the cortex of a cat (Hoffman and Stone 1971; Stone and Dreher 1973; Ikeda and Wright 1974). Is the independence of the two types of detectors maintained at the human visual cortex? The answer to this question could also be relevant to a large body of research involving the role of the extrageniculostriate system in luminance detection (Pasik and Pasik 1971) and to the concept of 'two visual systems' (Trevarthen 1968; Schneider 1969). Studies in normals have not been able to answer this question. If a purely cortical lesion could be shown to produce a dissociation between the two types of detector, this would establish two selectively vulnerable sets of human cortical neurones.

Among the patients in our study with signs of dissociated functions, S.V. had no definite diagnosis and her findings rather suggested a subcortical lesion, while a second, V.M., had a well demonstrated parieto-occipital lesion. This suggests that dissociation may occur in the presence of a cortical lesion. However, we cannot exclude the possibility that V.M.'s lesion was exerting pressure on subcortical structures, including the visual pathways. His field defect was also characterized by a dissociation rather than by anopia. It is interesting to compare this case with M.F., who also presented a tumour in the parieto-occipital region but had intact central vision without any sign of dissociation. She had a real homonymous hemianopia. A third patient with signs of dissociation, F.C., probably had distinct metastatic lesions in his occipital lobes, but we cannot exclude the possibility that there were dysfunctions and/or metatases in other areas of the brain. Nor do the clinical data of the other patients with dissociated visual functions prove beyond doubt that a parallel organization exists at the human visual cortex.

Contrast detection versus contrast-modulation detection

If the detection of spatial contrast and local luminance changes was mediated by the human analogues of sustained and transient cells, it is worth considering the role of these cells in contrast detection. Our suprathreshold modulation data agree with the findings of Kulikowski (see Chapter 8 of this book) on the detectability of gratings to suggest that low- and mid-range spatial frequencies gratings are preferred by the transient mechanism and higher-range spatial frequencies by the sustained mechanism. These two mechanisms overlap, but their spatial-frequency optima are different. The loss of one of these channels would mean that all gratings, regardless of spatial frequency, should be detected by the remaining mechanism whose features would be revealed by the contrast-sensitivity curve. Along this line one could predict that losing the spatial-contrast mechanism should result in a visuogram gradually dropping by at least 6 dB as the spatial frequency increases from 1·8 cycles per degree to 10 cycles per degree. The gradient of the rest of the visuogram is not easy to predict. A high-frequency-loss visuogram suggests the existence of a transient mechanism, which does not cover high frequencies. However, most of our patients had rather flat visuograms which could be interpreted in several ways. For example a loss in the sustained mechanism may have been only partial, and unequally affecting different spatial frequencies, or else the dissociation could be due, not to a loss of one of the two mechanisms, but rather to a defect in their interaction. Bodis-Wollner and Diamond (1973) also considered the possibility that a flat visuogram might be caused by a general rise of the threshold criteria, but found no such evidence and interpreted their patient's flat visuograms by using the notion of specific visual deficits rather than multimodal elevation of sensory thresholds.

Diagnostic applications of VEP

The use of VEP for clinical diagnosis has often produced disappointing results. VEPs are rarely needed in the diagnosis of patients with gross deficits. In patients with more subtle disorders of vision, the VEP tests should have a resolution at least as good as other objective methods of neurological diagnosis. This raises the problem of adequate pattern VEP methodologies.

Our results suggest that parallel pathways with selective vulnerabilities are involved in the processing of visual information. They also suggest that the appropriateness of photic stimuli for clinical applications must be carefully assessed on the basis of their physiological significance. Another point is the usefulness of VEP-amplitude measurements which allow quantitative correlations of psychophysical and VEP functions. Rigorous psychophysical measurements are admittedly not suitable for the routine testing of all patients. However VEP to contrast-modulated stimuli can easily be investigated, once the basic data have been established. VEP amplitudes for a variety of mean contrast levels can be fitted with a single ΔC function in some patients, but not in normals. This functional relationship results from a deficit in the normal pattern of interaction between spatial contrast and local luminance detectors and it is associated with subjective visual complaints. Our data show that a small set of modulation depths and mean contrasts may be adequate to reveal, in a given patient, whether VEP-amplitude functions do or do not correlate with luminance detection. Such a convenient standard test should help in the diagnosis of dissociated disorders in the human visual system.

Summary

Some patients with cerebral lesions complain of blurred vision even though their acuity and contrast detection seem relatively intact. In a number of these patients, we found a dissociation in the detection of spatial contrast and local luminance of a 6 cycles per degree grating pattern. This was demonstrated both by psychophysical and by VEP methods. This dissociation is thought to reveal an impairment in the balance of sustained and transient pathways of the human visual system. A simple test of VEP to contrast modulation is described for diagnostic investigations of patients with cerebral lesions.

Acknowledgements

We thank Miss Laura Balsam and Mr. Amos Orlofsky for help and Prof. B. Cohen for lending of equipment. Dr. I. Bodis-Wollner is recipient of NINDS individual research fellowship IF 22NS-02803-01. This work was supported in part by Grant NS-11631-03 from the National Institutes of Health.

Bibliography

Adams, R. D., and Kubik, C. S. (1952). The morbid anatomy of the demyelinative diseases. *Am. J. Med.* **12**, 510–46.

Adams, W. L., Arden, G. B., and Behrman, J. (1969). Responses of human visual cortex following excitation of peripheral retinal rods. *Br. J. Ophthal.* **53**, 439–52.

Adey, W. R., and Noda, H. (1973). Influence of eye movements on geniculo-striate excitability in the cat. *J. Physiol., Lond.* **235**, 805–21.

Anders, T., Emde, R., and Parmelee, A. (eds.) (1971). *A manual of standardized terminology, techniques and criteria for scoring of states of sleep and wakefulness in newborn infants.* UCLA Information Service, Los Angeles.

Andrews, D. P. (1965). Perception of contours in the central fovea. *Nature, Lond.* **205**, 1218–20.

Anstis, S. M. (1970). Phi movement as a substraction process. *Vision Res.* **10**, 1411–30.

Arden, G. B. (ed.) (1972). The visual system. Neurophysiology, biophysics and their clinical applications. In *Advances in experimental medicine and biology*, Vol. 24. Plenum, London.

——(1973). The visual evoked response in ophthalmology. *Proc. R. Soc. Med.* **66**, 1037–43.

——, and Weale, R. A. (1954). Variations of the latent period of vision. *Proc. R. Soc. Med.* **142**, 258–67.

Armington, J. C. (1964). Relations between electroretinograms and occipital potentials elicited by flickering stimuli. *Documenta opth.* **18**, 194–206.

——(1966). Spectral sensitivity of simultaneous electroretinograms and occipital responses. *Vision Res.*, Suppl. **1**, 225–33.

——(1968). The electroretinogram, the visual evoked potential and the area–luminance relation. *Vision Res.* **8**, 263–76.

——(1970). Simultaneous electroretinograms and evoked potentials. *Am. J. Optom.* **47**, 450–9.

——(1972). Using the Lab-8 for experimentation with the human visual system. *Behav. Res. Meth. Instrum.* **4**, 61–3.

——(1974). *The electroretinogram.* Academic Press, New York.

——, and Bloom, M. B. (1974). Relations between amplitudes of spontaneous saccades and visual responses. *J. opt. Soc. Am.* **64**, 1263–71.

——, Corwin, T. R., and Marsetta, R. (1971). Simultaneously recorded retinal and cortical responses to pattern stimuli. *J. opt. Soc. Am.* **61**, 1514–21.

——, Gaarder, K., and Schick, A. M. L. (1967). Variations of spontaneous ocular and occipital responses with stimulus patterns. *J. opt. Soc. Am.* **57**, 1534–9.

——, Marsetta, R., and Schick, A. M. L. (1970). Stimulus alternation and low level response. *Vision Res.* **10**, 227–36.

Asselman, P., Chadwick, D. W., and Marsden, C. D. (1975). Visual evoked responses in the diagnosis and management of patients suspected of multiple sclerosis. *Brain* **98**, 261–82.

Atkinson, J., Braddick, O., and Braddick, F. (1974). Acuity and contrast sensitivity of infant vision. *Nature, Lond.* **247**, 403–4.

Bagrash, F. M. (1973). Size-selective adaptation: psychological evidence for size-tuning and the effects of stimulus contour and adapting flux. *Vision Res.* **13**, 575–98.

Baker, H. D. and Rushton, W. A. H. (1965). The red-sensitive pigment in normal cones. *J. Physiol., Lond.* **176**, 56–72.

Baker, J. B., Larson, S. J., Sances, A., and White, B. T. (1968). Evoked potentials as an aid to the diagnosis of multiple sclerosis. *Neurology, Minneap.* **18**, 286.

Barlow, H. B., Blakemore, C., and Pettigrew, J. D. (1967). The neural mechanism of binocular depth discrimination. *J. Physiol., Lond.* **193**, 327–42.

Barlow, J. S. (1962). The relationship among "photic driving" responses to single flashes and the resting EEG. *Quarterly Report of the Research Laboratory of Electronics* No. 64. M.I.T., Cambridge, Massachusetts.

Barlow, J. S. and Ciganek, L. (1969). Lambda responses in relation to visual evoked responses in man. *Electroenceph. clin. Neurophysiol.* **26**, 183–92.

Barrett, G., Halliday, A. M., Halliday, E., and Michael, W. F. (1974). A four-dimensional display of the potential field of evoked responses on the head. *Electroenceph. clin. Neurophysiol.* **37**, 106.

Bartlett, J. R., and Doty, R. W. (1974). Influence of mesencephalic stimulation on unit activity in striate cortex of squirrel monkeys. *J. Neurophysiol.* **37**, 642–52.

———, Pecci-Saavedra, J., and P. D. Wilson (1973). Mesencephalic control of lateral geniculate nucleus in primates. III. Modifications with state of alertness. *Exp. Brain Res.* **18**, 214–24.

Bartlett, N. R., Eason, R. G., and White, C. T. (1968). Binocular summation in the evoked cortical potential. *Percept. Psychophys.* **3**, 75–6.

Bartley, S. H. (1941). *Vision: a study of its basis.* Van Nostrand, New York.

Beck, E. C., and Dustman, R. E. (1975). Changes in evoked responses during maturation and aging in man and macaque. In *Behavior and brain electrical activity* (ed. N. R. Burch). Plenum, New York.

Becker, W., Hoehne, O., Iwase, K., and Kornhuber, H. H. (1972). Bereitschaftspotential, Prämotorische Positivierung und andere Hirnpotentiale bei sakkadischen Augenbewegungen. *Vision Res.* **12**, 421–36.

Behrman, J., Halliday, A. M., and McDonald, W. I. (1972). Visual evoked responses to flash and pattern in patients with retrobulbar neuritis. *Electroenceph. clin. Neurophysiol.* **33**, 445.

———, Nissim, S., and Arden, G. B. (1972). A clinical method for obtaining pattern visual evoked responses. In *Experimental medicine and biology* (ed. G. B. Arden), Vol. 24, pp. 199–206. Plenum, London.

Bement, S. L., and Ranck, J. B. (1969). A quantitative study of electrical stimulation of central myelinated fibres. *Expl. Neurol.* **24**, 147–70.

Bendat, J. S. (1958). *Principles and applications of random noise theory.* Wiley, London.

Bender, M. B. (1964). Disorders in visual perception. In *Problems of dynamic neurology* (ed. Lo Halpern), pp. 319–75. Grune and Stratton, New York.

Benton, A. L., and Hecaen, H. (1970). Stereoscopic vision in patients with unilateral cerebral disease. *Neurology, Minneap.* **20**, 1084–8.

Berlucchi, G., and Strata, P. (1965). Ocular phenomena during synchronized and desynchronized sleep. In *Aspects anatomo-fonctionnels de la physiologie du sommeil* (ed. M. Jouvet), pp. 282–98. Centre National de la Recherche Scientifique, Paris.

Berlyne, D. E. (1958). The influence of the albedo and complexity of stimuli on visual fixation in the human infant. *Br. J. Psychol.* **49**, 315–18.

Beverley, K. I., and Regan, D. (1973). Evidence for the existence of neural mechanisms selectively sensitive to the direction of motion in space. *J. Physiol., Lond.* **235**, 17–29.

——, and —— (1974). Visual sensitivity to disparity pulses: evidence for directional selectivity. *Vision Res.* **14**, 357–61.

Biersdorf, W. R., and Nakamura, Z. (1971). Electroencephalogram potentials evoked by hemi-retinal stimulation. *Experientia* **27**, 402–3.

Bigum, H. B., Dustman, R. E., and Beck, E. C. (1970). Visual and somatosensory evoked responses from mongoloid and normal children. *Electroenceph. clin. Neurophysiol.* **28**, 202–5.

Bilge, M., Bingle, A., Seneviratne, K. N., and Whitteridge, D. (1967). A map of the visual cortex in the cat. *J. Physiol., Lond.* **191**, 116–118P.

——, Seneviratne, K. N., and Whitteridge, D. (1963). The primary visual receptive area of the cerebral cortex in the cat. *J. Physiol., Lond.* **169**, 36P.

Birren, J. E. (1959). Sensation perception and modification of behavior in relation to the process of aging. In *The process of aging in the nervous system*, (ed. J. E. Birren, H. A. Imus, and W. F. Windle), pp. 143–64. C. C. Thomas, Springfield, Illinois.

Bishop, P. O., Henry, G. H., and Smith, C. J. (1971). Binocular interaction fields of single units in the cat striate cortex. *J. Physiol., Lond.* **261**, 39–68.

Bizzi, E. (1968). Discharge of frontal eye field neurons during saccadic and following movements in unanesthetized monkeys. *Exp. Brain Res.* **6**, 69–80.

——, and Brooks, D. C. (1963). Functional connections between pontine reticular formation and lateral geniculate neurons during sleep. *Archs. ital. Biol.* **101**, 666–80.

——, and Schiller, P. H. (1970). Single unit activity in the frontal eye fields of unanesthetized monkeys during eye and head movement. *Exp. Brain Res.* **10**, 151–8.

Blake, R., and Fox, R. (1973). The psychological inquiry into binocular summation. *Percept. Psychophys.* **14**, 161–85.

Blakemore, C., and Campbell, F. W. (1969). On the existence in the human visual system of neurones selectively sensitive to the orientation and size of retinal images. *J. Physiol., Lond.* **203**, 237–60.

——, Muncey, J. P. J., and Ridley, R. M. (1973). Stimulus specificity in the human visual system. *Vision Res.* **13**, 1915–31.

Bodis-Wollner, I. (1972). Visual acuity and contrast sensitivity in patients with cerebral lesion. *Science, N.Y.* **178**, 769–71.

—— (1974). On dissociated visual functions. *J. Mt Sinai Hosp.* **41**, 38–45.

——, and Diamond, S. P. (1973). A method of testing and evaluating blurred vision in cerebral lesions. *Trans. Am. neurol. Ass.* **98**, 57–60.

——, Hendley, C. D., and Kulikowski, J. J. (1972). Electrophysiological and psychological response to modulation of contrast of a grating pattern. *Perception* **1**, 341–9.

——, ——, and Tajfel, L. (1973). Contrast-modulation thresholds as a function of spatial frequency. *J. opt. Soc. Am.* **63**, 1297.

de Boer, E., and Kuyper, P. (1968). Triggered correlation. *IEEE Trans. Bio-med. Electron. (Inst. elec. electron. Eng.)* **15**, 169–79.

Bondareff, W. (1959). Morphology of the aging nervous system. In *Handbook of aging and the individual* (ed. J. E. Birren), pp. 136–72. University of Chicago Press.

Borish, I. (1970). *Clinical refraction.* Professional Press, Chicago.

Bowsher, R. M. (1970). Reticular projections to lateral geniculate in cat. *Brain Res.* **23**, 247–9.

Box, G. E., and Jenkins, G. M. (1970). *Time series analysis, forecasting and control.* Holden Day, San Francisco.

Boyton, R. M. (1973). Discrimination of homogeneous double pulses of light. In *Handbook of sensory physiology* (ed. R. Jung), Vol. 8/4, pp. 202–32. Springer, Berlin.

Braddick, O. (1973). The masking of apparent motion in random dot patterns. *Vision Res.* **13**, 355–69.

Breitmeyer, B. G. and Cooper, L. A. (1972). Frequency-specific color adaptation in the human visual system. *Percept. Psychophys.* **11**, 95–6.

Brennan, W. M., Ames, E. W., and Moore, R. W. (1966). Age differences in infants' attention to patterns of different complexity. *Science, N.Y.* **151**, 354–6.

Brindley, G. S., and Lewin, W. S. (1968). The sensation produced by electrical stimulation of the visual cortex. *J. Physiol., Lond.* **196**, 479–93.

Brooks, B. A., and Fuchs, A. F. (1976). Influence of stimulus parameters on visual sensitivity during saccadic eye movement. *Vision Res.* **15**, 1389–98.

Brooks, D. C. (1967). Effect of bilateral optic nerve section on visual system monophasic wave acticity in the cat. *Electroenceph. clin. Neurophysiol.* **23**, 134–41.

——(1968*a*). Localization and characteristics of cortical waves associated with eye movement in the cat. *Expl. Neurol.* **22**, 603–13.

——(1968*b*). Waves associated with eye movement in the awake or sleeping cat. *Electroenceph. clin. Neurophysiol.* **24**, 532–41.

——, and Bizzi, E. (1963). Brain stem electrical activity during deep sleep. *Archs. ital. Biol.* **101**, 648–65.

——, and Gershon, M. D. (1971). Eye movement potentials in the oculomotor and visual systems of the cat: a comparison of reserpine induced waves with those present during wakefulness and rapid eye movement sleep. *Brain Res.* **27**, 223–39.

Brown, P. K., and Wald, G. (1964). Visual pigments in single rods and cones of the human retina. *Science, N.Y.* **144**, 45–52.

Bunge, R. P. (1968). Glial cells and the central myelin sheath. *Physiol. Rev.* **48**, 197–251.

Bürger, M. (1952). *Alter und Krankheit* (2nd edn.), Georg Thieme, Stuttgart.

Buss, A. R. (1973). An extension of developmental models that separate ontogenetic changes and cohort differences. *Psychol. Bull.* **80**, 466–79.

Bussgang, J. J. (1952). Cross correlations functions of amplitude distorted Gaussian signals. *Research Laboratory Electronics Technical Report* No. 216. M.I.T. Cambridge, Massachusetts.

Butler, B. V., and Engel, R. (1969). Mental and motor scores at 8 months in relation to neonatal photic response. *Develop. Med. Child Neurol.* **11**, 77–82.

Butler, S. R. and Glass, A. (1974). Asymmetries in the electroencephalogram associated with cerebral dominance. *Electroenceph. clin. Neurophysiol.* **36**, 481–91.

Callaway, E. (1973). Correlations between averaged evoked potentials and measures of intelligence. *Arch. gen. Psychiat.* **29**, 553–8.

Campbell, F. W. (1974). The transmission of spatial information through the visual system. In *The neurosciences third study program* (ed. F. O. Schmitt and F. G. Worden), pp. 95–103. M.I.T. Press, Cambridge, Massachusetts.

——, Cleland, B. G., Cooper, G. F., and Enroth-Cugell, C. (1968). The angular selectivity of visual cortical cells to moving gratings. *J. Physiol., Lond.* **198**, 237–50.

——, Cooper, G. F., and Enroth-Cugell, C. (1969). The spatial selectivity of the visual cells of the cat. *J. Physiol., Lond.* **203**, 223–35.

——, ——, Robson, J. G., and Sachs, M. B. (1969). The spatial selectivity of visual cells of the cat and the squirrel monkey. *J. Physiol., Lond.* **204**, 120–1.

——, and Green, D. G. (1965). Optical and retinal factors affecting visual resolution. *J. Physiol., Lond.* **181**, 576–93.

——, and Kulikowski, J. J. (1966). Orientational selectivity of the human visual system. *J. Physiol., Lond.* **187**, 437–45.

——, and —— (1971). An electrophysiological measure of the psychophysical contrast threshold. *J. Physiol., Lond.* **217**, 54P–55P.

——and —— (1972). The visual evoked potential as a function of contrast of a grating pattern. *J. Physiol., Lond.* **222**, 345–56.

——, ——, and Levinson, J. (1966). The effect of orientation on the visual resolution of gratings. *J. Physiol., Lond.* **187**, 427–36.

——, and Maffei, L. (1970). Electrophysiological evidence for the existence of orientation and size detectors in the human visual system. *J. Physiol., Lond.* **207**, 635–52.

——, ——, and Piccolino, M. (1973). The contrast sensitivity of the cat. *J. Physiol., Lond.* **229**, 719–31.

——, and Robson, J. G. (1968). Application of Fourier analysis to the visibility of gratings. *J. Physiol., Lond.* **197**, 551–66.

Cappin, J. and Nissim, S. (1975). Visual evoked responses in the detection of field defects in glaucoma. *Archs. Ophthal., N.Y.* **93**, 9–18.

Carmon, A., Harishana, Y., Lowinger, E., and Lavy, S. (1972). Asymmetries in hemispheric blood volume and cerebral dominance. *Behav. Biol.* **7**, 853–9.

Cartwright, R. F., and Regan, D. (1974). Semi-automatic, multi-channel Fourier analyser for evoked potential analysis. *Electroenceph. clin. Neurophysiol.* **36**, 547–50.

Cavonius, C. R. (1965). Evoked response of the human visual cortex: spectral sensitivity. *Psychon. Sci.* **2**, 185–6.

——, and Estévez, O. (1975). Sensitivity of human color mechanisms to gratings and flicker. *J. opt. Soc. Am.* **65**, 7.

——(1972). Comments. *Trace* **6**, 70.

Cederlöf, R., Frieberg, L., Jonsson, E., and Kaij, L. (1961). Studies on similarity diagnosis in twins with the aid of mailed questionnaires. *Acta genet. Statist. med.* **11**, 338–62.

Chacko, L. W. (1948). Analysis of fibre size in the human optic nerve. *Br. J. Ophthal.* **32**, 457–61.

Chase, R., and Kalil, R. (1972). Suppression of visual evoked responses to flashes and pattern shifts during voluntary saccades. *Vision Res.* **12**, 215–20.

Chatrian, G. E. (1975). The lambda waves. In *Handbook of electroencephalography and clinical neurophysiology* (ed. A. Remond) Elsevier, Amsterdam.

Chow, K. L. (1970). Integrative functions of the thalamocortical visual system of the cat. In *The biology of memory* (ed. K. H. Pribram and D. Broadbent), pp. 273–92. Academic Press, New York.

Churchill, J. A., Grisell, J., and Darnley, J. D. (1966). Rhythmic activity in the EEG of newborns. *Electroenceph. clin. Neurophysiol.* **21**, 131–9.

Ciganek, L. (1961). *Die elektroencephalographische lichtreizantwort der menschlichen Hirnrinde.* Slovenskej Adademie Vied, Bratislava.

—— (1971). Binocular addition of the visual response evoked by dichoptic patterned stimuli. *Vision Res.* **11**, 1289–97.

——, and Ingvar, D. H. (1969). Colour specific features of visual cortical responses in man evoked by monochromatic features. *Acta physiol. scand.* **76**, 82–92.

—— (1970). Binocular addition of the visually evoked response with different stimulus intensities in man. *Vision Res.* **10**, 479–87.

——, and Shipley, T. (1970). Color evoked brain responses in man. *Vision Res.* **10**, 917–19.

Clarke, P. G. H. (1973). Comparison of visual evoked potentials to stationary and moving patterns. *Exp. Brain Res.* **18**, 145–55.

Cleland, B. G., Dubin, M. W., and Levick, W. R. (1971). Sustained and transient neurones in the cat's retina and lateral geniculate nucleus. *J. Physiol., Lond.* **217**, 473–96.

Clynes, M., Kohn, M., and Lifshitz, K. (1964). Dynamic and spatial behaviour of light evoked potentials, their modification under hypnosis and on-line correlation in relation to rhythmic components. *Ann. N.Y. Acad. Sci.* **112**, 468–509.

Cobb, W. A., Ettlinger, G., and Morton, H. B. (1967). Visual evoked potentials in binocular rivalry. *Electroenceph. clin. Neurophysiol.*, Suppl. 26, 100–7.

——, Morton, H. B., and Ettlinger, G. (1967). Cerebral potentials evoked by pattern reversal and their suppression in visual rivalry. *Nature, Lond.* **216**, 1123–5.

——, and Pampiglione, G. (1952). Occipital sharp waves responsive to visual stimuli. *Electroenceph. clin. Neurophysiol.* **4**, 110–11.

Cohen, B. and Feldman, M. (1968). Relationship of electrical activity in pontine reticular formation and lateral geniculate body to rapid eye movements. *J. Neurophysiol.* **31**, 806–17.

——, and —— (1971). Potential changes associated with rapid eye movement in the calcarine cortex. *Expl. Neurol.* **31**, 100–13.

——, ——, and Diamond, S. P. (1969). Effect of eye movement, brainstem stimulation and alertness on transmission through lateral geniculate body of monkey. *J. Neurophysiol.* **32**, 583–94.

——, and Henn, V. (1972). Unit activity in the pontine reticular formation associated with eye movements. *Brain Res.* **46**, 403–10.

Cohn, R. (1963). Evoked visual cortical response in homonymous hemianopic defects in man. *Electroenceph. clin. Neurophysiol.* **15**, 922.

—— (1964). Rhythmic after-activity in visual evoked responses. *Ann. N.Y. Acad. Sci.* **281**, 281–91.

Coltheart, M. (1973). Colour-specificity and monocularity in the visual cortex. *Vision Res.* **13**, 2595–8.

Conel, J. L. (1939, 1941, 1947, 1951, 1959). *The postnatal development of the human cerebral cortex*, Vols. I–IV. Harvard University Press, Cambridge, Massachusetts.

Cook, R. C., and Glasscock, R. E. (1951). Refractive and ocular findings in the newborn. *Am. J. Ophthal.* **34**, 1407–13.

Copenhaver, R. M., and Perry, N. W. (1964). Factors affecting visually evoked cortical potentials such as impaired vision of varying etiology. *Invest. Ophthalmol.* **3**, 665–75.

Coppa, G. V., Nichols, B. L., Singh, J., and Di Ferrante, N. (1973). Urinary excretion of disulfated disaccharides in Hunter syndrome: correction by infusion of a serum fraction. *Analyt. Lett.* **6**, 225–33.

Cowey, A. (1964). Projection of the retina onto striate and pre-striate cortex in the squirrel monkey. *J. Neurophysiol.* **27**, 366–93.

——(1973). Brain damage and seeing: a new look at some old problems. *Trans. ophthal. Soc. U.K.* **93**, 409–16.

Cragg, B. G. (1969). The topography of the afferent projections in the circumstriate visual cortex of the monkey studied by the Nauta method. *Vision Res.* **9**, 733–47.

Crelin, E. S. (1973). *Functional anatomy of the newborn.* Yale University Press, New Haven.

Creutzfeldt, O. D. and Kuhnt, U. (1967). The visual evoked potential: physiological developmental and clinical aspects. *Electroenceph. clin. Neurophysiol.* **26**, 29–41.

Critchley, M. (1956). Neurological changes in the aged. *Res. Publs. Ass. Res. nerv. ment. Dis.* **35**, 198–223.

Crosby, E. C. (1953). Relations of brain centers to normal and abnormal eye movements in the horizontal plane. *J. comp. Neurol.* **99**, 437–79.

—— and Henderson, J. W. (1948). The mammalian midbrain and isthmus regions. II. Fiber connections of the superior colliculus. B. Pathways concerned in automatic eye movements. *J. comp. Neurol.* **88**, 53–91.

Crosby, E. C., Yoss, R. E., and Henderson, J. W. (1952). The mammalian midbrain and isthmus regions. II: The fiber connections, D. The pattern for eye movements on the frontal eye field and the discharge of specific portions of this field to and through midbrain levels. *J. comp. Neurol.* **97**, 357–83.

Crowell, D. H., Jones, R. J., Kapuniai, L. E., and Nakagawa, J. K. (1973). Unilateral cortical activity in newborn humans: An early index of cerebral dominance? *Science, N.Y.* **180**, 205–8.

Daniel, P. M., and Whitteridge, D. (1961). The representation of the visual field on the cerebral cortex in monkeys. *J. Physiol., Lond.* **159**, 203–21.

Davis, F. A. (1972). Impairment of repetitive impulse conduction in experimentally demyelinated and pressure-injured nerves. *J. Neurol. Neurosurg. Psychiat.* **35**, 537–44.

——, and Schauf, C. L. (1974). The pathophysiology of multiple sclerosis a theoretical model. In *Models of human neurological diseases* (ed. H. L. Klawans, Jr), Chapter 3, pp. 87–107. *Excerpta med.*, Amsterdam.

Dawson, G. D. (1947). Central responses to electrical stimulation of peripheral nerve in man. *J. Neurol. Neurosurg. Psychiat.* **10**, 137–40.

——(1951). A summation technique for detecting small signals in a large irregular background. *J. Physiol., Lond.* **115**, 2P.

Dawson, W. W., Perry, N. W., and Childers, D. G. (1972). Variations in human cortical responses to patterns and image quality. *Invest. Ophthalmol.* **11**, 789–99.

Dayton, G., Jones, M. H., Aiu, P. Rawson, R. A., Steele, B., and Rose, M. (1964). Developmental study of coordinated eye-movements. I. Visual acuity in the newborn human. *Archs. Ophthal., N.Y.* **71**, 871–5.

Desmedt, J. E. (1971). Somatosensory cerebral evoked potentials in man. In *Handbook of EEG and clinical neurophysiology* (ed. A. Rémond), Vol. 9, pp. 55–82. Elsevier, Amsterdam.

——, Brunko, E., and Debecker, J. (1976). Maturation of the somatosensory evoked potentials in normal infants and children, with special reference to the early N_1 component. *Electroenceph. clin. Neurophysiol.* **40**, 43–58.

——, and Noël, P. (1973). Average cerebral evoked potentials in the evaluation of lesions of the sensory nerves and of the central somatosensory pathway. In

New developments in electromyography and clinical neurophysiology (ed. J. E. Desmedt), Vol. 2, pp. 352–71. Karger, Basel.

Deutsch, R. (1962). *Nonlinear transformations of random processes.* Prentice Hall, Englewood Cliffs, New Jersey.

De Valois, R. L., Smith, C. J., Karoly, A. J., and Kitai, S. T. (1958). Electrical responses of primate visual system. I. Different layers of macaque lateral geniculate nucleus. *J. comp. physiol. Psychol.* **51**, 662–8.

DeVoe, R. G., Ripps, H., and Vaughan, H. G., Jr (1968). Cortical responses to stimulation of the human fovea. *Vision Res.* **8**, 135–47.

Dewan, E. M. (1964). Nonlinear oscillations and electroencephalography. *J. theor. Biol.* **7**, 141.

Ditchburn, R. W. (1955). Eye-movements in relation to retinal action. *Optica Acta* **1**, 171–6.

Doris, J., Casper, M., and Poresky, R. (1967). Differential brightness thresholds in infancy. *J. exp. Child. Psychol.* **5**, 522–35.

——, and Cooper, L. (1966). Brightness discrimination in infancy. *J. exp. Child Psychol.* **3**, 31–9.

Doty, R. W., and Negrao, N. (1973). Forebrain commissures and vision. In *Handbook of sensory physiology* (ed. R. Jung), pp. 543–82, Vol. VII/3B. Springer, Berlin.

——, Wilson, P. D., Bartlett, J. R., and Pecci-Saavedra, J. (1973). Mesencephalic control of lateral geniculate nucleus in primates. I. Electrophysiology. *Exp. Brain Res.* **18**, 189–203.

Dubowitz, L. M. S., Dubowitz, V., and Goldberg, C. (1970). Clinical assessment of gestational age in the newborn infant. *J. Pediat.* **77**, 1–10.

Duffy, F. H., and Burchfield, J. L. (1975). Eye movement-related inhibition of primate visual neurons. *Brain Res.* **89**, 121–32.

——, and Lombroso, C. T. (1968). Electrophysiological evidence for visual suppression prior to the onset of a voluntary saccadic eye movement. *Nature, Lond.* **218**, 1074–5.

——, and Rengstorff, R. H. (1971). Ametropia measurements from the visual evoked response. *Am. J. Optom.* **48**, 717.

Duke-Elder, S. (1963). *Systems of ophthalmology*, Vol. III: *Normal and abnormal development*, Part I: Embryology. Mosby, St Louis.

—— (1969). *The practice of refraction* (8th edn). Mosby, St Louis.

——, and Abrams, D. (1970). Ophthalmic optics and refraction. In *System of ophthalmology* (ed. S. Duke-Elder), Vol. 5, pp. 286–88. Kimpton, London.

Dustman, R. E., and Beck, E. C. (1965). The visually evoked potential in twins. *Electroenceph. clin. Neurophysiol.* **19**, 570–5.

——, and —— (1966). Visually evoked potentials: amplitude changes with age. *Science, N.Y.* **151**, 1013–15.

——, and —— (1969). The effects of maturation and aging on the waveform of visually evoked potentials. *Electroenceph. clin. Neurophysiol.* **26**, 2–11.

Ebersole, J. S., and Galambos, R. (1973). Lambda waves evoked by retinal stimulation in the absence of eye movement. *Electroenceph. clin. Neurophysiol.* **35**, 39–47.

Efron, R. (1970). The minimum duration of a perception. *Neuropsychologia* **8**, 57–63.

Ellingson, R. J. (1960). Cortical electrical responses to visual stimulation in the human infant. *Electroenceph. clin. Neurophysiol.* **12**, 663–77.

—— (1968). Clinical applications of evoked potential techniques in Infants and

children. *Electroenceph. clin. Neurophysiol.* **24**, 293.
—— (1970). Variability of visual evoked responses in the human newborn. *Electroenceph. clin. Neurophysiol.* **29**, 10–19.
——, Danahy, T., Nelson, B., and Lathrop, G. H. (1974). Variability of auditory evoked potentials in human infants and adults. *Electroenceph. clin. Neurophysiol.* **34**, 155–62.
——, Lathrop, G. H., Danahy, T., and Nelson, B. (1973). Variability of visual evoked potentials in human infants and adults. *Electroenceph. clin. Neurophysiol.* **34**, 113–24.
——, and Schain, R. J. (1969). EEG patterns in juvenile cerebral lipidosis. *Electroenceph. clin. Neurophysiol.* **27**, 191–4.
Emsley, H. H. (1963). *Visual optics.* Hatton Press, London.
Engel, R., and Fay, W., (1972). Visual evoked responses at birth, verbal scores at three years, and IQ at four years. *Develop. Med. Child Neurol.* **14**, 283–9.
——, and Henderson, N. B. (1973). Visual evoked responses and IQ scores at school age. *Develop. Med. Child Neurol.* **15**, 136–45.
Enroth-Cugell, C., and Robson, J. G. (1966). The contrast sensitivity of retinal ganglion cells of the cat. *J. Physiol., Lond.* **187**, 517–52.
Estevez, O., and Spekreijse, H. (1974*a*). Relationship between pattern appearance–disappearance and pattern reversal responses. *Exp. Brain Res.* **19**, 233–8.
——, and —— (1974*b*). A spectral compensation method for determining the flicker characteristics of the human colour mechanisms. *Vision Res.* **14**, 823–30.
——, ——, Van den Berg, T. J. T. P., and Cavonius, C. R. (1975). The spectral sensitivities of the isolated human color mechanisms determined from contrast evoked potential measurements. *Vision Res.* **15**, 1205–12.
Evans, C. C. (1952). Comments on "occipital sharp waves responsive to visual stimuli". *Electroenceph. clin. Neurophysiol.* **4**, 111.
—— (1953). Spontaneous excitation of the visual cortex and association areas – Lambda waves. *Electroenceph. clin. Neurophysiol.* **5**, 69–74.
Evans, B. T., Binnie, C. D., and Lloyd, D. S. L. (1974). A simple visual pattern stimulator. *Electroenceph. clin. Neurophysiol.* **37**, 403–6.
Fantz, R. L. (1963). Pattern vision in newborn infants. *Science, N.Y.* **140**, 296–7.
——, Ordy, J. M., and Udelf, M. S. (1962). Maturation of pattern vision in infants during the first six months. *J. comp. Physiol. Psychol.* **55**, 907–17.
Favreau, O. E., Emerson, V. F., and Corballis, M. O. (1972). Motion perception: a color-contingent after-effect. *Science, N.Y.* **176**, 78–9.
Feinsod, M., Abramsky, O., and Auerbach, E. (1973). Electrophysiological examinations of the visual system in multiple sclerosis. *J. neurol. Sci.* **20**, 161–75.
Ferris, G. S., Davis, C. D., Dorsen, M., and Hackett, E. R. (1967). Changes in latency and form of the photically induced average evoked response in human infants. *Electroenceph. clin. Neurophysiol.* **22**, 305–12.
Fidell, L. S. (1970). Orientation specificity in chromatic adaptation of human "edge-detectors". *Percept. Psychophys.* **8**, 235–7.
Finney, D. J. (1971). *Probit analysis.* pp. 50–80. Cambridge University Press, London.
Fiorentini, A., and Maffei, L. (1970*a*). Transfer characteristics of excitation and inhibition in the human visual system. *J. Neurophysiol.* **33**, 285–92.
——, and —— (1970*b*). Electrophysiological evidence for binocular disparity detectors in human visual system. *Science, N.Y.* **169**, 208–9.
——, and —— (1973). Contrast perception and electrophysiological correlates.

J. Physiol., Lond. **231**, 61–9.

——, and —— (1974). Evoked potentials in astigmatic subjects. *Vision Res.* **13**, 1781–3.

Fisher, R. A. (1934). *Statistical methods for research workers* (5th edn). Oliver and Boyd, Edinburgh.

Fishman, R. S., and Copenhaver, R. M. (1967). Macular disease and amblyopia. *Archs. Ophthalmol.* **77**, 303–725.

Flamm, L. E. (1971). The electroretinogram and visual evoked potential associated with paced saccadic displacement of the stimulus. Ph.D. Thesis. Northeastern University, Boston.

Flynn, J. T. (1967). Spatial summation in amblyopia. *Archs. Ophthalmol.* **78**, 470–4.

Franceschetti, A., and Burian, H. M. (1971). Visually responses in alternating strabismus. *Am. J. Ophthal.* **71**, 1292–7.

Françon, M., and Mallick, S. (1971). *Polarisation interferometer.* Wiley-Interscience, New York.

Freeman, R. D., Mitchell, D. E., and Millodot, M. (1972). A neural effect of partial visual deprivation in humans. *Science, N.Y.* **175**, 1384–6.

——, and Thibos, L. N. (1973). Electrophysiological evidence that abnormal early visual experience can modify the human brain. *Science, N.Y.* **180**, 876–8.

Freund, H-J. (1973). Neuronal mechanisms of the lateral geniculate body. In *Handbook of sensory physiology*, Vol. 8/3B, pp. 178–246: Central processing of visual information, Part B (ed. R. Jung). Springer, Berlin.

Frisén, L., and Hoyt, W. F. (1974). Insidious atrophy of retinal nerve fibers in multiple sclerosis. *Arch. Ophthal., N.Y.* **92**, 91–7.

Fry, G. A., and Bartley, S. H. (1935). The relation of stray light in the eye to the retinal action potential. *Am. J. Physiol.* **3**, 335–40.

Fuchs, A. F., and Luschei, E. S. (1971). The activity of single trochlear nerve fibres during eye movements in the alert monkey. *Exp. Brain Res.* **13**, 78–89.

Fukada, Y. (1971). Receptive field organization of cat optic nerve fibres with special reference to conduction velocity. *Vision Res.* **11**, 209–26.

Gaarder, K., Krauskopf, J., Graf, V., Kropel, W., and Armington, J. C. (1964). Averaged brain activity following saccadic eye movement. *Science, N.Y.* **146**, 1481–3.

Galambos, R., Norton, T. T., and Frommer, C. P. (1967). Optic tract lesions sparing pattern vision in cats. *Exp. Neurol.* **18**, 8–25.

Ganong, W. F. (1969). *Review of medical physiology* (4th edn). Lange Medical Publications, Los Altos, California.

Gazzaniga, M. S. (1970). *The bisected brain.* Appleton–Century–Crofts, New York.

Giannitrapani, D. (1967). Developing concepts of lateralization of cerebral functions. *Cortex* **3**, 353–70.

Gibson, J. E. (1963). *Nonlinear automatic control.* McGraw-Hill, New York.

Giles, G. H. (1960). *The principles and practice of refraction.* Hammon, London.

Gilliatt, R. W., and Hjorth, R. J. (1972). Nerve conduction during Wallerian degeneration in the baboon. *J. Neurol. Neurosurg. Psychiat.* **35**, 335–41.

—— and Taylor, J. C. (1959). Electrical changes following section of the facial nerve. *Proc. R. Soc. Med.* **52**, 1080–3.

Gills, J. P., Hobson, R., Hanley, W. B., and McKusick, V. A. (1965). Electroretinography and fundus oculi findings in Hunter's disease and allied mucopolysaccharidoses. *Archs. Ophthal., N.Y.* **74**, 596–603.

Gledhill, R. F., Harrison, B. M., and McDonald, W. I. (1973). Demyelination and remyelination after acute spinal cord compression. *Exp. Neurol.* **38**, 472–87.

Glickstein, M., and Millodot, M. (1970). Retinoscopy and eye size. *Science, N.Y.* **168**, 605–6.

Goldman, H. (1972). Examination of the function of the cataractous eye. *Am. J. Ophthal.* **73**, 309–20.

Gorman, J. J., Gogen, D. G., and Gellis, S. S. (1967). Testing the visual acuity of infants. In *Behavior in infancy and early childhood* (eds Y. Brackbill and G. C. Thompson), pp. 173–8. The Free Press, New York.

Gouras, P. (1968). Identification of cone mechanisms in monkey ganglion cells. *J. Physiol., Lond.* **199**, 533–47.

Grader, J., and Heller, G. L. (1964). Photic stimulation and the EEG in macular disease. *Archs. Ophthal, N.Y.* **72**, 763.

Graham, C. (1965). *Vision and visual perception.* Wiley, New York.

Graham, N. (1972). Spatial frequency channels in the human visual system: effects of luminance and pattern drift rate. *Vision Res.* **12**, 53–68.

Graziani, L. J., Weitzman, E. D., and Pineda, G. (1972). Visual evoked responses during neonatal respiratory disorders in low birth weight infants. *Pediat. Res.* **6**, 203–10.

Green, D. G. (1968). The contrast sensitivity of the colour mechanisms of the human eye. *J. Physiol., Lond.* **196**, 415–29.

—— (1969). Sinusoidal flicker characteristics of the colour sensitive mechanisms of the eye. *Vision Res.* **9**, 591–601.

—— (1970). Testing the vision of cataract patients by means of laser generated interference fringes. *Science, N.Y.* **168**, 1240–2.

——, and Cohen, M. M. (1971). Laser interferometry in the evaluation of potential macular function in the presence of opacities in the ocular media. *Trans. Am. Acad. Ophthal. Otol.* **75**, 629–7.

Green, J. B. (1969). Photosensitive epilepsy. The electroretinogram and visually evoked response. *Archs. Neurol., Chicago* **20**, 191–8.

Greenfield, J. G. (1963). *Greenfield's neuropathology* (eds W. Blackwood, W. H. McMenemey, A. Meyer, R. M. Norman, and D. S. Russell). Arnold, London.

——, and King, L. S. (1936). Observations on the histopathology of the cerebral lesions in disseminated sclerosis. *Brain* **52**, 445–57.

Groethuysen, U. C., and Bickford, R. G. (1956). Study of the lambda wave response of human beings. *Electroenceph. clin. Neurophysiol.* **8**, 344–5.

Gross, E. G., Vaughan, G. H., Jr, and Valenstein, E. (1967). Inhibition of visual evoked responses to patterned stimuli during voluntary eye movements. *Electroenceph. clin. Neurophysiol.* **22**, 204–9.

Gutmann, E., and Holubar, J. (1950). The degeneration of peripheral nerve fibres. *J. Neurol. Neurosurg. Psychiat.* **13**, 89–105.

Haber, R. N., and Standing, L. G. (1970). Direct estimates of the apparent duration of a flash. *Can. J. Psychol.* **24**, 216–29.

Hall, J. I. (1967). Studies on demyelinated peripheral nerves in guinea pigs with experimental allergic neuritis. A histological and electrical study. II. Electrophysiological observations. *Brain* **90**, 313–32.

Halliday, A. M. (1972*a*). Discussion on component analysis and topology. *Trace* **6**, 39–46.

—— (1972*b*). Evoked responses in organic and functional sensory loss. In *Activités évoquées et leur conditionement chez l'Homme normal et en pathologie mentale* (eds A. Fessard, and G. Lelord), pp. 189–212. INSERM, Paris.

——, McDonald, W. I., and Mushin, J. (1972). Delayed visual evoked responses in optic neuritis. *Lancet* **1**, 982–5.

——, ——, and —— (1973*a*). Delayed pattern-evoked responses in optic neuritis in relation to visual acuity. *Trans. ophthal. Soc. U.K.* **93**, 315–24.

——, ——, and —— (1973*b*). The visual evoked response in the diagnosis of multiple sclerosis. *Br. med. J.* **4**, 661–4.

——, ——, and —— (1974*a*). The dissociation of amplitude and latency changes in the pattern-evoked response following optic neuritis. *Electroenceph. clin. Neurophysiol.* **36**, 218.

——, ——, and —— (1974*b*). Delayed visual evoked response in progressive spastic paraplegia. *Electroenceph. clin. Neurophysiol.* **37**, 328.

——, and Michael, W. F. (1970). Changes in pattern-evoked responses in man associated with the vertical and horizontal meridians of the visual field. *J. Physiol., Lond.* **208**, 499–513.

——, and Wakefield, G. W. (1963). Cerebral evoked potentials in patients with dissociated sensory loss. *J. Neurol. Neurosurg. Psychiat.* **26**, 211–19.

Hanefeld, F., and Pampiglione, G. (1972). EEGs in 18 cases of mucopolysaccharidoses. *Electroenceph. clin. Neurophysiol.* **33**, 447.

Harden, A. (1974). The non-corneal electro-retinogram: parameters in normal children. *Br. J. Ophthal.* **58**, 811–16.

——, and Pampiglione, G. (1970). Neurophysiological approach to disorders of vision. *Lancet* (i), 805–9.

——, ——, and Picton-Robinson, N. (1973). Electroretinogram and visual evoked response in a form of 'neuronal lipidosis' with diagnostic EEG features. *J. Neurol. Neurosurg. Psychiat.* **36**, 61–7.

Harding, G. F. A. (1974). The visual evoked response. *Adv. Ophthal.* **28**, 2–28.

——, Thompson, C. R. S., and Panayiopoulos, C. R. (1970). Evoked response diagnosis in visual field defects. *Proc. electrophysiol. Technol. Ass.* **16**, 159–63.

Harris, C. S. (1969). Retinal localization of orientation-specific color after-effects. *J. opt. Soc. Am.* **59**, 504.

—— (1970). Effect of viewing distance on a colour after-effect specific to spatial frequency. *Psychon. Sci.* **21**, 350.

——, and Gibson, A. R. (1968). Is orientation-specific color adaptation in human vision due to edge-detectors after-images or "dipoles"? *Science, N.Y.* **162**, 1406–507.

Harris, E. K. and Woody, C. D. (1969). Use of an adaptative filter to characterize signal-noise relationships. *Comput. Biomed. Res.* **2**, 242–73.

Harter, M. R. (1970). Evoked cortical responses to checkerboard patterns: effects of check size as a function of retinal eccentricity. *Vision Res.* **10**, 1365–76.

—— (1971*a*). Visually evoked cortical responses to the on- and off-set of patterned light in humans. *Vision Res.* **11**, 685–95.

—— (1971*b*). Visually evoked cortical responses to checkerboard patterns: effect of check-size as a function of retinal eccentricity. *Electroenceph. clin. Neurophysiol.* **28**, 48–54.

——, and Salmon, L. E. (1971). Evoked cortical responses to patterned light flashes: effects of ocular convergence and accommodation. *Electroenceph. clin. Neurophysiol.* **30**, 527–33.

——, Seiple, W. H., and Musso, M. (1974). Binocular summation and suppression; Visually evoked cortical responses to dichoptically presented patterns of different spatial frequencies. *Vision Res.* **14**, 1169–80.

——, ——, and Salmon, L. E. (1972). Evoked cortical responses to dichoptically

presented light flashes: interocular interaction. *J. Life Sci.* 2, 27–33.
——,——, and —— (1973). Binocular summation of visually evoked responses to pattern stimuli in humans. *Vision Res.* **13**, 1433–46.
——, and Suitt, C. D. (1970). Visually-evoked cortical responses and pattern vision in the infant: a longitudinal study. *Psychon. Sci.* **18**, 235–7.
——, and White, C. T. (1968). Effects of contour sharpness and check-size on visually evoked cortical potentials. *Vision Res.* **8**, 701–11.
——, and —— (1970). Evoked cortical responses to checkerboard patterns: effect of check size as a function of visual acuity. *Electroenceph. clin. Neurophysiol.* **28**, 48–54.
——, White, B. L., and Held, R. (1965). Visual accommodation in human infants. *Science, N.Y.* **148**, 528–30.
Held, R., and Shattuck, S. R. (1971). Color- and edge-sensitive channels in the human visual system: tuning for orientation. *Science, N.Y.* **174**, 314–16.
Helmholtz, H. von (1866). *Physiological optics* 1962 translation by Dover Publications, New York.
Helper, N. (1968). A motion contingent after-effect. *Science, N.Y.* **162**, 376–7.
Henderson, N. B., and Engel, R. (1974). Neonatal visual evoked potentials as predictors of psycho-educational tests at age seven. *Develop. Psychol.* **10**, 269–76.
Heron, J. R., Regan, D., and Milner, B. A. (1974). Delay in visual perception in unilateral optic atrophy after retrobulbar neuritis. *Brain* **97**, 69–78.
Hershenson, M. (1964). Visual discrimination in the human newborn. *J. comp. Physiol. Psychol.* **58**, 270–6.
—— (1967). Development of the perception of form. *Psychol. Bull.* **67**, 326–36.
Hess, A., and Young, J. Z. (1949). Correlation of internodal length and fibre diameter in the central nervous system. *Nature, Lond.* **164**, 490–1.
Hewitt, W. (1962). The development of the human corpus callosum. *J. Anat.* **96**, 355–8.
Hirsch, H. V. B., and Spinelli, D. N. (1970). Visual experience modifies distribution of horizontally and vertically oriented receptive fields in cats. *Science, N.Y.* **168**, 869–71.
Hishikawa, Y., Yamamoto, J., Furuya, E., Yamada, Y., Miyazaki, K., and Kanedo, Z. (1967). Photosensitive epilepsy: relationships between the visual evoked responses and the epileptiform discharges induced by intermittent photic stimulation. *Electroenceph. clin. Neurophysiol.* **23**, 320–34.
Hoffman, K. P., and Stone, J. (1971). Conduction velocity of afferents to cat visual cortex: a correlation with cortical receptive field properties. *Brain Res.* **32**, 460–6.
——, ——, and Sherman, S. M. (1972). The relay of receptive field properties in the dorsal lateral geniculate nucleus of the cat. *J. Neurophysiol.* **35**, 518–31.
Holmes, G. (1918). Disturbance of vision by cerebral lesions. *Br. J. Ophthal.* **2**, 353–84.
—— (1945). The organization of the visual cortex in man. *Proc. R. Soc. B* **132**, 348–61.
von Holst, E., and Mittelstaedt, H. (1950). Das Reafferenzprinzip. Wechselwirkungen zwischen Zentralnervensystem und Peripherie. *Naturwissenschaften* **37**, 464–76.
Hopkins, H. H., and Tiziani, H. (1970). Speckling in diffraction patterns and optical images formed with the laser. In *C.R. International Symposium* on *applications de l'holographie* (eds J. C. Vienot, J. Bulabois, and J. Pasteur). Basançon.

Horowitz, F. D., Tims, S. M., and McCluskey, K. A. (1974). Duration of visual fixation to different black and white checkerboard stimuli. In Visual attention, auditory stimulation and language discrimination in young infants (ed. F. D. Horowitz). *Monogr. Soc. Res. Child Develop.* **39**, 116–20.

Howard, I. P., and Templeton, W. B. (1966). *Human spatial orientation.* Wiley New York.

Hrbek, A., Karlberg, P., and Olsson, T. (1973). Development of visual and somatosensory evoked responses in pre-term newborn infants. *Electroenceph. clin. Neurophysiol.* **34**, 225–32.

Hrbek, A., and Mares, P. (1964). Cortical evoked responses to visual stimulation in full-term and premature newborns. *Electroenceph. clin. Neurophysiol.* **16**, 575–81.

Hubel, D. H., and Wiesel, T. N. (1959). Receptive fields of single neurones in the cat's striate cortex. *J. Physiol., Lond.* **148**, 574–91.

——, and —— (1962). Receptive fields, binocular interaction and functional architecture in the cat's visual cortex. *J. Physiol., Lond.* **160**, 106–54.

——, and —— (1965). Receptive fields and functional architecture in two non-striate visual areas of the cat (areas 18 and 19). *J. Neurophysiol.* **28**, 229–89.

——, and —— (1967). Cortical and callosal connexions concerned with the vertical meridian of visual fields in the cat. *J. Neurophysiol.* **30**, 1561–73.

——, and —— (1968). Receptive fields and functional architecture of monkey striate cortex. *J. Physiol., Lond.* **195**, 215–43.

——, and —— (1970). Stereoscopic vision in the macaque monkey. *Nature, Lond.* **225**, 41–2.

Huber, C. (1972). Visual evoked responses during exposure to strong colored lights. *Ophthal. Res.* **3**, 55–62.

Huxley, A. F., and Stämpfli, R. (1949). Evidence for saltatory conduction in peripheral myelinated nerve fibres. *J. Physiol., Lond.* **108**, 315–39.

Ikeda, H., and Wright, M. J. (1972*a*). Functional organization of the periphery effect on retinal ganglion cells. *Vision Res.* **12**, 1857–79.

——, and —— (1972*b*). Receptive field organization of 'sustained' and 'transient' retinal ganglion cells which subserve different functional roles. *J. Physiol., Lond.* **227**, 769–800.

Ikeda, H., and Wright, M. J. (1974). Evidence for 'sustained' and 'transient' neurones in the cats visual cortex. *Vision Res.* **14**, 133–6.

Jacobson, J. H., Hirose, T., and Suzuke, T. A. (1968). Simultaneous ERG and VER in lesions of the optic pathway. *Invest. Ophthal.* **7**, 279–92.

Jasper, H. H. (1958). Report of a Committee on methods of clinical examination in electroencephalography. *Electroenceph. clin. Neurophysiol.* **10**, 370–5.

Jeannerod, M., and Chouvet, G. (1973). Saccadic displacements of the retinal image: effects on the visual system in the cat. *Vision Res.* **13**, 161–9.

——, and Sakai, K. (1971). Potentials related to visual field motions as compared to eye movement potentials in the cat's visual system. *Vision Res.* **11**, 161–5.

Jeavons, P. M. (1972). Television epilepsy. *Nursing Mirror* (August).

——, and Harding, G. F. A. (1970). Television epilepsy. Letter to the Editor. *Lancet* ii, 926.

——, and —— (1975). *Photosensitive epilepsy.* Heinemann, London.

——, and ——, and Panayiotopoulos, C. R. (1971). Photosensitive epilepsy and driving. *Lancet* i, 1125.

——, ——, ——, and Drasdo, N. (1972). The effect of geometric patterns

combined with intermittent photoc stimulation in photosensitive epilepsy. *Electroenceph. clin. Neurophysiol.* **33**, 221–4.
Jeffreys, D. A. (1968). Separable components of human evoked responses to spatially patterned visual fields. *Electroenceph. clin. Neurophysiol.* **24**, 596.
Jeffreys, D. A. (1969). Characteristics of visual and auditory evoked potentials. *Neurosci. Res. Prog. Bull.* **7**, 205–27.
——— (1971*a*). Striate and extra-striate origins of pattern-related visual evoked potential (VEP) components. *J. Physiol., Lond.* **211**, 29P–30P.
——— (1971*b*). Cortical source locations of pattern-related visual evoked potentials recorded from the human scalp. *Nature, Lond.* **229**, 502–4.
——— (1972). Component analysis of the spatial contrast EP. *Trace* **6**, 30–8.
———, and Axford, J. G. (1972*a*). Source location of pattern-specific components of human visual evoked potentials. I. Components of striate cortical origin. *Exp. Brain Res.* **16**, 1–21.
———, and ——— (1972*b*). Source locations of pattern-specific components of human visual evoked potentials. II. Component of extrastriate cortical origin. *Exp. Brain Res.* **16**, 22–40.
Jenkins, C. M., and Watts, D. C. (1968). *Spectral analysis and its applications.* Holden Day, San Francisco.
Johnson, E. P., Riggs, L. A., and Schick, A. M. L. (1966). Photopic retinal potentials evoked by phase alternation of a barred pattern. *Vision Res.*, Suppl. **1**, 75–91.
Jones, R. H., Crowell, D. H., and Kapuniai, L. E. (1969). A method for detecting change in a time series applied to newborn EEG. *Electroenceph. clin. Neurophysiol.* **27**: 436–40.
———, ———, and, ——— (1970). Change detection model for serially correlated multivariate data. *Biometrics* **26**, 269–80.
Julesz, B. (1960). Binocular depth perception of computer-generated patterns. *Bell Syst. tech. J.* **39**, 1125–62.
——— (1971). *Foundations of cyclopean perception.* University of Chicago Press, Chicago.
Kaeser, H. E., and Lambert, E. H. (1962). Nerve function studies in experimental polyneuritis. *Electroenceph. clin. Neurophysiol.*, Suppl. **22**, 29–35.
Kahana, E., Leibowitz, U., Fishback, N., and Alter, M. (1973). Slowly progressive and acute visual impairment in multiple sclerosis. *Neurology, Minneap.* **23**, 729–33.
Kahneman, D. (1968). Method, findings and theory in studies of visual masking. *Psychol. Bull.* **70**, 404–25.
Karmel, B. Z. (1969*a*). Complexity, amount of contour and visually dependent preference behavior in hooded rats, domestic chicks and human infants. *J. comp. Physiol. Psychol.* **69**, 649–57.
——— (1969*b*). The effects of age, complexity and amount of contour on pattern preferences in human infants. *J. exp. Child Psychol.* **7**, 339–54.
———, Hoffman, R. F., and Fegy, M. J. (1974). Processing of contour information by human infants evidenced by pattern-dependent evoked potentials. *Child Develop.* **45**, 39–48.
Kawasaki, K., Hirose, T., Jacobson, J. H., and Cordella, M. (1970). Binocular fusion: effect of breaking on the human visual evoked response. *Archs. Ophthal. Chicago* **84**, 25–8.
Kayama, Y. (1974). Evoked potentials of the central visual system during and after hypoxia in cats. *Electroenceph. clin. Neurophysiol.* **36**, 619–28.

Keeney, A. H. (1966). Development of the eye. In *Human development* (ed. F. Falkner). Saunders, Philadelphia.

Keesey, V. T. (1972). Flicker and pattern detection: a comparison of thresholds. *J. opt. Soc. Am.* **61**, 632–40.

Kelly, D. H. (1959). Effects of sharp edges in a flickering field. *J. opt. Soc. Am.* **49**, 730–2.

—— (1961). Visual responses to time-dependent stimuli. I. Amplitude sensitivity measurements. *J. opt. Soc. Am.* **51**, 422–9.

—— (1971). Theory of flicker and transient responses. II. Counterphase gratings. *J. opt. Soc. Am.* **61**, 632–40.

—— (1974). Spatio-temporal characteristics of color-vision mechanisms. *J. opt. Soc. Am.* **64**, 983–90.

Kelly, J. P., and Van Essen, D. C. (1974). Cell structure and function in the visual cortex of the rat. *J. Physiol., Lond.* **238**, 515–47.

Kennard, M. A., and Ectors, L. (1938). Forced circling in monkeys following lesions of the frontal lobes. *J. Neurophysiol.* **1**, 45–54.

King-Smith, P. E., and Kulikowski, J. J. (1973). Spatial arrangement of the flicker and pattern detectors for a fine line. *J. Physiol., Lond.* **234**, 33P–35P.

Kinney, J. A. S., McKay, C. L., Mensch, A. J., and Luria, S. M. (1972). Techniques for analysing differences in VERs to colored and patterned stimuli. *Vision Res.* **12**, 1733–47.

Koles, Z. J., and Rasminsky, M. (1972). A computer simulation of conduction in demyelinated nerve fibres. *J. Physiol., Lond.* **227**, 351–64.

Kooi, K. A., and Bagchi, B. K. (1964). Visual evoked responses in man: normative data. *Ann. N.Y. Acad. Sci.* **112**, 254–69.

——, Yamada, T., and Marshall, R. E. (1973). Field studies of monocularly evoked cerebral potentials in bitemporal hemianopsia. *Neurology, Minneap.* **23**, 1217–25.

Krauskopf, J. (1973). Contributions of the primary chromatic mechanisms to the generation of visual evoked potentials. *Vision Res.* **13**, 2289–98.

——, Graf, V., and Gaarder, K. (1966). Lack of inhibition during involuntary saccades. *Am. J. Psychol.* **79**, 73–81.

Kuffler, S. W. (1953). Discharge patterns and functional organization of mammalian retina. *J. Neurophysiol.* **16**, 37–68.

Kulikowski, J. J. (1969). Limiting conditions of visual perception. *Pr. Inst. Auto. P.A.N.* **77**, 1–133.

—— (1971). Effect of eye movements on the contrast sensitivity of spatiotemporal patterns. *Vision Res.* **11**, 261–73.

—— (1972). Relation of psychophysics and electrophysiology. *Trace* **6**, 64–9.

—— (1974). Human averaged occipital potentials evoked by pattern and movement. *J. Physiol., Lond.* **242**, 70P–71P.

——, and Kozak, W. (1967). ERG, visual evoked responses and pattern detection in man. In *Advances in electrophysiology and pathology of the visual system: 6th International Symposium of Electro-retinography*. G. Thieme, Leipzig.

——, and Leisman, G. (1973). The effect of nitrous oxide on the relation between the evoked potential and contrast threshold. *Vision Res.* **13**, 2079–86.

——, and Tolhurst, D. J. (1973). Psychophysical evidence for sustained and transient detectors in human vision. *J. Physiol., Lond.* **232**, 149–62.

Kurtzberg, D., and Vaughan, H. G. (1973). Electrocortical potentials associated with eye movements. In *The oculomotor system and brain functions* (ed. V. Zikmund), pp. 137–46. Butterworths, London.

Landau, W. M. (1953). The duration of neuromuscular function after nerve section in man. *J. Neurosurg.* **10**, 64–8.

Lansing, R. W. (1964). Electroencephalographic correlates of binocular rivalry in man. *Science, N.Y.* **146**, 1325–7.

Latto, R., and Cowey, A. (1971*a*). Visual field defects after frontal eye-field lesions in monkeys. *Brain Res.* **30**, 1–24.

——, and —— (1971*b*). Fixation changes after frontal eye-field lesions in monkeys. *Brain Res.* **30**, 25–36.

Lawwill, T., and Biersdorf, W. (1968). Binocular rivalry and visual evoked responses. *Invest. Ophthal.* **7**, 378–85.

——, Cox, W. E., Tuttle, D., Meur, G., and Burian, H. M. (1973). Lateral inhibition and the VER in the central field of an amblyopic subject. *Invest. Ophthal.* **12**, 154–6.

Le Grand, Y. (1956). *Optique physiologique.* Tome 3, *L'espace visuel*, pp. 392. Masson et Cie, Paris.

Lehmann, D., and Fender, D. H. (1967). Monocularly evoked electroencephalogram potentials: influence of target structure presented to the other eye. *Nature, Lond.* **215**, 204–5.

——, and —— (1968). Component analysis of human averaged evoked potentials: dichoptic stimuli using different target structure. *Electroenceph. clin. Neurophysiol.* **24**, 542–53.

——, and —— (1969). Averaged visual evoked potentials in humans: mechanism of dichoptic interaction studies in a subject with a split chiasma. *Electroenceph. clin. Neurophysiol.* **27**, 142–5.

——, and Tackmann, W. (1971). Refraktärperiode und Übermittlung von Serienimpulsen im N.tibialis des Meerschweichens bei experimentaller allergischer Neuritis. *Z. Neurol.* **199**, 67–85.

——, and Tackmann, W. (1970). Die Uebermittlung frequenter Impulsserien in demyelinisierten und degenerierenden Nervenfasern. *Arch. Psychiat. Nervenkrankh.* **213**, 215–27.

Lennox, W. G., Gibbs, E. L., and Gibbs, F. A. (1945). The brain-wave pattern, an hereditary trait. *J. Hered.* **36**, 233–43.

Lenz, W. (1961). *Medizinische Genetik: eine Einführung in ihre Grundlagen und Probleme.* G. Thieme, Stuttgart.

Lesèvre, N. (1973). Potentiels évoqués par des patterns chez l'homme: influence de variables caractérisant le stimulus et sa position dans le champ visuel. In *Activités évoquées et leur conditionnement chez l'homme normal et en pathologie mentale* (eds A. Fessard and G. Lelord), pp. 1–22. INSERM, Paris.

——, and Rémond, A. (1972). Chronotopographical study of the various components of the pattern response. *Trace* **6**, 47–61.

——, and —— (1973). Effects of contrasts on the visual evoked potentials related to eye movements. In *The oculomotor system and brain functions* (ed. V. Zikmund), pp. 119–34. Butterworths, London.

Levick, W. R., Cleland, B. E., and Combes, J. S. (1972). On the apparent orbit of the Pulfrich Pendulum. *Vision Res.* **12**, 1381–8.

Lewis, E. G., and Sears, T. A. (1970). The effects of alcohol on visual and somato-sensory evoked responses. *Electroenceph. clin. Neurophysiol.* **28**, 202–5.

——, Dustman, R. E., and Beck, E. C. (1970). The effects of alcohol on visual and somato-sensory evoked responses. *Electroenceph. clin. Neurophysiol.* **28**, 202–5.

——, Dustman, R. E., and Beck, E. C. (1972). Evoked response similarity in monozygotic, dizygotic and unrelated individuals: a comparative study. *Electroenceph. clin. Neurophysiol.* **32**, 309–16.

Lewkonia, I. (1969). Objective assessment of visual acuity by induction of optokinetic nystagmus. *Br. J. Ophthal.* **53**, 641–4.

Lindquist, E. F. (1953). *Design and analysis of experiments in psychology and education.* Houghton Mifflin Company, Boston, Massachusetts.

Linsk, A. (1973). Visual acuity in the newborn with notes on some objective methods to determine visual acuity. *Documenta Ophth.* **34**, 259–70.

Lissak, K., Dempsey, D. W., and Rosenbluth, A. (1939). The failure of transmission of motor nerve impulses in the course of Wallerian degeneration. *Am. J. Physiol.* **128**, 45–56.

Lombroso, C. T., Duffy, F. H., and Robb, R. M. (1969). Selective suppression of cerebral evoked potentials to patterned light in amblyopia ex anopsia. *Electroenceph. clin. Neurophysiol.* **27**, 238–47.

Lopes da Silva, F. H. (1970). Dynamic characteristics of visual evoked potentials. Thesis, University of Utrecht.

——, Rotterdam, A. van, Storm van Leeuwen, W., and Tielen, A. M. (1970). Dynamic characteristics of visual evoked potentials in the dog. II. Beta frequency selectivity in evoked potentials and background activity. *Electroenceph. clin. Neurophysiol.* **29**, 260–8.

Lovegrove, W. J., and Over, R. (1973). Colour selectivity in orientation masking and after-effect. *Vision Res.* **13**, 895–902.

Lowenthal, S., and Arsenault, H. (1970). Image formation for coherent diffuse objects: statistical properties. *J. opt. Soc. Am.* **60**, 1478–83.

——, and Joyeux, D. (1971). Speckle removal by a slowly moving diffuser associated with a motionless diffuser. *J. opt. Soc. Am.* **61**, 847–51.

Ludlam, W. M., and Meyers, R. R. (1972). The use of visual evoked responses in objective refraction. *Trans. N.Y. Acad. Sci.* **34**, 154–70.

Lumsden, C. E. (1955). Pathology. In *Multiple sclerosis* (eds D. McAlpine, N. D. Compston, and C. E. Lumsden). Livingstone, Edinburgh.

MacKay, D. M. (1968). Evoked potentials reflecting interocular and monocular suppression. *Nature, Lond.* **217**, 81–3.

—— (ed.) (1969). Evoked brain potentials as indicators of sensory information processing. *Neurosci. Res. Prog. Bull.* **7**, 1–276.

—— (1970). Elevation of visual threshold by displacement of retinal image. *Nature, Lond.* **225**, 90–2.

——, and Jeffreys, D. A. (1973). Visual evoked potentials and visual perception in man VII/3B. In *Handbook of sensory physiology* (ed. R. Jung), pp. 647–78. Springer, Berlin.

——, and MacKay, V. (1973) Orientation-sensitivity after-effects of dichoptically presented colour and form. *Nature, Lond.* **242**, 477–9.

Maffei, L., and Campbell, F. W. (1970). Neurophysiological localization of the vertical and horizontal coordinates in man. *Science, N.Y.* **167**, 386–7.

——, and Fiorentini, A. (1972). Retinogeniculate convergence and analysis of contrast. *J. Neurophysiol.* **35**, 65–72.

——, and —— (1973). The visual cortex as a spatial frequency analyser. *Vision Res.* **13**, 1255–67.

——, ——, and Bisti, S. (1973). Neural correlate of perceptual adaptation to gratings. *Science, N.Y.* **182**, 1036–8.

Magladery, J. W. (1959). Neurophysiology and aging. In *Handbook of aging and*

the individual (ed. J. E. Birren). University of Chicago Press.
Mansfield, R. J. W. (1974). Neural basis of orientation perceptoin in primate vision. *Science, N.Y.* **186**, 1133–5.
Marcus, M. M. (1970). Visual evoked responses to pattern in normals and mental retardates. *Clin. Res.* **18**, 206.
——— (1971). Developmental change and age-related waveforms in the visual evoked response. *Psychophysiology* **8**, 271.
Marg, E., Adams, J. E., and Rutkin, B. (1968). Receptive fields of cells in human visual cortex. *Experientia* **24**, 348–50.
Marks, W. B., Dobelle, W. H., and MacNichol, E. F. (1964). Visual pigments of single primate cones. *Science, N.Y.* **143**, 1181–3.
Marsden, C. D., Meadows, J. C., and Merton, P. A. (1971). Isolated single motor units in human muscle and their rate of discharge during maximal voluntary effort. *J. Physiol., Lond.* **217**, 12P–13P.
Marshall, C., and Harden, C. (1952). Use of rhythmically varying patterns for photic stimulation. *Electroenceph. clin. Neurophysiol.* **4**, 283–7.
Martin, G. (1890). Amblyopie astigmatique. Condition du développement parfait de la vision. *Bull. Soc. fr. Opht.* **8**, 217.
Martin, J. I. (1970). Effects of binocular fusion and binocular rivalry on cortically evoked potentials. *Electroenceph. clin. Neurophysiol.* **28**, 190–201.
Mastropaolo, C., Pampiglione, G., and Stephens, R. (1971). EEG studies in 22 children with sulphatide lipidosis (metachromatic leucodystrophy) *Develop. Med. Child Neurol.* **13**, 20–31.
Matthews, W. B., Beauchamp, M., and Small, D. G. (1974). Cervical somatosensory evoked responses in man. *Nature, Lond.* **252**, 230–2.
Maumenee, A. E. (1971). Report and discussion at the end of the paper by Green and Cohen. *Trans. Am. Acad. Ophthal. Otol.* **75**, 635.
May, J. G. (1972). Chromatic adaptation of orientation- and size-specific visual processes inman. *Vision Res.* **12**, 1509–17.
———, Forbes, W. B., and Piantanida, T. P. (1971). The visual evoked responses obtained with an alternating barred pattern: rate, spatial frequency and wavelength. *Electroenceph. clin. Neurophysiol.* **30**, 222–8.
———, Leftwich, D. A., and Aptaker, P. (1974). Evoked potential correlates of adaptation to wavelength and orientation. *Vision Res.* **14**, 143–6.
———, and Siegfried, J. B. (1970). Spectral sensitivity of the human VER obtained with an alternating barred pattern. *Vision Res.* **10**, 1339–40.
Mayer, R. F., and Denny-Brown, D. (1964). Conduction velocity in peripheral nerve during experimental demyelination in the cat. *Neurology, Minneap.* **14**, 714–26.
Mayhew, J. E. W., and Anstis, S. M. (1972). Movement after-effects contingent on color, intensity, and pattern. *Percept. Psychophys.* **12**, 77–85.
McAlpine, D., Lumsden, C. E., and Acheson, E. D. (1972). *Multiple sclerosis: a reappraisal.* Churchill–Livingstone, Edinburgh.
McCollough, C. (1965). Color adaptation of edge-detectors in the human visual system. *Science, N.Y.* **149**, 1115–16.
McCormack, G. and Marg, E. (1973). Computer-assisted eye examination II. Visual evoked response meridional refractometry. *Am. J. Optom.* **50**, 889–902.
McDonald, W. I. (1962). Conduction in muscle afferent fibres during experimental demyelination in cat nerve. *Acta Neuorpath.* **1**, 425–32.
——— (1963). The effects of experimental demyelination on conduction in peripheral nerve. A histological and electrophysiological study. II. Electro-

physiological observations. *Brain* **86**, 501–24.
——(1972). The time course of conduction failure during degeneration of a central tract. *Exp. Brain Res.* **14**, 550–6.
——(1973). Experimental Neuropathy. The use of diphtheria toxin. In *New developments in electromyography and clinical neurophysiology* (ed. J. E. Desmedt), pp. 129–44). Karger, Basel.
——(1974). Remyelination in relation to clinical lesions of the central nervous system. *Br. med. Bull.* **30**, 186–9.
——, and Ohlrich, G. D. (1971). Quantitative anatomical measurements on single isolated fibres from the cat spinal cord. *J. Anat.* **110**, 191–202.
——, and Robertson, M. A. H. (1972). Changes in conduction during nerve fibre degeneration in the spinal cord. *Brain*, 151–62.
——, and Sears, T. A. (1969). Effect of demyelination on conduction in the central nervous system. *Nature, Lond.* **221**, 182–3.
——, and—— (1970*a*). Focal experimental demyelination in the central nervous system. *Brain* **93**, 575–82.
——, and—— (1970*b*). The effects of experimental demyelination on conduction in the central nervous system. *Brain* **93**, 583–98.
McFadden, D., and Gummerman, K. (1973). Monoptic and dichoptic metacontrast across the vertical meridian. *Vision Res.* **13**, 185–96.
Meikle, T. H., and Sprague, J. M. (1964). The neural organization of the visual pathway in the cat. *Int. Rev. Neurobiol.* **6**, 149–89.
Meyer, D. L., and Schwassmann, H. O. (1970). Electrophysiological methods for determination of refractive state in fish eyes. *Vision Res.* **10**, 1301–3.
Michael, W. F., and Halliday, A. M. (1971). Differences between the occipital distribution of upper and lower field pattern-evoked responses in man. *Brain Res.* **32**, 311–24.
Michael, J. A., and Stark, L. (1967). Electrophysiological correlates of saccadic suppression. *Expl. Neurol.* **17**, 233–46.
Michel, F., Jeannerod, M., Mouret, J., Rechtschaffen, A., and Jouvet, M. (1964). Sur les mécanismes de l'activité de pointes au niveau du système visuel au cours de la phase paradoxale du sommeil. *C.r. Soc. Biol.*, Paris **158**, 103–6.
Mikiten, T. M., Niebyl, P. H., and Hendley, C. D. (1961). EEG desynchronization during behavioral sleep associated with spike discharge from the thalamus of the cat. *Fedn. Proc. Fedn. Am. Soc. exp. Biol.* **20**, 327.
Miller, E. F. (1954). The nature and cause of impaired vision in the amblyopic eye of a squinter. *Am. J. Optom.* **31**, 615–23.
Millodot, M. (1971*a*). Measurement of the refractive state of the eye frogs (*Rana pipiens*). *Rev. Can. Biol.* **30**, 249–52.
—— (1971*b*). New method of objective refraction: electrophysiology. *Can. J. Optom.* **33**, 64–8.
——(1972). Retinoscopy and the ametropia of infants. *Ophthal. Opt.* **12**, 1130–2.
——(1973). A centenary of retinoscopy. *J. Am. Optom. Ass.* **44**, 1057–9.
——, Miller, D., and Jernigan, M. (1973). Evaluation of an objective visual acuity device. *Archs. Ophthal., N.Y.* **90**, 449–52.
——, and Riggs, L. A. (1970). Refraction determined electrophysiologically. *Archs. Ophthal., N.Y.* **84**, 272–8.
Milner, B. A., Regan, D., and Heron, J. R. (1974). Differential diagnosis of multiple sclerosis by visual evoked potential recording. *Brain* **97**, 755–72.

Minke, B. and Auerbach, E. (1972). Latencies and correlation in single units and visual evoked potentials in the cat striate cortex following monocular and binocular stimulation. *Exp. Brain Res.* **14**, 409–22.

Miranda, S. (1970). Visual abilities and pattern preferences of premature infants and full-term neonates. *J. exp. Child Psychol.* **10**, 189–205.

Mitchell, D. E., Freeman, R. D., Millodot, M., and Haegerstrom, G. (1972). Meridional amblyopia: evidence for modification of the human visual system by early visual experience. *Vision Res.* **13**, 535–58.

Mitrani, L., Mateeff, St., and Yakimoff, N. (1971). Is saccadic suppression really saccadic? *Vision Res.* **11**, 1157–61.

Mohler, C. W. (1975). *The effect of saccadic eye movements on the visual response of lateral geniculate neurones in monkey.* Association for Research on Vision and Ophthalmology, Sarasota, Florida.

——, Goldberg, H. E., and Wurtz, R. H. (1973). Visual receptive fields of frontal eye field neurons. *Brain Res.* **61**, 385–9.

Mollon, J. D., and Krauskopf, J. (1973). Reaction time as a measure of the temporal response properties of individual colour mechanism. *Vision Res.* **13**, 27–40.

Montagu, J. D. (1967). The relationship between the intensity of repetitive photic stimulation and the cerebral response. *Electroenceph. clin. Neurophysiol.* **23**, 152–61.

Morrell, F. (1967). Electrical signs of sensory coding. In *Neurosciences: a study program* (eds G. C. Quarton, T. Melnechuk, and F. O. Schmitt), pp. 452–69. Rockefeller University Press, New York.

Moser, E. A., and Krueger, H. (1972). Retinoscopic and neurophysiological refractometry in *Rana temporaria. Pflüger's Arch. ges. Physiol.* **335**, 235–42.

Morton, H. B., and Cobb, W. A. (1973). Lambda waves and visual suppression. *Electroenceph. clin. Neurophysiol.* **34**, 694.

Moskowitz, A. F., Armington, J. C., and Timberlake, G. (1974). Corners, receptive fields and visually evoked cortical potentials. *Percept. Psychophys.* **15**, 325–30.

Mountcastle, V. B., Lynch, J. C., Georgopoulos, A., Sakata, H., and Acuna, C. (1975). Posterior parietal association cortex of the monkey: command functions for operations within the extrapersonal space. *J. Neurophysiol.* **38**: 871–909.

Murch, G. M. (1968). McCollough after-images and Emmert's law. *Proceeding of the 76th annual Convention of the American Psychological Association* **3**, 103–4.

—— (1969). Size judgments of McCollough after-images. *J. exp. Psychol.* **81**, 44–8.

—— (1972). Binocular relationships in a size and color orientation specific after-effect. *J. exp. Psychol.* **93**, 30–4.

——, and Hirsch, J. (1972). The McCollough effect created by complementary after-images. *Am. J. Psychol.* **85**, 241–7.

Mussen, P. H., Conger, J. J., and Kagan, J. (1969). *Child development and personality.* Harper and Row, New York.

Musso, M. F., and Harter, M. R. (1975). Visually evoked potentials and selective masking with patterned flashes of different spatial frequencies. *Vision Res.* **15**, 231–8.

Myers, R. E. (1962). Commissural connections between occipital lobes of the monkey. *J. comp. Neurol.* **118**, 1–16.

Nakamura, Z., and Biersdorf, W. F. (1971). Localization of the human visual evoked response: early components specific to visual stimulation. *Am. J.*

Ophthal. **72**, 988–97.
———, and Roberts, D. J. (1972). Line length detectors in the human visual system: evidence from selective adaptation. *Vision Res.* **12**, 1709–13.
Namerow, N. S. (1968). Somatosensory evoked responses in multiple sclerosis patients with varying sensory loss. *Neurology, Minneap.* **18**, 1197–204.
——— (1970). Somatosensory recovery functions in multiple sclerosis patients. *Neurology, Minneap.* **20**, 813–17.
——— (1971). Temperature effects on critical fusion frequency in multiple sclerosis. *Arch. Neurol., Chicago* **25**, 269–75.
———, and Enns, N. (1972). Visual evoked responses in patients with multiple sclerosis. *J. Neurol. Neurosurg. Psychiat.* **35**, 269–75.
Nichols, R. C., and Bilbro, W. C. (1966). The diagnosis of twin zygosity. *Acta genet. Statist. med.* **16**, 265–75.
Norton, A. L., Spekreijse, H., Wolbarsht, M. L., and Wagner, H. G. (1968). Receptive field organization of the *S*-potential. *Science, N.Y.* **160**, 1021–2.
Ogden, T. E., and Miller, R. F. (1966). Studies of the optic nerve of the rhesus monkey: nerve fiber spectrum and physiological properties. *Vision Res.* **6**, 485–506.
Oosterhuis, H. J. G. H., Ponsen, L., Jonkman, E. G., and Magnus, O. (1969). The average visual response in patients with cerebrovascular disease. *Electroenceph. clin. Neurophysiol.* **27**, 23–34.
Padmos, P., Haaijman, J. J., and Spekreijse, H. (1973). Visually evoked potentials to patterned stimuli in monkey and man. *Electroenceph. clin. Neurophysiol.* **35**, 153–63.
Pampiglione, G., and Harden, A. (1973). Neurophysiological identification of a late infantile form of 'neuronal lipidosis'. *J. Neurol. Neurosurg. Psychiat.* **36**, 68–74.
———, and ——— (1974). An infantile form of neuronal 'storage' disease with characteristic evolution of neurophysiological features. *Brain* **97**, 355–60.
———, and Lehovsky, M. (1968). The evolution of EEG features in Tay–Sachs' disease and amaurotic family idiocy in 24 children. In *Clinical electro-encephalography of children* (eds P. Kellaway and I. Petersen), pp. 287–306. Greene and Stratton, New York.
———, Privett, G., and Harden, A. (1974). Tay–Sachs' disease: neurophysiological studies in 20 children. *Develop. Med. Child Neurol.* **16**, 201–8.
Panayiotopoulos, C. R., Jeavons, P. M., and Harding, G. F. A. (1972). Occipital spikes and their relation to visual evoked responses in epilepsy with particular reference to photosensitive epilepsy. *Electroenceph. clin. Neurophysiol.* **32**, 179–90.
Pantle, A., and Sekuler, R. (1968). Size-detecting mechanisms in human vision. *Science, N.Y.* **162**, 1146–8.
Pasik, T., and Pasik, P. (1971). The visual world of monkeys deprived of striate cortex: effective stimulus parameter and the importance of the accessory optic system. *Vision Res.*, Suppl. **3**, 419–35.
Pearson, R. M. (1966). The objective determination of vision and visual acuity. *Br. J. Physiol. Opt.* **23**, 107–28.
——— (1970). An evaluation of Wagner's method of objective determination of visual acuity. *Ophthal. Optician* **10**, 1229–33.
Penfield, W., and Boldrey, E. (1937). Somatic motor and sensory representation in the cerebral cortex of man as studied by electrical stimulation. *Brain* **60**, 389–443.

Perez-Borja, C., Chatrian, G. E., Tyce, F. A., and Rivers, M. H. (1962). Electrographic patterns of the occipital lobe in man: a topogrraphic study based on use of implanted electrodes. *Electroenceph. clin. Neurophysiol.* **14**, 171–82.

Perry, N. W., Childers, D. G., and McCoy, J. G. (1968). Binocular addition at different cortical locations. *Vision Res.* **8**, 567–73.

Pettigrew, J. D. (1973). Binocular neurons which signal change of disparity in area 18 of cat visual cortex. *Nature New Biol.* **241**, 123–4.

——, Nikara, T., and Bishop, P. O. (1968). Binocular interaction on single units in cat striate cortex: simultaneous stimulation with single moving slits with receptive fields in correspondance. *Exp. Brain Res.* **6**, 391–410.

Piéron, H. (1952). *The sensations. Their functions, processes and mechanisms.* Muller, London.

Poggio, G. F. (1968). Central neural mechanism in vision. In *Medical physiology* (ed. V. B. Mountcastle), Vol. 2, pp. 1592–625. Mosby, St. Louis.

Pollen, D., and Ronner, S. F. (1975). Periodic excitability changes across the receptive fields of complex cells in the striate and parastriate cortex of the cat. *J. Physiol., Lond.* 245, 667–97.

Pollen, D., and Taylor, J. H. (1974). The striate cortex and the spatial analysis of visual space. In *The neurosciences 3rd study program* (eds F. O. Schmitt and F. G. Worden), pp. 239–47. M.I.T. Press, Cambridge, Massachusetts.

Polyak, S. (1957). *The vertebrate visual system.* University of Chicago Press, Chicago.

Potts, A. M., Hodges, D., Shelman, C. B., Fritz, K. S., Levy, N. S., and Magnall, Y. (1972). Morphology of the primate optic nerve. II. Total fiber size, distribution and fiber density distribution. *Invest. Ophthal.* **11**, 989–1003.

Pribram, K. H. (1971). *Languages of the brain. Experimental paradoxes and principles in neuropsychology.* Prentice Hall, London.

Price, R. A. (1958). A useful theorem for nonlinear devices having Gaussian inputs. I.R.E. Trans. *Inf. Theory* **IT-4**, 69–76.

Pulfrich, D. (1922). Die Stereoskopie im Dienst der Isochromen und Heterchromen Photometrie. *Naturwissenschaften* **10**, 553.

Raab, D. H. (1963). Backward masking. *Psychol. Bull.* **60**, 118–29.

Ramon y Cajal, S. (1955). *Histologie du système nerveux de l'homme et des vertébrés.* Vol. 2. Instituto Ramon y Cajal, Madrid.

Raney, E. T. (1939). Brain potentials and lateral dominance in identical twins. *J. exp. Psychol.* **24**, 21.

Rashbass, C. (1968). Spatio-temporal interaction in visual resolution. *J. Physiol., Lond.* **196**, 102P–103P.

Rasminsky, M., and Sears, T. A. (1972). Internodal conduction in undissected demyelinated nerve fibres. *J. Physiol., Lond.* **227**, 323–50.

Rassow, B., and Wolf, D. (1973). Erfahrungen mit dem Laser-Interferenz-streifen-Test bei der Messung des retinalen Auflösungsvermögens. A. von Graefes *Arch. klin. exp. Ophthal.* **187**, 61–6.

Ratliff, F., Knight, B. W., and Graham, N. (1969). On tuning and amplification by lateral inhibition. *Proc. natn. Acad. Sci. U.S.A.* **62**, 733–40.

Reese, H. W., and Lipsitt, L. P. (1970). *Experimental child psychology.* Academic Press, New York.

Regan, D. (1966*a*). Some characteristics of average steady state and transient responses evoked by modulated light. *Electroenceph. clin. Neurophysiol.* **20**, 238–48.

—— (1966*b*). Apparatus for the correlation of evoked potentials and repetitive

stimuli. *Med. Electron. biol. Engng.* **4**, 169–77.
——— (1968*a*). Chromatic adaptation and steady-state evoked potentials. *Vision Res.* **8**, 149–58.
——— (1968*b*). Evoked potentials and sensation. *Percept. Psychophys.* **4**, 347–50.
——— (1968*c*). A high frequency mechanism that underlies visual evoked potentials. *Electroenceph. clin. Neurophysiol.* **25**, 231–37.
——— (1969). Evoked potentials and colour vision. *Proceedings of the International Symposium of Clinical Electro-retinography*, Istanbul 1969. Medical Faculty, University of Istanbul.
——— (1970*a*). An objective method of measuring the relative spectral luminosity curve in man. *J. opt. Soc. Am.* **60**, 856–9.
——— (1970*b*). Evoked potential and psychophysical Correlates of changes in stimulus colour and intensity. *Vision Res.* **10**, 163–78.
——— (1972*a*). *Evoked potentials in psychology, sensory physiology and clinical medicine.* Chapman and Hall, London.
——— (1972*b*). Evoked potentials to changes in the chromatic contrast and luminance contrast of checkerboard stimulus patterns. *Adv. exp. Med. Biol.* **24**, 171–87.
——— (1973*a*). Evoked potentials specific to spatial patterns of luminance and colour. *Vision Res.* **13**, 2381–402.
——— (1973*b*). An evoked potential correlate of colour: evoked potential findings and single-cell speculations. *Vision Res.* **13**, 1933–41.
——— (1973*c*). Objective refraction using evoked brain potentials. *Invest. Ophthal.* **12**, 669–79.
——— (1974*a*). Electrophysiological evidence for colour channels in human pattern vision. *Nature, Lond.* **250**, 401–7.
——— (1974*b*). Visually evoked potentials method with clinical applications. *Proceedings of the 2nd ISCERG Symposium Bad Nauheim 1973.* Documenta Ophtalmologica.
——— (1975*a*). Recent advances in electrical recording from the brain. *Nature, Lond.* **253**, 401–7.
——— (1975*b*). Colour coding of pattern evoked potentials investigated by direct plot and evoked potential feed-back techniques. *Vision Res.* **15**, 175–83.
———, and Beverley, K. I. (1973*a*). The dissociation of sideways movements from movements in depth: psychophysics. *Vision Res.* **13**, 2403–15.
———, and ——— (1973*b*). Electrophysiological evidence for neurones sensitive to direction of depth movement. *Nature, Lond.* **246**, 504–6.
———, and ——— (1973*c*). Relation between the magnitude of flicker sensation and evoked potential amplitude in man. *Perception* **2**, 61–5.
———, and Cartwright, R. F. (1970). A method of simultaneous stimulation of the left and right half fields. *Electroenceph. clin. Neurophysiol.* **28**, 314–19.
———, and Richards, W. (1971). Independence of evoked potentials and apparent size. *Vision Res.* **11**, 679–84.
———, and ——— (1973). Brightness contrast and evoked potentials. *J. opt. Soc. Am.* **63**, 606–11.
———, Schellart, N. A. M., Spekreijse, H., and Van der Berg, T. J. T. P. (1975). Photometry in goldfish by electrophysiological recording: comparison of criterion response method with heterochromatic flicker photometry. *Vision Res.* **15**, 799–807.
———, and Spekreijse, H. (1970). Electrophysiological correlate of binocular depth perception in man. *Nature, Lond.* **225**, 92–4.

——, and —— (1974). Evoked potentials indications of colour blindness. *Vision Res.* **14**, 89–95.

——, and Sperling, H. G. (1971). A method of evoking contour-specific scalp potentials by chromatic checkerboard patterns. *Vision Res.* **11**, 173–6.

Reits, D. (1975). Cortical potentials in man evoked by noise modulated light. Thesis, University of Utrecht.

Rémond, A. (1969). Evoked brain potentials as indicators of sensory information processing. *Neurosci. Res. Prog. Bull.* **7**, 240–2.

——, and Lesèvre, N. (1956). Remarques sur les conditions d'apparition et l'importance statistique des ondes Lambda chez les individus normaux. *Revue neurol.* **94**, 160–1.

——, and —— (1971). Etude de la fonction du regard par l'analyse des potentiels évoqués visuels (lumière, patterns complexes et mouvements des yeux). In *La fonction du regard* (eds A. D. Poulsen, G. C. Lairy, and A. Rémond), pp. 127–75. Colloques INSERM, Paris.

——, ——, and Torres, F. (1965). Etude chronotopographiques de l'activite occipitale moyenne recueillie sur scalp chez l'homme en relation avec les déplacements du regard (complex lambda). *Revue neurol.* **113**, 195–226.

Rhodes, L. E., Dustman, R. E., and Beck, E. C. (1969). The visual evoked response: a comparison of bright and dull children. *Electroenceph. clin. Neurophysiol.* **27**, 364–72.

Richards, W. (1968). Visual suppression during passive eye movement. *J. opt. Soc. Am.* **58**, 1159–60.

——(1969). Saccadic suppression. *J. opt. Soc. Am.* **59**, 617–23.

——(1970). Stereopsis and stereo-blindness. *Exp. Brain Res.* **10**, 380–8.

Richey, E. T., Kooi, K. A., and Tourtellotte, W. W. (1971). Visually evoked responses in multiple sclerosis. *J. Neurol. Neurosurg. Psychiat.* **34**, 275–80.

Richlin, M., Weisinger, M., Weinstein, S., Giannini, M., and Morganstern, M. (1971). Interhemispheric asymmetries of evoked cortical responses in retarded and children. *Cortex* **7**, 98–105.

Riddoch, G. (1917). Disorders of visual perception due to occipital injuries with special reference to appreciation of movement. *Brain* **40**, 15–57.

Rietveld, W. J., Tordoir, W. E., and Duyff, J. W. (1965). Contribution of fovea and parafovea to the visual evoked response. *Acta physiol. pharmacol. neerl.* **13**, 330–9.

——, ——, Hagenouw, J. R. B., and van Dongen, W. K. J. (1965). Contribution of foveo-parafoveal quadrants to the visual evoked response. *Acta physiol. pharmac. neerl.* **13**, 340–7.

——, ——, ——, Lubbers, J. A., and Spoor, A. C. (1967). Visual evoked responses to blank and to checkerboard patterned flashes. *Acta physiol. pharmac. neerl.* **14**, 259–85.

Rife, D. C. (1933). Genetic studies of monozygotic twins, diagnostic formula. *J. Hered.* **24**, 339–45.

Riggs, L. A. (1965). Visual acuity. In *Vision and visual perception* (ed. C. H. Graham), pp. 321–49. Wiley, New York.

—— (1973). Curvature as a feature of pattern vision. *Science, N.Y.* **181**, 1070–2.

——, Johnson, E. P., and Schick, A. M. L. (1966). Electrical responses of the human eye to changes in the wavelength of the stimulating light. *J. opt. Soc. Am.* **56**, 1621–7.

——, Merton, P. A., and Morton, H. B. (1974). Suppression of visual phosphenes during saccadic eye movements. *Vision Res.* **14**, 997–1011.

——, and Sternheim, C. E. (1969). Human retinal and occipital potentials evoked by changes of the wavelength of the stimulating light. *J. opt. Soc. Am.* **59**, 635–40.

——, White, K. D., and Eimis, P. D. (1973). Encoding and decay of orientation contingent after effects of color. *J. opt. Soc. Am.* **63**, 287.

——, and Whittle, P. (1967). Human occipital and retinal potentials evoked by subjectively faded visual stimuli. *Vision Res.* **7**, 441–51.

——, and Wooten, B. R. (1973). Electrical measures and psychophysical data on human vision. In *Handbook of sensory physiology* (eds D. Jameson and L. M. Hurvich), VII/4, pp. 690–731. Springer-Verlag, Berlin.

Robinson, D. A. (1972). Eye movements evoked by collicular stimulation in the alert monkey. *Vision Res.* **12**, 1795–808.

——, and Fuchs, A. F. (1969). Eye movements evoked by stimulation of frontal eye fields. *J. Neurophysiol.* **32**, 637–48.

Robinson, D. N., and Strandburg, R. (1973). Differences in inter-hemispheric variance in brain responses of attentive and inattentive human subjects. *Percept. Motor Skills* **36**, 1099–1102.

Robson, J. G. (1966). Spatial and temporal contrast sensitivity functions of the visual system. *J. opt. Soc. Am.* **56**, 1141–2.

Rodin, E. A., Grisell, J. L., Gudobba, R. D., and Zachary, G. (1965). Relationship of EEG background rhythms to photic evoked responses. *Electroenceph. clin. Neurophysiol.* **19**, 301–4.

Ronchi, L., and Castellini, C. (1973). On the influence of contrast depth on VER elicited by Jo patterns. *Atti Fond. Giorgio Ronchi* **28**, 461–77.

——, and Millodot, M. (1974). The cortical counterpart of the chromatic aberration of the eye. *Am. J. Optom.* **51**, 635–41.

Roth, M., and Green, J. (1953). The lambda wave as a normal physiological phenomenon in the human electroencephalogram. *Nature, Lond.* **172**, 864–6.

Sanderson, K. J., Bishop, P. O., and Darian-Smith, I. (1971). The properties of the binocular receptive fields of lateral geniculate neurons. *Exp. Brain Res.* **13**, 178–207.

Santavuori, P. (1973). EEG in the infantile type of so-called neuronal ceroidlipofuscinosis. *Neuropädiatrie* **4**, 375–87.

Santavuori, P., Haltia, M., Rapola, J., and Raitta, C. (1973). Infantile type of so-called neuronal ceroid-lipofuscinosis. Part I. A clinical study of 15 patients. *J. neurol. Sci.* **18**, 257–67.

Schaie, K. W. (1965). A general model for the study of developmental problems. *Psychol. Bull.* **64**, 92–107.

Scheie, H. G., and Albert, D. M. (1969). *Adler's textbook of ophthalmology*, pp. 158–9. Saunders, Philadelphia.

Schiller, P. H. (1970). Discharge characteristics of single units in the oculomotor and abducens nuclei of the unanesthetized monkey. *Exp. Brain Res.* **10**, 347–62.

——, and Koerner, F. (1971). Discharge characteristics of single units in superior colliculus of the alert rhesus monkey. *J. Neurophysiol.* **34**, 920–36.

——, and Stryker, M. (1972). Single-unit recording and stimulation in superior colliculus of the alert rhesus monkey. *J. Neurophysiol.* **35**, 915–24.

Schneider, G. E. (1969). Two visual systems: brain mechanisms for localization and discrimination are dissociated by tectal and cortical lesions. *Science, N.Y.* **163**, 895–902.

Schreinemachers, H. P., and Henkes, H. E. (1968). Relation between localized retinal stimuli and the visual evoked response in man. *Ophthalmologica (Basel)* **155**, 17–27.

Scott, D. F., and Bickford, R. G. (1967). Electrophysiologic studies during scanning and passive movements in human. *Science, N.Y.* **155**, 101.

———, and ——— (1969). Stimulus indicators of summated human lambda responses. *Archs Neurol., Chicago* **21**, 277–84.

———, Groethuysen, U. C., and Bickford, R. G. (1967). Lambda responses in the human electroencephalogram. *Neurology, Minneap.* **17**, 770–8.

Sears, T. A., and Stagg, D. (1967). Methods used for the recording and subsequent analysis of spontaneous efferent and afferent activity in intact intercostal nerve filaments. *J. Physiol., Lond.* **191**, 108P–109P.

Sekuler, R. W., Rubin, E. L., and Cushman, W. H. (1968). Selectivities of human visual mechanisms for direction of movement and contour orientation. *J. opt. Soc. Am.* **58**, 1146–50.

Shagass, C. (1972). *Evoked brain potentials in psychiatry.* Plenum, New York.

———, Schartz, M., and Straumanis, J. J. (1966). Subject factors related to variability of averaged evoked responses. *Electroenceph. clin. Neurophysiol.* **20**, 97.

Shaw, J. C., and Roth, M. (1955). Potential distribution analysis. II. A theoretical consideration of its significance in terms of electrical field theory. *Electroenceph. clin. Neurophysiol.* **7**, 285–92.

Sheppard, J. J. (1968). *Human color perception: a critical study of the experimental foundation.* American Elsevier, New York.

Shipley, T. (1969). The visually evoked occipitogram, in strabismic amblyopia under direct view ophthalmology. *J. Pediat. Ophthalmol.* **6**, 97–112.

———, Jones, R. W., and Fry, A. (1965). Evoked visual potentials and human color vision. *Science, N.Y.* **150**, 1162–4.

———, ———, and ——— (1968). Spectral analysis of the visually evoked occipitogram in man. *Vision Res.* **8**, 409–31.

Shuttlesworth, D. E. (1974). Visually evoked responses and reaction time: inter-ocular and intra-ocular lateral inhibitory effects. Unpublished doctoral Dissertation, University of North Carolina, Greensboro.

Siegel, J. M., Coleman, P. D., and Reisen, A. H. (1973). Visual attention and neurological organization in neonates. *Electroenceph. clin. Neurophysiol.* **35**, 569–73.

Siegel, S. (1956). *Nonparametric statistics for the behavioral sciences.* McGraw-Hill, New York.

———, Tepas, D., Sperling, H. G., and Hess, R. H. (1965). Evoked brain potential correlates of psychophysical responses: heterochromatic flicker photometry. *Science, N.Y.* **149**, 321–3.

Sigman, M., Kopp, C. B., Parmelee, A. H., and Jeffreys, W. E. (1973). Visual attention and neurological organization in neonates. *Child Dev.* **44**, 461–6.

Singer, W. (1973). Brain stem stimulation and the concept of presynaptic inhibition in the cat LGN. *Brain Res.* **61**, 55–68.

———, and Bedford, N. (1974). Correlation between the effects of brain stem stimulation and saccadic eye movements on transmission in the cat lateral geniculate nucleus. *Brain Res.* **72**, 185–202.

———, and Drager, U. (1972). Postsynaptic potentials in relay neurons of the cat lateral geniculate neurons after stimulation of the mesencephalic reticular formation. *Brain Res.* **41**, 214–20.

Sivak, J. (1974). The refractive error of the fish eye. *Vision Res.* **14**, 209–13.

Sloan, L. (1957). Measurement of visual acuity. *Archs Ophthal, N.Y.* **45**, 704–25.
Small, D. H., Beauchamp, M., and Matthews, W. B. (1975). Subcortical somatosensory evoked potentials in man. *Electroenceph. clin. Neurophysiol.* **38**, 215.
Sokol, S. (1972). An electrodiagnostic index of macular degeneration. *Archs. Ophthal., N.Y.* **88**, 619–24.
——, and Bloom, B. (1973). Visually evoked cortical responses of amblyopes to a spatially alternating stimulus. *Invest. Ophthal.* **12**, 936–9.
——; and Dobson, V. (1976). Pattern reversal visually evoked potentials in infants. *Investig. Ophtalm.* **15**, 58–62.
——, and Shatterian, E. T. (1976). The pattern evoked cortical potential in amblyopia as an index of visual function. In: *Orthoptics, past, present, future.* (S. Moore, J. Mein and L. Stockbridge, eds). Symposia Specialists, Miami, pp. 59–67.
Spalding, J. M. K. (1952). Wounds of the visual pathway. Part II: the striate cortex. *J. Neurol. Neurosurg. Psychiat.* **15**, 169–83.
Spehlmann, R. (1965). The averaged electrical responses to diffuse and to patterned light in the human. *Electroenceph. clin. Neurophysiol.* **19**, 560–9.
Spekreijse, H. (1966). *Analysis of EEG responses to diffuse and to patterned light in the human* (Thesis) D. W. Junk, The Hague.
——, (1969). Rectification in the goldfish retina: analysis by sinusoidal and auxilliary stimulation. *Vision Res.* **9**, 1461–72.
——, and Van den Berg, T. J. T. P. (1971). Interaction between colour and spatial coded processes converging to retinal ganglion cells in goldfish. *J. Physiol., Lond.* **215**, 679–92.
——, and Estevez, O. (1972). The pattern appearance–disappearance response. *Trace* **6**, 13–19.
——, Khoe, L. H., and Van der Tweel, L. H. (1972). A case of amblyopia: electrophysiology and psychophysics of luminance and contrast. In *The visual system* (ed. G. B. Arden), pp. 141–56. Plenum, New York.
——, Van Norren, D., and Van den Berg, T. J. T. P. (1971). Flicker responses in monkey lateral geniculate nucleus and human perception of flicker. *Proc. natn. Acad. Sci. U.S.A.* **68**, 2802–5.
——; and Oosting, J. (1970). Linearizing: A method for analysing and synthesizing nonlinear systems. *Kybernetik* **7**, 23–31.
——, Van der Tweel, L. H., and Regan, D. (1972). Interocular sustained suppression: correlations with evoked potential amplitude and distribution. *Vision Res.* **12**, 521–6.
——, ——, and Zuidema, T. (1973). Contrast evoked responses in man. *Vision Res.* **13**, 1577–601.
——, Wagner, H. G., and Wolbarsht, M. L. (1972). Spectral and spatial coding of ganglion cell responses in goldfish retina. *J. Neurophysiol.* **35**, 73–86.
Sperry, R. W. (1950). Neural basis of the spontaneous optokinetic response produced by visual inversion. *J. comp. Physiol. Psychol.* **43**, 482–9.
Steinman, R. M., Haddad, G. M., Skavenski, A. A., and Wyman, D. (1973). Miniature eye movement. *Science, N.Y.* **181**, 810–19.
Stiles, W. S. (1939). The directional sensitivity of the retina and the spectral sensitivity of rods and cones. *Proc. R. Soc. B* **127**, 64–105.
—— (1959). Colour vision: the approach through increment threshold sensitivity. *Proc. natn. Acad. Sci. U.S.A.* **45**, 100–14.
Stone, J. (1972). Morphology and physiology of the genicilocortical synapse in the cat: the question of parallel input to the striate cortex. *Invest. Ophthal.*

11, 338–46.
——, and Dreher, B. (1973). Projections of X- and Y-cells of the cat's lateral geniculate nucleus to areas 17 and 18 of the visual cortex. *J. Neurophysiol.* **36**, 551–67.

Stromeyer, C. F. (1969). Further studies of the McCollough effect. *Percept. Psychophys.* **6**, 109–10.

——— (1972). Contour-contingent, color after-effects: retinal area specificity. *Am. J. Psychol.* 85, 227–35.

———, and Mansfield, R. (1970). Colored after-effects produced with moving edges. *Percept. Psychophys.* 7, 108–14.

Sullivan, G. D., Georgeson, M. A., and Oatley, K. (1972). Channels for spatial frequency selection and the detection of single bars by the human visual system. *Vision Res.* **12**, 383–94.

Suzuki, K., Andrews, J. M., Waltz, J. M., and Terry, R. D. (1969). Ultrastructural studies of multiple sclerosis. *Lab. Invest.* **20**, 444–54.

Talbot, S. A. (1942). Lateral localisation in cat's cortex. *Fedn. Proc. Fedn. Am. Socs. exp. Biol.* **1**, 84.

———, and Marshall, W. H. (1941). Physiological studies on neural mechanisms of visual localization and discrimination. *Am. J. Ophthal.* **24**, 1255–64.

Tamura, K., and Kuroiwa, Y. (1972). Somatosensory evoked responses in patients with multiple sclerosis. *Folia psychiat. neurol. jap.* **26**, 269–74.

Tasaki, I. (1952). Properties of myelinated fibres in frog sciatic nerve and in spinal cord as examined with microelectrodes. *Jap. J. Physiol.* **3**, 73–94.

Teft, D. Y., Morse, R., Borton, R., and Regan, D. (1974). Visual acuity for vertical and diagonal gratings in human infants. *Vision Res.* **14**, 1433–9.

Teft, L. W., and Clark, F. T. (1968). The effects of stimulus density on orientation specific after effects of color adaption. *Psychon. Sci.* **11**, 265–6.

Teuber, H. L. (1961). Neuere Beobachtungen über Sehstrahlung und Sehrinde. In *Neurophysiology and psychophysics. Freiburg Symposium 1960.* (ed. H. Kornhuber). Springer, Berlin.

———, Battersby, W. S., and Bender, M. B. (1960). *Visual field defects after penetrating missile wounds of brain.* Harvard University Press, Cambridge, Mass.

Thomas, G. (1965). Refraction of the newborn. *Archivos Oftal. hisp.-am.* **25**, 666–75.

Timney, B. N., Gentry, T. A., Skowbo, D., and Morant, R. B. (1974). Chromatic grating thresholds and the McCollough effect. *Vision Res.* **14**, 1033–5.

Tolhurst, D. J. (1972). On the possible existence of edge detector neurones in the human visual system. *Vision Res.* **12**, 797–804.

——— (1973). Separate channels for the analysis of the shape and the movement of a moving visual stimulus. *J. Physiol. Lond.* **232**, 149–62.

Towers, T. D. (1967). Colour receiver techniques. *Wireless Wld.* **73**, 8–12.

Toyama, K., Maekawa, K., and Takeda, T. (1973). An analysis of neuronal circuitry for two types of visual cortical neurones classified on the basis of their responses to photic stimuli. *Brain Res.* **61**, 395–9.

Trevarthen, C. B. (1968). Two mechanisms of vision in primates. *Psychol. Forsch.* **31**, 299–337.

———, and Sperry, R. W. (1973). Perceptual unity of the ambient visual field in human commissurotomy patients. *Brain* **96**, 547–70.

Trincker, D. and Trincker, E. (1967). Development of brightness vision in infants. In *Behavior in infancy and early childhood* (eds Y. Brackbill, and G. G. Thompson). The Free Press, New York.

Turner, O. A. (1948). Growth and development of the cerebral cortical pattern in man. *Archs. Neurol. Psychiat., Chicago* **59**, 1.

Van der Tweel, L. H. (1961). Some problems in vision regarded with respect to linearity and frequency response. *Ann. N.Y. Acad. Sci.* **89**, 829.

——— (1964). Relation between psychophysics and electrophysiology of flicker. *Documenta Opthal.* **18**, 287–304.

———, and Boon, P. (1970). Small signal influences upon a sawtooth oscillator. *Electroenceph. clin. Neurophysiol.* **28**, 423.

———, and Estevez-Uscanga, O. (1972). Significations of the stimulus in human pattern evoked potentials. *Trace* **6**, 8–12.

———, and Verduyn Lunel, H. F. E. (1965). Human visual responses to sinusoidally modulated light. *Electroenceph. clin. Neurophysiol.* **18**, 587–98.

———, and Spekreijse, H. (1966). Visual evoked responses: clinical value of electro-retinography. *International Symposium on Clinical Electro-retinography Ghent*, pp. 83–94.

———, and ——— (1969). Signal transport and rectification in the human evoked-response system. *Ann. N.Y. Acad. Sci.* **156**, 678–95.

Umezaki, H., and Morrell, F. (1970). Developmental study of photic evoked responses in premature infants. *Electroenceph. clin. Neurophysiol.* **28**, 55–63.

Van Balen, A. (1964). The influence of suppression on the flicker ERG. In *Proceedings of the symposia on physiology of flicker and flicker electro-retinography* (eds H. E. Henkes and L. H. van der Tweel). D. W. Junk, The Hague.

Van Hof, M. W., Van der Mark, F., and Rietveld, W. J. (1962). Influence of formation of retinal image on occipito-cortical response to photostimulation. *Acta physiol. pharmac. néerl.* **10**, 317–26.

Van Nes, F. M., Koenderick, J. J., Nas, H., and Bouman, M. A. (1967). Spatio-temporal modulation transfer in the human eye. *J. opt. Soc. Am.* **57**, 1087–8.

Vaughan, H. G. (1966). The perceptual and physiologic significance of visual evoked responses recorded from the scalp in man. Clin. Electroret. Suppl. to *Vision Res.* 203–23.

——— (1969). The relationship of brain activity to scalp recordings of event-related potentials. In *Averaged evoked potentials: methods, results, evaluations* (eds E. Donchin and D. B. Lindsley), pp. 45–94. SP 191, NASA, Washington.

——— (1972). A note on the visual neurosensorium. *Adv. Behav. Biol.* **5**, 167–76.

——— (1973). The role of stimulus pattern in suppression of vision during eye movements. In *The oculomotor system and brain functions* (ed. V. Zikmund), pp. 149–55. Butterworths, London.

——— (1974). The analysis of scalp recorded brain potentials. In *Bioelectric recordings techniques.* Part B: *electroencephalography and human brain potentials* (eds R. F. Thompson and M. M. Patterson), pp. 157–207. Academic Press, New York.

———, and Katzman, R. (1964). Evoked responses in visual disorders. *Ann. N. Y. Acad. Sci.* **112**, 305–19.

———, ———, and Taylor, J. (1963). Alterations of visual evoked responses in the presence of homonymous field defects. *Electroenceph. clin. Neurophysiol.* **15**, 737–46.

———, and Silverstein, L. (1968). Metacontrast and evoked potentials: a reappraisal. *Science, N.Y.* **160**, 207–8.

Volkmann, F. C., Schick, A. M. L., and Riggs, L. A. (1968). Time course of visual inhibition during voluntary saccades. *J. opt. Soc. Am.* **58**, 562–9.

von Holst, E., and Mittelstaedt, H. (1950). Das Reafferenzprincip (Wechselwirkungen zwischen Zentralnervensystem und Peripherie). *Naturwissenschaften* **37**, 464–76.

de Vries, H. (1948). The fundamental response curves of normal and abnormal dichromatic and trichromatic eyes. *Physica*, **14**, 367–80.

Wald, L. G. (1964). The receptors of human color vision. *Science, N.Y.* **145**, 1007–16.

Walter, W. G. (1962). Oscillatory activity in the nervous system. In *Neural physiopathology* (ed. R. Grenell). Harper and Row, New York.

——— (1964). Slow potential waves in the human brain associated with expectancy, attention and decision. *Arch. Psychiat. Nerv Krankh.* **206**, 309–22.

Watanabe, K., Iwase, K., and Hara, K. (1972). Maturation of visual evoked responses in low-birthweight infants. *Dev. Med. Child Neurol.* **14**, 425–35.

Weale, R. A. (1954). The theory of the Pulfrich effect. *Ophthalmologica, Basel* **128**, 380–8.

Weiss, A. D. (1959). Sensory functions. In *Handbook of aging and the individual* (ed. J. E. Birren), pp. 503–42. University of Chicago Press.

Welford, W. T. (1969). Some application of projected interference fringes. *Optica Acta* **16**, 371–6.

Westheimer, G. (1966). The Maxwellian view. *Vision Res.* **6**, 669–82.

White, C. T. (1969). Evoked cortical responses and patterned stimuli. *Am. J. Psychol.* **24**, 211–14.

———, and Eason, R. G. (1966). Evoked cortical potentials in relation to certain aspects of visual perception. *Psychol. Monogr.* **80**, no. 24.

———, and Bonelli, L. (1970). Binocular summation in the evoked potentials as a function of image quality. *Am. J. Optom.* **47**, 304–9.

Whitteridge, D. (1973). Projection of optic pathways to the visual cortex. In *Handbook of sensory physiology* (ed. R. Jung), VII/3B, pp. 247–68. Springer-Verlag, Berlin.

———, and Walsh, E. G. (1963). The physiological basis of the electroencephalogram. In *Electroencephalography* (eds J. D. N. Hill and G. Parr). Macmillan, New York.

Wilson, P. D., Pecci-Saavedra, J. P., and Doty, R. W. (1973). Mesencephalic control of lateral geniculate nucleus in primates II. Effective Loci. *Exp. Brain Res.* **18**, 204–13.

Winer, B. J. (1962). Statistical principles. In *Experimental design.* McGraw-Hill, New York.

Wooten, B. R. (1972). Photopic and scotopic contribution to the human visually evoked cortical potential. *Vision Res.* **12**, 1647–60.

Wurtz, R. H. (1968). Visual cortex neurons: response to stimuli during rapid eye movements. *Science, N.Y.* **162**, 1148–150.

——— (1969*a*). Visual receptive fields of striate cortex neurons in awake monkeys. *J. Neurophysiol.* **32**, 727–42.

——— (1969*b*). Comparison of effects of eye movements and stimulus movements on striate cortex neurones of the monkey. *J. Neurophysiol.* **32**, 987–94.

———, and Goldberg, M. E. (1972). Activity of superior colliculus in behaving monkey. III. Cells discharging before eye movements. *J. Neurophysiol.* **35**, 587–96.

Wyszecki, G., and Stiles, W. S. (1967). *Colour science, concepts and methods: quantitative data and formulas.* Wiley, New York.

Yakovlev, P. I. (1962). Morphological criteria of growth and maturation of the nervous system in man. In *Mental retardation* (eds L. C. Kalb, R. L. Masland, and R. E. Cooke), pp. 3–46. William and Wilkins, Baltimore.

——, and Lecours, A. (1967). The myelogenetic cycles of regional maturation of the brain. In *Regional development of the brain in early life* (ed. A. Minkowski), pp. 3–70. Davis, Philadelphia.

Yinon, U., Jakobovitz, L., and Auerbach, E. (1974). The visually evoked response to stationary checkerboard patterns in children with strabismic amblyopia. *Invest. Ophthal.* **13**, 293–6.

Zeki, S. M. (1969). Representation of central visual fields in pre-striate cortex of monkey. *Brain Res.* **14**, 271–91.

—— (1971). Convergent input from the striate cottex (area 17) to the cortex of the superior temporal sulcus in the rhesus monkey. *Brain Res.* **28**, 338–40.

—— (1974*a*). Functional organization of a visual area in the posterior bank of the superior temporal sulcus of the rhesus monkey. *J. Physiol. Lond.* **236**, 549–73.

—— (1974*b*). Cells responding to changing image size and disparity in the cortex of rhesus monkey. *J. Physiol., Lond.* **242**, 827–41.

Zeman, W., and Dyken, P. (1969). Neuronal ceroid-lipofuscinosis (Batten's disease). Relationship to amaurotic family idiocy. *Pediatrics,* **44**, 570–83.

Zuber, B. L., Stark, L., and Lorber, M. (1966). Saccadic suppression of the pupillary light reflex. *Expl. Neurol.* **14**. 351–70.

Index